Contemporary Nursing

ISSUES, TRENDS, & MANAGEMENT

Contemporary Nursing

Nursing

ISSUES, TRENDS, & MANAGEMENT

8th Edition

Barbara Cherry, DNSc, MBA, RN, NEA-BC
Professor, Associate Dean and Department Chair
  for Leadership Studies
Texas Tech University Health Sciences Center
School of Nursing
Lubbock, Texas

Susan R. Jacob, PhD, MSN, RN
Professor and Assistant Dean of Quality and Strategic Affairs
The University of Tennessee Health Science Center,
  College of Nursing
Education Consultant for Faith Community Nursing
Westberg Institute, Church Health
Memphis, Tennessee

ELSEVIER

ELSEVIER

3251 Riverport Lane
St. Louis, Missouri 63043

CONTEMPORARY NURSING: ISSUES, TRENDS, & MANAGEMENT,
EIGHTH EDITON   ISBN: 978-0-323-55420-6

NOTICES

Previous editions copyrighted 2017, 2014, 2011, 2008, 2005, 2002, 1999.

Library of Congress Control Number: 2018957299

Senior Content Strategist: Sandy Clark
Content Development Manager: Lisa P. Newton
Publishing Services Manager: Julie Eddy
Senior Project Manager: Cindy Thoms
Senior Book Designer: Amy Buxton

Working together
to grow libraries in
developing countries

www.elsevier.com • www.bookaid.org

Printed in Canada.

Last digit is the print number: 9 8 7 6 5 4

To all the student nurses whose curiosity and enthusiasm for nursing will provide strong leadership for the profession far into the future and to all practicing nurses who face serious challenges but reap great rewards for providing high-quality health care for individuals, families, and communities.

Being a Nurse Means . . .

You will never be bored,
You will always be frustrated,
You will be surrounded by challenges,
So much to do and so little time.
You will carry immense responsibility
And very little authority.
You will step into people's lives,
And you will make a difference.
Some will bless you.
Some will curse you.
You will see people at their worst,
And at their best.
You will never cease to be amazed at people's capacity
For love, courage, and endurance.
You will see life begin
and end.
You will experience resounding triumphs
And devastating failures.
You will cry a lot.
You will laugh a lot.
You will know what it is to be human
And to be humane.

Melodie Chenevert, RN

CONTRIBUTORS

Jeri Ashley, MSN, RN, AOCNS, CHPN
System Director, Life Planning/Palliative Medicine
    Services
Palliative Care
Baptist Trinity Home Care and Hospice
Memphis, Tennessee

Mary Jo Assi, DNP, RN, NEA-BC, FNP-BC, FAAN
Associate Chief Nursing Officer
Clinical Consulting
Press Ganey
South Bend, Indiana

**L. Antoinette (Toni) Bargagliotti, PhD, RN, ANEF,
    FAAN**
Professor, Loewenberg School of Nursing
The University of Memphis
Memphis, Tennessee

Barbara Cherry, DNSc, MBA, RN, NEA-BC
Professor, Associate Dean and Department Chair for
    Leadership Studies
Texas Tech University Health Sciences Center, School
    of Nursing
Lubbock, Texas

**Genevieve J. Conlin, DNP, Med, MS/MBA,
    RN, NEA-BC**
Associate Chief Nursing Officer
Ambulatory Services
Boston Medical Center
Boston, Massachusetts

Charlotte Eliopoulos, PhD, RN, MPH, ND
Consultant, Educator, Author
Nursing
Health Education Network
Glen Arm, Maryland

Debra D. Hatmaker, PhD, RN, FAAN
Executive Director
American Nurses Association
Silver Spring, Maryland

Susan R. Jacob, PhD, MSN, RN
Professor and Assistant Dean of Quality and Strategic
    Affairs
The University of Tennessee Health Science Center,
    College of Nursing
Education Consultant for Faith Community Nursing
Westberg Institute, Church Health
Memphis, Tennessee

Rebecca R. Keck, DNP, RN, NEA-BC
Senior Associate Dean for Administration &
    Operations; Chief Administrative Officer
Administration: Vanderbilt School of Nursing
Vanderbilt University School of Nursing
Nashville, Tennessee

Patricia R. Keene, DNP, ACNP-BC, ACHPN
Nurse Practitioner, Hospice
Baptist Trinity Hospice
Collierville, Tennessee

Laura R. Mahlmeister, PhD, MSN, RN
Lecturer, Nursing
University of California, San Francisco
San Francisco, California;
President, Mahlmeister & Associates
Nursing Quality and Patient Safety
Belmont, California

Rosemary A. McLaughlin, PhD, CNE, RN-NIC
Clinical Associate Professor
University of Memphis
Memphis, Tennessee

Carole R. Myers, PhD, RN
Associate Professor
College of Nursing
University of Tennessee
Knoxville, Tennessee

Tommie L. Norris, DNS, RN
Dean, School of Nursing
Miami Dade College
Miami, Florida

Cheryl Peterson, MSN, RN
Executive Director/EVP
ANA Executive Director
American Nurses Association
Silver Spring, Maryland

Patricia Reid Ponte, DNSc, RN, FAAN, NEA-BC
Associate Clinical Professor
School of Nursing
Boston College
Boston, Massachusetts

Anna Marie Sallee, PhD, MSN, RN
Adjunct Faculty
Nursing
University of Mary Hardin Baylor
Belton, Texas

Zoila V. Sanchez, PhD, FNP
Consultant
Jackson, Tennessee

Carla D. Sanderson, PhD, RN
Provost, Academics
Chamberlain College of Nursing
Downers Grove, Illinois

Teresa M. Stephens, PhD, RN, CNE
Associate Professor
College of Nursing
Medical University of South Carolina
Charleston, South Carolina

Margaret Elizabeth Strong, DNP, RN, NE-BC
Visiting Professor, Nursing
Chamberlain University
Chicago, Illinois

Dawn Vanderhoef, PhD, DNP, RN, PMHNP, BC, FAANP
Assistant Professor and PMHNP Program Director
School of Nursing, Vanderbilt University
Nashville, Tennessee

Elizabeth E. Weiner, PhD, RN-BC, FACMI, FAAN
Senior Associate Dean for Informatics
Frist Nursing Informatics Center
Vanderbilt University School of Nursing
Centennial Independence Foundation Professor of Nursing
Vanderbilt University School of Nursing
Nashville, Tennessee

Kathleen M. Werner, MS, BSN, RN, CPHQ
Director
Performance Improvement
UnityPoint Health – Meriter
Madison, Wisconsin

Tami H. Wyatt, PhD, RN, CNE, ANEF, FAAN
Associate Professor
College of Nursing
University of Tennessee
Knoxville, Tennessee

REVIEWERS

Tamara Bryant, RN, MSN
Program Chair
Associate of Science in Nursing Program
Southern Regional Technical College
Thomasville, Georgia

Lori Dambaugh DNP, CNS, RN, PCCN, ACCNS-AG
Assistant Professor of Nursing
Wegmans School of Nursing
St. John Fisher College Rochester Regional Health
    System
Rochester, New York

Marcee C. Everly, RN, CNM, DNP
Doctor
Baccalaureate Nursing
Indiana State University, School of Nursing
Terre Haute, Indiana

Debrayh Gaylle, RN, MS, EdD
Assistant Professor
Nursing
San Jose State University
San Jose, California

Kimberly A. Head, BA, BS, DC
Director of Continuing Education
Continuing Education, Health Sciences
Collin College
Plano, Texas

Renee Norberg, MPA, MSN, RN-BC
Adjunct Faculty
Nursing
Saint Xavier University
Chicago, Illinois

In today's rapidly evolving health care system, nurses have tremendous opportunities to improve health care and advance the nursing profession. By understanding and providing leadership to address the serious issues currently facing the U.S. health care system, nurses can advance health care to promote the health and well-being of individuals and populations in our society. These important issues include patient safety and quality care, health care reform and the uninsured population, nursing workforce challenges, advancing technology, changing legal and ethical concerns, care at the end of life, evolving nursing education trends, rising health care costs, and working within a multicultural and multigenerational society.

WHO WILL BENEFIT FROM THIS BOOK?

The eighth edition of *Contemporary Nursing: Issues, Trends, & Management* is an excellent resource to help nursing students and practicing nurses understand the complex issues facing today's health care systems and implement strategies from the direct patient care level to the national legislative arena that can significantly improve patient care, population health, the health care system, and the nursing profession.

ORGANIZATION

Unit 1: The Development of Nursing

The book opens with a presentation about the exciting evolution of nursing, its very visible public image, and its core foundations, which include nursing education, licensure and certification, nursing theory, and nursing research and evidence-based practice. These opening chapters provide the reader with a solid background for understanding and studying current and future trends.

Unit 2: Current Issues in Health Care

This unit provides a comprehensive overview of the most current trends and issues occurring today in nursing and health care, including health care financing and economics, legal and ethical issues, cultural and social issues, complementary and alternative healing, workplace issues and nursing workforce challenges, collective bargaining and unions, technology in the clinical setting, end-of-life care, and emergency preparedness. Students, faculty, and seasoned nurses will be challenged to critically examine each of these significant issues that are shaping the practice of professional nursing and the health care delivery system.

Unit 3: Leadership and Management in Nursing

This unit offers a foundation of knowledge in nursing leadership and management, with a focus on the basic skills that are necessary for all nurses, regardless of the setting or position in which they work, to function effectively in the professional nursing role. Chapters examine leadership and management theory and roles, budgeting basics, effective communication, delegation and supervision, staffing and nursing care delivery models, quality improvement and patient safety, and health policy and politics. The updated content in this unit provides the most current information available related to nursing leadership and management and will serve as both a valuable educational tool for students and a useful resource for practicing nurses.

Unit 4: Career Management

The final unit prepares the student to embark on a career in nursing. Making the transition from student to professional, managing time, understanding career opportunities, finding a good match between the nurse and the employer, and passing the NCLEX-RN® examination are all presented with practical, useful advice that will serve as an excellent resource for both students and novice nurses as they build their careers in professional nursing.

LEARNING AIDS

Each chapter in the eighth edition contains the same features that made the previous editions so successful:
- A **Professional/Ethical Issue** is included in every chapter as an interesting, real-life dilemma that will test the reader's ability to think critically and apply

ethical and professional standards to address issues or concerns the reader may face in his or her nursing practice.

- Real-life **Vignettes** and **Questions to Consider** at the beginning of each chapter, which pique the reader's interest in the chapter content and stimulate critical thinking
- **Key Terms** that contain clear and concise definitions of terms that are critical to enhance readers' understanding of the topics and expand their vocabulary related to health care issues
- Integrated **Learning Outcomes** that provide instructors and students with a clear understanding of what behaviors can be expected after a study of the chapter is completed
- **Chapter Overview,** which is an overall perspective and guide to the chapter content
- **Case Studies,** included as appropriate, that apply theory to clinical practice
- **Summary** at the end of each chapter that provides a wrap-up and helps students focus on points to remember
- **References** related to chapter content that help students explore further the issues that were covered

NEW TO THIS EDITION

Every chapter in the eighth edition has been updated to include the most current and relevant information available. New and expanded content in this edition includes the following:

- Marginalized Groups and LGBT2QIA Health Issues
- The enhanced Nurse Licensure Compact (eNLC)
- The **Nursys**' program, a unique service that allows nurses, employers, and boards of nursing to verify that nursing licenses are current and in good standing.
- Current legal cases involving nurses
- Hospice care
- Evolution of the nation's healthcare system based on healthcare reform
- Alternative models of healthcare reimbursement to promote quality and cost effectiveness with new opportunities for nursing practice
- Emphasis on every nurses' responsibility to serve as a leader to promote healthier patients and healthier work environments
- Integration of advanced technology into all aspects of clinical care "Hand-offs" in the clinical setting

- Response to active shooter events
- The *Culture of Health* initiative along with the evidence-based *County Health Rankings Model* for population health
- Technology used for job interviews

TEACHING AND LEARNING RESOURCES

For Instructors

Instructor Resources on Evolve, available at http://evolve.elsevier.com/Cherry/, provide a wealth of material to help you make your nursing instruction a success. In addition to all of the Student Resources, the following are provided for Faculty:

- **TEACH for Nurses Lesson Plans,** based on textbook chapter Learning Outcomes, serve as ready-made, modifiable lesson plans and a complete roadmap to link all parts of the educational package. These concise and straightforward lesson plans can be modified or combined to meet your particular scheduling and teaching needs.
- **PowerPoint Presentations** are organized by chapter, with more than 1000 slides for in-class lectures. These are detailed and include customizable text and image lecture slides to enhance learning in the classroom or in Web-based course modules. If you share them with students, they can use the note feature to help them with your lectures.
- The **Test Bank** has more than 500 test items, complete with the correct answer, rationale, cognitive level of each question, corresponding step of the nursing process, appropriate NCLEX format, and text page reference(s).
- **Image Collection** includes all the images from the book.

For Students

Student Resources on Evolve, available at http://evolve.elsevier.com/Cherry/, provide a wealth of valuable learning resources. The Evolve Resources page near the front of the book gives login instructions and a description of each resource.

- **Resumé Builder** offers templates and samples of resumés and cover letters.
- **Case Studies** provide detailed case studies covering the major content in the chapters.
- **Review Questions** assist in preparing for the NCLEX® examination.

ABOUT THE AUTHORS

Barbara Cherry, DNSc, MBA, RN, NEA-BC, received her diploma in nursing from Methodist Hospital School of Nursing, her BSN from West Texas A&M University, her MBA from Texas Tech University, her MSN from Texas Tech University Health Sciences Center, and her Doctor of Nursing Science from the University of Tennessee Health Science Center. Dr. Cherry's clinical background is in critical care, medical-surgical, and nephrology nursing. Her research is focused on the long-term care nursing workforce and technology. She has more than 25 years of clinical and nursing leadership experience followed by 20 years as a nurse educator and academic administrator. She is currently Professor, Associate Dean and Department Chair for Leadership Studies at Texas Tech University Health Sciences Center School of Nursing in Lubbock, Texas.

Susan R. Jacob, PhD, MSN, RN, received her BSN from West Virginia University, her MSN from San Jose State University, and her PhD from the University of Tennessee, Memphis. Her extensive experience as a clinician, educator, and researcher has been focused in the community health arena, specifically home health and hospice. She has been an educator for more than 30 years and has taught at both the undergraduate and graduate levels. She has been in academic administration for approximately 20 years. Dr. Jacob's research has addressed the bereavement experience of older adults and enhanced models of home health care delivery. Dr. Jacob, Professor and Assistant Dean of Quality and Strategic Affairs in the College of Nursing at the University of Tennessee, Health Science Center, Memphis, Tennessee, serves as the educational consultant for faith community nursing for Westberg Institute, a ministry of Church Health and schools of nursing preparing for accreditation.

ACKNOWLEDGMENTS

Our contributors deserve our most sincere thanks for their high-quality, timely work that demonstrates genuine expertise and professionalism. Their contributions have made this book a truly first-rate text that will be invaluable to nursing students and faculty and will serve as an outstanding resource for practicing nurses. We extend a special thanks to our reviewers, who gave us helpful suggestions and insights as we developed the eighth edition.

We would like to express our grateful appreciation to the Elsevier staff—Sandra Clark, Senior Content Strategist; Lisa Newton, Content Development Manager; and Cindy Thoms, Project Manager—for their very capable and professional support, guidance, and calm reassurance.

Our deepest appreciation goes to the most important people in our lives—our husbands, Mike and Dick, our families, and our friends. Their enduring support and extreme patience have allowed us to accomplish what sometimes seemed to be the impossible.

CONTENTS

UNIT 1 The Development of Nursing

1 **The Evolution of Professional Nursing,** 1
Susan R. Jacob, PhD, MSN, RN

2 **The Contemporary Image of Professional Nursing,** 21
L. Antoinette (Toni) Bargagliotti, PhD, RN, ANEF, FAAN

3 **The Influence of Contemporary Trends and Issues on Nursing Education,** 37
Dawn Vanderhoef, PhD, DNP, RN, PMHNP -BC, FAANP

4 **Nursing Licensure and Certification,** 62
Susan R. Jacob, PhD, MSN, RN

5 **Theories of Nursing Practice,** 75
Susan R. Jacob, PhD, MSN, RN

6 **Nursing Research and Evidence-Based Practice,** 88
Rosemary A. McLaughlin, PhD, CNE, RN-NIC,
Zoila V. Sanchez, PhD, FNP

UNIT 2 Current Issues in Health Care

7 **Paying for Health Care in America: Rising Costs and Challenges,** 106
Barbara Cherry, DNSc, MBA, RN, NEA-BC

8 **Legal Issues in Nursing and Health Care,** 119
Laura R. Mahlmeister, PhD, MSN, RN

9 **Ethical and Bioethical Issues in Nursing and Health Care,** 161
Carla D. Sanderson, PhD, RN

10 **Cultural Competency and Social Issues in Nursing and Health Care,** 179
Susan R. Jacob, PhD, MSN, RN

11 **Complementary and Alternative Healing,** 199
Charlotte Eliopoulos, PhD, RN, MPH, ND

12 **Palliative Care,** 216
Jeri Ashley, MSN, RN, AOCNS, CHPN,
Patricia R. Keene, DNP, ACNP-BC, ACHPN

13 **Workforce Advocacy for a Professional Nursing Practice Environment,** 232
Mary Jo Assi, DNP, RN, NEA-BC, FNP-BC, FAAN,
Cheryl Peterson, MSN, RN, Debra D. Hatmaker, PhD, RN, FAAN

14 **Collective Bargaining and Unions in Today's Workplace,** 251
Barbara Cherry, DNSc, MBA, RN, NEA-BC

15 **Information Technology in the Clinical Setting,** 261
Teresa M. Stephens, PhD, RN, CNE,
Tami H. Wyatt, PhD, RN, CNE, ANEF, FAAN

16 **Emergency Preparedness and Response for Today's World,** 274
Rebecca R. Keck, DNP, RN, NEA-BC,
Elizabeth E. Weiner, PhD, RN-BC, FACMI, FAAN

UNIT 3 Leadership and Management in Nursing

17 **Nursing Leadership and Management,** 288
Barbara Cherry, DNSc, MBA, RN, NEA-BC

18 **Budgeting Basics for Nurses,** 309
Barbara Cherry, DNSc, MBA, RN, NEA-BC

19 **Effective Communication and Conflict Resolution,** 322
Anna Marie Sallee, PhD, MSN, RN

20 **Effective Delegation and Supervision,** 345
Barbara Cherry, DNSc, MBA, RN, NEA-BC,
Margaret Elizabeth Strong, DNP, RN, NE-BC

21 **Staffing and Nursing Care Delivery Models,** 359
Barbara Cherry, DNSc, MBA, RN, NEA-BC

22 **Quality Improvement and Patient Safety,** 372
Kathleen M. Werner, MS, BSN, RN, CPHQ

23 **Health Policy and Politics: Get Involved!,** 392
Barbara Cherry, DNSc, MBA, RN, NEA-BC,
Carole R. Myers, PhD, RN

UNIT 4 Career Management

24 **Making the Transition from Student to Professional Nurse,** 409
Tommie L. Norris, DNS, RN

25 **Managing Time: The Path to High Self-Performance,** 431
Genevieve J. Conlin, DNP, MEd, MS/MBA, RN, NEA-BC,
Patricia Reid Ponte, DNSc, RN, FAAN, NEA-BC

26 **Contemporary Nursing Roles and Career Opportunities,** 445
Susan R. Jacob, PhD, MSN, RN

27 **Job Search: Finding Your Match,** 463
Susan R. Jacob, PhD, MSN, RN

28 **The NCLEX-RN® Examination,** 482
Tommie L. Norris, DNS, RN

Index, 495

1

Building on a strong foundation for a bright future.

The Evolution of Professional Nursing

Susan R. Jacob, PhD, MSN, RN

ⓔ Additional resources are available online at: *http://evolve.elsevier.com/Cherry/*

LEARNING OUTCOMES

After studying this chapter, the reader will be able to:

1. Summarize health practices throughout the course of history.
2. Analyze the effect of historic, political, social, and economic events on the development of nursing.
3. Describe the evolution of professional challenges experienced by nurses of diverse ethnic, racial, and educational backgrounds.

KEY TERMS

Florence Nightingale (1820 to 1910) Considered the founder of organized, professional nursing. She is best known for her contributions to the reforms in the British Army Medical Corps, improved sanitation in India, improved public health in Great Britain, use of statistics to document health outcomes, and the development of organized training for nurses.

Professional nurse A specially trained professional who addresses the humanistic and holistic needs of patients, families, and environments and provides responses to patterns and/or needs of patients, families, and communities to actual and potential health problems. The professional nurse has diverse roles, such as health care provider, client advocate, educator, care coordinator, primary care practitioner, and change agent (Katz et al, 2009).

PROFESSIONAL/ETHICAL ISSUE

Gretchen Ornish graduated from nursing school last year and became active in the local nurses association. She volunteered for the program planning committee

We thank Shiphrah A. Williams-Evans, PhD, APRN, BC, for her contribution to this chapter in the fourth edition.

because her friend, Beth Aaron, was also on the committee. The committee decided to plan a program for Nurses Week that would highlight pioneers in nursing. Beth agreed to pull a list of famous nurses together for the committee. When the committee met to start planning the program Beth presented her list, which included **Florence Nightingale**, Clara Barton, Dorothea

Dix, Lillian Wald, Mary Breckenridge, and many others. When Gretchen realized that all of the nurses on Beth's list were white, she suggested that Beth add names of nurses such as Harriet Tubman, Sojourner Truth, Mary Mahoney, Beverly Malone, and Elizabeth Carnegie. Beth was very reluctant to add other nurses to the list she had already developed, saying that there would not be enough time to feature more nurses than she already had on the list. She also stated that the names she had already come up with were widely known, and in her opinion the most significant. Gretchen was very disappointed because she remembered so many black nurses of distinction and felt that they should be honored as well. She feared that the program planning committee would be criticized for overlooking some very important black nursing leaders. Gretchen did not want to be part of providing what might be considered a biased program. She voiced her concerns to Beth and the committee, stating that she felt that it would be so much better if a more diverse group of nursing pioneers was highlighted. In spite of Gretchen's concerns Beth persuaded the committee to proceed with planning the program to include the list of nursing pioneers she presented.

What are some strategies that Gretchen might use to persuade Beth and the committee to present a more diverse group of nursing pioneers at the Nurses Week program?

VIGNETTE

My mother and grandmother, who are both nurses, were very excited when I decided to pursue nursing as a career. They love to talk about their experiences in nursing school in the 70s and 90s. They shared with me what they were taught about Florence Nightingale, who began the work of organized nursing. My class on the evolution of nursing covers much of the same history that my mother and grandmother were taught in their nursing programs. However, since the time when they received their education, nursing has evolved into a profession that is focused on meeting the complex needs of the diverse people it serves and preparing providers who can think critically to meet those needs. Nursing education today involves interprofessional experiences and the use of technologies such as vSim for Nursing and Shadow Health, which were unheard of in their day. Although my grandmother, mother, and I have a lot in common when it comes to our desire to

help individuals achieve optimal health outcomes, our nursing education and career opportunities are vastly different.

Questions to Consider While Reading this Chapter

1. What were the challenges faced by nurses historically?
2. How has access to care and managed care affected professional nursing practice?
3. What are the challenges facing nurses in the twenty-first century?
4. What areas of nursing specialization enhance patient care?

CHAPTER OVERVIEW

Throughout the pages of recorded history, nursing has been integrated into every facet of life. A legacy of human caring was initiated when, according to the book of Exodus, two midwives, Shiphrah and Puah, rescued the baby Moses and hid him to save his life. This legacy of caring has progressed throughout the years, responding to psychological, social, environmental, and physiologic needs of society. Nurses of the past and present have struggled for recognition as knowledgeable professionals. The evolution of this struggle is reflected in political, cultural, environmental, and economic events that have sculpted our nation and world history (Catalano, 2012).

Traditionally, society recognized men as healers. Women challenged the status quo and transformed nursing from a mystical phenomenon to a respected profession (Catalano, 2012). Florence Nightingale played a major role in bringing about changes in nursing. Using the concept of role modeling, she and other nursing leaders demonstrated the value of their worth through their work in fighting for the cause of health and healing. During the twentieth century, nurses made tremendous advancements in the areas of education, practice, research, and technology. Nursing as a science progressed through education, clinical practice, development of theory, and rigorous research. Today nurses continue to be challenged to expand their roles and explore new areas of practice and leadership. This chapter provides a brief glimpse of health care practices and nursing care in the prehistoric period and early civilization and then describes the evolution of professional nursing practice. Box 1.1 summarizes some of the important events in the evolution of nursing.

BOX 1.1 Important Events in the Evolution of Nursing

1751—The Pennsylvania Hospital is the first hospital established in America.

1798—The U.S. Marine Hospital Service comes into being by an act of Congress on July 16. It is renamed the U.S. Public Health Service in 1912.

1840—Two black women, Mary Williams and Frances Rose, who founded Nursing Sisters of the Holy Cross, are listed as nurses in the City of Baltimore Directory.

1851—Florence Nightingale (1820-1910) attends Kaiserswerth to train as a nurse.

1854—During the Crimean War, Florence Nightingale transforms the image of nursing.

1861—The outbreak of the Civil War causes black women to volunteer as nurses. Among these women are Harriet Tubman, Sojourner Truth, and Susie King Taylor.

1872—Another school of nursing opens in the United States: the New England Hospital for Women and Children in Boston, Massachusetts.

1873—Linda Richards is responsible for designing a written patient record and physician's order system—the first in a hospital.

1879—Mary Mahoney, the first trained black nurse, graduates from the New England Hospital for Women and Children in Boston, Massachusetts.

1881—The American Red Cross is established by Clara Barton.

1886—The Visiting Nurse Association (VNA) is started in Philadelphia, Pennsylvania; Spelman College, Atlanta, Georgia, establishes the first diploma-granting nursing program for African-Americans.

1893—Lillian Wald and Mary Brewster establish the Henry Street Visiting Nurse Service in New York.

1896—The Nurses' Associated Alumnae of the United States and Canada is established.

1898—Namahyoke Curtis, an untrained black nurse, is assigned by the War Department as a contract nurse in the Spanish-American War.

1899—The International Council of Nurses (ICN) is founded.

1900—The first issue of the *American Journal of Nursing* is published.

1901—The Army Nurse Corps is established under the Army Reorganization Act.

1902—School nursing is established in New York City by Linda Rogers.

1903—The first nurse practice acts are passed, and North Carolina is the first state to implement registration of nurses.

1908—The National Association of Colored Graduate Nurses is founded; it is dissolved in 1951.

1909—Ludie Andrews sues the Georgia State Board of Nurse Examiners to secure black nurses the right to take the state board examination and become licensed; she wins in 1920.

1911—The American Nurses Association (ANA) is established.

1912—The U.S. Public Health Service and the National League for Nursing (NLN) are established.

1918—Eighteen black nurses are admitted to the Army Nurse Corps after the armistice ending World War I is signed.

1919—*Public Health Nursing* is written by Mary S. Gardner. A public health nursing program is started at the University of Michigan.

1921—The Sheppard-Towner Act is passed providing federal aid for maternal and child health care.

1922—Sigma Theta Tau is founded (becomes the International Honor Society of Nursing in 1985).

1923—The Goldmark Report criticizes the inadequacies of hospital-based nursing schools and recommends increased educational standards.

1924—The U.S. Indian Bureau Nursing Service is founded by Elinor Gregg.

1925—The Frontier Nursing Service is founded by Mary Breckenridge.

1935—The Social Security Act is passed.

1937—Federal appropriations for cancer, venereal diseases, tuberculosis, and mental health begin.

1939—World War II begins.

1943—The U.S. Army establishes a quota of 56 black nurses for admission to the Army Nurse Corps. The Nurse Training Act is passed.

1943—An amendment to the Nurse Training Act is passed that bars racial bias.

1945—The U.S. Navy drops the color bar and admits four black nurses.

1946—Nurses are classified as professionals by the U.S. Civil Service Commission. The Hospital Survey and Construction Act (Hill-Burton) is passed.

1948—The Brown Report discusses the future of nursing.

1948—Estelle Osborne is the first black nurse elected to the board of the ANA. The ANA votes individual membership to all black nurses excluded from any state association.

1949—M. Elizabeth Carnegie is the first black nurse to be elected to the board of a state association (Florida).

1950—The Code for Professional Nurses is published by the ANA.

1952—National nursing organizations are reorganized from six to two: ANA and NLN.

Continued

BOX 1.1 Important Events in the Evolution of Nursing—cont'd

1954—The Supreme Court decision Brown v. Board of Education asserts that "separate educational facilities are inherently unequal."

1965—The Social Security Amendment includes Medicare and Medicaid.

1971—The National Black Nurses Association is organized.

1973—The ANA forms the American Academy of Nursing.

1974—Luther Christman helps establish the National Male Nurse Association, which becomes the American Assembly for Men in Nursing in 1981.

1978—Barbara Nichols is the first black nurse elected president of the ANA. M. Elizabeth Carnegie, a black nurse, is elected president of the American Academy of Nursing.

1979—Brigadier General Hazel Johnson Brown is the first black chief of the Army Nurse Corps.

1983—The American Academy of Nursing (AAN) Task Force on Nursing Practice in Hospitals identifies work environment characteristics known to this day as the "Forces of Magnetism."

1985—Vernice Ferguson, a black nurse, is elected president of Sigma Theta Tau International.

1986—The Association of Black Nursing Faculty is founded by Dr. Sally Tucker Allen.

1990—Congress proclaims March 10 as Harriet Tubman Day in the United States, honoring her as a brave black freedom fighter and nurse during the Civil War.

1990—The Bloodborne Pathogen Standard is established by the Occupational Safety and Health Administration (OSHA).

1991—*Healthy People 2000* is published.

1993—The National Center for Nursing Research is upgraded to the National Institute of Nursing Research within the National Institutes of Health.

1994—NCLEX-RN, a computerized nurse-licensing examination, is introduced.

1996—The Commission on Collegiate Nursing Education is established as an agency devoted exclusively to the accreditation of baccalaureate and graduate-degree nursing programs.

1999—Beverly Malone, the second black president of the ANA, is named Deputy Assistant Secretary for Health, Department of Health and Human Services, Office of Public Health and Science.

1999—The Institute of Medicine (IOM) releases its landmark report: *To Err Is Human: Building a Safer Health System.*

2000—M. Elizabeth Carnegie is inducted into the ANA Hall of Fame. The American Nurses Credentialing Center gives its first psychiatric mental health nurse practitioner examination. *Healthy People 2010* is published.

2001—Beverly Malone is appointed General Secretary, Royal College of Nursing, London. The Health Care Financing Administration (HCFA) becomes the Centers for Medicare & Medicaid Services (CMS).

2002—Johnson & Johnson Health Care Systems, Inc. launches The Future of Nursing, a national publicity campaign to address the nursing shortage.

2002—To address the nursing shortage, the Nurse Reinvestment Act is signed into law by President George W. Bush.

2002—Significant funding is obtained for geriatric nursing initiatives.

2003—The American Nurses Foundation launches an "Investment in Nursing" campaign to deal with the nursing shortage.

2003—The IOM report *Keeping Patients Safe: Transforming the Work Environment of Nurses* is released.

2003—The AACN White Paper on the Role of the Clinical Nurse Leader is published.

2005—The CCNE decides that only programs that offer practice doctoral degrees with the Doctor of Nursing Practice (DNP) title will be eligible for CCNE accreditation.

2005—The NLN offers and certifies the first national certification for nurse educators; the initials CNE may be placed behind the names of those certified.

2006—The AACN approves essentials of doctoral education for advanced nursing practice (DNP).

2007—The Commission on Nurse Certification, an autonomous arm of the AACN, begins certifying clinical nurse leaders (CNLs).

2007—American Nurses Credentialing Center acquires the Texas Nurses Association's Nurse Friendly Program and renames it Pathway to Excellence.

2008—The Commission on Collegiate Nursing Education begins accrediting DNP programs.

2010—*Healthy People 2020* is launched by the Department of Health and Human Services.

2010—The Patient Protection and Affordable Care Act (Public Law 111-152) is passed.

2010—The Health Care and Education Affordability Reconciliation Act is passed.

2011—The IOM report *The Future of Nursing: Leading Change, Advancing Health* is released.

2016 - *Advancing Healthcare Transformation: A New Era for Academic Nursing*, commissioned by the American Association of Colleges of Nursing (AACN) is released.

From AACN, 2006; Carnegie, 1995; Deloughery, 1998; Donahue, 1999; Kalisch and Kalisch, 1995; IOM, 2003, 2011.

PREHISTORIC PERIOD

Nursing in the prehistoric period was delineated by health practices that were strongly guided by beliefs of magic, religion, and superstition. Individuals who were ill were considered to be cursed by evil spirits and evil gods that entered the human body and caused suffering and death if not cast out. These beliefs dictated the behavior of primitive people, who sought to scare away the evil gods and spirits. Members of tribes participated in rituals, wore masks, and engaged in demonstrative dances to rid the sick of demonic possession of the body. Sacrifices and offerings, sometimes including human sacrifices, were made to rid the body of evil gods, demons, and spirits. Many tribes used special herbs, roots, and vegetables to cast out the "curse" of illness.

EARLY CIVILIZATION

Egypt

Ancient Egyptians are noted for their accomplishments in health care at an early period in civilization. They were the first to use the concept of suture in repairing wounds. They also were the first to be recorded as developing community planning that resulted in a decrease in public health problems. One of the main early public health problems was the spread of disease through contaminated water sources. Specific laws on cleanliness, food use and preservation, drinking, exercise, and sexual relations were developed. Health beliefs of Egyptians determined preventive measures taken and personal health behaviors practiced. These health behaviors were usually carried out to accommodate the gods. Some behaviors were also practiced expressly to appease the spirits of the dead (Catalano, 2012). The Egyptians developed the calendar and writing, which initiated recorded history. The oldest records date back to the sixteenth century BC in Egypt. A pharmacopoeia that classified more than 700 drugs was written to assist in the care and management of disease (Ellis and Hartley, 2012). As in the case of Shiphrah and Puah, the midwives who saved baby Moses, nurses were used by kings and other aristocrats to deliver babies and care for the young, older adults, and those who were sick.

Palestine

From 1400 to 1200 BC, the Hebrews migrated from the Arabian Desert and gradually settled in Palestine, where they became an agricultural society. Under the leadership of Moses, the Hebrews developed a system of laws called the Mosaic Code. This code, one of the first organized methods of disease control and prevention, contained public health laws that dictated personal, family, and public hygiene. For instance, laws were written to prohibit the eating of animals that were dead longer than 3 days and to isolate individuals who were thought to have communicable diseases. Hebrew priests took on the role of health inspectors (Ellis and Hartley, 2012).

Greece

From 1500 to 100 BC, Greek philosophers sought to understand man and his relationship with the gods, nature, and other men. They believed that the gods and goddesses of Greek mythology controlled health and illness. Temples built to honor Aesculapius, the god of medicine, were designated to care for the sick. Aesculapius carried a staff that was intertwined with serpents or snakes, representing wisdom and immortality. This staff is thought to be the model of today's medical caduceus. Hippocrates (460 to 362 BC), considered the "Father of Medicine," paved the way in establishing scientific knowledge in medicine. Hippocrates was the first to attribute disease to natural causes rather than supernatural causes and curses of the gods. His teachings also emphasized the patient-centered approach and use of the scientific method for solving problems (Catalano, 2012).

India

Dating from 3000 to 1500 BC, the earliest cultures of India were Hindu. The sacred book of Brahmanism (also known as Hinduism), the Vedas, was used to guide health care practices. The Vedas, considered by some to be the oldest written material, emphasized hygiene and prevention of sickness and described major and minor surgical procedures. The Indian practice of surgery was very well developed. The importance of prenatal care to mother and infant was also well understood. Public hospitals were constructed from 274 to 236 BC and were staffed by male nurses with qualifications and duties similar to those of the twentieth-century practical nurse (Ellis and Hartley, 2012).

China

The teachings of the Chinese scholar Confucius (551 to 479 BC) had a powerful effect on the customs and practices of the people of ancient China. Confucius taught a moral philosophy that addressed one's obligation to society. Several hundred years after his death, this philosophy became the basis for Chinese education and government. Central to his teachings were service to the community and the value of the family as a unit. However, women were considered inferior to men.

The early Chinese also placed great value on solving life's problems. Their belief about health and illness was based on the yin and yang philosophy. The yin represented the feminine forces, which were considered negative and passive. The yang represented the masculine forces, which were positive and active. The Chinese believed that an imbalance between these two forces would result in illness, whereas balance between the yin and yang represented good health (Ellis and Hartley, 2012). The ancient Chinese used a variety of treatments believed to promote health and harmony, including acupuncture. Acupuncture involves insertion of hot and cold needles into the skin and underlying tissues to manage or cure conditions (such as pain, stroke, and breathing difficulty) and ultimately to affect the balance of yin and yang. Hydrotherapy, massage, and exercise were used as preventive health measures (Giger and Davidhizar, 2008). Baths were used to reduce fever, and bloodletting was used to release evil spirits from the body (Ellis and Hartley, 2012).

Rome

The Roman Empire (27 BC to 476 AD), a military dictatorship, adapted medical practices from the countries they conquered and the physicians they enslaved. At the end of the Dark Ages, there were a series of holy wars, including the Crusades. The first military hospital in Europe was established in Rome to care for the injured. Military nursing orders that were made up exclusively of men were also developed. They were very well organized and dedicated, and they wore suits of armor for protection with the emblem of a red cross (Catalano, 2012; Walton et al, 1994). The Romans practiced advanced hygiene and sanitation and emphasized bathing (Ellis and Hartley, 2012).

THE MIDDLE AGES

The Middle Ages (476 to 1450) followed the demise of the Roman Empire (Walton et al, 1994). Women began using herbs and new methods of healing, whereas men continued to use purging, leeching, and mercury. This period also saw the Roman Catholic Church become a central figure in the organization and management of health care. Most of the changes in health care were based on the Church's emphasis on charity and the sanctity of human life. Wives of emperors and other women considered to be noble became nurses. These women devoted themselves to caring for the sick, often carrying baskets of food and medicine as they journeyed from house to house (Bahr and Johnson, 1997). Widows and unmarried women became nuns and deaconesses. Two of these deaconesses, Dorcas and Phoebe, are mentioned in the Bible as outstanding for the care they provided to the sick (Freedman, 1995).

During the Middle Ages, physicians spent most of their time translating medical essays and provided little actual medical care. Poorly trained barbers, who lacked any formal medical education, performed surgery and medical treatments that were considered "bloody" or "messy." Nurses also provided some medical care, although in most hospitals and monasteries, female nurses who were not midwives were forbidden to witness childbirth, help with gynecologic examinations, or even diaper male infants (Kalisch and Kalisch, 1986). During the Crusades, which lasted for almost 200 years (from 1096 to 1291), military nursing orders, known as Templars and Hospitalers, were founded. Monks and Christian knights provided nursing care and defended the hospitals during battle, wearing suits of armor under their religious habits. The habits were distinguished by the Maltese cross to identify the monks and knights as Christian warriors. The same cross was used years later on a badge designed for the first school of nursing and became a forerunner for the design of nursing pins (Ellis and Hartley, 2012).

THE RENAISSANCE AND THE REFORMATION PERIOD

Following the Middle Ages came the Renaissance and the Reformation, also known as the rebirth of Europe (the fourteenth to sixteenth centuries). Major advancements were made in pharmacology, chemistry, and medical knowledge, including anatomy, physiology, and surgery. During the Renaissance, new emphasis was given to medical education, but nursing education was practically nonexistent.

The Reformation, which began in Germany in 1517, was a religious movement that resulted in a dissention between Roman Catholics and Protestants. During this period, religious facilities that provided health care closed. Women were encouraged toward charitable services, but their main duties included bearing and caring for children in their homes. Furthermore, hospital work was no longer appealing to women of high economic status, and the individuals who worked as nurses in hospitals were often female prisoners, prostitutes, and alcoholics. Nursing was no longer the respected profession it had once been. This period is referred to as the "Dark Ages" of nursing (Ellis and Hartley, 2012).

During the sixteenth and seventeenth centuries, famine, plague, filth, and crime ravaged Europe. King Henry VII eliminated the organized monastic relief programs that aided the orphans, poor, and other displaced people. Out of great concern for social welfare, several nursing groups, such as the Order of the Visitation of St. Mary, the Daughters of Charity of St. Vincent de Paul, and the Sisters of Charity, were organized to give time, service, and money to the poor and sick. The Sisters of Charity recruited intelligent young women for training in nursing, developed educational programs, and cared for abandoned children (Ellis and Hartley, 2012).

THE COLONIAL AMERICAN PERIOD

The first hospital and the first medical school in North America were founded in Mexico—the Hospital of the Immaculate Conception in Mexico City and the medical school at the University of Mexico. During this time in the American colonies, individuals with infectious diseases were isolated in almshouses or "pesthouses" (Ellis and Hartley, 2012). Procedures such as purgatives and bleeding were widely used, leading to shortened life expectancy. Plagues, such as scarlet fever, dysentery, and smallpox, caused thousands of deaths. Benjamin Franklin, who was outspoken regarding the care of the sick, insisted that a hospital be built in the colonies. He believed that the community should be responsible for the management and treatment of those who were ill. Through his efforts, the first hospital, called the Pennsylvania Hospital, was built in the United States in Philadelphia in 1751 (Ellis and Hartley, 2012).

FLORENCE NIGHTINGALE

Florence Nightingale was born in Florence, Italy, on May 12, 1820. Her family was wealthy, well-traveled, and well educated. Nightingale was an intelligent, talented, and attractive woman. From an early age, she demonstrated a deep concern for the poor and suffering. At 25 years of age, she became interested in training as a nurse. However, her family was strongly opposed to this choice and preferred that she marry and take her place in society (Joel, 2006). In 1851, her parents finally permitted her to pursue training as a nurse. At 31 years of age, Nightingale attended a 3-month nursing training program at the Institution of Deaconesses at Kaiserswerth, Germany. In 1854, she began training nurses at the Harley Street Nursing Home and served as superintendent of nurses at King's College Hospital in London (Ellis and Hartley, 2012). The outbreak of the Crimean War marked a turning point in Nightingale's career. In October 1854, Sidney Herbert, British Secretary of War and an old friend of the Nightingale family, wrote to Nightingale and asked her to lead a group of nurses to the Crimea to work at one of the military hospitals under government authority and expense. Nightingale accepted his offer and assembled 38 nurses who were sisters and nuns from various Catholic and Anglican orders (Ellis and Hartley, 2012).

Nightingale and her team were assigned to the Barracks Hospital at Scutari. When Nightingale arrived, she found deplorable conditions. Between 3000 and 4000 sick and wounded men were packed into the hospital, which was originally designed to accommodate 1700 patients. There were no beds, blankets, food, or medicine. Many of the wounded soldiers had been placed on the floor, where lice, maggots, vermin, rodents, and blood covered their bodies. There were no candles or lanterns. All medical care had to be rendered during the light of day (Ellis and Hartley, 2012).

Despite the distressing conditions at the Barracks Hospital, the army physicians and surgeons at first refused Nightingale's assistance. However, within a week and faced with scurvy, starvation, dysentery, and the eruption of more fighting, the physicians, in desperation, called her to help. Nightingale immediately purchased medical supplies, food, linens, and hospital equipment, using her own money and that of the Times Relief Fund. Within 10 days, she had set up a kitchen for special diets and had rented a house that she converted into a laundry (Gill, 2004; Small, 2002). The wives of soldiers were hired to manage and operate the laundry service. She assigned soldiers to make repairs and clean up the building. Just weeks later, she initiated social services, reading classes, and even coffeehouses where soldiers could enjoy music and recreation (Nies and McEwen, 2015).

Nightingale worked long, hard hours to care for these soldiers. She spent up to 20 hours each day caring for wounds, comforting soldiers, assisting in surgery, directing staff, and keeping records. Nightingale introduced principles of infection control, a system for transcribing physicians' orders, and a procedure to maintain patient records.

Nightingale is credited with using public health principles and statistical methods to advocate for improved health conditions for British soldiers. Through carefully recorded statistics, Nightingale was able to document that the soldiers' death rate decreased from 42% to 2% as a result of health care reforms that emphasized sanitary conditions. Because of her remarkable work in using statistics to demonstrate cause and effect and improve the health of British soldiers, Nightingale is recognized for her contributions to nursing research (Nies and McEwen, 2015).

Nightingale also demonstrated the power of political activism to effect health care reform by writing letters of criticism accompanied by constructive recommendations to British army leaders. Nightingale's ability to overthrow the British army's management method, which had allowed the deplorable conditions to exist in the army hospitals, was considered one of her greatest achievements (Nies and McEwen, 2015).

After her return from the Crimea, Nightingale experienced ongoing health problems. Early writers suggest that she retreated to her bedroom for the next 43 years and continued her involvement in health care from her secluded apartment. More recent research, however, indicates a more active involvement (Ellis and Hartley, 2012).

Florence Nightingale's work, from the Crimean War to the establishment of formal nursing education programs, was a catapult for the reorganization and advancement of professional nursing. Nightingale wrote extensively about hospitals, sanitation, health and health statistics (creating the first pie chart), and nursing education. Among her most popular books is *Notes on Nursing,* published in 1859.

In 1860, Nightingale established the first nursing school in England, St. Thomas' Hospital of London. By 1873, graduates of Nightingale's nurse training program in England migrated to the United States, where they became supervisors in the first of the hospital-based (diploma) nursing schools: Massachusetts General Hospital in Boston, Bellevue Hospital in New York, and the New Haven Hospital in Connecticut.

Until her death in August 1910, Nightingale demonstrated the powerful effect that well-educated, creative, skilled, and competent individuals have in the provision of health care. She is honored as the founder of professional nursing (Ellis and Hartley, 2012). Nightingale had the means to support her work and the stamina to drive forward in her belief concerning health care. Even though Louis Pasteur's germ theory was not widely known and was very controversial at the time, her theory of environmental cleanliness is still applicable today.

NURSING IN THE UNITED STATES

The Civil War Period

During the United States Civil War, or the War Between the States (1861 to 1865), health care conditions in the United States were similar to those encountered by Nightingale. Numerous epidemics plagued the country, including syphilis, gonorrhea, malaria, smallpox, and typhoid (Nelson, 2001; Oermann, 1997).

The Civil War was initiated by the attack on Fort Sumter, South Carolina, April 17, 1861. At this time, there were no nurses formally trained to care for the sick. However, thousands of men and women from the South and North volunteered to care for the wounded. Hospitals were set up in the field, and transports were put in place to carry the wounded to hospitals (Carnegie, 1995).

Secretary of War Simon Cameron appointed a schoolteacher named Dorothea Dix to organize military hospitals and provide medical supplies to the Union Army soldiers. Dix received no official status and no salary for this position.

Women providing nursing care during the Civil War worked under very primitive conditions. Maintaining sanitary conditions was an overwhelming challenge and often not possible. More than 6 million patients were admitted to hospitals. Approximately 500,000 surgical procedures were performed. Unfortunately, there were only about 2000 individuals who served as nurses, far fewer than the number needed to provide adequate care (Fitzpatrick, 1997; Kalisch and Kalisch, 1995). According to records kept at three hospitals, 181 male and female black nurses served between July 16, 1863, and June 14,

1864. White nurses were paid $12 per month; black nurses received $10 per month (Carnegie, 1995).

Three black nurses made particularly important contributions to nursing efforts during the Civil War: Harriet Tubman cared for the sick as a nurse in the Sea Islands off the coast of South Carolina and was later known as the "conductor of the Underground Railroad." It is also reported that she was the first woman to lead American troops into battle (Carnegie, 1995). So-journer Truth, known for her abolitionist and nursing efforts, was an advocate of clean and sanitary conditions for patients. She insisted that these conditions were needed for patients to heal. Susie King Taylor, although hired to work in the laundry, served as a nurse because of the growing number of wounded who needed care. Having learned to read and write, which was against the law for blacks at the time, she also taught many of her comrades in Company E to read and write (Carnegie, 1995).

Many other volunteer nurses made important contributions during the Civil War: Clara Barton served on the front line during the Civil War and operated a war relief program to provide supplies to the battlefields and hospitals. Barton also set up a postwar service to find missing soldiers and is credited with founding the American Red Cross (Nies and McEwen, 2015). Louisa May Alcott, who served as a nurse for 6 weeks until stopped by ill health, authored detailed accounts of the experiences encountered by nurses during the war for a newspaper publication titled *Hospital Sketches* (Kalisch and Kalisch, 1995, 2003).

When the Civil War ended, the number of nurse training schools increased. The war had proven the need for more nurses to be formally trained. These early nursing programs offered little or no classroom education, and on-the-job training occurred in the hospital wards. The students learned routine patient care duties, worked long hours 6 days a week, and were used as supplemental hospital staff. After graduation, most of the nurses practiced as private duty nurses or hospital staff (Lindeman and McAthie, 1990). The first nursing textbook, titled *A Manual of Nursing,* was published in 1876 and was used by the New York Training School for Nurses at Bellevue Hospital (Kalisch and Kalisch, 1995).

During the 1890s, the nationwide establishment of hospitals and nursing schools for blacks gained momentum as black musicians, educators, and community leaders became alarmed at the high rates of morbidity and mortality among black Americans. Because of segregation and discrimination, African-Americans had to establish their own health care institutions to provide black patients with access to quality health care and to provide black men and women with opportunities to enter the nursing profession. However, in 1886, John D. Rockefeller, a white philanthropist, funded the establishment of the first school of nursing for black women at the Atlanta Baptist Seminary—now known as Spelman College (Jones, 2004). (Box 1.2.)

BOX 1.2 Duties of the Hospital Floor Nurse in 1887

In addition to caring for your 60 patients, each nurse will follow these regulations:

1. Daily sweep and mop the floors of your ward; dust the patient's furniture and windowsill.
2. Maintain an even temperature on your ward by bringing in a scuttle of coal for the day's business.
3. Light is important to observe the patient's condition; therefore, each day fill kerosene lamps, clean chimneys, and trim wicks. Wash the windows once a week.
4. The nurse's notes are important in aiding the physician's work. Make your pens carefully; you may whittle nibs to your individual taste.
5. Each nurse on day duty will report every day at 7 AM and will leave at 8 PM except on Sabbath, on which day you will be off from 12 noon to 2 PM.
6. Graduate nurses in good standing with the director of nurses will be given an evening off each week if you regularly attend church.
7. Each nurse should lay aside from each payday a good sum of her earning for her benefits during her declining years so that she will not become a burden. For example, if you earn $20 a month, you should set aside $10.
8. Any nurse who smokes, uses liquor in any form, gets her hair done at a beauty shop, or frequents dance halls will have given the director of nurses good reason to suspect her worth, intentions, and integrity.
9. The nurse who performs her labors, serves her patients and physicians faithfully and without fault for a period of 5 years will be given an increase by the hospital administration of 5 cents per day, providing there are no hospital debts that are outstanding.

1900 to World War I

In the 1900s, states began to require nurses to become registered before entering practice. By 1910, most states had upgraded education requirements to high school, upgraded training, and required registration before practice (Deloughery, 1998; Donahue, 1999). The Army and Navy Nurse Corps were created in 1901 and 1908, respectively, and an estimated 30,000 nurses served in World War I (Ellis and Hartley, 2012).

Lillian Wald, a pioneer in public health nursing, is best known for the development and establishment of the first viable practice for public health nurses. The main location for this practice was the Henry Street Settlement House, located in the Lower East Side of New York City. Its purpose was to provide well-baby care, health education, disease prevention, and treatment of patients with minor illnesses. Nursing practice based at the Henry Street Settlement House formed the basis of public health nursing for the entire country. Instead of relying on patients to visit the clinic, public health nurses made their way to the various tenements located around Henry Street (Nies and McEwen, 2015).

Wald also developed the first nursing service for occupational health. She believed that prevention of disease among workers would improve productivity and was able to persuade the Metropolitan Life Insurance Company that her ideas had merit. As a result, nursing agencies, such as those in place at the Henry Street Settlement House, provided skilled nursing services to employees. Another innovation that emerged from this program was the sliding fee scale, by which patients were billed according to their income or their ability to pay. In 1911, Wald chaired a committee formed by members of the Associated Alumnae of Training Schools for Nurses, later to become the American Nurses Association (ANA), and the Society of Superintendents of Training Schools for Nurses, the precursor of the National League for Nursing (NLN). The purpose of the committee was to develop standards for nursing services performed outside the hospital environment. The committee determined that a new organization was necessary to meet the needs of community health nurses. The result of the committee's recommendation was the formation of the National Organization for Public Health Nursing, whose goals were to establish educational and practice standards for community health nursing (Stanhope and Lancaster, 2015).

The ANA and the NLN are still leading nursing organizations today. The ANA has focused primarily on professional aspects of nursing, and the NLN was the only accrediting body for nursing schools until 1996, when the Commission on Collegiate Nursing Education (CCNE), an autonomous arm of the American Association of Colleges of Nursing (AACN), was established as an agency devoted exclusively to the accreditation of baccalaureate and graduate degree nursing programs (Ellis and Hartley, 2012).

In 2013 the National League for Nursing Accreditation Commission (NLNAC) changed its name and is now the Accreditation Commission for Education in Nursing (ACEN). This organization accredits practical, diploma, baccalaureate, and graduate degree nursing programs.

World War I and the 1920s

During the early 1900s, the world was rapidly changing and moving toward global conflict. Germany was arming, and the rest of Europe was trying to ignore the threat. "Prosperous" was the word used to describe the U.S. economy. Women were granted the right to vote and were moving into the workforce on a regular basis.

Advancements in medical care and public health were being made. The primary site for medical care moved from the home to the hospital, and surgical and diagnostic techniques were improved. Pneumonia management was the focus of scientific study. Insulin was discovered in 1922, and in 1928 Alexander Fleming discovered the precursor of penicillin, which would eventually be used to successfully treat patients with pneumonia and other infections (Kalisch and Kalisch, 1995). (See Box 1.2.)

Environmental conditions improved, and the serious epidemics of the previous century became nonexistent. Lillian Wald, in *The House on Henry Street*, linked poor environmental and social conditions to prevalent illnesses and poverty and used this information to lead the fight for better sanitation and housing conditions (Nies and McEwen, 2015).

With the outbreak of World War I in 1914, nurses were desperately needed to care for the soldiers who were injured or who suffered from the many illnesses resulting from trench warfare (Nies and McEwen, 2015). The war offered nurses a chance to advance into new fields of specialization. For example, nurse anesthetists made their first appearance as part of the surgical teams at the front lines. More than 20,000 U.S.-trained nurses served in World War I (Oermann, 1997).

Because many nurses volunteered to provide services during the war, the community health nursing movement in the United States stalled. However, the American Red Cross, founded by Clara Barton in 1882, assisted in efforts to continue public health nursing. The Red Cross nurses originally focused on members of rural communities who were not able to access health care services. As the war continued, however, the Red Cross nurses also moved into urban areas to provide health care services (Stanhope and Lancaster, 2015).

During World War I, the U.S. Public Health Service, founded in 1798 to provide health care services to merchant seamen, was charged with the responsibility to provide health services at military posts located within the United States. A nurse, who was "loaned" by the National Organization for Public Health Nursing, established nursing services at U.S. military outposts. The responsibilities of the U.S. Public Health Service continued to grow; eventually it was composed of physicians, nurses, and other allied health professionals, who provided indigent care and practiced in community health programs (Stanhope and Lancaster, 2015).

Further changes were in store for nursing during World War I. In 1918, the Vassar Camp School for Nurses was established. Its purpose was to provide an intensive 2-year nurses' training program for college graduates. Graduates of the program were given an army reserve commission and would be activated during times of war to meet increased nursing needs. Sponsored by the American Red Cross and the Council of National Defense, the school graduated 435 nurses. The Vassar Camp School for Nurses was a short-lived enterprise. When peace was declared in 1919, the program was permanently disbanded (Snodgrass, 2004; Stanhope and Lancaster, 2015).

In 1921, the federal government recognized the need to improve the health of women and children and passed the Sheppard-Towner Act, one of the first pieces of federal legislation to provide funds to assist in the care of special populations (Nies and McEwen, 2015). This funding provided public health nurses with resources to promote the health and well-being of women, infants, and children.

Following these improvements, the Frontier Nursing Service (FNS) was established in 1925 by Mary Breckenridge of Kentucky. Born into a wealthy family,

Breckenridge learned the value of providing care to others from her grandmother. Breckenridge began her career at St. Luke's Hospital School of Nursing in New York. After serving as a nurse during World War I, she returned to Columbia University to learn more about community health nursing. Armed with her new knowledge and a passion to assist disadvantaged women and children, Breckenridge returned to Kentucky and the rural Appalachian Mountains (Stanhope and Lancaster, 2015).

Breckenridge believed that the rural mountain area of Kentucky, cut off from many modern conveniences, was an excellent place to prove the value of community health nursing. She established the FNS in a five-room cabin in Hyden, Kentucky. After serious obstacles such as no water supply or sewage disposal were overcome, six other nursing outposts were constructed in the rural mountains from 1927 to 1930. The FNS based its hospital in Hyden and eventually attracted physicians and nurses to provide medical, dental, surgical, nursing, and midwifery services to the rural poor. Financial support for the FNS ranged from fees for labor and supplies to funds raised through annual family dues to donations and fundraising efforts. Nurses working for the FNS traveled a 700-square mile area, often on horseback, to provide services to approximately 10,000 patients (Stanhope and Lancaster, 2015).

Breckenridge established an important health care service for rural Kentucky communities. Equally important was her documentation of the results of community health nursing in rural communities. Breckenridge followed the advice of a consulting physician and collected mortality data on the communities before nursing services actually were started. The results were startling; mortality was significantly reduced, and the need for the nursing services was clearly documented. Breckenridge proved that even in appalling environmental conditions without heat, electricity, or running water, nursing services could make a substantial positive impact on the health of the community (Stanhope and Lancaster, 2015). The FNS is still in operation today and provides vital service to the rural communities of Kentucky.

The Great Depression (1930 to 1940)

The U.S. economy prospered during World War I and well into the 1920s. However, after the stock market crash in October 1929, economic prosperity quickly dissipated. Millions of men and women became unemployed. Before the Depression, many people had private duty nurses. However, during the Depression, many nurses found themselves unemployed because most families could no longer afford private duty nurses.

Franklin D. Roosevelt, elected president of the United States in 1932, faced a country in shambles. He responded with several innovative and necessary interventions and ushered in the first major social legislation enacted in U.S. history. Titled the "New Deal," the legislation had several social components that affected the provision of medical care and other services for indigent people across the country (Karger, 2005).

The piece of legislation that had the greatest effect on health care in the United States was the Social Security Act of 1935, which set the precedent for the passage of the Medicare and Medicaid acts in 1965. The main purposes of the 1935 Social Security Act were to provide (1) a national old-age insurance system, (2) federal grants to states for maternal and child welfare services, (3) vocational rehabilitation services for the handicapped, (4) medical care for crippled children and blind people, (5) a plan to strengthen public health services, and (6) a federal-state unemployment system (Karger and Stoesz, 2005).

The passage of the 1935 Social Security Act provided avenues for nursing care, and nursing jobs were created. With funds from the Social Security Act, public health nursing became the major source of health care for dependent mothers and children, the blind, and crippled children. Nurses found employment as public health nurses for county or state health departments (Stanhope and Lancaster, 2015). Hospital job opportunities also were created for nurses, and the hospital became the usual employment setting for graduate nurses.

World War II (1940 to 1945)

The United States officially entered World War II after the bombing of Pearl Harbor in December 1941. At that time, the nursing divisions of all of the military branches had inadequate numbers of nurses. Congress passed legislation to provide needed funds to expand nursing education. A committee of six national nursing organizations, called the National Nursing Council, received $1 million to accomplish the needed expansion. The U.S. Public Health Service became the administrator of the funds, further strengthening the tie between the U.S. Public Health Service and nursing (Stanhope and Lancaster, 2015).

The war was considered a global conflict, and nursing became an essential part of the military advance. Nurses were required to function under combat conditions and had to adapt nursing care to meet the challenges of different climates, facilities, and supplies. As a result of their service during World War II, nurses finally were recognized as an integral part of the military and attained the ranks of officers in the army and navy. Colonel Julie O. Flikke was the first army nurse to be promoted to colonel in the U.S. Army and served as Superintendent of the Army Nurse Corps from 1937 to 1942 (Deloughery, 1998; Robinson and Perry, 2001).

Post–World War II Period (1945 to 1950)

The period after World War II was a time of prosperity for the average American. The GI Bill enabled returning veterans to complete their interrupted education. The unemployment rate dropped to an all-time low in the United States. In an effort to provide more areas of employment for the returning men, the federal government mounted a massive campaign to encourage women to return to the more traditional roles of wife and mother. Consequently, numerous women in all professions, including nursing, chose to return to marriage and childrearing rather than continue employment outside the home.

After World War II the Soviet Union began invading and taking over Eastern European countries. With support from China, the North Koreans made a grab for South Korea, resulting in the Korean War. Again, nurses volunteered for the armed services to provide care to patients near the battlefields in Korea. This time they worked in mobile army surgical hospitals, better known as MASH units, where medical and surgical techniques were further refined.

The two decades after World War II saw the emergence of nursing as a true profession. National standards for nursing education were established by the National Nursing Accrediting Service. By 1950, all state boards were participating in the test pool; they continue to do so today. Nursing continued to improve the quality and quantity of educational programs as the number of nursing baccalaureate programs increased and associate degree programs developed in community or junior colleges (Ellis and Hartley, 2012) (see Box 1.1).

The end of World War II and the early 1950s marked the beginning of significant federal intervention in health care. The Nurse Training Act of 1943 was the first

BOX 1.3 Qualities of Good Nurses During Post–World War II

1. Tidy and loyal to the hospital and its personnel
2. Compliant with the orders of the physicians and directives of nursing management
3. Always busy
4. If census was low, fold laundry, clean shelves, prepare supplies to be sterilized
5. Ability to get work done no matter how many patients assigned

From Martell, L.K. (1999). Maternity care during the post–World War II baby boom: the experience of general duty nurses, *West J Nurs Res, 96*(3), 387-391.

instance of federal funding being used to support nurse training. The passage of the Hill-Burton Act, or the Hospital Survey and Construction Act of 1946, marked the largest commitment of federal dollars to health care in the country's history. The purpose of the act was to provide funding to construct hospitals and to assist states in planning for other health care facilities based on the needs of the communities. Nearly 40% of the hospitals constructed in the late 1940s and the early 1950s were built with Hill-Burton funds. The hospital construction boom created by the Hill-Burton Act led to an increased demand for professional nurses to provide care in hospitals (Nies and McEwen, 2015) (Box 1.3.)

It was also in the early 1950s that the National Association of Colored Graduate Nurses (NACGN) went out of existence. This was the organization that had fought for integration of the black nurse into the ANA. From 1916 to 1948, black nurses in the South were barred from membership in the ANA because of segregation laws in the Southern states. In the 1940s, the NACGN began to wage an all-out war against discrimination by the Southern constituents of the ANA. The NACGN chose as its central issue the route to membership in ANA. This issue was raised by the NACGN on the floor at every national convention of the ANA, and it evoked strong opposition from the Southern state constituents. Speaking from the floor of the House of Delegates at the 1946 convention in Atlantic City, a white nurse from Georgia referred to black nurses as "our darkies." Immediately a motion was passed to strike the reference from the record. However, this comment caused an uproar, and the black nurses who were barred from membership in the Southern states started the wheels turning to

bypass the states and join ANA directly. This arrangement, known as *individual membership,* was put into effect in 1948. With the establishment of individual membership, black nurses in the South could bypass their states and become members of the ANA. This type of individual membership continued until all barriers had been dropped in the early 1960s (Carnegie, 1995).

Nursing in the 1960s

Federal legislation enacted during the 1960s had a major and lasting effect on nursing and health care. The Community Mental Health Centers Act of 1963 provided funds for the construction of community outpatient mental health centers; opportunities for mental health nursing were expanded when funds to staff these centers were appropriated in 1965 with the passage of the Medicare and Medicaid acts (Nies and McEwen, 2015). Medicaid, Title XIX of the Social Security Act, was enacted and replaced all programs previously instituted for medical assistance. The purpose of the Medicaid program, which was jointly sponsored and financed with matching funds from federal and state governments, was to serve as medical insurance for those families, primarily women and children, with an income at or below the federal poverty level. Medicaid quickly became the largest public assistance program in the nation.

Health departments employed public health nurses to provide the bulk of the care needed by children and pregnant women in the Medicaid population. Services provided by these nurses included family planning, well-child assessments, immunizations, and prenatal care. A physician assigned as the district health officer supervised the nurses. Without the public health nurses and local health departments, many women and children in the inner city areas and rural communities would have been without access to basic health care.

Another important amendment to the Social Security Act was Title XVIII, or Medicare, passed in 1965. The Medicare program provides hospital insurance, part A, and medical insurance, part B, to all people 65 years of age and older who are eligible to receive Social Security benefits; people with total, permanent disabilities; and people with end-stage renal disease. As a result of Medicare reimbursement, many hospitals began catering to physicians who treated Medicare patients. Medicare patients were attractive to the hospitals because all hospital charges, regardless of amount or appropriateness of services, were reimbursed through the Medicare program (Nies and McEwen, 2015).

As a result of Medicare reimbursement, hospital-bed occupancy increased, which led to the need for increased numbers of nurses to staff hospitals. Nursing embraced the hospital setting as the usual practice area and moved away from the community as the preferred practice site. Nursing schools also followed the trend by reducing the number of curriculum hours devoted to community health and concentrating their efforts on hospital-based nursing (Stanhope and Lancaster, 2015).

Another outcome of the Medicare legislation was the home health movement. To receive Medicare reimbursement for home health services, patients had to have (1) home-bound status; (2) a need for part-time or intermittent, skilled nursing care; (3) a medically reasonably and necessary need for treatment; and (4) a plan of care authorized by a physician. Home health agencies were established and began to employ increasing numbers of nurses. The number of home health agencies began to grow in the mid-1960s, and the home health industry continued unprecedented growth into the 1990s as a result of Medicare reimbursement and other influences, including a growing older adult population, advances in medical technology, and public demand for increased access to health care. Home health was one of the first employment settings that provided nurses the opportunity to work weekdays only.

Nursing in the 1970s

The women's movement of the 1970s greatly influenced nursing. Nurses began to focus not only on providing quality care to patients but also on enhancing the economic benefits of the profession. Hospitals were receiving significant reimbursements for patient care; however, nurses' salaries did not reflect an adequate percentage of that reimbursement. Health care costs soared. This increase in health care costs built the framework for mandated changes in reimbursement. Nursing practice and the educational focus remained in the hospital setting.

During this time, nurses played a major role in providing health care to communities and were instrumental in developing hospice programs, birthing centers, and daycare centers for older adults (Nies and McEwen, 2015). Although basic educational programs for nurse practitioners expanded during the 1970s and master's-level preparation was developed as the requirement for

graduation and practice, certification was also required for practice as a nurse practitioner. Before this time, only certification was required. State nursing practice acts were amended to provide for monitoring and licensing of advanced practice nurses. The numbers of men participating in this female-dominated profession also began to increase (Ellis and Hartley, 2012).

In 1974, the ANA conducted research in the area of ethnic minorities and submitted a proposal to the National Institute of Mental Health to fund a project to permit minority nurses—African-Americans, Hispanics, Asians, and American Indians—to earn PhDs. Of the graduates of the project, the vast majority serves on faculties of universities and is conducting research on factors in mental health and illness related to ethnicity and cross-cultural conflict, thereby fulfilling their commitment to advance the cause of quality health care for people of all ethnicities.

Despite past laxity, the ANA House of Delegates at its 1972 convention passed an affirmative action resolution calling for a task force to develop and implement a program to correct inequities. The house also provided for the position of an ombudsman to evaluate involvement of minorities in leadership roles within the organization and to treat complaints by applicants for membership or by members of the association who had been discriminated against because of nationality, race, creed, lifestyle, color, age, or sex. It was also in the 1970s that the ANA elected its first black president, Barbara Nichols, who served two terms.

Within the structure of many professional organizations is a unit referred to as an *academy,* which is composed of a cadre of scholars who deal with issues that concern the profession and take positions in the name of the academy. The American Academy of Nursing (AAN) was created by the ANA board in 1973. An elected group of highly accomplished leaders across all sectors of nursing (education, research, and practice), it uses the credential FAAN (Fellow, American Academy of Nursing). Through the application of visionary leadership, the intent of the AAN is to transform health care policy through nursing knowledge to optimize the well-being of the American people.

At its convention in Atlantic City in 1976, the ANA launched its Hall of Fame to pay tribute to those nurses who have paved the way for others to follow or who have made outstanding contributions to the profession.

Nursing in the 1980s

The types of patients needing health care changed in the 1980s. Homelessness became a common problem in large cities. Unstable economic developments contributed to an increase in indigent populations (Nies and McEwen, 2015). Acquired immunodeficiency syndrome (AIDS) emerged as a frightening, fatal epidemic.

Runaway health care costs became a national issue in the 1980s. Medicare was still reimbursing for any and all hospital services provided to recipients. In 1983, in an attempt to restrain hospital costs, Congress passed the Diagnosis-Related Group system for reimbursement, better known as the DRG system.

Before 1983, Medicare payments were made to the hospital after the patient received services. Although there were restrictions, the entire bill generally was paid without question. DRGs were implemented to provide prospective payment for hospital services on the basis of the patient's admitting diagnosis and thereby to reduce the overall cost to Medicare. Hospitals now were to be reimbursed one amount based on the patient's diagnosis, not on hospital charges. The system was developed by physicians at the Yale–New Haven Hospital and addressed approximately 468 diagnoses classified according to length of stay and cost of procedures associated with the diagnosis (Nies and McEwen, 2015).

As a result of the DRG reimbursement system, hospitals were forced to increase efficiency and more closely manage hospital services, including the patient's length of stay, laboratory and radiographic testing, and diagnostic procedures. Case management and critical pathways were developed to more efficiently manage patient care, and case management became a new area of specialization for the professional nurse.

Despite the high cost of health care, medicine prospered. Medical care advanced in areas such as organ transplantation, resuscitation and support of premature infants, and critical care techniques. Physician specialization and advances in medical technology flourished. Medical specialties, such as nephrology, cardiology, endocrinology, orthopedics, neurosurgery, cardiovascular surgery, and advanced practices for obstetrics, all led to improved health care services. Costs in the hospital setting increased with increased specialization and technology. The advanced technology also led to the development of outpatient surgery units.

Outpatient surgery services blossomed and provided a quick and efficient site for surgery that did not require extended hospital stays. Costs were greatly reduced because of the need for fewer staff members needed for coverage, fewer supplies, and reduced facility costs. Nurses were interested in employment opportunities in outpatient facilities because they afforded a chance to work only during the day with no weekend assignments.

As the concern over increasing health care costs heightened, use of ambulatory services increased and enrollment in health maintenance organizations grew. Advanced nurse practitioners rose in popularity as cost-effective providers of primary and preventive health care. A growing number of nurses moved from the hospital setting into the community to practice in programs such as hospice and home health. Consumers began to demand bans on unhealthy activities, such as smoking in public. Health education became more important as consumers were encouraged to take responsibility for their own care (Stanhope and Lancaster, 2015). Even the terminology changed; the individual once known as the *patient* became known as the *client* or *consumer* and was afforded respect as a person who purchases a service.

Public health programs struggled to survive as counties and states cut health department budgets. A landmark study conducted by the Institute of Medicine (IOM) in 1988, titled *Who Will Keep the Public Healthy?* (IOM, 2003), painted a dismal picture for public health. The study determined that public health had moved away from its traditional role and core functions and that no strategy was in place to bring public health back to its original purpose (Stanhope and Lancaster, 2015). Inadequate funding for public health continues to be a problem; however, it is hoped that soon public health will be restored to its original function and purpose.

Nursing enrollments dropped drastically in the late 1980s. This drop in enrollment occurred as the complexity of health care was rapidly increasing and more nurses were assuming expanded roles. As a result of these trends, a serious national shortage of nurses occurred across all settings (Ellis and Hartley, 2012).

In the late 1980s, several nursing scholars suggested that nursing research be firmly focused on the substantive information required to guide practice, rather than on philosophical and methodologic dilemmas of scientific inquiry. In 1985 the creation of the National Center for Nursing Research at the National Institutes of Health brought with it an increase in federal resources for nursing research and research training (LoBiondo-Wood & Haber, 2017).

Nursing in the 1990s

The 1990s began with alarm over the state of the U.S. economy. Government statisticians reported an alarming increase in the national debt complicated by slow economic growth. In the early 1990s, average household incomes were stagnating. More women with families entered the workforce to afford the increasing cost of living. More nurses selected jobs in which they could work more hours in fewer days for more money, sometimes sacrificing the fringe benefits, allowing them to work a second job or earn higher pay through shift differential for working evening and night shifts. Creative shifts, such as the 10-hour day, 4-day workweek or the 12-hour day, 3-day workweek became commonplace in health care facilities. Just as in the 1980s, the cost of health care continued to rise with the technologic advancements in medical care. Men were considered a minority in nursing, and salaries were thought to be on the increase as a result of male presence in the profession (O'Lynn and Tranbarger, 2006).

There also were growing concerns in the 1990s about the health of the nation, which prompted the *Healthy People 2000* initiative. Many diseases associated with preventable causes characterized mortality in the United States. In 1990, more than 2 million U.S. residents died from causes such as heart disease, cancer, cerebral vascular disease, accidents, chronic obstructive pulmonary disease, liver cirrhosis, tuberculosis, and human immunodeficiency virus infection. Disparities in rates of these diseases in the inner city due to issues related to access and quality of care became a concern (Nies and McEwen, 2015). Factors contributing to these common disease states related to lifestyle patterns, behaviors, and habits (modifiable risk factors). More youth were at risk because of behavior such as smoking cigarettes, using abusive drug substances, eating poorly balanced diets, failing to exercise, having sex with multiple partners, and being subjected to acts of violence. *Healthy People 2000: National Health Promotion and Disease Prevention Objectives* was published in 1991 by the U.S. Department of Health and Human Services as a nationwide effort to help states, cities, and communities identify health promotion and disease prevention strategies to address these health risk problems.

The AIDS epidemic radically changed the process for infection control among health care workers in health care institutions across the nation. Recapping needles, wearing latex gloves, and using isolation precautions were issues that triggered much dialogue and debate among health care workers. Health care workers were mandated to use preventive measures in the form of Universal Precautions; all contact with blood and body fluids from all patients was considered potentially infectious.

Exposure to hazardous materials became a major issue of concern for not only health care workers but also the general public. Chemical and radioactive substances that created dangerous exposure and health risks were increasingly used in the workplace. Employers were held legally accountable for informing their employees of the actual or potential hazards and for reducing their exposure risk through training and the use of protective equipment. The hazardous materials issue was especially important in nursing and medicine, particularly with regard to exposure to carcinogenic chemicals used in drug therapy and in environmental infection control.

In 1990, the rising costs of Medicaid and Medicare triggered political action for health care reform. Findings of a federal commission appointed to evaluate the American health care system included the following (Chitty and Black, 2014):

- Fifteen percent of the gross national product was related to health care expenditures (this amounts to approximately $1 trillion annually).
- The United States spent more than twice as much as any industrialized nation for health care services.
- Americans were living longer, accounting for a growing demand for home health and nursing home care in addition to increased Medicare expenditures.

It became apparent that if health care spending continued to increase, the U.S. economy would be in danger of collapse. Thus the health care system moved toward managed care in an attempt to control health care expenditures. The managed care movement has had a tremendous effect on nursing.

The focus of managed care was on providing more preventive and primary care, using outpatient and home settings when possible, and limiting expensive hospitalizations. Massive downsizing of hospital nursing staff occurred, with a greater use of unlicensed assistive personnel to provide care in hospitals. There was an increasing demand for community health nurses and advanced practice nurses to provide primary care services. The nurse of the 1990s had to be focused on delivering health care services that (1) encompassed health risk assessment based on family and environmental factors, (2) supported health promotion and disease prevention, and (3) advanced counseling and health education (Nies and McEwen, 2015).

In June 1993, the National Center for Nursing Research was renamed the National Institute of Nursing Research. Moving nursing research into the National Institutes of Health enhanced the interprofessional possibilities for collaborative investigation. As a result, nursing research grew rapidly during the 1990s. Multiple research programs focused on important health issues, such as health promotion across the lifespan. Nursing research began to inform health care policy through federal commissions and agency programs (LoBiondo-Wood & Haber, 2017).

In the 1990s, mandatory state licensure authorities (which set practice standards at the level of entering associate-degree graduates) and national nongovernmental bodies (which certify graduate-prepared specialists) forged a partnership. These national certifying agencies were intensely engaged in improving methods for determining the continual competence of certified nurse practitioners within the swift current of health care change. The consumer's voice in the partnership was heard via collaboration with advocacy organizations and the appointment of more public members to licensing, certifying, and accreditation boards. Voluntary credentialing bodies recognized that if they were to serve effectively, they had to engage in active public information campaigns to inform consumers about their health care choices (Buhler-Wilkerson, 2001).

Nursing in the Twenty-First Century

It is frequently claimed that nursing is vital to the safe provision of health care and health service to our populations. It is also recognized, however, that nursing is a costly health care resource that must be used effectively and efficiently. Therefore, there is growing recognition, from within the nursing profession as well as by health care policy makers and society, of the need to analyze the contribution of nursing to health care and its costs. This issue becomes increasingly important in an era of staff cuts and staffing deficits, combined with higher patient expectation, escalating health care costs, and a health care system restructuring and reform agenda. Such factors make the identification and effective use of

the nursing contribution to health care an issue of critical importance (Scott et al, 2014).

Professional nurses in the twenty-first century are faced with many challenges within the dynamic state of health care. In addition to the issues of access, cost, quality, safety, and accountability in health care, nurses today are challenged by an aging population, a serious nursing shortage, generational differences in an aging workforce with poor prospects for replacements, high acuity and short staffing, conflict in the workplace, expanding technology, complex consumer health values, and an increasingly intercultural society. Nurses have identified numerous areas of concern, including insufficient staffing, inadequate salaries, effects of stress and overwork, violence in the workplace, lack of participation in decision making, and dissatisfaction with the quality of their own nursing care.

Changing duties, responsibilities, and conflicts amid nursing shortages and public concern over patient safety and quality of care characterize present-day practice. These changes require professional nurses to have core competency in critical thinking, communication, interprofessional collaboration, assessment, leadership, and technical skills, in addition to knowledge of health promotion and disease prevention, information technology, health systems, and public policy.

In 2008, the Robert Wood Johnson Foundation (RWJF) proposed a partnership with the IOM to assess and respond to the need to transform the nursing profession. The RWJF and the IOM established a 2-year Initiative on the Future of Nursing. The IOM report released in 2011 had the following four key messages: (1) Nurses should practice to the full extent of their education and training; (2) nurses should achieve higher levels of education and training through an improved education system that promotes seamless academic progression; (3) nurses should be full partners with physicians and other health professionals in redesigning health care in the United States; and (4) effective workforce planning and policy making require better data collection and an improved information infrastructure (IOM, 2011). These recommendations focus on the intersection between the health needs of diverse populations across the lifespan and the actions of the nursing workforce.

In 2010, Congress passed and President Barak Obama signed into law comprehensive health legislation. These laws, the Patient Protection and Affordable Care Act (Public Law 111-148) and the Health Care and Education

Affordability Reconciliation Act (Public Law 111-152), are collectively referred to as the Affordable Care Act (ACA). The ACA represents the broadest changes to the health care system since the creation of Medicare and Medicaid programs in 1965. The ACA is expected to provide insurance coverage for 32 million previously uninsured Americans. This new demand on the health care system has significant implications for nursing, the nation's largest health care profession with more than 3 million RNs nationwide. Nurses have the potential to effect significant changes in the health care system that will meet the demand for safe, quality, patient-centered, accessible, and affordable care (IOM, 2011).

The U.S. is projected to experience a shortage of Registered Nurses (RNs) that is expected to intensify as Baby Boomers age and the need for health care grows. Compounding the problem is the fact that nursing schools across the country are struggling to expand capacity to meet the rising demand for care, given the national move toward healthcare reform.

High nurse retirement and turnover rates are affecting access to health care. A 2015 study has found that almost 40% of registered nurses are over the age of 50 (Auerbach et al, 2015). The number of nurses leaving the workforce each year has grown steadily from around 40,000 in 2010 to an expected nearly 80,000 by 2020. Meanwhile, the study observed, the dramatic growth in nursing school enrollment since 2000 has begun to level off (Auerbach et al, 2015).

A wave of faculty retirements is expected across the United States over the next decade. Master's and doctoral programs in nursing are not producing a large enough pool of potential nurse educators to meet the demand. Higher compensation in clinical and private-sector settings is luring current and potential nurse educators away from teaching. According to the American Academy of Nurse Practitioners, the average salary of a nurse practitioner, across settings and specialties, was $97,083 in 2015 (American Academy of Nurse Practitioners, 2015). By contrast, AACN reported in March 2016 that master's-prepared faculty earned an annual average salary of $77,022 (American Association of Colleges of Nursing Research and Data Center, 2016).

March 2016 marked the release of the report *Advancing Healthcare Transformation: A New Era for Academic Nursing,* commissioned by the AACN. This report calls for enhanced partnerships to advance integrated systems of health care, achieve improved health outcomes, and foster new models for innovation.

▍SUMMARY

Nursing is a dynamic profession that has evolved into a theory-, research-, and evidence-based practice. From its unorganized and variably defined beginnings, a profession based on the framework of competence, autonomy, determination, and human caring has developed. The challenges and opportunities have paralleled the path of world history and have brought about significant changes in the profession. From the men who opened the path, to the women who brought dignity and respect to their philosophy of caring, to the pioneers who brought unity to a profession plagued by a history of racism, sexism, and sometimes disgrace, nursing has become recognized as critical to the health of the nation. Despite myriad challenges, the practice of nursing has been distinguished and qualified by the intellect, skill, commitment, and contribution of countless nuns, deaconesses, and individuals such as Dix, Barton, Wald, Breckenridge, and Nightingale.

The nursing profession has the capacity to effect far-reaching changes in the health care system. Close proximity to patients and scientific understanding of care across the health care continuum from health promotion to disease prevention to coordination of care give nurses the unique ability to lead in the improvement and redesign of the health care system. Research has linked nursing care to the safety of patients. Nurses will continue to increase knowledge, manage technology, and maintain ethical standards to provide high-quality, patient-centered, safe care to individuals, families, communities, and populations throughout the world.

Nurses are crucial in preventing medication errors, reducing infection rates, and facilitating patients' transition from hospital to home. Significant nursing contributions to the creation of a quality, patient-centered health care system that is accessible, equitable, evidence based, and sustainable will require transforming the work environment, scope of practice, education, and numbers of nurses in the United States.

Through periods of war, socioeconomic change, and health care reform, nurses have played a vital role in initiating change to improve the health care arena. Nurses have provided the integrity to maintain the quality of care in all health care settings. The evolution of the practice from the treatment of disease to health promotion and disease prevention has led the way in determining the type of providers needed to care for patients in the future. This evolution will continue to provide the foundation for the scope of practice, educational curricula, scholarship, and research necessary for nurses to lead and manage the health care environment of the future (Catalano, 2012).

REFERENCES

American Academy of Nurse Practitioners. (2015). *Annual Income For Full-time Nurse Practitioners Up 10% Since 2011: AANP Releases 2015 National Nurse Practitioner Compensation Survey.* https://www.aanp.org/166-press-room/2015-press-releases/1803-annual-income-for-full-time-nurse-practitioners-up-10-since-2011.

American Association of Colleges of Nursing. (2006). *The Essentials of Doctoral Education for Advanced Nursing Practice.* http://www.aacn.nche.edu/DNP/pdf/Essentials.pdf

American Association of Colleges of Nursing Research and Data Center. (2016). 2016-2017 *Salaries of Instructional and Administrative Nursing Faculty in Baccalaureate and Graduate Programs in Nursing.* http://www.aacnnursing.org/news-information/research-data

Auerbach, D. I., Buerhaus, P. I., & Staiger, D. O. (2015). Will the RN Workforce Weather the Retirement of the Baby Boomers? *Medical Care, 53*(10), 850. doi:10.1097/MLR.0000000000000415.

Bahr, L., & Johnson, B. (1997). *Collier's encyclopedia (Vol. 18).* New York: Simon and Schuster.

Buhler-Wilkerson, K. (2001). *No place like home: a history of nursing and home care in the United States.* Baltimore: Johns Hopkins University Press.

Carnegie, M. E. (1995). *The path we tread: blacks in nursing worldwide, 1854–1994* (3rd ed.). New York: National League for Nursing, Jones and Bartlett.

Catalano, J. T. (2012). *Nursing now: today's issues, tomorrow's trends* (6th ed.). Philadelphia, 2012, FA Davis.

Chitty, K. B., & Black, B. P. (2014). *Professional nursing: concepts and challenges* (7th ed.). St Louis: Elsevier/Saunders.

Delougherty, G. L. (1998). *Issues and trends in nursing* (3rd ed.). St Louis: Mosby.

Donahue, M. P. (1999). *Nursing: the finest art—an illustrated history.* St Louis: Mosby.

Ellis, J. R., & Hartley, C. L. (2012). *Nursing in today's world: challenges, issues and trends* (10th ed.) Philadelphia: Wolters Kluwer/Lippincott Williams & Wilkins.

Fitzpatrick, M. F. (1997). The mercy brigade. *Civil War Times Illustrated, 36*(5), 34–40.

Freedman, D. (1995). *The Anchor bible dictionary.* New York: Doubleday.

Giger, J., & Davidhizar, R. (2008). *Transcultural nursing: assessment and intervention* (5th ed.). St Louis: Mosby.

Gill, G. (2004). *Nightingales: the extraordinary upbringing and curious life of Miss Florence Nightingale.* New York: Ballantine Books.

Institute of Medicine. (2003). Who will keep the public healthy? Educating public health professionals for the 21st century. Workshop summary. In K. Gebbie, L. Rosenstock, LM Hernandez (Eds.), *Committee on Educating Public Health Professionals for the 21st Century, 2003, Board on Health Promotion and Disease Prevention, Institute of Medicine of the National Academies.* Washington, DC: The National Academies Press.

Institute of Medicine. (2011). *The future of nursing: Leading change, advancing nurse.* Washington, DC: The Academies Press. http://www.thefutureofnursing.org/IOM.Report.

Joel, L. (2006). *The nursing experience: trends, challenges and transition* (5th ed.). New York: McGraw-Hill.

Jones, Z. O. (2004). Knowledge systems in conflict: the regulation of African American midwifery. *Nursing History Review: Official Journal of the American Association for the History of Nursing, 12,* 167–184.

Kalisch, P., & Kalisch, B. (1986). *The advance of American nursing* (2nd ed.). Philadelphia: JB Lippincott.

Kalisch, P., & Kalisch, B. (1995). *The advance of American nursing* (3rd ed.). Philadelphia: JB Lippincott.

Kalisch, B., & Kalisch, P. (2003). *American nursing: A history* (4th ed.). Philadelphia: Lippincott Williams & Wilkins.

Karger, H. J., & Stoesz, D. (2005). *American social welfare policy: A pluralist approach* (5th ed.). New York: Allyn and Bacon.

Katz, J. R., Carter, C., Bishop, J., & Kravits, S. L. (2009). *Keys to nursing success* (3rd ed.). Columbus, OH: Pearson/Prentice-Hall.

Lindeman, C., & McAthie, M. (1990). *Nursing trends and issues.* Springhouse, PA: Springhouse.

Nelson, S. (2001). *"Say Little, Do Much": Nineteenth century religious women and care of the sick.* Philadelphia: University of Pennsylvania Press.

Nies, M. A., & McEwen, M. (2015). *Community/public health nursing: promoting the health of populations.* (6th ed.). St Louis: Elsevier Saunders.

Oermann, M. H. (1997). *Professional nursing practice.* Stamford, CT: Prentice-Hall.

O'Lynn, C. O., & Tranbarger, R. (2006). *Men in nursing: history, challenges, and opportunities.* New York: Springer.

LoBiondo-Wood, G., & Haber, J. (2017). *Nursing research: methods and critical appraisal for evidence-based practice* (9th ed.). St. Louis: Elsevier.

Robinson, T. M., & Perry, P. M. (2001). *Cadet nurse stories: The call for and response of women during World War II.* Indianapolis: Center Nursing Press.

Scott, P. A., Matthews, A., & Kirwan, M. (January 2014). What is nursing in the 21st century and what does the 21st century health system require of nursing? *Nursing Philosophy, 15,* 23–34.

Small, H. (2002). *Florence Nightingale: Avenging angel.* London: Constable and Robinson.

Snodgrass, M. E. (2004). *Historical encyclopedia of nursing.* Santa Barbara, CA: Diane Publishing.

Stanhope, M., & Lancaster, J. (2015). *Public health nursing; population-centered health care in the community* (9th ed.). St Louis: Elsevier.

Walton, J., Barondess, J., & Locke, S. (1994). *The Oxford medical companion.* New York: Oxford University Press.

2

Each nurse forms the image of nursing every day.

The Contemporary Image of Professional Nursing

L. Antoinette (Toni) Bargagliotti, PhD, RN, ANEF, FAAN

ⓔ Additional resources are available online at: *http://evolve.elsevier.com/Cherry/*

"People are always blaming their circumstances for what they are. I don't believe in circumstances. The people who get on in this world are the people who get up and look for the circumstances they want, and if they can't find them, make them."

George Bernard Shaw

LEARNING OUTCOMES

After studying this chapter, the reader will be able to:

1. Describe the image of nursing in art, media, and literature over time.
2. Recognize nursing actions that convey a negative image of nursing.
3. Recommend strategies to enhance the image of nursing.
4. Explain how the IOM *Future of Nursing* report is shaping nursing's image.
5. Create a plan to promote a positive image of nursing in practice.

KEY TERMS

Antiestablishment Opposition to the conventional social, political, and economic principles of society.

Art Any branch of creative work, especially painting and drawing, that displays form, beauty, and any unusual perception.

Literature All writings in prose or verse.

Media All the means of communication, such as newspapers, radio, and television.

Stereotype A fixed or conventional conception of a person or group held by many people that allows for no individuality.

PROFESSIONAL/ETHICAL ISSUE

John is asked to join a health care mission trip to a remote area of South Sudan that has no health care. John, the only nurse, will be joining a physician's assistant, a dentist, and multiple laypersons who will "help." They will be taking donated out-of-date medications (fourth-generation antibiotics, vials of multi-dose vaccines) as well as syringes and sterile supplies that were to be discarded because of their age and questionable sterility. When John asks whom he needs to contact in this country about a temporary license to practice, the team assures him that a license isn't necessary because it would be such "a hassle" and they will only be there for 10 days. There will be minimal water and no electricity in the target village.

Response 1

Because there is no health care, the team reasons that the medications and syringes are probably fine. Following this line of reasoning, John would provide unsafe care that would place people at risk who have no idea of the risk that they are taking. There would be no follow-up care or referral resources. Highly sophisticated antibiotics would be introduced into an "antibiotic-naïve" region to people who may not finish a course of treatment because they give the remaining pills to a needy family member or trade them for food.

Response 2

John reasons that he would be violating the ANA Code of Ethics and cannot participate in unsafe care that is disrespectful of human rights. He cannot practice without a license or the knowledge and consent of the government or bring drugs into the country in suitcases without any permission to do so. Once reconstituted, the vaccines would be unrefrigerated.

VIGNETTE

Mary, a senior nursing student, asks a faculty member, "Why can't we wear different scrubs and jewelry to clinical? Have you seen what nurses wear? Patients don't care what we're wearing. They care that we know how to take care of them. Two months after we graduate, we'll be wearing what everyone else does. Why should we look better than everyone else does?"

Questions to Consider While Reading This Chapter:

1. How does the image of a nurse differ from that of a physician?
2. How does the nurse's appearance affect the patient's opinion of the quality of care the nurse provides?

CHAPTER OVERVIEW

This chapter describes how the image of nursing has been shaped and suggests strategies that nurses can use to forge a positive public and professional image of their practice. Because nurses have been the subjects of artists, sculptors, and writers for thousands of years, an historic perspective is used to illustrate the contextual background for the evolving image of the profession.

IMAGES OF NURSING

When you imagine a nurse, what mental picture comes to mind? Do you think of *LIFE* magazine's 1942 cover picture of a nurse in a starched white uniform with a cap, the nurses portrayed in Johnson & Johnson's Campaign for Nursing's Future (2017), or your colleagues with whom you practiced yesterday? All of them are architects of healing.

The contemporary image of professional nursing in the United States is an ever-changing kaleidoscope created by the 4.73 million men and women of all ages, races, and religious beliefs who have active licensure as registered nurses (RNs) (National Council of State Boards of Nursing [NCSBN], 2017). Adding to this multifaceted collage are the numerous snapshots of nurses and nursing as portrayed in television commercials, bumper stickers, art, poetry, architecture, postage stamps, television dramas, television series, movies, newspaper comic strips, stained-glass windows, and statues. Nurses, whose profession is second in size to that of teaching, have been alternatively described as either saints or sinners, powerless or powerful, admired or ignored, and those who dare to care. Their practice has captured the attention of historians, economists, and sociologists who have studied this unusual group of people.

To whatever your image of nursing is, first add the many heroic nurses who served in Afghanistan and Iraq and in every U.S. war. In July 1775 after the United States established the Continental Army, General George Washington requested the Second Continental Congress to provide one nurse for every 10 patients and one matron for every 100 patients to supervise the care of wounded and sick soldiers. His confidence was well placed.

In 2007, Captain Maria Ortiz, a 40-year-old clinic nurse manager, became the first nursing casualty in Iraq, dying from mortar fire to her clinic in Baghdad. Captain Jennifer Moreno was a 25-year-old University of San Francisco nursing graduate who was commissioned in the U.S. Army upon graduation. A medical-surgical nurse, she volunteered and was selected from thousands of female officers to a Special Operations Cultural Support team that included multinational, multi-branch soldiers. For the first time, women were included on these male Ranger or Green Beret teams to obtain information from Afghan women unavailable to male soldiers. Every mission would be highly dangerous, especially for women. The first nurse to serve on a team, Captain

Fig. 2.1 Captain Jennifer Moreno.

Moreno, served in Afghanistan with the 3rd Battalion, 75th Ranger Regiment (see Fig. 2.1).

In October 2013, while Moreno was on a night mission to prevent a high-profile suicide attack in Kandahar that would have killed hundreds of civilians, an Afghan woman walked out of the compound, detonating her suicide vest and wounding six Rangers, followed by an insurgent detonating another bomb that injured others. Receiving a wounded staff sergeant's call for help and the ground commander's order for everyone to stay put to avoid detonating other bombs, Moreno heeded the call for help and ran through a heavily mined village to rescue wounded Rangers. Her Bronze Star commendation reads, "Disregarding her own well-being, Moreno unhesitatingly moved to assist (the soldiers) upon realizing the severity of the wounds sustained by her fellow teammates. While in transit, Moreno detonated Device No. 5 and was killed in action" (Associated Press, 2013; The last moments, 2014). More than a thread in the rich tapestry of the heroic work of all nurses, Ortiz's and Moreno's courage and sacrifice illuminate the timeless commitment of all nurses to save lives and advance health.

The July 26, 2017, the arrest and assault of burn center charge nurse Alex Wubbels by Salt Lake City, Utah, Detective Payne, a 27-year veteran of the police department, enraged the American public. The body camera video released September 1, 2017, reveals Nurse Wubbels calmly explaining and providing the written protocol that the blood draw Payne was demanding from an unconscious patient required meeting one of three conditions: patient consent, a warrant, or arrest of the patient. Responding with, "I either go away with blood in vials or body in tow" (Mele and Victor, 2017) and "We're done," Payne pushed her against a wall, held and handcuffed her, and dragged her from the hospital. Wubbels was released after being confined in a closed police car for 20 minutes. The unconscious patient, a reserve police officer with an Idaho police department involved in a crash, was not at fault in the accident. Following the film's release on September 1, the mayor and police chief apologized.

Since Florence Nightingale reduced mortality rates from 42% to 2% in a Crimean hospital constructed over an open sewer, nurses have been reformers who use limited resources to address unlimited "wants" for health care and to protect patients. The request for Nightingale's nursing services in the Crimea was borne out of newspaper reports about the devastating health care conditions in the Crimean War. However, the outcome that Nightingale and these nurses achieved changed conditions in the British Army, forged a system of nursing education, and continues to strongly influence the profession.

Although nurses are concerned with their public image and media portrayal, Kalisch and Kalisch's (1995) extensive work outlining the image of nursing in film and media over time permanently etched the image issue into the professional radar screen.

WHY IMAGE IS IMPORTANT

Registered nurses (RNs), who account for 59% of the entire health professional workforce, are the "glue" that binds the health care of many into a more seamless experience for the patient. Safe patient care demands coordination of the armada of health professionals using many technologies and handoffs to provide care to a single person in intensive care and other technology-driven areas. How nursing is perceived inside and outside the health care system directly affects how successful nurses will be in providing and coordinating patient care.

The requirement for health care usually comes unexpectedly and without warning. When patients seek health care in a hospital, they are entrusting their life and well-being to the one person who has 24/7 direct responsibility for their care and their environment—the RN. Unlike their personal physician, with whom patients may have had a long-term relationship, or a hospitalist or intensivist the patient and family just met, it is the RN, the coordinator of their care, who is new to them and changes every 8 to 12 hours. It is important that the public trusts and believes in this nurse and the profession the nurse represents.

REGISTERED NURSE SUPPLY

The United States averted a projected 20% shortfall (400,000 RNs) in 2020 because of the importance of nurses in health care. A combination of factors forestalled the 2020 national shortfall (Buerhaus et al, 2017). The combined effects of the Johnson & Johnson Campaign for Nursing, followed closely by other foundation initiatives, and the Institute of Medicine (IOM) *Future of Nursing* report changed the image of nursing for both millennials entering college and the public. Underscoring these events were the unprecedented job losses (8.8 million) of the Great Recession (2007-2009) that happened in other fields (Goodman and Mance, 2011) as nursing saw record increases in new job growth. RN graduates increased by more than 222% between 2002 (70,692) and 2016 (157,073) (National Council of State Boards of Nursing [NCSBN], 2003, 2017). However, the greatest growth, between 2002 and 2012, with annual increases of 7% in National Council Licensure Examination for RN (NCLEX-RN) test-takers for Associate of Science in Nursing (ASN) degrees and of 8% in test-takers for Bachelor of Science in Nursing (BSN) degrees, has leveled off to a 5% BSN annual increase and 1% ASN increase (Buerhaus et al, 2017a). Modifying the increases in new nurses is the projected retirement of one third of the nursing workforce between 2017 and 2027 (Buerhaus et al, 2017). In part, this change will occur because almost 24% of registered nurses remained in the workforce full time until age 69, a trend that was mirrored among men in

other professions as well (Auerbach et al, 2014). Later retirement ages have converted a gradual workforce loss over several years to larger losses at one time when the Baby Boomer majority reaches age 70. As Buerhaus and colleagues (2017a) noted, the significant loss when one third of the nursing workforce retires is not one of numbers because of growth increases but rather a loss of experience and know-how. Nursing lost 1.7 million experience years to retirement in 2015 and will lose an additional 2 million experience years in 2020.

Although it is important to know why an unprecedented nursing shortage was averted, the crucial issue is how it was reversed. Multiple legislative efforts began with the 2002 Nurse Reinvestment Act (Public Law 107-205), which provided nursing scholarships, public service announcements promoting nursing as a career, faculty loan cancellation programs, geriatric training grants, and nurse retention and safety enhancement grants. In 2010, the Patient Protection and Affordable Care Act increased the nursing student loan amounts, provided $50 million per year to fund nurse-managed health centers (Title V, Section 330A-1), funded gerontology nursing fellowship programs (Title V, Section 5305), provided up to $40,000 in educational loan repayment for nurse faculty and $80,000 for PhD-prepared nurse faculty, and significantly strengthened Title VIII advanced nursing education grants. Additionally, funding was made available for graduate nursing demonstration grants (Section 5509) to hospitals providing advanced nursing education clinical training to advanced practice nurses (nurse anesthetists, clinical nurse specialists, nurse practitioners, and nurse-midwives).

The image of nursing as a job growth profession continues with an expected new job growth rate from 2016-2026 of 15% or twice the average of all occupations (7%) (U.S. Bureau of Labor Statistics [USBLS], 2017).

NURSING IN ART AND LITERATURE

Although the way that nursing has been portrayed in art and literature over time may seem to be unrelated to the contemporary image of nursing, the mental image of contemporary nursing is enmeshed with the earlier images.

Art and literature have been the way in which people describe the human condition and cultural values of their time. In these earliest descriptions of nurses and nursing are found the enduring fundamental and essential tensions that exist within the profession today. Found within art and literature is the eternal question asked by those who know they will one day require nursing care, "Can I trust and entrust my life to this nurse?"

Antiquity's Image of Nursing

The earliest literary reference to nursing chronicles the actions of two nurse-midwives in approximately 1900 BC in Exodus 1 of the Old Testament, which indicates that the practice of two midwives became the vehicle through which the Israelites, the Jewish race, and the resultant Judeo-Christian heritage survived. From the sixth century until the 1800s, nurses were imaged as untrained servants, soldiers, women of religious orders, or wealthy people performing acts of Christian charity (Kalisch and Kalisch, 1995; Kampen, 1988). These meager artistic renderings of nurses convey images that continue to be familiar to contemporary nurses.

Victorian Image of Nursing

In 1844 when Florence Nightingale was "called" to become a nurse, Charles Dickens immortalized a different kind of nurse through Sairy Gamp, who nursed the sick because of the lack of other opportunities. For Sairy Gamp, a drunken, physically unkempt, uncaring nurse in *The Life and Adventures of Martin Chuzzlewit,* nursing provided a way to profit from the sick and dying. Reflecting the concern of Victorian England for untrained caregivers, Dickens writes that Sairy should be advised of the advantages of "a little less liquor, and a little more humanity, and a little less regard for herself, and a little more regard for her patients, and perhaps a trifle of additional honesty" (Dickens, 1910).

Fortunately, Sairy's literary arrival was followed by Longfellow's portrayal of the heroic Nightingale in *Santa Filomena* (1857). As important as Nightingale was to the improved health care of British soldiers and the development of modern nursing, the ever-increasing positive images of Nightingale occurred solely because she succinctly demonstrated aggregated outcomes of nursing practice. Nightingale was one of the earliest users of the emerging body of knowledge called *statistics* and developed the pie chart that remains in common use. Notably, nursing emerged at a time of turbulent social change and reform in Great Britain.

Early Twentieth-Century Nursing

Toward the end of the Nightingale period at the turn of the century, nurses in war settings vividly captured the attention of artists. The most compelling image is George Bellows' 1918 canvas, *Edith Cavell Directing the Escape of Soldiers from Prison Camp* (Donahue, 1910). World War I Germany shocked the world with its 1915 firing squad execution of Edith Cavell, founder of the first nursing school in Belgium, who aided soldiers escaping prison camps. The art of heroic nursing expressed in several famous paintings reflected the reality of World War I nurses, who were also the recipients of three Distinguished Service Crosses, 23 Distinguished Service Medals, 28 French Croix de Guerres, 69 British Military Medals, and 4 U.S. Navy Crosses (Donahue, 2010). Notably, American nurses who served in World War I were not commissioned in the military services.

The 1930s Nurse as Angel of Mercy

On a grander scale, Warner Brothers' film *The White Angel* (1936) chronicled the professional life of Florence Nightingale (Jones, 1988). Endorsed by the American Nurses Association (ANA), *The White Angel* clearly portrayed Nightingale's persistence and head-to-head confrontation with medicine. Anticipating that the medical staff would deny rations for the nurses, she brought provisions for them. When the medical staff locked her out of the hospital, Nightingale sat outside in the snow until patients and soldiers required physicians to admit the nurses. *The White Angel* conveyed to the public that nursing is a holy vocation, nurses have professional credentials, and their career choice is opposed because popular opinion held that women belong at home (Jones, 1988).

In 1938, Francis Rich's tall and imposing white limestone statue, *The Nurses Memorial,* sometimes referred to as the *Spirit of Nursing,* was placed in Arlington National Cemetery to honor military nurses. Similarly, Germany's postage stamp issued in 1936 commemorated nursing with a larger-than-life nurse compassionately overlooking people (Donahue, 2010).

The 1940s Nurse as Heroine

Considered to be the most positive movie about nursing, *So Proudly We Hail* is the 1942 story of nurses in Bataan and Corregidor. The film, starring Claudette Colbert, portrayed a small group of nurses rerouted to the Philippines after the attack on Pearl Harbor. Soon cut off from supplies and replacements as the Japanese captured the Philippines, these nurses provided care with few supplies and no staff to the thousands of soldiers in the Philippines. When the last nurses were to be evacuated from the occupied islands, 78 nurses (Army, Navy, and 1 Certified Registered Nurse Anesthetist [CRNA]) voluntarily stayed behind, made the march to Bataan, and were prisoners of war until 1945. Norman's *We Band of Angels: the Untold Story of American Nurses Trapped on Bataan by the Japanese* (1999) tells their gritty, difficult, and heroic story from their diaries and interviews.

Nursing was depicted positively on a 1940 Australian postage stamp as a larger-than-life figure looking over a soldier, a sailor, and an aviator; on Costa Rica's 1945 postage stamp of Florence Nightingale and Edith Cavell; and in the 1945 commissioning of the USS *Higbee,* a navy destroyer named to honor a navy nurse (Donahue, 2010).

After nursing's glorious contributions to World War II, in which one in three nurses served, nurses returned home to low salaries, long hours, too few staff, and too many patients. However, the Cherry Ames book series, the Sue Barton series, and other romance novels glamorized nursing.

Nursing in the Antiestablishment Era of the 1960s

Ken Kesey developed the modern version of Sairy Gamp through the character of Nurse Ratched in *One Flew Over the Cuckoo's Nest* (1962). This best-selling novel later became a play and motion picture (1975) that won six Oscars, including Best Picture. Entrusted with the care of the mentally ill, Nurse Ratched, a militaristic nurse in a starched white uniform, was the ultimate power figure who punished patients to cure their psychosis through conformity to a "system" (Jones, 1988). However, the reality of the turbulent, antiestablishment period of the 1960s is that nursing was one of President Lyndon Johnson's first salvos in the war on poverty. The Nurse Training Act of 1964 was funded at $250 million ($1.99 billion in 2017 dollars). Although nurses also dramatically shaped the future of health care through the development of coronary care units, intensive care units, hemodialysis, and Silver and Ford's first nurse practitioner program in Colorado, a U.S. Bureau of Labor Statistics study indicated that nursing salaries at the time were woefully inadequate in comparison with those of other, far less trained American workers (Kalisch and Kalisch, 1995).

Nursing in the Sexual Revolution of the 1970s

Media images of the nurse in the 1970s were formed amid a sexual revolution and a growing antimilitary American culture. War provided the media backdrop. The 1976 postage stamp Clara Maas, She Gave Her Life commemorated the 100th birthday of a 25-year-old nurse who died after deliberately obtaining two carrier mosquito bites so that she could continue providing care to soldiers with yellow fever in the Spanish-American War (Donahue, 2010). Her modern-day counterparts would be nurses in *M*A*S*H*, the hit television series from 1972 to 1983.

The nursing profession viewed *M*A*S*H* as professionally destructive because of the negative portrayal of Major Margaret "Hot Lips" Hoolihan and the nurses of the 4077th Army MASH (Mobile Army Surgical Hospital) unit in Korea. The sexual exploits of nurses and physicians and Margaret's uncaring attitude provided few positive images. However, for the American public who were receiving a daily dose of Vietnam footage on nightly news, *M*A*S*H* presented a glimmer of reality.

The continuous frontline exposure to the massive trauma of young men did not immunize the more than 5000 army nurses who served in Vietnam from the horrors of what they were seeing or prevent them from caring. These nurses were young (average age 23), newly graduated (only 35% having 2 years of experience, 60% having less than 6 months), and 21% were men. From 15 Army nurses in Vietnam in 1965, their numbers quickly expanded to a maximum of 900 nurses in 1969, who provided care for 5283 beds (58 patients to 1 nurse), working 12-hour shifts, 6 days a week (West, 2014). Lieutenant Sharon Lane, who was killed by mortar fire to her nursing ward, was the only nurse killed by direct enemy fire. At the end of the war, Captain Mary Klinker, a flight nurse, was killed when her plane carrying 128 people, mostly Vietnamese orphans, was downed by enemy fire near Saigon (History Channel, n.d.).

Nurses serving in Vietnam would later be imaged in the television series *China Beach* (1988-1991).

Nursing in the 1980s to 1990s

The complexities of nursing are realistically described in the play and television movie *Miss Evers' Boys*. The character Miss Evers tells the story of actual nurse Eunice Rivers, who was hired to recruit and retain young African-American men in the infamous Tuskegee experiment designed to describe the long-term effects of untreated syphilis. Although the study began in 1932, penicillin became the treatment of choice for syphilis in 1947 in the civilian population. When subjects asked Nurse Evers to obtain the new treatment of penicillin for them and she sought to do so, the physician investigators required her to discourage them from treatment. Subjects were told they would be dropped from the study and forgo the benefits of free treatment: a free ride to the clinic, one hot meal per day, and, in case of dying, $50 for the funeral. Subjects were never told they had syphilis, only that they had "bad blood." The study, which was funded for 40 years by the U.S. Public Health Service, ended in 1972 only because it became publicly known through the press. Ironically, Nurse Rivers was the only consistent staff person throughout the 40 years of the study. As the narrator of the story, Nurse Evers introduces non-nurses to the dilemmas of nursing practice during that era and the consequences of failing to protect patients and their descendants because of misplaced faith and trust in other health care disciplines. An outcome of the Tuskegee study was the requirement for institutional review boards to prevent this from occurring again.

In 1997, three films used war and nursing as a backdrop: *The English Patient, Love and War,* and *Paradise Road.* In these films, the nurse is knowledgeable and nonjudgmental.

Artistic views of nursing during this period focused on caring. In the Vietnam War Women's Memorial, in Washington, DC, the central figure is the nurse in battle fatigues cradling the head of a soldier. Evident in the bronze statue is the fatigue of the nurse and her care for this dying soldier.

Millennial Media

Stanley's (2008) study of nurses in film from 1900 to 2007 found that later films portrayed nurses as thoughtful, independent, intelligent professionals. The nurses in *Pearl Harbor* (2001) heroically provide care and order to the chaos following the bombing attack on Pearl Harbor. The character Greg Focker, RN, in the movies *Meet the Parents* (2000), *Meet the Fockers* (2004), and *The Little Fockers* (2010), endured his father-in-law's stereotyped views about men who are nurses. Several successful television series took place in hospitals, such as NBC's *ER* (1994-2009), ABC's *Grey's Anatomy* (2005-), Fox's *House* (2004-2012), and ABC's *Scrubs* (2001-2010), with physicians as central characters who

often provide nursing care. Because their primary storylines portray physicians negatively, the scriptwriters' neglect of nursing may be professionally helpful.

Weaver and colleagues' (2013) study of the image of men in nursing in *Grey's Anatomy, Hawthorne, Mercy, Nurse Jackie,* and *Private Practice* (2007-2010) found that the men in nursing were in minor, often comedic roles in all of these shows. Questions about their sexuality and why they chose nursing reinforced every negative stereotype about men in nursing.

NBC's *Night Shift* (2014-2017) featured Kenny, an African-American nurse in a San Antonio emergency department who managed physician logistics rather than sophisticated nursing practice in emergency situations (Truth about Nursing, n.d.). NBCs *Chicago Med* (2015-) portrays three African-American nurses positively, highlighting their nursing judgment and the safety net that nurses provide to patients.

On April 6, 2014, CBS television's *60 Minutes* traveled with two West Virginia nurse practitioners, Teresa Gardner and Paula Meade, in their Health Wagon as they provided primary care to rural Appalachian people who cannot afford health care in six West Virginia counties. Originally begun by Sr. Bernie Kenny from a Volkswagen Beetle, the Health Wagon is now a mobile primary care clinic in a 13-year-old Winnebago van that is funded by federal grants, donations, and the support of pharmaceutical suppliers, who provide needed medications.

Social Media

Nurses portray nursing through their use of the social media platforms Facebook, Snapchat, Instagram, and Twitter. Although it provides asynchronous communication medium among friends, the connection offered by "friending" or following on such platforms is often extended to unknown persons. Nurses and student nurses who have self-identified as nurses or students have posted comments about their practices, managers, or patients (whether named or not), creating serious professional issues for nursing. Thirty-three state boards of nursing (SBNs) reported receiving complaints about nurses' use of social media, and twenty-six of these SBNs reported having disciplined the licenses of nurses (NCSBN, 2011). Nursing students have been expelled from nursing programs because of both positive and negative online postings about patients. The courts have upheld those decisions because of the significant breach of professional boundaries such postings make. Regrettably, nurses have "friended" patients and their families, leading to significant professional concerns about maintaining professional boundaries (Cronquist and Spector, 2011; NCSBN, 2011).

The widespread use of candid cell phone camera pictures and video clips produces images amusing to friends but not as amusing to human resource personnel hiring nurses, to nurse managers, or to a courtroom when an error with serious consequences brings the nurse's professional judgment into question. Nurses have been terminated from positions and had their licenses disciplined or removed because they have posted pictures of patients on a social media site. They have been similarly disciplined for receiving patient pictures and not immediately reporting the problem. Removing a posting or a picture from a website does not make it unavailable because it remains retrievable (Cronquist and Spector, 2011).

Nurses can positively use electronic social media to share workplace concerns or events that are emotionally charged for support and guidance, but they must always be mindful of not providing names, explicit details, or patient identifiers, including photographs, to protect patient and nurse privacy. For more information, review *Social Media Guidelines for Nurses* at https://www.ncsbn.org/347.htm.

Nursing's Response

Nursing students are the future of nursing. Taking this responsibility seriously, students began two similar programs directed toward the image of nursing: the National Student Nurses' Association's (NSNA) Image of Nursing (1993-) program and the Johns Hopkins Center for Nursing Advocacy, which has been rebranded as Truth About Nursing.org. With the theme "Healthy nurse, healthy patient", NSNA annually awards outstanding Image of Nursing projects and provides information to students. An important part of the program is the media surveillance information furnished to students. How to contact the television networks, how to most effectively transmit information to them, and sample letters are offered to enable student voices to be heard when there is negative nursing media or advertisements (NSNA, 2017). NSNA has adopted a policy on social media that includes important examples of boundary violations.

In April 2001, seven graduate students at the Johns Hopkins University School of Nursing founded the Center for Nursing Advocacy (http://www.nursingadvocacy.org),

which in 2008 became Truth About Nursing. Designed to challenge stereotypes and to monitor and positively influence the portrayal of nurses in all media venues, the organization successfully changed many negative nurse images. Skechers, Schick, Dentyne Ice, and the Lung Cancer Alliance all were persuaded by this organization to remove "naughty nurse" televised advertisements (Truth About Nursing, n.d.).

Media Campaigns for Nursing

In 1990, the Tri-Council of Nursing with funding from the Pew Foundation implemented the Nurses of America (NOA) media campaign to convey to the public that nurses are expert clinicians who interpret technical data in usable ways as well as coordinate and negotiate health care. A strategically important part of the NOA campaign raised consciousness among nurses about the lack of visibility of nursing in the news media. A study of sources quoted by health coverage journalists in *The New York Times, The Los Angeles Times,* and *The Boston Globe* indicated that nurses accounted for only 10 of more than 900 citations, ranking nurses last after patients (Buresch et al, 1991). Sigma Theta Tau International's Woodhull study (1998) of 20,000 articles published in 16 newspapers, magazines, and other health care publications indicated that nurses were cited only 4% of the time in the more than 2000 articles about health care.

Seeking to stem the nursing shortage and enhance the image of nursing, the pharmaceutical company Johnson & Johnson (2013) launched a $50 million multiyear media campaign (Campaign for Nursing's Future) in 2002. This project has included the issuing of more than 32 million pieces of recruitment posters, brochures, and videos in English and Spanish to junior high schools and career and community centers as well as many television advertisements that are also available on YouTube (http://www.youtube.com). These have influenced 24% of 18- to 24-year-olds to consider nursing as a career. Additionally, there is the Nursing Notes by Johnson & Johnson Facebook fan page that launches two nursing videos per month, a comprehensive website (*Discover Nursing*) with information about nursing, an interactive program (*Your Future in Nursing*) for new graduates, and a Twitter handle (@JNJNursingNotes) (Johnson & Johnson, 2013, 2016). To commemorate the tenth year of this campaign, Johnson & Johnson invited nurses and nursing students to send pictures that became the *Art of Nursing: A Portrait of Thanks Mosaic project*. For every picture they received, Johnson & Johnson donated $1 to the NSNA Foundation Scholarship Fund. Accompanying their marketing campaign for nursing, the ongoing Promise of Nursing galas have raised more than $20 million for nursing faculty scholarships for students planning to be nursing faculty in the states where the galas are held (Johnson & Johnson, 2016).

THE ENDURING PUBLIC CONCERN WITH NURSING

Against this backdrop of nursing images that extend from antiquity to the latest news broadcast is the question of the image that nurses will create today.

The Institute of Medicine's Future of Nursing

In 2010, The Institute of Medicine (IOM) issued a landmark report, *The Future of Nursing*, that has significantly affected the image and future of nursing. This report included four main recommendations: (1) higher levels of nursing education (80% bachelor's of science degrees [BSNs] by 2020 and doubling the number of doctorates) through seamless academic progression; (2) removal of barriers to enable nurses to perform to their full scope of practice based on their educational preparation; (3) inclusion of nurses as full partners with physicians and other professionals in redesigning the health care system in the United States; and (4) improved data collection and information infrastructure to facilitate more effective workforce planning and information infrastructure (IOM, 2010). The IOM also recommended nurse residency programs that would be funded through redirection, by the Secretary of Health and Human Services, of all graduate medical education funds from diploma schools to residency programs in rural and critical access areas; a change in accreditation standards to require an assessment of clinical competency; and seamless access to higher levels of nursing education that extends beyond an articulation agreement, insuring that nurses engage in lifelong learning and prepare and enable nurses to lead change to advance health (IOM, 2010).

What the Public Believes About Nursing

Since 1999, when the Gallup Company began including nursing in its annual December public opinion poll on ethics, the public has rated nursing higher than all other professions for every year except 2001, when firefighting outranked nursing—likely representing a response to firefighters' work during and after the 9/11 attacks. In the 2016 Gallup poll on ethical professions, 84% of the public rated nurses as the most ethical profession followed by pharmacist at 67%, physician at 65%, dentist at 59%, and psychiatrist at 38% (Gallup Poll, 2016).

THE REALITY OF THE CONTEMPORARY STAFF NURSE

"The reason for the existence of the modern health care institution—the hospital, the nursing home, the mental hospital, the home care agency—is to deliver nursing. If surgery could be done safely and economically on the kitchen table, and if people could survive it, it would be. If diagnosis and management of serious medical illness could be done in office practices in 8.5-minute visits, it would be. If the chronically mentally ill could be taken care of at home, and protected from the world and from themselves, they would be. If the demented, the frail, the paralyzed, the very old could be cared for at home, they would be and it would be a whole lot cheaper because public policy would not contemplate channeling the money to family caregivers: they're supposed to want to do it anyway" (Diers, 1988).

Logically it could be inferred that nurses' satisfaction with the work setting should be high because their practice settings exist to deliver their services, and new practice settings are emerging daily. The public highly values their profession. The last National Sample Survey of Registered Nurses (NSSR) found that 79.8% of practicing RNs were satisfied with their job and 88.4% were with the same employer in the preceding year (U.S. Department of Health and Human Services [USDHHS], 2010). Among all RNs, nursing faculty are the most satisfied (86.6%). A later survey found that 90% of RNs were satisfied with their career choice (AMN Healthcare, 2013).

FACTS ABOUT TODAY'S REGISTERED NURSE

Fifty-nine percent of all health care professionals (health diagnosing and treating occupations) in the United States are registered nurses, making nursing the largest health care professional group (USDHHS, 2017). *U.S. News and World Report*'s 2017 list of the 100 best jobs ranked dentist as first, nurse practitioner as fourth, and nurse anesthetist as sixth. Nurse anesthetists, who are 58% of anesthesia providers in the US (n=42,260 CRNAs [USBLS, 2018a] and n=30,590 anesthesiologists [USBLS, 2018b]), are the major providers of anesthesia care to rural, medically underserved, and military personnel (American Association of Nurse Anesthetists [AANA], 2018a). In many rural hospitals, CRNAs are the sole anesthesia providers (AANA, 2018b). They rank thirteenth, slightly above general dentists, in the top 20 highest-paying occupations in the United States (USBLS, 2017).

Although nursing is a profession for all people, only 12% in 2017 were men (Buerhaus et al, 2017b). The numbers of men entering the field are growing, however. Prior to 2000, men constituted only 5% of the nursing workforce; between 2013 and 2015 they accounted for 14.1% of new nurses entering the workforce. Men make up almost half (41.1%) of CRNAs (U.S. Census Bureau, 2013), 12% of nurse practitioners (NPs), 7% of nurse managers, and 7% of staff nurses (Budden et al, 2016). Former U.S. Surgeon General Dr. Richard Carmona entered health care as a nurse. Interestingly, men are as equally likely as women to obtain a baccalaureate degree in nursing.

Nursing's workforce racial diversity closely mirrors that of the U.S. workforce and U.S. population. A 2015 comparison of the diversity of the nursing workforce and total U.S. workforce found the following percentages, respectively: 76% and 79% White; 11% and 12% African-American; 10% and 6% Asian; 7% and 17% Hispanic (Buerhaus et al, 2017b); 0.4% and 0.6% American Indian/Alaska Native; 0.1% and 0.2% Hawaiian/Pacific Islander; and 1.5% and 1.8% other (USDHHS, 2017). The 2016 enrollment data of the American Association of Colleges of Nursing (AACN) (2017) predicts an increasingly diverse nursing workforce. The percentages of White enrollees are lower and similar at the BSN (67%), master of science in nursing (MSN; 66%), and PhD (67%) levels (AACN, 2017). The percentages of African-Americans increased from 9.7% for BSN enrollees to 14.7% MSN to 16.5% PhD. However, the precipitous drop in percentages of Hispanic students, from 11% for BSN to 7.6% for MSN, and 5.8% for PhD, is troubling. These differences may reflect differences in the initial pipeline of students or cultural differences.

In 2016, 46% of new graduates entered nursing with a BSN (NCSBN, 2017). Regardless of the initial preparation of nurses, 62% of the nursing workforce have a BSN or graduate degree. From the 1980s to 2015, graduate degrees earned per year in nursing increased 571% (from 7,000 per year to 40,000 per year) (Buerhaus et al, 2017b).

Slightly more than half (61%) of all nurses practice in hospitals, 18% in ambulatory health care, 7% in long-term care and extended care facilities, 5% in government, and 3% education (USBLS, 2017). Most nurses (64%) are staff nurses, 4% are nurse managers, 7% are advanced practice registered nurses (APRNs), 2% are faculty, and in the less than 1% category are researchers and nurse executives. Interestingly, 85% of younger nurses (<30 years old) practice in hospitals (Budden et al, 2016).

According to the USBLS (2017), the majority (76%) of practicing APRNs are NPs, 21% are CRNAs, and 3% are clinical nurse-midwives (CNMs). In 2015, clinical nurse specialists were 13% of APRNs (Budden et al, 2016). From 2008 to 2013, the numbers of APRNs rose by 29%, with increases of 33% for NPs, 46% for CRNAs, 26% for CNMs, and 19% for clinical nurse specialists (CNSs) (Budden et al, 2016).

Men are still the minority in nursing. As Coleman's 2013 book title demands, it is past time for nursing to *Man Up!* Nurses are the problem and the solution to the low percentages of men in nursing. As Kouta and Kaite (2011) noted, women do not have female "privilege" as sole owners of empathy or caring, and we can change the subtle and not so subtle gender bias in nursing education and practice. A good place to begin is to recognize that men in nursing are nurses, not "male" nurses. What men think about being called a "male" nurse and how often it occurs is captured by the nurse who reported that he jokingly responds with "no, actually I started nursing school as an iguana and they put me out as a male nurse" (Rajecich et al. 2013, p. 77). The American Assembly for Men in Nursing (AAMN) is an organization dedicated to shaping the "practice, education, research, and leadership for men in nursing and advancing men's health" (AAMN, 2018). The barriers encountered by men entering nursing have been well documented (Roth and Coleman, 2008). A small study of male nursing students older than 25 years of age in a community college program (n = 29) indicated that gender did not interfere with their opportunities as students, although they did report a lack of locker facilities, absence of male faculty, and a feminine gender bias in nursing textbooks. All subjects described problems in maternity clinical rotation regarding patients who refused their care on the basis of gender. Although describing the events as being uncomfortable for both patients and themselves, these students believed they had other life experiences that ameliorated any possible negative effects (Smith, 2006).

CREATING THE IMAGE OF TWENTY-FIRST CENTURY NURSING

The twenty-first century image of nursing is one that nurses create every day as they practice and describe nursing to others. Conceptually, nursing is first and foremost "knowledge work" (Bargagliotti, 2003), and a profession for all people, not "just" a woman's profession. Knowledge workers are people who require specialized education to do work that requires judgment (Drucker, 2002). When nursing practice is conceptualized as knowledge work in which nursing judgment counts, other images of nursing fade away. For example, a randomized national study of primary care physicians (n = 505) and primary care NPs (n = 467) found that primary care physicians were more likely to advise a high ability high school student to be a nurse practitioner than a primary care physician (DesRoches et al, 2015).

Consider the following data about the potential benefits of nursing judgment to patients. A meta-analysis of all mortality/morbidity/nurse staffing studies since 1990 indicated that decreasing the nurse-patient ratio in the evening was accompanied by a 90% increase in mortality and that 47% of deaths from abdominal aortic surgery were due to nursing staffing (Kane et al, 2007). Hospitals with higher percentages of BSN nurses (36%) reported a 19% to 34% lower mortality rate than hospitals with lower percentages (11%). Nurses who worked shifts lasting 12.5 hours or longer were three times more likely to make medication and other procedural mistakes. The data clearly indicate that decreased nurse-patient ratios have been associated with higher rates of mortality, shock, urinary tract infections, sepsis, hospital-acquired pneumonia, and failure to rescue, especially among surgical patients (Kane et al, 2007).

Aiken and colleagues' 2011 study of all hospital admissions in four of the largest states in the United States in one calendar year found that simply increasing the number of RNs is not the sole answer to reducing patient mortality. Rather, it is the educational level of the nurses and a positive work environment of the nurse, along with increasing the numbers of nurses, that matters. A "positive work environment" was defined as one in which there are positive physician-nurse relationships, management listens to the patient concerns of bedside nurses, nurses are engaged in

hospital affairs, and hospitals invest in improving quality and in the continuing educational development of nurses. Nursing education matters because for every 10% increase in the percentage of BSN nurses, mortality rates decreased by 4%. These are cumulative, multiplicative effects. Similarly, increasing nurse-patient ratios in hospitals with positive work environments reduced mortality by 12% and failure to rescue by 14%.

There are tangible ways that the knowledge work of nurses is being portrayed to the public. Kalisch and associates (2007) found that on 70% of the Internet sites examined in 2001 and 2004, nurses were being imaged as intelligent and educated health professionals who are committed to patient care.

THE BASICS

At the simplest level, 4.73 million RNs create their image by ensuring that only an RN is referred to as "the nurse." Although the International Council of Nurses reserved the title of "nurse" for the RN in 1985, it is the responsibility of every nurse to ensure that the housekeeper, the untrained caregiver, the nursing assistant, and everyone else are not referred to as "the nurse." Imagine how confusing this is for patients and their families. Ensuring that patient teaching and questions about patient care are referred to "the nurse," rather than the assistant to the nurse, ensures that patients and families receive the best information possible.

A second and equally important image issue is how nurses refer to themselves and what they do. Nurses are not "medical professionals," do not practice in the "medical field," and do not provide medical care. Physicians provide medical care. Nurses practice nursing and they practice in health care, not medical care. Medicine is not the entirety of all health care, as 4.73 million RNs and a host of pharmacists, occupational therapists, physical therapists, and many other health professionals indicate. Aside from being legally incorrect, referring to nurses as medical professionals is misleading to the public.

Changing Nurse-Physician Interactions

An enduring mystery and common experience for nurses is how to address a medical problem with the primary customer of the hospital, the physician. Physicians generate revenue for hospitals and, in exchange for hospital privileges, agree to be self-governing and to abide by a set of medical staff bylaws, as do all advanced practice nurses in hospital practice. All medical staff bylaws include a disciplinary process that begins with the section chief, who is required to address documented patient care problems.

Too often, when nurses practice with a physician whose practice is substandard or who is highly volatile, they believe that this behavior is a nursing problem. Rather it is a medical problem that must be addressed by medicine via their staff bylaws. The problem can be resolved only when nurses disengage, factually document the problem in patient care terms rather than as a personality issue, and forward this documentation in writing to a nurse manager and the appropriate section chief.

Just as nursing's involvement with medical problems is confined to appropriate notification, medicine's involvement with nursing must be similarly confined. When a physician notifies a nurse about a nursing problem, a more positive answer is, "Thank you. Let me investigate the problem and get back to you." Lengthy detailed discussions are unhelpful. When the nurse makes an error, a simple apology and sincere statement of corrective action is sufficient. Consider the following actual clinical situations (Case Studies 2.1 and 2.2).

CASE STUDY 2.1

A nephrologist complained in a meeting with a nursing service administrator, the chief of medical staff, and the physician liaison that he was not being notified by nursing about his patients and that nurses did not know how to take care of his dialysis patients.

Response 1
Nurse 1 told the nephrologist how well prepared the nursing staff is and that his was the first complaint of this type that had been received. (The problem was denied.) However, she indicated that nursing is short-staffed and that there are a lot of agency nurses. (Two excuses were provided.) She will investigate. (This was the first positive response.) However, without a specific incident and patient, she might not be able to correct the problem. (This was the third excuse.)

Response 2
Nurse 2 carefully took notes and limited his comments to clarifying questions while the physician became increasingly more derogatory. He concluded that there was a

need to investigate, indicated that a written report would be sent to all parties, and thanked the physician for bringing this matter to his attention.

The nurse's investigation indicated that multiple nurses over time and in different units telephoned the nephrologist, who loudly announced that they had awakened his baby and abruptly hung up the phone. Second, the nurse learned that the complainer was a difficult physician who never had time to discuss his patients when making rounds. The nurse obtained specific examples of unanswered questions nurses had asked the nephrologist.

The written findings were prepared, and nurse 2 posed only one question: "Since the physician was not able to 'take calls' after 5:30 PM, the patient care issue that concerned nursing is the question of who would be covering his patients."

Outcome
Within 2 weeks, the nephrologist's hospital privileges were quietly rescinded.

CASE STUDY 2.2

The nurses on a pediatric unit thought additional nursing staff was needed.

Response 1
The nurses and nurse manager "made their case" by describing how stressed the nursing staff was to the medical staff and to nursing administration. They insisted that they could not provide safe nursing care with their current level of staffing. Nothing happened.

Response 2
The nurse manager requested data from the pharmacy about the number of medications administered by

nurses on this 24-bed unit for a specified period. The data indicated that nurses on the unit had administered 84,000 medications over 3 months. The only unit administering more medications was a 96-bed Neonatal Intensive Care Unit, which had administered only 10,000 more medications. Additionally, the laboratory data revealed that the pediatric unit usually administered 12 units of blood products daily, necessitating 48 additional sets of vital signs and assessments per day.

Outcome
Additional nursing staff positions were provided to the unit.

THE LOOK OF NURSING

Somewhere between the gleaming white uniform, hose, shoes, and cap of the past and the Mickey Mouse T-shirts, wrinkled scrubs, tattoos, and nose rings often seen today (which seem better for going to a "come as you are" party) there is a professional image for nurses. Fogle and Ream (2014) suggest that nursing attire is now directed more toward reflecting the nurse's individual preferences than projecting a professional image. Nurses are realizing that the "grunge" look encourages no one to take them seriously and are finding more appropriate ways to express their individuality. The work attire of any professional says to the world how significant the task at hand is to that professional. The wrinkled, mismatched scrubs or tank-top-over-tank-top look is far more appropriate for gardening than the knowledge work of nursing.

When some nurses and nursing students design and wear T-shirts that are sexually demeaning to the profession and to themselves, economic demand and economic support are provided to companies to demean the profession. We all must find a better way to express humor.

More recently, the nursing attire of hospital nurses has become an issue of safety for two important reasons. Patients and families have expressed their concerns about being unable to identify who the nurse is in a hospital. When time may be a critical factor, patients and/or family members may relay critical information about a patient's condition to a housekeeper believing that person to be a knowledgeable nurse or may waste valuable time asking multiple people whether they are the nurse (Fogle and Reams, 2014; Tolbert and Beilstein, 2010).

The second safety issue is found in the possible transmission of infectious organisms via nursing clothing that is worn in public places. Elizabeth (Betsy) McCaughey, former lieutenant governor of New York and chair of a committee on infectious diseases, wrote a commentary in the *Wall Street Journal* that began as follows:

You see them everywhere—nurses, doctors and medical technicians in scrubs or lab coats. They shop in them, take buses and trains in them, go to restaurants in them, and wear them home. What you can't see on these garments are the bacteria that could kill you.

Dirty scrubs spread bacteria to patients in the hospital and allow hospital superbugs to escape into public places such as restaurants.

Her warning was later supported by a study that cultured nurse and physician scrubs and lab coats and found pathogenic bacteria on 65% of nursing clothing. Notably, the highest colony counts were found for *Staphylococcus aureus,* with a higher colony count for methicillin-resistant *S. aureus* (MRSA) than for methicillin-sensitive *S. aureus* (Weiner-Well et al, 2011). When the public sees nurses in scrubs in public places, such as grocery stores, restaurants, and department stores, they are rightfully concerned.

Although "inking" or tattoos are popular today, many health care organizations have decided that tattoos cannot be made visible to patients. A study of health care providers and medical and nursing students (n = 513) found that no respondent group had positive attitudes toward tattooed individuals. Women's attitudes were more negative than those of their male counterparts and were extremely negative toward tattooed professional women (Stuppy et al, 1998).

Collectively, the voices of nurses are heard through nursing professional associations, and nursing is imaged through participation rates in professional organizations. There are approximately 60,000 members of the National Student Nurses Association (NSNA, 2014). Because 157,073 first-time takers took the NCLEX-RN in 2016 (NCSBN, 2016), it's reasonable to estimate there are at least 320,000 to 400,000 registered nursing students in the United States today. Where are the other 82% of nursing students?

These rates of participation in NSNA mirror the membership rate in the American Nurses Association (ANA). The influence that nursing could have in health policy and health legislation could be phenomenal if nurses participated more fully in their primary professional organization—the ANA. There are 61 or more specialty nursing organizations; however, the primary professional association is the ANA. At the International Council of Nursing, the national representative for the United States is the ANA.

CREATING A NEW IMAGE

Envision a new world in which nurses value nursing and image it daily. Nurses take themselves seriously and dress the part. Nurses are highly visible to patients, families, and physicians because they have reclaimed their practice. Nurses are clear about the role boundaries between themselves and those who extend their practice, and others are also. Nurses are "stuck like glue" together. Negative comments about a colleague are made to the colleague and to no one else. Professional nurses recognize that their greatest benefit is the less than 1% of their salary they spend for membership in the ANA, Sigma Theta Tau International, and their specialty organization. They look forward to annual meetings because such meetings provide an excellent opportunity to meet colleagues and discuss issues and practice innovations.

Because all nursing is valued, nurses recognize the value of caring, health promotion, and health teaching in addition to that of illness care. They celebrate that nurses save lives every day. In contemporary practice, nurses supervise assistive personnel and use their authority to ensure that patient care delivery is excellent. Nurses value the caring, knowledgeable role of the nurse because it is worn with style. To this legacy, they add the astute businessperson, advanced practice role, researcher, policymaker, legislator, and entrepreneur.

In this new world, nurses believe in nursing, in themselves, and in their colleagues. When nurses safeguard the image of nursing in local newspapers, television, media dramas, and daily practice, they protect the image of nursing.

SUMMARY

This chapter describes the major factors that have influenced the image of nursing and how society has viewed the profession during different periods throughout history. Nursing actions that contribute to a negative view are described, as well as strategies that enhance our public image.

Ensuring the public that nursing is a caring, scientifically based, safety-driven profession is essential. Everyone can care, but not everyone can be a nurse. When nurses recognize and convey to others the knowledge work they do, nursing's role as the architect of healing is enhanced.

REFERENCES

Aides relieve nursing shortage. (1942). Life, 12(1), 32–34, 36.

Aiken, L. H., Cimiotti, J. P., Sloane, D. M., Smith, H. L., Flynn, L., & Neff, D. F. (2011). Effects of nurse staffing and nurse education on patient deaths in hospitals with different nurse work environments. Medical Care, 49, 1047–1053.

American Assembly of Men in Nursing (2018). About us. Retrieved from http://aamn.org/about-us.

American Association of Colleges of Nursing. (2017). Race/ethnicity of students enrolled in generic (entry-level) baccalaureate, master's, and doctoral (research-focused) programs in nursing 2007-2016. Retrieved from http://www.aacnnursing.org/Portals/42/News/Surveys-Data/EthnicityTbl.pdf.

American Association of Nurse Anesthetists [AANA] (2018a). Certified registered nurse anesthetists fact sheet. Retrieved from https://www.aana.com/patients/certified-registered-nurse-anesthetists-fact-sheet.

American Association of Nurse Anesthetists (2018b). Protect access to rural anesthesia services. Retrieved from https://www.aana.com/docs/default-source/fga-aana-com-web-documents-(all)/1-pager-rural-anesthesia–final.pdf?sfvrsn=245d49b1_4.

AMN Healthcare. 2013 survey of registered nurses. San Diego, CA: Author. Retrieved from http://www.amnhealth care.com/uploadedFiles/MainSite/Content/Healthcare_Industry_Insights/Industry_Research/2013_RNSurvey.pdf.

Auerbach, D. I., Buerhaus, P. I., & Staiger, D. O. (2014). Registered nurses are delaying retirement, a shift that has contributed to recent growth in the nurse workforce. Health affairs, 33(8), 1474–1480. doi:10.1377/hlthaff.2014.0128. Retrieved from http://content.healthaffairs.org/content/early/2014/07/23/hlthaff.

Associated Press. Madigan Army nurse killed in action in Afghanistan, KOMO News.com. Retrieved from http://www.komonews.com/news/local/Madigan-Army-nurse-killed-in-Afghanistan-226919901.html.

Bargagliotti, L. A. (2003). Reframing nursing to renew the profession. Nursing Education Perspectives, 24(1), 12–16.

Budden, J. S., Moulton, P., Haroe, K. J., Brunell, M. L., & Smiley, R. Supplement. (2016). The 2015 national workforce survey of registered nurses. Journal of Nursing Regulation, 7(1S), S2–S90.

Buerhaus, P. I., Auerbach, D. I., & Staiger, D. O. (2016). Data watch: Recent changes in the numbers of nurses graduating from undergraduate and graduate programs. Nursing Economic$, 34(1), 46–48.

Buerhaus, P. I., Skinner, L. E., Auerbach, D. I., & Staiger, D. O. (2017). Four challenges facing the nursing workforce in the United States. Journal of Nursing Regulation, 8(2), 40–46.

Buerhaus, P. I., Skinner, L. E., Auerbach, D. I., & Staiger, D. O. (2017). State of the Registered Nurse workforce as a new era of health reform emerges. *Nursing Economic$*, *35*(5), 229–237.

Buresh, B., Gordon, S., & Bell, N. (1991). Who counts in news coverage of health care? *Nursing Outlook*, *39*(5), 204–208.

Coleman, C. L. (2013). Man Up! A practical guide for men in nursing. Indianapolis, IN: Sigma Theta Tau.

Cronquist, R., & Spector, N. (2011). Social media: regulatory concerns and guidelines. *Journal of Nursing Regulation*, *2*(3), 37–40.

DesRoches, C. M., Buerhaus, P. I., Dittus, R. S., & Donelan, S. (2015). Primary care workforce shortages and career recommendations from practicing clinicians. *Academic Medicine*, *90*(5), 671–677.

Dickens, C. (1910). Martin Chuzzlewit. New York: Macmillan.

Diers, D. (1988). The mystery of nursing: Secretary's Commission on Nursing: Support studies and background information (vol 2, pp VIII-1–VIII-10). Rockville, MD: Department of Health and Human Services.

Donahue, M. P. (2010). Nursing: The finest art: An illustrated history. St Louis: Mosby.

Drucker, P. (2002). Managing in the next society. New York: St Peter's Press.

Fagan, J. (2014, April 6). Executive Producer: 60 Minutes Affordable health care for those still uninsured [television broadcast]. New York: CBS News.

Fogle, C. and Reams, P. (2014). Taking a uniform approach to nursing attire. Nursing 44(6), 50-54.

Gallup poll. Honesty, ethics in professions. Retrieved from http://news.gallup.com/poll/1654/honesty-ethics-professions.aspx.

Goodman, C. J. & Mance, S.W. (2011, April). Employment loss and the 2007-2009 recession: An overview. Monthly Labor Review. Retrieved from https://www.bls.gov/opub/mlr/2011/04/art1full.pdf.

Institute of Medicine. The future of nursing: Leading change to advance health. Washington, DC: The National Academies Press. Retrieved from http://www.iom.edu/Reports/2010/the-future-of-nursing-leading-change-advancing-health.aspx.

Johnson & Johnson. Meet the future. Meet the next generation of nurses. Retrieved from http://www.discovernursing.com.

Johnson & Johnson. About the Johnson & Johnson Campaign for Nursing's Future. Retrieved from https://www.discovernursing.com/sites/default/files/media/press1796178328/Campaign%20for%20Nursing%27s%20Future_Overview_5%203%2016.pdf.

Jones, A. H. (1988). The White Angel (1936): Hollywood's image of Florence Nightingale. In A. H. Jones (Ed.), Images of nurses: Perspectives from history, art, and literature, Philadelphia: University of Pennsylvania Press.

Kalisch, B. J., Begeny, S., & Neumann, S. (2007). The image of the nurse on the internet. *Nursing Outlook*, *55*(4), 182–188.

Kalisch, P. A., Kalisch, B. J. (1995). The advance of American nursing (3rd ed.). Philadelphia: Lippincott.

Kampen, M. B. (1988). Before Florence Nightingale: A prehistory of nursing in painting and sculpture. In A. H. Jones (Ed.), Images of nurses: Perspectives from history, art, and literature. Philadelphia: University of Pennsylvania Press.

Kane, R. L., Shamliyan, T., Mueller, C., Duval, S., & Wilt, T. J. (2007). Nurse staffing and quality of patient care. Rockville, MD: U.S. Department of Health and Human Services, Evidence Report/Technology Assessment, Number 151, Agency for Healthcare Research and Quality Publication No. 07-E005.

Kesey, K. (1962). One flew over the cuckoo's nest. New York: New American Library/Signet.

Kouta, C., & Kaite, C. P. (2011). Gender discrimination and nursing: A literature review. *Journal of Professional Nursing*, *27*(1), 59–63.

Longfellow, H. W. (1857). Santa Filomena. *Atlantic Monthly*, *1*(11), 22–23.

McCaughey, B. (2009, January 8). Hospital scrubs are a germy, deadly mess. *Wall Street Journal*. Retrieved from http://online.wsj.com/news/articles/SB123137245971962641.

Mele, C., Victor, D. (2017, September 1). Utah nurse handcuffed and arrested after refusing to draw patient's blood. *New York Times*. Retrieved from https://www.nytimes.com/2017/09/01/us/utah-nurse-arrested-blood.html?emc=edit_tnt_20170901&nlid=10672999&tntemail0=y.

National Council of State Boards of Nursing. (2003). 2002 Nurse licensee volume and NCLEX examination statistics (Vol. 13). Retrieved from https://www.ncsbn.org/1236.htm.

National Council of State Boards of Nursing (2011). White paper: A nurse's guide to the use of social media. Retrieved from https://www.ncsbn.org/Social_Media.pdf.

National Council of State Boards of Nursing. (2017). Number of active RN licenses by state. Retrieved from https://www.ncbsn.org/Aggregate-RNActiveLicensessTable.pdf.

National Council of State Boards of Nursing. (2016). NCLEX Examination Statistics & Pass Rates 2016. Retrieved from https://www.ncsbn.org/exam-statistics-and-publications.htm.

National Student Nurses Association (2017). Image of nursing. Retrieved from http://www.nsna.org/image-of-nursing-committee.html.

Norman, E. M. (1999). We band of angels: The untold story of American nurses trapped on Bataan by the Japanese. New York: Random House.

Rajacich, D., Kane, D., Williston, C., & Cameron, S. (2013). If they do call you a nurse, it is always "male nurse": experiences of men in the nursing profession. *Nursing Forum*, *48*(1), 71–80.

Sigma Theta Tau International. (1998). The Woodhull study on nursing and the media: Health care's invisible partner. Indianapolis: STT Center Nursing Press.

Smith, J. S. (2006). Exploring the challenges for nontraditional male students transitioning into a nursing program. *The Journal of Nursing Education*, *45*(7), 263–269.

Stanley, D. J. (2008). Celluloid angels: a research study of nurses in feature films 1900-2007. *Journal of Advanced Nursing*, *64*(1), 84–95.

Stuppy, D. J., Armstrong, M. L., & Casals-Ariet, C. (1998). Attitudes of health care providers and students toward tattooed people. *Journal of Advanced Nursing*, *27*(6), 1165–1170.

The History Channel. Women in the Vietnam War. Retrieved from http://www.history.com/topics/vietnam-war/women-in-the-vietnam-war.

The last moments of Jennifer Moreno, an Army nurse killed in Afghanistan. (2014, April 29). Army Times. Retrieved from http://www.armytimes.com/article/20140429/NEWS/304290068/The-last-moments-Jennifer-Moreno-an-Army-nurse-killed-Afghanistan.

The Truth About Nursing. Retrieved from http://www.truthaboutnursing.org.

Tolbert, C., & Beilstein, L. (2010). Nurses attire: Choosing the right answer. *Nursing Leadership*, *12*(5), 55–58.

U.S. Bureau of Labor Statistics. Highest paying occupations. Occupational Outlook Handbook. Retrieved from https://www.bls.gov/ooh/highest-paying.htm. US Bureau of Labor Statistics. Occupational outlook handbook 2017. Retrieved from https://www.bls.gov/ooh/healthcare/registered-nurses.htm#tab-5.

U.S. Bureau of Labor Statistics, (2016). Registered Nurses. Retrieved from https://www.bls.gov/ooh/healthcare/registered-nurses.htm.

U.S. Bureau of Labor Statistics (2018a). Occupational employment and wages, 2017. Nurse anesthetists. Retrieved from https://www.bls.gov/oes/current/oes291151.htm.

U.S. Bureau of Labor Statistics (2018b). Occupational employment and wages, May 2017. Anesthesiologists. Retrieved from https://www.bls.gov/oes/current/oes291061.htm.

U.S. Census Bureau (2013). Men in nursing occupations. Retrieved from https://www.census.gov/content/dam/Census/library/working-papers/2013/acs/2013_Landivar_02.pdf

U.S. Department of Health and Human Services. (2010). The registered nurse population: findings from the 2008 national sample survey of registered nurses. Rockville, MD: Author.

U.S. Department of Health and Human Services, Bureau of Health Workforce. (2017). Sex, race, and ethnic diversity of US health occupations (2011-2015). Rockville, MD.

U.S. News and World Report (2017, January 11). US News and World Reports announces the 2017 best jobs. Retrieved from https://www.usnews.com/info/blogs/press-room/articles/2017-01-11/us-news-announces-the-2017-best-jobs.

Weaver, R., Ferguson, C., Wilbourn, M., & Salamonson, Y. (2013). Men in nursing on television: Exposing and reinforcing sterotypes. *Journal of Advanced Nursing* 70(4), 843-841.

Weiner-Well, Y., Galuty, M., Rudensky, B., Schlesinger, Y., Attias, D., & Yinnon, A. M. (2011). Nursing and physician attire as possible source of nosocomial infections. *American Journal of Infection Control*, *39*, 555–559.

West, I. J. The women of the Army Nurse Corps during the Vietnam War, Vietnam War Memorial. Retrieved from http://www.vietnamwomensmemorial.org/pdf/iwest.pdf.

Educational diversity promotes access and career development.

3

The Influence of Contemporary Trends and Issues on Nursing Education

Dawn Vanderhoef, PhD, DNP, RN, PMHNP-BC, FAANP

ⓔ Additional resources are available online at: *http://evolve.elsevier.com/Cherry/*

LEARNING OUTCOMES

After studying this chapter, the reader will be able to:

1. Integrate knowledge of 10 current trends and issues in society and health care into a more holistic perception of their influence on nursing education, students, faculty, and nursing practice.
2. Create a personal philosophy and plan for ongoing professional development and practice that integrates knowledge of current trends and issues.
3. Access current information resources from the Internet related to evolving trends and issues as a component of ongoing learning and preparation for practice.
4. Differentiate among various types of conventional, mobility, and new nursing education programs and the issues associated with them.

KEY TERMS

Competency outcomes The results, or end products, of planned study and experience that are focused on specific abilities required for practice.

Contemporary issues The problems, changes, and concerns that are current for the present time.

Core competencies The essential cluster of abilities and skills required for competent nursing practice.

Educational mobility The progressive movement from one type or level of education to another, often based on flexible, self-directed, or advanced placement options. Examples are progression from diploma preparation to an academic degree, such as RN to BSN or MSN; BSN to doctoral degree; and non-nursing degree to BSN, MSN, or doctoral degree.

Education trends Shifts in conditions and concerns that emerge from and influence various aspects of society; broad changes in the United States and the world that influence the education and practice of nurses and other providers.

Performance examinations Standardized evaluation based on objective demonstration of specific required competencies; used in conjunction with written tests of knowledge about those abilities. They may require performance in actual or simulated situations, related to physical psychomotor skills or the observable evidence of other skills such as critical thinking, communication, teaching, planning, writing, and analysis and integration of data.

We thank Carrie B. Lenburg, EdD, RN, FAAN, for her contribution to this chapter in the first through fifth editions and Susan R. Jacob, PhD, RN, for her contribution to the sixth edition.

PROFESSIONAL/ETHICAL ISSUE

Amy, a pre-licensure nursing student, was in her first year of clinical, and excited to begin her 5-week inpatient psychiatric rotation. Amy was considering becoming a psychiatric nurse, like her father and grandmother, and was looking forward to this clinical rotation, which she was sure would help her make a decision about psychiatric nursing. During her fourth week on the psychiatric unit, Amy was assigned to work with Sandy, an RN on the psychiatric intensive care unit (PIC-U). During morning report, Amy learned that a female patient was placed in four-point restraints about 1 hour before the day shift nurses started. The patient, "Lindsay," was assigned to Sandy, and Amy was interested in working with a very ill psychiatric patient, but also very anxious.

After completion of her 15-minute checks, Sandy asked Amy to stay in the room with the patient while she went to the medication room to prepare Lindsay's medications, and Amy agreed. As soon as Sandy left the room, Lindsay asked Amy if she had her cell phone in her pocket, and Amy felt her face get beet red, her heart race, and her palms become sweaty; she did not know how to answer the question because she did have her cell phone in her pocket. Lindsay noticed Amy's anxiety and asked her to take her cell phone out of her pocket to take a picture of her in restraints so she could show it to her attorney. Lindsay explained how the night shift had mistreated her, and said she was abused and needed documentation. She told Amy that it was okay to take the picture, that it would only be used if necessary, and if she didn't need it she could delete the photo. Lindsay made a very logical compelling case for needing a photo, so Amy took out her cell phone and took two photos of Lindsay. Quickly, Lindsay said, "Oh, just text the photos to me at 999-999-9999. Don't worry, you are really being a great help and I know you will make an excellent psychiatric nurse. Once you send me the pictures, you can delete them." Amy hesitated, felt uncomfortable, but sent the pictures to Lindsay.

Amy continued the shift with Sandy, and Lindsay was taken out of restraints and doing much better when Amy left for the day. Lindsay thanked Amy for her care and told her that she was doing much better and would delete the pictures from her cell when she was allowed to get her personal belongs back. Amy said good-bye to Sandy and her assigned patients, and went to post conference. Amy did not tell her nursing instructor or Sandy about the pictures and deleted them from her camera as soon as she got into post conference. Amy was embarrassed that a psychiatric patient persuaded her to take her cell phone out and take pictures, and feared she would be dismissed from the nursing program if she told anyone.

What ethical considerations need to be considered in the clinical experience just described? What ethical principles can be applied to this case? Provide examples.

VIGNETTE

Three students were having an animated discussion after class.

Mark: I'm tired of all this lecturing! I just want to DO nursing! Why do we always have to discuss things like EBP and critical thinking? What is it anyway? And we're always having to analyze a situation when it's perfectly clear what needs to be done! I don't get it. Just do what the doc orders or what's in the procedure book. I don't need to keep looking up stuff when I've done it before. Besides, we already have way too much to read for every class!

Katelyn: But listen to this. I heard about a student several days ago who really got into trouble because of a big mistake she made. She did just what you said, followed the provider's orders, and gave digoxin to an 80-year-old patient. She had already written a note that he was complaining of anorexia, nausea, and visual disturbances, but she didn't take time to look up "dig" toxicity or to really think things through. And guess what? The patient got into a really bad situation. It was lucky that the nurse practitioner read the note, checked the patient, put the pieces together, and got a stat serum "dig" level. She had to administer Digibind! It was so life threatening and really scary! He's not out of the woods yet. The student said the NP was nice and helped her understand what she should have done, but the instructor pulled her off the unit and gave her a serious dressing-down because she had not taken a couple of minutes to analyze the situation, to think about what things are danger signs, or to just look up the meds and the patient's condition at the time—she just followed the provider's orders. I'd be scared to be the one being grilled at the risk management meeting! She may even fail the course.

Audrey: That sounds like a good example of what our instructors keep telling us. Nursing is about thinking as well as doing. We can seriously harm a patient if we don't know what actually needs to be done. We have to learn enough so we're competent and know how to use best practices for all kinds of situations, and where to get the information fast. We have to really study resources, use our e-books, and medical software to check things out first, and then figure out what we need to do, and fast. Even if we're busy or just don't want to stop and look up something.

Katelyn: Why don't we start our own little study group, to learn how to get a better understanding of each class? Nursing is a lot more than just "doing" skills. We've got to be competent in the thinking that goes with the doing. And, there's got to be a way to organize all this information and learn how to put it together for different situations. Whaddaya say? I don't want to get into trouble like that other student! Come on; let's get started on those study questions.

Questions to Consider While Reading This Chapter:

1. What are the major current trends in society and health care, and how do they influence nursing education and practice?
2. What are the most compelling reasons that nurses require ongoing development and validation of competencies for licensure and continuing practice?
3. What local, state, and national resources and Internet websites are available to learn about the trends and issues that influence nursing education?
4. What are the pros and cons of the many different types of nursing education programs that prepare students for current nursing practice?
5. What educational opportunities exist for graduates of various programs to advance beyond their current preparation, including traditional, mobility, and distance-learning programs?

CHAPTER OVERVIEW

Society as a whole is going through many significant changes, and all of them influence nursing education and health care. Nursing care is more complex, and the role of the registered nurse (RN) is more demanding, requiring nurses to be active participants in health care decisions. Nurses need to be effective and efficient in understanding how societal, political, educational, and health care systems influence health outcomes. Our knowledge, skills, and abilities are critical to the kind of nursing care we provide, and they influence how we respond to changes in patients, families, and communities. Nurse educators must be vigilant in learning about these changes and integrating trends and changes into nursing curricula. Students also need to be aware of evolving trends and issues and must learn how they influence learning and practice.

As American society becomes increasingly diverse and complex, new trends precipitate different issues. This chapter describes 10 contemporary trends that influence the way students (and nurses) learn, become competent practitioners, and meet the needs of patients. Competent nurses integrate these changes into their way of being, to become "thinking" nurses as well as "doing" nurses. Thinking nurses learn to integrate essential knowledge, skills, and abilities to provide care using best practices, evidence-based practices that promote patient safety and quality. Some of these trends and related issues include the following: the extreme and rapid changes of technology in patient care and education, significant changes in the demographics of our society, the economic crisis and its consequences, the globalization of knowledge and diseases, the demand for competent health care providers, the increase in domestic abuse and violence of all sorts, the complexity of physical and mental health conditions including suicide and substance use disorders, ethical issues, and the shortage of nursing faculty and nurses. This chapter also describes the types of nursing education programs, their contribution to the profession, the expansion of innovative nursing programs, the degrees and specialties available, and the multiple technologic advances that inform learning and patient care. Tables and boxes contain online resources, important organizations and associations, and some statistics related to types of programs.

INTRODUCTION

New nursing programs, courses, and experiences as well as changing requirements for the development of clinical skills and critical thinking pave the way for different opportunities for students to prepare for initial and continuing nursing practice in a rapidly changing society, amidst a rapidly changing health care delivery system. These trends influence the number and types of nursing programs for basic and experienced students at the undergraduate and graduate levels. In this chapter, essential differences among basic education programs, innovations in new degree programs, majors, and courses, and mobility and distance-learning programs are reviewed in the context of changes in national organizations and accrediting and regulatory bodies. Students who study and comprehend these trends are better prepared to cope with rapidly changing nursing education models and health care systems. It is critical that nursing students at all levels stay abreast of changes in nursing education and the health care landscape so they may become competent health care practitioners and can meet the complex needs of patients from diverse multicultural and demographic backgrounds. Lenburg (2008) identified trends and issues related to nursing education, which are used as the framework to organize this chapter (Table 3.1).

TABLE 3.1 **Summary of Trends and Issues That Influence Nursing Education**	
Major Contemporary Trends	**Related Issues for Students**
Rapid knowledge expansion; increasing use of technology and informatics in education and practice	Choosing the most effective electronic and technology options Information overload; virtually unlimited global resources, global research opportunities, issues Identifying current and accurate information; material rapidly outdated Expanded expectations, limited time, rapid response expected; little time for reflection Expansion of nursing informatics, content, and skills development
Practice-based competency; outcomes- and evidence-based content	Learning focused on core practice competency outcomes, professional skills beyond technical psychomotor skills; core practice competencies; multiple conflicting versions; which to use? Integration of evidence-based standards, research findings into practice; emphasis on critical thinking, problem solving Changes in standards; ensuring patient safety
Performance-based competency; learning and objective assessment methods	Multiple teaching-learning methods: interactive collaborative, in-class and out-of-class projects; problem-based learning; increasing self-responsibility; accountability for learning and competence; interprofessional learning; using electronic devices, media to access resources Competency assessment based on performance examinations, specified portfolio documentation; standards-based assessment methods; emphasis on patient safety
Sociodemographics, cultural, diversity, economic, and political changes	Larger aging population; increasing multicultural, ethnic diversity requires greater learning, respect for differences, preferences, customs; generational issues Immigration conflicts, protests; consequences for access and health care Community, faith-based projects, service-learning projects Social, economic, and political changes influence health care delivery and access to clinical experiences; influence disrespect, conflict, abuse, violence; greater poverty and need Multidimensional content, client care, clinical learning sites
Community-focused interdisciplinary approaches	Interprofessional collaborative learning Diverse alternative health practices, influence of cultures Broad scope of nursing; clinical approach; increasing use of diverse experiences throughout community; continuum from acute care to health promotion, from hospitals to home to rural to global settings Requires more planning, travel time, expenses, arrangements; different skills, communications; critical thinking, problem-solving strategies Multiple teachers, preceptors, staff instructors, part-time, with varying abilities; time constraints

TABLE 3.1 Summary of Trends and Issues That Influence Nursing Education—cont'd	
Major Contemporary Trends	**Related Issues for Students**
Global health	Extensive global travel and commerce Illness can arrive on any airplane, ship, or bus and spread throughout the country Threat of epidemics Nurses are connected globally through shared networks and technology
Patient-centered care: engagement, safety, and privacy	All expect value, quality, individual respect, consideration, attention; privacy issues Patient initiatives for involvement and protection; balance standards and preferences Increased litigation, medical-nursing errors; focus on safe, competent patient care Increased individual responsibility, accountability for learning and practice
Ethics and bioethical concerns	Alternative solutions to ethical dilemmas; issues regarding diverse beliefs; disputes regarding biotechnology and bioengineering in health care Many gray zones instead of black-and-white absolutes; separation of professional practice responsibilities from personal opinions, consequences for competence, and patient safety Integrate into professional practice an acceptance of the individual's right of choice regarding life and death issues, health care methods; respect, tolerance for patient's decisions, ethical competencies for students Standards of quality care, patient's rights issues
Increasing shortage of nurses and faculty	Shortage of staff results in limitations in clinical learning; heavy workload; using preceptors, part-time instructors; less one-to-one help for students; consequences for learning and patient safety Shortage of qualified faculty; aging, retiring; increased part-time instructors, clinical staff, national and global problems, influence quality education and future nursing staff; need for more educational funding Students need more clinical learning; more responsibility for self-directed learning, seek assistance from others Increased use of simulation; required to validate initial and continuing competence
Disasters, violence, and terrorism	New learning skills required for major natural disaster events; new program options, new courses, and new skills needed for emergency responders Violence in society, homes, workplace, schools; abuse against women and children Preparedness for terrorism; skills, programs for first responders; increased anxiety, uncertainty
Increasing professional and personal responsibility	Lifelong learning to meet professional expectations; certification requirements Increasing competency assessment in workplace Changes in standards for quality care practice High stress from competing demands of school, home, meeting competency requirements

TRENDS AND ISSUES IN CONTEMPORARY NURSING EDUCATION

Knowledge Expansion and Use of Technology and the Internet

With ever-expanding developments in electronic information and communication technology, the volume of information is growing exponentially on a global level. Nurses have been interacting with technology for decades. In 1994, the American Nurses Association (ANA) published nursing informatics standards, understanding that nurses interact with technology at high rates (Darvish et al, 2014). Informatics has become a major part of education and practice (Cipriano and Murphy, 2011) and is part of the American Association of Colleges of Nursing (AACN) Essentials for all levels of nursing education (AACN, 2017). The ability to create, access, and disseminate unlimited information rapidly has enormous benefits. Individuals from across the globe use various forms of social media, including blogs, Twitter, Facebook, YouTube, and LinkedIn. Millennials grew up using technology and are the main generation in many undergraduate nursing programs. Nursing educators must be sensitive to the learning needs of their students and incorporate innovative technologies into learning (Hay et al, 2017; Ross and Myers, 2017). Use of social media has become so common in nursing that guidelines and code of ethics statements for it are being developed by employers and by national nursing organizations (ANA, 2017a; National Council of State Boards of Nursing [NCSBN], 2014). The use of social media has become a concern for nurses, nursing students, and educators. Using digital forums to communicate requires an understanding of policies and potential legal implications because few understand the implications and health systems lack policies for its use (Burton et al, 2017).

Websites allow for rapid access to online and printed material. Digital health-related materials can be updated quickly, allowing educators to create and revise online course content, assignments, and examinations. Nursing educators are using TED (Technology, Entertainment and Design) Talks to cover a variety of topics from science to global issues. Nursing is also engaged in various technologies that impact care. For example, nurses are now challenged with having an understanding of genetics and genomics, digital diagnostics and treatments, robotics, biometrics, and electronic health records (Huston, 2013).

Using computerized testing prepares students for computerized licensure examinations. A study conducted by Brodersen and Mills (2014) found that using the RN-Comprehensive Predictor examination or Exit Evaluation at the end of a basic RN program predicts a student's success on the National Council Licensure Examination for Registered Nurse (NCLEX-RN). Information technology and computer use have become larger parts of patient care and nursing workflow process but do not take away from direct patient care time and allow nurses to access and analyze information (Cornell et al, 2010). Further, the Healthcare Information and Management Systems Society (HIMSS) identified that nurses at all levels of education need health informatics competencies (Sensmeier, 2011).

Increasingly versatile smart phones help students, faculty, and nurses access valuable current information to manage complex patient data and thus reduce emotional stress and error (Farrell, 2016). Furthermore, smart phone use in acute care settings quickly connects the nurse with the provider, allowing critical information to be sent and patient care needs to be expeditiously addressed (Whitlow et al, 2014). Nurses receive real-time patient data using model devices and can access evidence-based resources at the point of care that lead to improved quality and outcomes (Farrell, 2016). Exposure to digital resources on mobile devices introduced early into the nursing curriculum and embedded throughout the program is effective (Zurmehly, 2010).

With almost unlimited information available, students may actually take more time to navigate online resources than traditional print-based resources and may become overly engaged in following links, networking, and using chat rooms. Faculty and students need to work together to promote efficient and effective use of electronic learning tools and networking; reducing overload and frustration requires disciplined focus and clear guidelines and outcomes. Learning from online resources can help students develop skills in analytic thinking, decision-making, and reflective judgment that are essential for selecting valid and reliable resources; these are difficult but essential competencies for evidence-based practice (Zurmehly, 2010). The use of blogs has been cited as a method to increase communication among nursing students and a forum to share medical information (Roland et al, 2011).

The Quality and Safety Education for Nurses (QSEN) project, funded by the Robert Wood Johnson Foundation, identified graduate and undergraduate informatics competency. The National Organization of Nurse Practitioner Faculty's (NONPF) core competencies also include information technology and information literacy (NONPF, 2017). Nurses, nursing students, and nursing educators must stay abreast of the rapid changes related to nursing informatics and information technology.

Practice-Based Competency Outcomes

One trend that has a powerful influence on nursing education and practice at all levels is the emphasis on competency outcomes and criteria that establish realistic expectations for clinical practice (Cronenwett et al, 2007). The National League for Nursing (NLN) has developed outcomes and competencies for graduates of nursing programs at all levels—licensed vocational nurse (LVN), associate degree in nursing (ADN) and diploma, bachelor of science in nursing (BSN), master of science in nursing (MSN), and practice and research doctorate programs (NLN, 2012). In 2008, the AACN (2008a) released *The Essentials of Baccalaureate Education for Professional Nursing Practice,* which serve as a guiding framework to build and transform nursing curriculum.

In recent years, nurse educator competencies have been developed, mirroring student competency evaluation. The NLN identified eight competencies: facilitate learning, facilitate learner development and socialization, use assessment and evaluation strategies, participate in curriculum design and evaluation of program outcomes, function as a change agent and leader, pursue continuous quality improvements in the nurse educator role, engage in scholarship, and function within the educational environment (NLN, 2018). Similarly, the World Health Organization (WHO, 2016) published eight nurse educator competencies: theories and principles of adult learning; curriculum and implementation, nursing practice; research and evidence; communication, collaboration, and partnership; ethical/legal principles and professionalism; monitoring and evaluation; and management, leadership, and advocacy. Nurse educators must stay current and must have a set of competencies to guide peer evaluation and professional development.

The NONPF has developed one set of core competencies for all graduating nurse practitioners (NONPF, 2017). Competency outcomes, with related criteria (critical elements), specify expected results, which are the measurable results of time and effort spent in learning. The ability to implement realistic practice-based abilities competently, therefore, is the essential outcome; competence is the target and the purpose of education.

The outcomes approach requires a mental shift from trying to memorize voluminous readings and class notes (resulting in frustration and the attitude of "just tell me what I need to know") to actually learning to think like a nurse, to integrate information in problem solving and decision making, and to provide competent patient care (DiVito-Thomas, 2005). Typical objectives begin with words like *describe, discuss, list,* and *recognize*; they are directions for learning, not what nurses do. Outcomes convert the meaning of the content objectives to actions that nurses actually perform, such as implement, integrate, plan, and conduct. Accrediting and certifying organizations must mandate demonstrated mastery of skills, managerial competencies, and

professional development at all levels (Institute of Medicine [IOM], 2012; NONPF, 2017).

In response to the Institute of Medicine report *To err is human: Building a safer health system* (IOM, 2000), the Robert Wood Johnson Foundation funded the national initiative, QSEN, as already mentioned, to help nursing programs reorganize curricula to focus on patient safety and quality care (Cronenwett et al, 2007). The QSEN competencies at both the pre-licensure level (AACN, 2007) and graduate level (AACN, 2012) assess the knowledge, skills, and attitudes of nurses within six areas: patient-centered care, teamwork and collaboration, evidence-based practice, quality improvement, safety, and informatics.

Performance-Based Learning and Assessment

Trends related to learning and evaluation methods are changing fundamentally, owing in part to changing technology and the greater focus on patient safety. The emphasis on competency outcomes and criteria for acceptable practice has prompted leaders in nursing education to promote innovative programs and learning methods (IOM, 2012) as well as more interactivity and engagement interspersed with lectures. Passively listening, reading, and passing written tests do not necessarily promote competence in the core performance skills expected in practice. Increased emphasis on critical thinking and learning to integrate principles is more effective than trying to remember "all the content," which often leads students to just want to pass the test. Competency-based learning creates an atmosphere that is focused on learning concepts and encourages collaboration between teacher and learner to achieve actual practice competencies (Lasater and Nielsen, 2009).

Practice-based competence uses terms like *interactive learning, collaborative learning,* and *competency-based learning.* This trend requires changes in the roles of teachers and students. The teacher is less a "lecturer" and more a facilitator and coach, providing direction for learning stated outcomes; the student is more actively accountable and responsible for achieving competence in designated knowledge and practice skills.

In this new paradigm, instructors focus on the most essential content; create practice-based case studies and simulations; and set the stage for students to engage in problem solving, critical thinking, and integration of concepts, knowledge, and evidence-based practice (Horan, 2009). Nursing faculty provide feedback and validation that cannot be gained through books or the Internet. Memorization of basic facts is still important but is insufficient when nursing practice emphasizes such skills as assessment, critical thinking, communication, patient teaching, and caring and advocating for patients. The focus on practice competence helps students learn how to access and integrate ever-changing information as required in actual practice, rather than trying to remember all the content.

The movement toward total adoption of competency-based nursing education is slow in part because of students' criticism that this model is expensive and requires active independent learning and faculty reports of increased workload and lack of metacognitive learning and critical thinking. Many colleges and universities have adopted a hybrid model of traditional teaching and learning pedagogies with some competency-based evaluations (Gravina, 2017).

A trend in many nursing programs is the development and incorporation of evidence-based practice (EBP) courses, in addition to traditional nursing research courses. Learning about EBP includes evaluation and translation of evidence into practice. The Academic Center for Evidence-Based Practice (ACE) at the University of Texas San Antonio, which was developed as a center for excellence, provides up-to-date information about evidence-based practice. In 1997, the Agency for Healthcare Research and Quality (AHRQ) developed an evidence-based practice center program.

Simulation, in various forms, is another major performance-based learning strategy. Shadow Health and vSim are technologies that use digital patient simulation to teach critical thinking. Shadow Health offers Digital Clinical Experiences such as concept labs, immersive tutorials that illustrate complex nursing subjects. Concept labs include examples of real body sounds and realistic, three-dimensional anatomic body models to compare and contrast normal and abnormal findings. The interactive interfaces of these concept labs can be used to explore body systems at an in-depth level. These experiences make classroom concepts come to life.

Designed to simulate real nursing scenarios, simulations allow students to interact with patients in a safe, realistic environment anytime, anywhere. This technology enables students to develop clinical reasoning skills, competence, and confidence in nursing. Mannequins have become more essential and incorporate sophisticated computerization to promote more realistic learning

and critical thinking (Unver et al, 2017). Another form of simulation is the use of standardized patients and telemedicine technology to achieve outcomes. The use of standardized patients has the ability to bring emotions to the simulation (Farra et al, 2017). A systematic review found the objective structured clinical examinations (OSCEs) to be the most valid assessment measurement in use (Cant and Cooper, 2010). The use of standardized patients as a competency-based summative assessment allows faculty to assess mastery of entry-level clinical skills, some of which the student may not have access to in the clinical setting. Other interactive learning strategies include portfolio learning (Lai & Wu, 2016) and peer-to-peer learning (Påisson et al, 2017). Interactive strategies are even more important when the location of clinical learning is considered. More and more diverse settings are used because these are places where nurses' expertise is needed. In addition to hospitals and extended care facilities, clinical learning often takes place in alternative settings, such as nurse-run clinics in schools, daycare and senior centers, and prisons. Over the past decade, service-learning projects have also helped students learn actual practice skills throughout the community (McGahee et al, 2017). Another form is faith-based learning projects that put nurses in churches and congregations. Many interactive clinical-related learning strategies and more traditional clinical assignments increasingly engage practicing nurses as preceptors (Matthew et al, 2018).

The change to competency outcomes and practice-based learning requires changes in evaluation methods that focus on valid, actual performance of required competencies in realistic scenarios; paper-and-pencil tests and inconsistent subjective clinical observations by instructors or preceptors are not adequate. Structured, objective validation of competence requires performance examinations that specify the core skills and related critical elements (the application of mandatory principles) that must be met according to established practice standards. In addition to performance of nursing skills, structured portfolios are used to document other competencies (Lai & Wu, 2016).

Needless to say, a more interactive approach in clinical and classroom courses is difficult for some students and creates issues; faculty and students have to change traditional habits and expectations of each other. Sometimes students think it is easier just to "figure out what the teacher wants" and "study for the test" rather than engage in learning to think and integrate best practices through teacher-assisted interactive exercises. Such exercises, however, help students learn to make effective decisions, to collaborate in the group process, and to manage time and resources. It may cause some anxiety, but performance examinations that require 100% accuracy of the mandatory critical elements (principles) provide more reliable evidence of practice competencies.

Sociodemographics, Cultural Diversity, and Economic and Political Changes

From rural to metropolitan areas throughout the United States, the population is undergoing significant changes in sociodemographic, cultural, and economic composition. These trends generate serious issues and consequences for education, health care, and many aspects of the socioeconomic-political systems. The following brief overview is a framework for learning how these trends and issues affect nursing education and practice.

- People are living longer, and the number of the very elderly is increasing more rapidly than other age groups. This means more people live with chronic disease and disability; many live in institutions, substandard conditions, or alone. All are subject to growing needs for health care and assistance. As a result, nursing and other provider programs have increased geriatric content and clinical experiences; geriatric patients require very different care from younger populations. The National Hartford Center of Gerontological Nursing Excellence, founded in 2000, has a mission to support research education, and practice to provide quality nursing care for our aging (https://www.nhcgne.org/). The Center has nine founding member institutions and has grown to over 60 institutions, providing a repository of resources, news, and updates about the care of older adults.
- The current political debate about health care reform is concerned about all age groups, and regardless of the outcome, nursing will continue to focus on quality care and competent practice (Bauer and Bodenheimer, 2017).
- The number of diverse ethnic minorities and illegal immigrants is expanding throughout the United States, with multiple socioeconomic consequences. The diversity often is unwanted and leads to disrespect, intolerance, conflicts, abuse, and violence. The Southern Poverty Law Center (SPLC) is a national organization that promotes tolerance in schools, monitors militant hate groups, and initiates lawsuits against violent offenders (SPLC, 2009). Increasingly, health care providers need to learn about different cultural values and

health practices and to integrate them into care to the extent possible. They need to incorporate and teach tolerance and understanding of cultural diversity as well as positive health practices (Fleckman et al, 2015). In 2008, the AACN (2008b) developed end-of-program competencies for graduates of baccalaureate nursing programs for integrating cultural competencies into undergraduate education. The AACN's *The Essentials of Baccalaureate Education for Professional Nursing Practice* (2008a) mandates the inclusion of culturally diverse nursing care concepts in the curriculum. Professional ethics requires that health care providers separate their personal values and beliefs from their professional responsibilities, even to those whose beliefs are different (Sanderson, 2018). The number of families who become uninsured, jobless, or homeless, and who survive in poverty is increasing. The economic crisis during the first decade of the twenty-first century has resulted in fewer financial resources for health care and ordinary expenses, and thus more people eat unhealthy diets, go without medicines or treatments, and obtain care in emergency departments. More than half of family bankruptcies are due to overwhelming health care debt. Dylan and associates (2017) describes the incredibly difficult circle of hunger, illness, theft, and incarcerations that poor people experience in the United States.

- Domestic abuse of women and children and various forms of violence are increasing in homes, schools, and public places (Stop Violence Against Women, 2010). The incidence of violence has increased even in nursing schools and in hospitals, including vertical abuse among nurses (ANA, 2017).
- Substance abuse, long a pervasive problem in society, has become a serious problem for college students and young adults (National Institute on Drug Abuse, 2018). *The CBHSQ Report,* published by the Center for Behavioral Health Statistics and Quality of the Substance Abuse and Mental Health Services Administration (SAMHSA, 2016), provides sobering statistics about the high rates of substance use in persons age 18 to 22 years of age. Substance use disorders have consequences for the safety and health of nurses, patients, and others; the increase in stress and anxiety often triggers violence and mental health and economic problems. The opioid epidemic in the United States affects more than 4.3 million Americans and leads to over 44 deaths a day (SAMSHA, 2016).

- In the United States suicide is the 10th leading cause of death in all age groups and the second cause of death in persons 10 to 34 years of age (Centers for Disease Control and Prevention [CDC], 2015). Persons who are discharged from behavioral health facilities are at 200 times greater risk of suicide (The Joint Commission [TJC], 2016). Nurses are frontline providers who can screen and provide care to high-risk populations, contributing to the Zero Suicide Initiative (Zero Suicide in Health, 2016).
- The United States is experiencing an epidemic of obesity, with major consequences for health and the health care system. Obesity leads to the most prevalent health problems that strain health care facilities and financial resources. It is paramount for health care providers to teach prevention of obesity and its consequences in schools. Learning to help people change their dietary habits is a major role for nurses (Obesity on the rise, 2009) and other health care workers.
- The traditional definition of family has changed, as evident in the number of single individuals living with other singles, single-parent households, and same-sex couples (with and without children). These nontraditional families often have limited finances and lack access to nursing and health care. They also may be resented by those with more traditional values and attitudes. Nurses must learn to respect and provide essential care regardless of differences.
- Disrespect for others, abuse of noisy mobile devices in public, and disregard for common courtesy have changed the nature of social interactions. Nursing students who use class time to send digital messages, use cell phones, or search the Internet are disrespectful of those who want to learn and the teacher who is trying to help them learn. This behavior is part of the larger trend of declining civility and integrity, with increased cheating and falsification in school and work (Lower, 2012). Such incidents trigger anger and retaliation when excessive. In health care facilities, abuse of patients is also increasing. Nurses often need to mediate health care–related situations, and effective communication skills are essential (Schlariet, 2009).
- As suggested, an important part of nursing education involves trends in society and the issues that result. Nurses work with people in all aspects of society, and thus, course content and interactive practice–based learning that incorporate these issues are essential. One of the most significant issues for students is learning to distinguish the meaningful differences in beliefs, values, and expectations among patients and their responses to illness, treatments, and caregivers. This is why nursing programs include, and students need to learn from, the areas of study that support effective nursing care, such as sociology, cultural diversity, psychology, ethics, religion, economics, history, and literature. Learning the experiences of diverse peoples, including patients and coworkers, their customs, beliefs, health practices, and expectations, not only is interesting but also expands human understanding, tolerance, compassion, and the creativity essential for effective professional practice (SPLC, 2009).

Community-Focused Interprofessional Approaches

The societal trends described here, along with the large-scale economic and political influences to reduce health care costs, may indirectly promote prevention and interprofessional initiatives. Many lay and professional health-conscious groups are working to change the national orientation from "illness care" to more efficient and effective "health care." Another contributing factor is the growing emphasis on health of the family as a whole and on entire communities and populations. *Healthy People 2020* has expanded on *Healthy People 2010,* with the current mission cited to identify health care initiatives, increase awareness of health, identify measurable objectives and outcomes, improve practice through evidence, and identify research, evaluation, and data collection methods.

As more citizens live longer and develop acute and chronic illnesses that can lead to disabilities, nurses work in a widening range of settings: acute care facilities, ambulatory clinics, nursing homes, hospices, home care, assisted living facilities, faith-based initiatives, and alternative integrated health care practices (Anastasi et al, 2009). Regardless of the setting, community health care involves an interprofessional team that is often coordinated by nurses. Nursing students are positioned to learn from and work with practicing nurses who function in diverse roles to understand the scope and role of a nurse and to begin to identify an area of nursing interest. Therefore, the concept of community care agencies has changed. Hospitals are only one of many community health care resources, along with wellness and senior centers. The changes in the health care landscape with a focus on preventive care and community care require a different philosophy of care and competencies that emphasize interprofessional and interagency collaboration. The rapidly changing and expanding health care culture incorporates concepts of shared responsibility for health promotion among individuals, family, community, and multiple care providers. Nursing education is influenced by these trends to promote family and community health and healthy lifestyles as well as increased interprofessional learning and collaboration (Holroyd et al, 2009; IOM, 2003).

In response to the paradigm shift to interprofessional care and the provision of care following the IOM's six aims for improvement—safe, effective, patient centered, timely, efficient, and equitable (IOM, 2001)—AACN developed core competencies for interprofessional collaborative practice. According to the AACN (2011) report, change is needed in the way health care professionals are trained, increasing didactic and clinical interprofessional collaboration. The four competency domains identified are values/ethics for professional practice, roles/responsibilities, interprofessional communication, and teams and teamwork. Although interprofessional educational experiences are encouraged for all health care disciplines, Delunas and Rouse (2014) cite the importance of preparation of students for interprofessional educational experiences and the need for regular meetings when students are engaged in learning as members of a health care team.

Global Health

With extensive global travel and commerce, the health community now encompasses the world. Illness can arrive on any airplane, ship, or bus and spread throughout the country. An example is the pandemic of the H1N1 "swine flu," which has spread to every continent and continues to cause illness and deaths. Nurses are on the front line of care and defense and have raised concerns about sufficient protection. Similarly, other infections, such as reemerging strains of tuberculosis and methicillin-resistant *Staphylococcus aureus* (MRSA), spread rapidly and are resistant to treatment; nurses and other providers need to become even more diligent in preventing the spread of organisms (WHO, 2017). With the recent identification of Ebola hemorrhagic fever in the United States among missionary health care providers, the CDC has reevaluated and updated the recommendations for health care providers working with patients who have symptoms of Ebola (CDC, 2016), with nurses often at the front line of care.

Consistent with the trend toward global health, nurses are engaged in the global health community through collaborative networks, research projects, and shared publications (Critchley et al, 2009). Programs incorporate global content, and students learn to participate in international health research projects and communication through the Internet and have direct learning experiences in countries abroad (Ramal, 2009). The International Council of Nurses (ICN, 2009) provides many opportunities for students to network and learn from each other; its periodic international conferences are a major resource for students and nurses to promote world health (ICN, 2009; see ICN website and student bulletin board).

These trends challenge students to prepare for a wide spectrum of nursing practice that depends on competencies such as clinical decision making (Flin et al, 2008), communication, collaboration, and leadership. Students need to learn how to manage illness and preventive health care for diverse clients dispersed throughout the community as well as to provide critical care to hospital patients who are sicker and go home sooner. Although very helpful, learning in diverse settings throughout the community presents some issues. For example, dispersed clinical learning requires more planning, travel, expense, and time; learning time is much shorter at each location; community-based group projects take more time; and students have less time with instructors because faculty can be at only one location at a time. In many settings, however, students work only with preceptors or staff who help them gain the competence and confidence they need but who also have other responsibilities. In addition, as students and health care leaders, nurses need to effectively communicate with other health care disciplines and to have a good understanding of their role and scope of practice, in order to practice at the highest level of their degree and licensure.

Patient-Centered Care: Engagement, Safety, and Privacy

As patients have become more knowledgeable about illness care, health promotion, and the consequences of errors in care, they have become more assertive about their right to competent care and privacy of information. The 2002 Health Insurance Portability and Accountability Act (HIPAA) mandates protection of an individual's privacy by health care providers and throughout society and has changed many previously careless and harmful practices. The economics and politics of health care and access to comprehensive information via the Internet have promoted more consumer activism through advocacy groups and Internet connections to influence health care policy and standards. Patients use Internet resources, sponsored by the government and private entities, to become more informed about illness and health care. As informed and engaged patients, they are better able to make effective decisions in collaboration with health care providers. This development makes critical thinking, communication, and teaching essential nursing competencies. It also means that student nurses need to change their approach from "giving patient care" to "working with the patient and family" as members of the health care team.

Another major issue affecting nursing education is the increasing number and consequences of serious medical errors, as reported in the IOM study *To Err is Human: Building a Safer Health System* (2000). These errors have led to an astonishing number of deaths and an increased number of expensive lawsuits, which further raise the cost of health care and tarnish the belief in the quality of available health care. Nursing faculty, administrators, and regulators therefore are increasingly concerned with ensuring the competence of students and nurses (Veltri and Barber, 2016). Medical-error issues have precipitated increased requirements for competency-based education and performance assessment in schools of nursing and other health disciplines, in annual employment evaluations, and in agency accreditation criteria, all for patient safety.

Many injuries and deaths in medical institutions are preventable, and Medicare will no longer pay for such preventable incidents, many of which are attributed to nurses. Thus, preventive care is being emphasized even more in nursing education. QSEN, Interprofessional Collaboration, and similar initiatives in every specialty organization are designed to change nursing education and practice to promote competence and patient safety (IOM, 2003).

Disasters, Violence, and Terrorism

Nurses have always worked in situations emanating from disasters, abuse, and violence in families and communities, and in military conflicts. Domestic violence, especially against women and children, has increased as has violence in the workplace and in schools. Greater violence has precipitated an increased emphasis in nursing education (SAMHSA, 2016]) and in state regulations for reporting and responding to violent incidents. Criminal acts and substance abuse have become more common in hospitals, other health care agencies, and schools of nursing, threatening the safety of patients and staff (ANA, 2017). As a consequence, criminal background checks are required for all students (and employees) by education programs as well as by agencies providing clinical experiences to students. Population expansion, especially in urban areas, and mass disasters, such as hurricanes, floods, and earthquakes, have precipitated the need for more nurses to become prepared to function effectively along with other first responders. Adelman and Legg (2009) describe details of preparedness and opportunities for nurses who want to learn more. See Chapter 16 for more information on emergency preparedness.

Since the terrorist attacks on September 11, 2001, in New York City, Washington, DC, and Pennsylvania, more nurses (and all other health care personnel and first responders) are more prepared to respond to acts of terrorism and disaster. Many nursing programs have added courses or even entire programs of study for specialized preparation as first responders, emergency nursing, and flight nursing (Adelman and Legg, 2009; Whitty and Burnett, 2009). Not all nurses will become first responders, but all nurses and students should gain enough knowledge to know their limitations, who and how to notify, and how they could work with more qualified responders. Chapter 15 also provides more information about disaster preparedness for nurses.

Ethics and Bioethical Concerns

Another trend affecting nursing education is related to the multicultural, multiethnic population and patients who have different ways of responding to illness, treatment, and care providers. This development raises ethical issues as to who "is right" and who "has the right to decide." As described, one difficult issue, particularly for students and novices, is the ethical necessity to differentiate personal beliefs, values, and preferences from professional practice responsibilities. Many ethical dilemmas require students, nurses, and other providers to accept the values of others and the concept of "a gray continuum of values" instead of the black-and-white interpretations based on one's own beliefs. Some of the most controversial issues relate to the right of individual choice regarding abortion, organ transplant, stem-cell research, preference in sexual partners, and the patient's right to a dignified death. Other issues emerge from the growing use of alternative health remedies outside the mainstream of traditional Western medicine, such as herbs and acupuncture (Anastasi et al, 2009).

Dishonesty among nursing students, nurses, and other professionals is increasing alarmingly and threatens patient safety (Klocko, 2014). The ANA's *Code of Ethics for Nurses with Interpretive Statements* (2015) provides a succinct statement of the ethical obligations and duties of every individual who enters the nursing profession. The code of ethics for nursing has nine provisions that outline the "ethical values, obligations, duties, and professional ideals of nurses individually and collectively"; they are a nonnegotiable ethic standard as well as an "expression of nursing's own understanding of its commitment to society" (ANA, 2015). Nurses are the largest health care workforce and for the last 16 years in a row have been identified as having the most trusted profession, with the highest level of honesty and ethics (Gallup Poll, 2016).

Chapter 9 presents a comprehensive discussion about ethics in health care and important issues students should be knowledgeable about for competent nursing practice.

Shortage of Nurses and Faculty

The nursing workforce shortage has challenges: aging of Baby Boomers, shortage and uneven distribution of physicians, accelerated rate of nurse retirements, and uncertainty of health care reform (Buerhaus et al, 2017). Buerhaus and Auerbach (2011) observed that during the 2008 recession, nurses older than 50 years reentered the hospital workforce. These writers assert that when this older hospital workforce retires, a hospital nursing shortage will reemerge. The nursing workforce is more than 90% female, 80% white, 47% prepared at the baccalaureate level, 64% employed in a hospital at rates of 64%, and 37% more than 50 years of age (Buerhaus et al, 2017a). The nursing workforce does not mirror the U.S population seeking care, in gender, ethnicity, or age. According to Buerhaus and Auerbach (2011), one area the RN workforce has advanced is in the percentage who have baccalaureate degrees, which now exceeds that of those with associate degrees. The percentage who enter BSN programs is up, but not enough to meet the workforce demands (AACN, 2017a).

Students are assigned to multiple and diverse community clinical settings, some of which may be short-staffed, making it difficult for them to find qualified preceptors. Staff nurses who act as clinical instructors or preceptors may or may not be prepared for these roles or have received adequate orientation. Students, therefore, need to learn to take more individual responsibility and initiative to gain essential core competencies. Online learning environments can be simulated to mimic real-world situations that allow for faculty to evaluate student learning from a distance (Phillips et al, 2010). New methods are created in partnership with agencies to promote more effective clinical learning opportunities for students without overburdening staff.

Education is the ladder to success.

Often the causative trends related to a shortage of faculty include a limited number of nurses prepared at advanced levels, space limitations, and other administrative constraints. For example, AACN's 2017a data report reveals that 64,065 qualified nursing applicants were denied admission to BSN programs because of faculty shortages, lack of clinical sites, and limited classroom space. According to a Special Survey on Vacant Faculty Positions released by AACN in October 2016, a total of 1567 faculty vacancies were identified in a survey of 821 nursing schools with baccalaureate and/or graduate programs across the country (85.7% response rate). Besides the vacancies, schools cited the need to create an additional 133 faculty positions to accommodate student demand. The data show a national nurse faculty vacancy rate of 7.9%. Most of the vacancies (92.8%) were faculty positions requiring or preferring a doctoral degree (AACN, 2017). According to AACN's report on 2016-2017 Salaries of Instructional and Administrative Nursing Faculty, the average ages of doctorally prepared nurse faculty holding the ranks of professor, associate professor, and assistant professor were 62.4, 57.2, 51.2, and 50.1 years, respectively; for master's degree–prepared nurse faculty, the average ages were 55.5, 56.4, and 50.6 respectively (AACN, 2017). Some schools are expanding enrollments by using more part-time, adjunct, and clinical faculty and by expanding the use of online courses and simulation. Moreover, the number of students in MSN or doctoral programs is not adequate to meet current needs. Nurse leaders and organizations are working vigorously with state and national governments and private entities to reverse these trends by seeking more funding and promoting recruitment and development efforts nationally (AACN, 2017c).

The nursing shortage and lack of nursing faculty present many hardships for students, faculty, and nurses; however, difficult situations promote creative and innovative initiatives and solutions. For example, many organizations and associations have initiated collaborative partnerships to improve education in all types and levels of nursing education. The NLN has implemented initiatives to improve nursing education and faculty development (see AACN and NLN websites for position statements regarding innovations and transitions in nursing education).

Increasing Professional and Personal Responsibilities

Given the complexity of health care delivery and need for health care team members to work as an interprofessional team, another trend with multiple issues has become evident. In the current health care environment, students, teachers, and nurses confront increasing life responsibilities and associated stressful demands on time and resources. Many cope simultaneously with the expansion of information and technology; changing health care systems; more interactive and out-of-class methods of learning; multiple care settings; higher expectations for competence; shortage of nurse preceptors and teachers; and multiple cultural, ethical, and legal aspects of an ever-changing society. Many also are responsible for the care of dependent children and aging parents.

At the same time, contemporary conditions require nurses to keep current through planned ongoing professional development. Complexities in practice, emphasis on reducing errors, and growing consumer activism increase the need for nurses to document continuing competence for initial licensure, relicensure, and recertification. Changes in state and multistate regulations increasingly focus on the need for initial and continuing competence (IOM, 2009). Current uniform licensure requirements facilitate nurses practicing in bordering states through the RN compact. As of 2015, 25 states are part of the licensure compact, and 10 states have enacted legislation for an Advanced Practice Registered Nurse (APRN) compact (NCSBN, 2018). See Chapter 4 for more information on nursing licensure. The high stress levels associated with these professional and personal demands have consequences for one's own health and that of those around one. It is important for everyone involved in the educational process to be more caring, understanding, respectful, and helpful to one another. Teachers, students, administrators, staff nurses, employers, family, and friends need to learn anew the meaning of "a caring community" in the context of rapid and complex change.

These trends in society, nursing, and academic programs present the problem of how to incorporate this additional knowledge into the already overloaded program of study. The issues for students include knowing how to access and use unlimited information, prioritize learning, implement evidence-based practice, deal with ethical dilemmas professionally, and develop competencies required for effective responses to contemporary issues. Above all, students must focus on learning to think critically, reflectively, ethically, and compassionately, which are essential professional skills (IOM, 2011).

DIVERSITY IN NURSING EDUCATION PROGRAMS

A brief review of the major types of education programs that prepare nurses for licensure and advanced practice sets the stage for summarizing some contemporary trends related to flexible, online, and other distance delivery methods in nursing education. A brief description of the types of programs is provided in Table 3.2.

Licensed Practical or Vocational Nurse Programs

Practical nurse (PN) or vocational nurse (VN) programs provide the shortest and most restricted option for individuals seeking a nursing license. The total number of PN licenses in the United States is 974,626, with more licenses in the Midwest, South, and Northeast regions of the country (NCSBN, 2017). Licensed practical nurse (LPN) programs, named licensed vocational nurses (LVN) in California and Texas, usually are 9 to 12 months in length and may be offered by high school adult education programs, community colleges, vocational and proprietary schools, and hospitals. The median earnings for female LPN/VNs was $38,000; the median earnings for male LPN/VNs was $43,200 (NCSBN, 2017).

Regardless of the increasing complexity of patient care, many individuals choose to begin a career in nursing as

TABLE 3.2 Types of Nursing Education Programs

Types of Program and Credential	Type of Institution	Length of Program	Purpose and Scope
Practical (LPN) or vocational (LVN) nurse program: prepares for LVN or LPN license	High school, hospitals, vocational-technical schools; some colleges	9 to 12 months	Basic technical bedside care; hospitals, nursing homes, home care, offices in LPN positions
Diploma program: prepares for registered nurse (RN) license	Hospitals, some in conjunction with colleges	2 to 3 years	Basic RN positions; hospitals and agency care
Associate degree in nursing (ADN): prepares for RN license	Community and junior colleges	2 years; some are 1 year bridge programs for LPN/LVN graduates	Basic technical care in RN positions, primarily in institutions
Bachelor's degree in nursing (BSN): prepares for RN license	Colleges and universities	2 to 4 years (depends on type of option); some are 1- to 2-year mobility options for graduates of PN or ADN programs or accelerated options for second-degree students	Basic professional practice as RN; management, community and public health settings; prepares for graduate school and certification; basic programs are 4 years; mobility options may be only 2 years
Master's degree in nursing (MSN)	Universities	1 to 2 years beyond BSN degree; some offer fast-track options	Advanced clinical practice, management, education, leadership positions
Doctoral degree in nursing	Universities	Varies: Doctor of Philosophy (in Nursing (PhD), DSN, Doctor of Nursing Practice (DNP), Doctor of Nursing Science (DNSc)	Advanced nursing for research, clinical practice, education, and leadership positions

LPNs/LVNs. The NLN's position statement supports the role and LPN/LVN workforce, citing that this level of provider is critical to health care redesign (NLN, 2014a). LPN/LVN nurses provide safe, quality, and cost-effective care (NLN). Once licensed, many graduates continue their education in mobility programs to become RNs. Many use "1 plus 1" type programs to earn an associate degree; others use the multiple entry-exit programs (MEEPs). For example, a MEEP is a program that allows students to enter with a ADN to obtain a MSN, or a student with a bachelor's degree to enter and obtain a Master's of Nursing or a MSN. Some BSN programs accept LPN graduates on the basis of outcomes of written and performance examinations for advanced placement.

Hospital Diploma Programs

The oldest, most traditional type of program that prepares for RN licensure is the hospital-based diploma program. These programs initially were developed in the United States in the late 1800s in general hospitals in cities such as Boston, New York, Hartford, and Philadelphia and subsequently spread across the country. They followed the Nightingale model and began as training programs taught by physicians, usually only several weeks in length. In time, nurse graduates began developing and teaching courses from the nursing perspective and subsequently obtained additional education as educators and administrators. Ultimately, the length of programs was extended, and by the mid-1900s most programs were 3 years long and had fairly uniform courses of study and clinical hours.

As the number of hospitals grew, the need for nurses likewise increased, and essentially, every hospital developed its own training program as its main source for nursing staff. At their peak from 1950 to 1960, more than 1300 diploma programs were operational. By 2014, only 67 diploma schools remained (NLN, 2012). Diploma programs now are more similar to associate degree programs, typically 2 years in length; many have arrangements with colleges so that students can simultaneously earn an associate or baccalaureate degree. The American Association of Colleges of Nurses report pre-licensure nursing programs at the diploma level to account for less than 10% of all basic RN programs, citing the transition from hospital instruction to college or university instruction (NLN, 2014b).

Associate Degree Programs

In the late 1950s, a very different trend in nursing education emerged in response to social, political, and educational changes in society and to a growing shortage of RNs. During World War II, the need for RNs who were prepared more quickly than in diploma programs became critical; the 2-year Cadet Nurse Corps was developed and proved to be very successful. From this experience, some educators realized that nurses and others could be prepared in less time and still meet RN licensure and practice requirements. After the war, Congress made funds available to publicly fund community colleges that offered 2-year associate degree programs in many technical fields. In addition, military benefits for college tuition allowed thousands of men and women to earn a 2-year college degree and fill jobs needed by burgeoning business and industry.

At the same time, the increasing complexity and expansion of medical care required more and better-prepared RNs. A few nurse educators began to create a new 2-year associate degree nursing program in community colleges, which required college courses in arts and sciences and a more integrated approach to nursing content and clinical learning. These pioneers reasoned that nursing belonged in a college setting, like other disciplines, to provide a better education for nurses and to establish more respect and recognition for nursing's contribution to the community's health. As the number of community colleges grew and the need for nurses increased, ADN programs became a logical program for development and expansion.

ADN education is a vivid example of how changes in society influence the evolution of nursing education; it was another significant "first" in nursing and an important part of the evolving professionalization of nursing as a discipline. For the first time, it was possible for all RNs to be educated in college settings and obtain college degrees.

In 2014, approximately 710 ADN programs were operational, a decrease of 338 programs since 2002 (NLN, 2014b). The majority of the ADN programs are found in the Midwestern and Southern regions of the United States (NLN, 2014). Of the qualified applicants to ADN programs, 45% are rejected due to difficulty with clinical placements (NLN, 2014). The trend of acceptance and growth of ADN programs along with the slow increase in 4-year BSN programs and progressive mobility options established the educational framework for current nursing education.

Baccalaureate Degree Nursing Programs

In 1924, Yale University offered the first separate department of nursing whose graduates earned the baccalaureate degree. The 28-month program required scientific studies and clinical work and had the prestige and authority of other departments, with its own dean and budget (Kalisch and Kalisch, 1995).

Generic BSN programs typically require 2 years of arts and sciences followed by 2 years of nursing courses. Currently 747 RN to BSN programs are available nationwide, including more than 600 programs that are offered at least partially online. Program length varies from 1 to 2 years depending upon the school's requirements, the program type, and the student's previous academic achievement (AACN, 2017a). The demographic of the degree-seeking student in this program, according to AACN, is "motivated, older, and has higher academic expectations than traditional entry-level students." As in other programs, BSN courses focus on the care of patients with medical, surgical, pediatric, obstetric, and psychiatric conditions, although course sequencing and names differ considerably from school to school. BSN programs focus more emphasis on the family and community and health promotion and illness prevention; a large part of clinical experience is in diverse community settings. These programs also require courses such as research, management, leadership, and statistics.

For the BSN programs in the United States the most common reason cited for denying an applicant is due to shortage of faculty (38%), followed by having a shortage of clinical placement sites (36%). The total number of BSN graduates in 2016 was 128,852, contrasted with the 2016 BSN program enrollment of 338,802 (AACN, 2017b). Graduates of BSN programs take the same NCLEX-RN licensure examination as diploma and ADN graduates. Most specialty areas require the BSN degree for practice and as preparation for specialty certification. Admission into masters programs usually requires a BSN or other degree. Current NCLEX-RN data, as of September 2017, indicate the following first-time pass rates by education type: diploma 90.65% (1,989), BSN 90.35% (69,353), and associate degree 85.37% (72,031). The median salary for female RNs was $64,000; the median salary for male RNs was $72,000 (NCSBN, 2017a).

Master's Degree Nursing Programs

In the 1960s and 1970s, the number of BSN graduates increased; however, in response to the complexity of health care, so did the need for more qualified clinicians, educators, and administrators. The federal government responded with support for the development of MSN and BSN degree programs. Nurse leaders lobbied for and obtained federal funding for building construction and increased student tuition. Traineeship and fellowship grants were made available to thousands of RNs that enabled them to earn BSN and advanced degrees to meet these needs. Different MSN program options are available; the most typical are for BSN graduates, although an increasing number are designed for graduates of non-nursing degree programs, called accelerated or second-degree programs. Second-degree graduate nursing programs, in which graduates do not receive a BSN but are eligible to sit for the NCLEX-RN licensure examination, are growing in number. Students in these programs have been described as self-directed adult learners who pass the RN licensure examination at high rates (Miller and Holm, 2011).

Until the late 1960s, MSN programs primarily focused on preparing educators and administrators, but then the curriculum shifted to an overwhelming emphasis on clinical practice. By the 1990s, the negative and positive consequences of this decision became apparent, with more competent clinicians but less well-prepared educators and administrators. Most MSN programs are designed to prepare advanced nurse practitioners and clinical specialists in various specialty areas. The extraordinary and rapid changes in health care since the early 1990s highlighted the cost-effective and quality care benefits of using advanced practice nurses in primary health care and other specialty areas. With intensive and persistent legal activities, nurses won battles to change state laws to permit nurse practitioners to write prescriptions, receive reimbursement for care, and operate independent nurse practices and health centers. As a result of this expanded scope of practice, a rising number of nurses have obtained MSN degrees and advanced practice certification. Most specialty practice nurses, managers, administrators, and educators now are required to have master's or doctoral degrees. The AACN and NLN offer descriptions and numbers of different types of programs on their websites. Additionally, the consensus model for advanced practice registered nurse regulation, which included licensure, accreditation, certification, and education, was published in 2008 (AACN, 2008d). *Consensus Model for APRN regulation: Licensure, Accreditation, Certification and Education* outlines four APRN roles—nurse anesthetist, nurse midwife, clinical nurse specialist, and nurse practitioner—followed by six population foci. This document provides data to guide nursing licensure, accreditation of programs, certification, and educational programs.

Clinical Nurse Leader

In 2000, the national movement to enhance quality and safety in health care inspired discussions among the AACN, nurse executives, and other health care leaders that led to the development of a new nursing role—the clinical nurse leader (CNL). In July 2002, the AACN board created the Task Force on Education and Regulation (TFER 2). Its focus was the nurse competencies needed in current and future health care systems to improve patient care and what the "new nurse" role might look like. This work resulted in the publication of the *White Paper on the Role of the Clinical Nurse Leader (CNL)* in 2007 (AACN, 2009a). The CNL is a master's-prepared generalist clinician, not an advanced practice nurse, who oversees the care coordination of a distinct group of patients, evaluates patient outcomes, and has the decision-making authority to change care plans when necessary. The CNL actively provides direct patient care in complex situations, serves as a lateral integrator who provides centralized care coordination for a distinct group of patients, and puts evidence-based care into practice to ensure that patients benefit from the latest innovations. A CNL is a leader in the health care delivery system with expertise in quality improvement and cost-effective resource utilization (Rosseter, 2009). The CNL is not an advanced practice nurse, nor is the CNL prepared in an area of clinical specialty; however, the CNL can consult with a Clinical Nurse Specialist as needed, and further, the CNL can provide evidence-based care to complex patients (Harris et al, 2011). The Commission on Nurse Certification, an autonomous arm of the AACN, began certifying CNLs in 2007.

Doctoral Programs

Changes in society and health care have necessitated an increase in the educational preparation of nurse leaders. Both clinical and research leaders are charged with the development, implementation, and leadership of nursing doctoral programs. In 1934, New York University offered a PhD program for nurses. More than 30 years elapsed before doctoral programs *in nursing* (instead of *for nurses*) were offered (e.g., the doctor of nursing science degree [DNS or DNSc]).

For the past few decades, three types of doctoral degrees in nursing have been available: (1) the doctor of philosophy (PhD) for those interested in research; (2) the DNS or DNSc for those interested in advanced clinical nursing practice; and (3) the doctor of nursing (ND) for those with BS or higher degrees in non-nursing fields who want to pursue a career in nursing leadership. The ND degree, which prepared nurses for basic licensure (NCLEX-RN), was first offered at Case Western Reserve University in 1979. Shortly thereafter, Rush University, the University of Colorado Health Sciences Center, and others offered this degree. Nursing schools have transitioned to Doctor of Nursing Practice or PhD programs.

Beginning in 2000, AACN leaders developed and implemented a new clinical-focused doctoral degree: the doctor of nursing practice (DNP) (AACN, 2017a). The DNP is conceived as preparation for contemporary advanced nurse practitioners; it is viewed as the clinical equivalent to the research-oriented PhD nursing degree. Although the DNP prepares clinicians and does not formally prepare nurse educators, many individuals who complete a DNP degree frequently shift from practice to a dual role and serve in faculty roles in addition to clinical roles. The AACN recommended that all advanced practice education programs move from the masters to the doctoral level by 2025. In 2017, the AACN reported that in the 874 schools that offer nursing degrees, the number of DNP programs increased from 53 in 2007 to 313 in 2016. The growth in programs is impressive, and this important trend is consistent with the NONPF statement that the entry into advanced practice nursing should be at the doctoral level.

FLEXIBLE EDUCATION, MOBILITY, AND DISTANCE-LEARNING PROGRAMS

Various and nontraditional educational mobility programs now are commonplace. The AACN and NLN websites attest to the growing number of programs that offer some form of flexible, alternative program in addition to position statements on technology in nursing education, distance-learning, and online programs. Distance or mobility programs include those for LPN or LVN to ADN and BSN; diploma and ADN graduates to BSN and MSN; and BSN to MSN and doctoral programs. Almost all use some form of Internet-based courses, and some are entirely online. Some require periods of intensive on-campus classes or assigned clinical experiences with preceptors. Distance nursing education at all levels is another important trend to track.

The most controversial but pace-setting distance-learning program in nursing was developed under the New York Board of Regents as "the external degree program." Initially named the NY Regents External Degree Program (NYREDP), it later was renamed Excelsior College. Its ADN program, initiated in 1972, and the BSN program, in 1976, were fully accredited by the NLN shortly thereafter. This innovative college provides quality degree programs in many disciplines for adult learners underserved by traditional programs by using assessment methods to document prior learning and theory and performance examinations to validate current knowledge and competence. The nursing programs enroll thousands of students and are accessible regardless of geographic location; the students are primarily LPNs or RNs, some of whom also have other degrees or health-related certificates. Over the years, many nursing programs have accepted and modified the distance-learning and assessment approach originally developed by the NYREDP and continued as Excelsior College. The integration of electronic learning technology with assessment methods makes nursing degrees accessible to an increasing number of nurses seeking additional preparation.

Career ladder programs designed as "1 plus 1" or "2 plus 2" options, which allow students to acquire two degrees at the same time, have been offered for many years by some schools and through several statewide programs. Multiple mobility programs are available for LPNs to obtain an ADN degree. Fortunately, an increasing number of registered nurses are recognizing the need to advance their education, and many employers are providing funding and support to facilitate academic progression. Enrollment in RN to BSN programs is increasing in response to calls for a more highly educated nursing workforce. From 2015 to 2016, enrollments in such programs increased by 1.0%, marking the 13th year of increases in RN to BSN programs (AACN, 2017a). To accommodate the growing demand, the number of RN to BSN programs also has increased dramatically over the last decade. Currently 747 RN to BSN programs are available nationwide, including more than 600 programs that are offered at least partially online. Program length varies from 1 to 2 years depending on the school's requirements, the program type, and the student's previous academic achievement (AACN, 2017a).

Changes in social, political, financial, and philosophic trends, the extensive use of communication and learning technology, verified success from past experiences, and the continuing shortage of nurses have combined to make education mobility and distance-learning opportunities a necessity and a reality both nationally and internationally. Whereas the NLN continues to support all levels of education programs, the AACN and other organizations vigorously support the BSN for "entry into practice" and the professionalization of nursing (IOM, 2010).

In October 2010, the IOM released the report *The Future of Nursing: Leading Change, Advancing Health,* which provides a blueprint for transforming the nursing profession. A key message of this IOM report was that nurses should achieve higher levels of education and training through an improved education system that promotes seamless academic progression (IOM, 2011). A variety of innovative strategies that include online education and simulation have been developed to create a seamless pathway from ADN to BSN, ADN to MSN, and BSN to DNP and PhD. On December 18, 2017, New York passed legislation (S6768/A1842B) that requires future RN graduates of associate degree and diploma nursing programs to finish a baccalaureate completion program in nursing within 10 years after initial licensure in New York State. This legislation took effect immediately, and the requirement that nurses obtain a baccalaureate degree in nursing within 10 years of licensure will take effect in June 2020, only 30 months after the legislation became law (ANA New York and New York Organization of Executives and Leaders, 2017).

The escalating nursing shortage and the aging of the current nursing workforce and nurse educators have prompted more schools to offer flexible mobility options and types of programs. Some target potentially underrepresented groups, such as men, minority groups, and those with existing academic degrees. It is estimated that more than 580,000 nurses would be needed by 2018 to replace the aging workforce who will be retiring. The most rapidly growing are the accelerated, fast-track, or second-degree programs, designed for non-nurses with other degrees. These programs are intended to try to meet the workforce need. In 2016, the AACN reported the availability of 272 accelerated BSN programs and 69 accelerated master's programs available at nursing schools nationwide. For a list of accelerated nursing programs, visit http://www.aacnnursing.org/Nursing-Education-Programs/Accelerated-Programs.

Trends and issues that influence nursing education make it even more important to comply with quality standards that emphasize competency outcomes. Educational trends include changes in number, diversity, and qualifications of students and shortage of faculty and finances make it necessary to develop more efficient and effective learning strategies for on-campus and distant students. Although mobility and electronic options are more convenient, they present issues. In addition to learning to access multiple digital resources, students also need discipline and determination to pursue courses and clinical learning when a teacher is not physically present or accessible. Regardless of methods, they must achieve required competencies in spite of other responsibilities and learn to integrate critical thinking, reflective judgment, and evidence-based practices in patient care. In contrast to previous decades, organizations and schools now require more creative, responsive programs and expect more documented competence from students and faculty. Nursing organizations (Box 3.1) set the standards and innovation that assist in the evolution of nursing education at all levels. Although these trends pose challenges for nursing students, faculties, and employers, they move nursing toward more competent professional practice and improved patient safety.

BOX 3.1   Selected Organizations Relevant to Nursing Education: General Description and Purpose

American Academy of Nursing (AAN)—The organization of leaders in all facets of nursing: practice, education, administration, research, organizations, and government; the think tank of the profession; promotes advancement of all aspects of nursing; and publishes position papers, conference proceedings, and documents to advance nursing.

American Association of Colleges of Nursing (AACN)—The organization of deans and directors of baccalaureate and higher-degree nursing programs: establishes standards for programs concerned with legislative issues that pertain to professional nursing education and publishes the *Journal of Professional Nursing*, *The Essentials of Baccalaureate Education* (2008), and other related documents pertaining to the BSN and higher-degree education.

American Nurses Association (ANA)—The major national nursing organization concerned with a broad scope of practice issues: standard of practice, scope of practice, ethics, legal, and employment issues; a federation of state nurses associations; and publications relate to an array of practice issues and standards.

Commission on Collegiate Nursing Education (CCNE)—A subsidiary of the AACN with responsibility for establishing and implementing standards and criteria and for accreditation of baccalaureate and graduate degree programs in nursing.

National Council of State Boards of Nursing (NCSBN)—The organization of all state boards: coordinates licensure activities on a national level; creates and administers licensure examinations (NCLEX); develops computerized licensure examinations; and works with other organizations to promote nursing standards and regulations and establish interstate licensure protocols.

National League for Nursing (NLN)—The national organization of nurse educators with long-standing commitment to four types of basic programs (LPN, diploma, ADN, and BSN): includes lay citizens concerned with nursing and health care on its board; has councils for nursing informatics, research in nursing education, wellness centers, and multiple types of print publications; initiated a certification program and examination to certify excellence of nursing educators; and established the Centers for Excellence for nursing programs that meet designated standards.

NLN Accreditation Commission (NLNAC)—Formed in 1997 as a subsidiary of the NLN with responsibility for establishing and implementing standards and criteria and for accrediting all types of schools of nursing.

National Organization of Nurse Practitioner Faculties (NONPF)—An organization of nurse practitioners in multiple specialties: sets national standards and criteria for programs and certification.

National Student Nurses Association (NSNA)—A national organization of statewide student nurse associations: concerned with education and career issues and provides student perspectives to other national nursing organizations.

SUMMARY

This chapter describes 10 major trends and related issues in nursing education programs and offers an overview of multiple types of nursing programs. The trends have a significant influence on the content, learning process, and evaluation methods used in all types of programs and have influenced the development of new degrees and majors. Additionally, they have had a remarkable effect on the persistence of various types of programs for entry into practice and on the increasing acceptance of diverse mobility and distance-learning programs. Regardless of the type of program, most students now use the Internet to access courses, electronic databases, and other e-learning resources and integrate evidence-based practice and critical thinking. As students integrate current trends and attempt to resolve issues, they create the trends for the next generation, and are participating in nursing history in the making. The most profound trend in nursing education is learning to learn, to reason, and to access relevant resources to solve problems. As American psychologist Carl Rogers said, "The only person who is educated is the one who has learned how to learn and change."

REFERENCES

Academic Center for Evidence Based Practice. (2016). *Star model research*. Retrieved from http://www.acestar.uthscsa.edu/.

Adelman, D. S., & Legg, T. J. (2009). *Disaster nursing: A handbook for practice*. Sudbury, MA: Jones and Bartlett.

Agency for Healthcare Research and Quality. *Evidenced based practice*. Retrieved from http://www.ahrq.gov/clinic/epcix.htm.

American Association of Colleges of Nursing. *Position statement: Baccalaureate degree in nursing as minimal preparation for professional practice*. Retrieved from http://www.aacn.nche.edu.

American Association of Colleges of Nursing. *Position statement on the practice doctorate in nursing*. Retrieved from http://www.aacn.nche.edu/DNP/DNPPosition Statement.htm.

American Association of Colleges of Nursing. *Issues bulletin: Accelerated baccalaureate and master's degrees in nursing*. Retrieved from http://www.aacn.nche.edu/media-relations/AccelProgsGlance.pdf.

American Association of Colleges of Nursing. (2017). *AACN Essentials*. Retrieved from http://www.aacnnursing.org/Education-Resources/AACN-Essentials.

American Association of Colleges of Nursing. (2017). *Key indicators and trends. Standard data reports*. Retrieved from http://www.aacnnursing.org/News-Information/Research-Data-Center/Standard-Data-Reports.

American Association of Colleges of Nursing. (2008a). *The essentials of baccalaureate education for professional nursing practice*. Retrieved from http://www.aacn.nche.edu/education-resources/BaccEssentials08.pdf.

American Association of Colleges of Nursing. (2008b). *Cultural competency in baccalaureate education*. Retrieved from http://www.aacn.nche.edu/education-resources/cultural-competency.

American Association of Colleges of Nursing. (2017a). *Nursing education programs*. Retrieved from http://www.aacnnursing.org/News-Information/Fact-Sheets.

American Association of Colleges of Nursing. (2008d). *Consensus model for APRN regulation: Licensure, accreditation, certification and education (LACE)*. Retrieved from http://www.aacn.nche.edu/education-resources/APRNReport.pdf.

American Association of Colleges of Nursing. (2009a). *The clinical nurse leader: Developing a new nurse*. Retrieved from http://www.aacn.nche.edu/cnl/index.htm.

American Association of Colleges of Nursing. *Clinical nurse leader certification*. Retrieved from http://www.aacn.nche.edu/cnl/cnl-certification/pdf/ExamHndbk.pdf.

American Association of Colleges of Nursing. (2017b). *Degree completion programs for registered nurses: RN to master's degree and RN to baccalaureate programs*. Retrieved from http://www.aacn.nche.edu/Media/FactSheets/Degree CompletionProg.htm.

American Association of Colleges of Nursing. (2009b). *End of life care*. Retrieved from http://www.aacn.nche.edu/elnec.

American Association of Colleges of Nursing. (2017c). *Nursing faculty shortage*. Retrieved from http://www.aacn.nche.edu/Media/FactSheets/FacultyShortage.htm.

American Association of Colleges of Nursing. (2011). *Core competencies for interprofessional collaborative practice*. Retrieved from http://www.aacn.nche.edu/education-resources/ipecreport.pdf.

American Association of Colleges of Nursing. (2017). *DNP Nursing fact sheet* (website). Retrieved from http://www.aacnnursing.org/News-Information/Fact-Sheets/Degree-Completion-Programs.

American Association of Colleges of Nursing. (2017). *Nursing fact sheet* (website). Retrieved from http://www.aacnnursing.org/News-Information/Fact-Sheets/DNP-Fact-Sheet

American Association of Colleges of Nursing. (2017). *2016-2017 Enrollment and graduations in baccalaureate and graduate programs in nursing.* Washington, DC: American Association of Colleges of Nursing.

American Association of Colleges of Nursing. (2012). *Knowledge, skills and attitudes.* Retrieved from http://www.aacn.nche.edu/faculty/qsen/competencies.pdf.

American Association of Colleges of Nursing. (2007). *Competencies.* Retrieved from http://qsen.org/competencies/.

American Nurses Association. (2006). *Bioterrorism and disaster response.* Retrieved from http://www.nursingworld.org/homepage/menu.

American Nurses Association. (2017a). *Code of ethics for nurses with interpretive statements.* Retrieved from http://www.nursingworld.org/about/01action.htm#code.

American Nurses Association. (2009b). *Nursing ethics: The center for ethics and human rights.* http://www.nursingworld.org/MainMenuCategories/EthicsStandards.aspx.

American Nurses Association. *On social media.* Retrieved from http://www.nursingworld.org/FunctionalMenuCategories/AboutANA/Social-Media.

American Nurses Association. (2017a). *Nurses rank #1 most trusted profession for the 15th year in a row.* Retrieved from http://www.nursingworld.org/HomepageCategory/NursingInsider/Archive-1/2016-NI/December-2016-NI/Nurses-Rank-1-Most-Trusted-Profession.html

American Nurses Association. (2017b). *Workplace violence.* Retrieved from http://www.nursingworld.org/workplaceviolence.

American Nurses Association New York, & New York Organization of Executives and Leaders. (2017). *Coaliton for advancement of nursing education.* Press Release: New York State Governor Cuomo signs legislation to strengthen educational requirements for future registered nurses. Retrieved from: https://www.foundationnysnurses.org/wp-content/uploads/2018/01/Nursing-Press-Release-final.pdf.

Anastasi, J. K., Capili, B., & Schenkman, F. (2009). Developing integrative therapies in primary care program. *Nurse Educator, 34*(6), 271–275.

Bauer, L., & Bodenheimer, T. (2017). Expanded roles of registered nurses in primary care delivery of the future. *Nursing Outlook, 65,* 624–632.

Brodersen, L. D., & Mills, A. C. (2014). A comparison of two nursing program exit exams that predict first-time NCLEX-RN outcome, computers, informatics. *Nursing, 32*(8), 404–412.

Buerhaus, P. I., & Auerbach, D. I. (2011). The recession's effect on hospital registered nurse employment growth. *Nursing Economic$, 29*(4), 163–167.

Buerhaus, P. I., Auerbach, D. I., & Staiger, D. O. (2009). The recent surge in nurse employment: causes and implications. *Health Affairs, 28*(4), 620–624.

Buerhaus, P. I., Skinner, L. E., Auerbach, D. I., et al. (2017a). Four challenges facing the nursing workforce in the United States. *J Nurs Regul, 8*(2), 40–46.

Buerhaus, P. I., Skinner, L., Auerbach, D., et al. (2017b). State of the registered nurse workforces as a new era of health reform emerges. *Nursing Economic$, 35*(5), 229–237.

Burton, C. W., McLemore, M. R., Perry, L., et al. (2017). Social media awareness and implications in nursing leadership: A pilot professional meeting campaign. *Policy, Politics, & Nursing Practice, 17*(4), 187–197.

Cant, R. P., & Cooper, S. J. (2010). Simulation-based learning in nurse education: Systematic review. *Journal of advanced nursing, 66*(1), 3–15.

Centers for Disease Control and Prevention. *About Ebola Virus Disease.* Updated February 18, 2016.

Centers for Disease Control and Prevention. (2015). *Suicide.* Retrieved from https://www.cdc.gov/violenceprevention/pdf/suicide-datasheet-a.pdf.

Cipriano, P. F., & Murphy, J. (2011). Nursing informatics. The future of nursing and health IT: The quality elixir. *Nursing Economic$, 29*(5), 286–282.

Cornell, P., Riordan, M., & Herrin-Griffith, D. (2010). Transforming nursing workflow, part 2 the impact of technology on nursing activities. *Journal of nursing administration, 40*(10), 432–439.

Critchley, K. A., Richardson, E., Aarts, C., et al. (2009). Student experiences with an international public health exchange project. *Nurse Educator, 34*(2), 69–74.

Cronenwett, L., Sherwood, G., Barnsteiner, J., et al. (2007). Quality and safety education for nurses. *Nursing Outlook, 55*(3), 122–131.

Darvish, A., Bahramnezhad, F., Keyhanian, S., et al. (2014). The role of nursing informatics on promoting quality of health care and the need for appropriate education. *Global Journal of Health Science, 6*(6), 11–18.

Delunas, L. R., & Rouse, S. (2014). Nursing and medical student attitudes about communication and collaboration before and after an interprofessional learning experience. *Nursing education perspectives, 35*(2), 100–105.

DiVito-Thomas, P. (2005). Nursing student stories on learning how to think like a nurse. *Nurse Educator, 30*(3), 133–136.

Dylan, B., Jackson, & Vaughn, M. (2017). Household food insecurity during childhood and adolescent misconduct. *Preventive Medicine, 96,* 113–111.

Farra, S. L., Smith, S. J., & Ulrich, D. (2017). The student experience with varying immersion levels of virtual reality simulation. *Nursing Education Perspectives.* doi:10.1097/01.NEP.0000000000000258.

Farrell, M. (2016). Use of iPhones by nurses in an acute care setting to improve communication and decision making processes: a qualitative analysis of nurses' perspectives on iPhone use. *JMIR mHealth and uHealth, 4*(2), e43.

Finkelman, A. W., & Kenner, C. (2009). *Teaching the IOM: Implications of the IOM reports for nursing education.* Silver Spring, MD: American Nurses Association.

Fleckman, J., Corso, M., Ramirez, S., et al. (2015). Intercultural competency in public health: A call for action to incorporate training into public health education. *Front Public Health, 3*, 210.

Flin, R., O'Connor, P., & Crichton, M. (2008). *Safety at the sharp end: A guide to non-technical skills.* Burlington, VT: Ashgate.

Gallup poll. Nurses ranked #1 most ethical profession. (2017). Retrieved from https://nurse.org/articles/ gallup-ethical-standards-poll-nurses-rank-highest/.

Gravina, E. (2017). Competency-based education and its effect on nursing education: A literature review. *Teaching & Learning in Nursing, 12*(2), 117–121.

Hay, B., Carr, P J., Dawe, L., & Clark-Burg, K. (2017). *I'm ready to learn: Undergraduate nursing students' knowledge, preferences, and practice of mobile technology and social media. Computers, Informatics, Nursing, 35*(1), 8–17.

Harris, J. L., Stanley, J., & Rosseter, R. (2011). The clinical nurse leader: Addressing health-care challenges through partnerships and innovation. *Journal of Nursing Regulation, 2*(2), 40–46.

Healthy People 2020. Retrieved from www.healthypeople. gov/2020/About-Healthy-People.

Matthew, S., Hockett, M., & Samek, L. (2018). Learning cultural humility through stories and global service-learning. *Journal of Christian Nursing, 35*(1), 33–37. doi:10.1097/ CNJ.0000000000000454.

Holroyd, A., Dahlke, S., Fehr, C., et al. (2009). Attitudes toward aging: Implications for a caring profession. *Journal of Nursing Education, 48*(7), 374–380.

Horan, K. M. (2009). Using the human patient simulator to foster critical thinking in critical situations. *Nursing Education Perspectives, 30*(1), 28–30.

Huston, C. (2013). The impact of emerging technology on nursing care: Warp speed ahead. *Online Journal of Issues in Nursing, 18*(2), 1–14.

Institute of Medicine. (2000). *To err is human: Building a safer health system.* Washington, DC: National Academies Press. Retrieved from http://www.iom.edu. See also Nursing response at www.aacn.nche.edu. and www. nursingworld.org.

Institute of Medicine. (2001). *Crossing the quality chasm a new health system for the 21st century.* Washington, DC: National Academies Press. Retrieved from http://www. iom.edu.

Institute of Medicine. (2003). *Health professions education: A bridge to quality.* Washington, DC: National Academies Press.

Institute of Medicine. (2009). *Redesigning continuing education in the health professions.* Washington, DC: National Academies Press.

Institute of Medicine. (2010). *The future of Nursing: Leading change, advancing health*, Washington, DC: National Academies Press.

Institute of Medicine. (2011). *The future of nursing: Leading change, advancing health*, Washington, DC: National Academies Press.

Institute of Medicine. (2012). The future of nursing: Accomplishments a year after the landmark report (Editorial). *Journal of Nursing Scholarship, 44*(1), 1.

International Council of Nurses (ICN). (2009). *Nurs Netw.* Retrieved from http://www.icn.ch/.

Kalisch, P. A., & Kalisch, B. J. (1995). *The advance of American nursing* (3rd ed.). Philadelphia: Lippincott.

Klocko, M. (2014). Academic dishonesty in schools of nursing: A literature review. *Journal of Nursing Education, 53*(3), 121–125.

Lai, C., & Wu, C. (2016). Promoting nursing students' clinical learning through a mobile e-Portfolio. *Computers, Informatics, Nursing, 34*(11), 535–543.

Lasater, K., & Nielsen, A. (2009). The influence of concept-based learning activities on students' clinical judgment development. *Journal of Nursing Education, 48*(8), 441–446.

Lenburg, C. B. (2008). The influence of contemporary trends and issues on nursing education. In B. Cherry & S. Jacob (Eds.), *Contemporary nursing: Issues, trends, and management* (4th ed.). St Louis: Mosby.

Lower, J. (2012). Civility starts with you. *American Nurse Today, 7*(5). Retrieved from https://www.americannurse today.com/civility-starts-with-you/

McGahee, T. W., Bravo, M., Simmons, L., & Reid, T. (2017). Nursing students and service learning: Research from a symbiotic community partnership with local schools and special Olympics. *Nurse Educator.* doi:10.1097/ NNE.0000000000000445.

Miller, J. F., & Holm, K. (2011). Graduate nursing programs for non-nurses: A national perspective. *Journal of Nursing Regulation, 2*(2), 4–9.

National Council of State Boards of Nursing. *NCLEX educational program codes.* Retrieved from https://www.ncsbn. org/NCLEX_Educational_Program_Codes.pdf.

National Council of State Boards of Nursing. (2011). *Social media guidelines for nurses.* Retrieved from https://www. ncsbn.org/347.htm.

National Council of State Boards of Nursing. (2017). *NCLEX examination pass rates.* 2017. Retrieved from https://www. ncsbn.org/Table_of_Pass_Rates_2017.pdf.

National Council of State Boards of Nursing. (2017a). National Nursing Workforce Study. Retrieved from: https:// www.ncsbn.org/workforce.htm

National Council of State Boards of Nursing. (2018). APRN Compact. Retrieved from https://www.ncsbn.org/ aprn-compact.htm

National League for Nursing. (2018). *Nurse educator core competency*. Retrieved from http://www.nln.org/professional-development-programs/competencies-for-nursing-education/nurse-educator-core-competency.

National League for Nursing. (2014a). *A vision recognition of the role of licensed practical/vocational nurses in advancing the nation's health*. Retrieved from http://www.nln.org/docs/default-source/about/nln-vision-series-%28position-statements%29/nlnvision_7.pdf?sfvrsn=4l.

National League for Nursing. (2014b). *Number of basic RN programs by program type: 2005–2014*. Retrieved from http://www.nln.org/docs/default-source/newsroom/nursing-education-statistics/number-of-basic-rn-programs-total-and-by-program-type-2005-to-2014.pdf?

National League for Nursing. (2009b). *Nursing shortage info*. Retrieved from http://www.nln.org/newsroom/nursing-education-statistics/nursing-shortage.

National League for Nursing. (2017). *Outcomes and competencies for graduates of practical/vocational, diploma, associate degree, baccalaureate, master's, practice doctorate, research doctorate programs in nursing*. Retrieved from http://www.nln.org/docs/default-source/professional-development-programs/program-outcomes-and-competencies2.pdf?sfvrsn=2.

National Institute on Drug Abuse. (2018). *College-Age & Young Adults*. Retrieved from https://www.drugabuse.gov/related-topics/college-age-young-adults.

National Organization of Nurse Practitioner Faculty. (2017). *Nurse practitioner core competencies with suggested curriculum content*. 2017_NPCoreComps_with_Curric.pdf. Retrieved from http://ncda.org.jm/.

Obesity on the rise: What can nurses do? (2009). Online Journal of Issues in Nursing. *Retrieved from* http://www.nursingworld.org/MainMenuCategories/ANAMarketplace/ANAPeriodicals/OJIN/JournalTopics/Obesity-on-the-Rise.aspx.

Påisson, Y., Mårtensson, G., Swenne, C. L., Ädel, E., & Engström M. (2017). A peer learning intervention for nursing students in clinical practice education: A quasi-experimental study. *Nurse Education Today, 51*, 81–87. doi:10.1016/j.nedt.2017.01.011.

Phillips, B., Shaw, R. J., Sullivan, D. T., & Johnson, C. (2010). Using virtual environments to enhance nursing distance education. *Creative Nursing, 16*(3), 132–135.

Quality and Safety Education for Nurses. (2012). *Informatics Competency*. Retrieved from http://qsen.org/competencies/.

Ramal, E. (2009). Integrating caring, scholarship and community engagement in Mexico. *Nurse Educator, 34*(1), 34–37.

Roland, E. J., Johnson, C., & Swain, D. (2011). "Blogging" as an educational enhancement tool for improved student performance: A pilot study in undergraduate nursing education. *New Review of Information Networking, 16*(2), 151–166.

Ross, G. J., & Myers, S. M. (2017). The current use of social media in undergraduate nursing education a review of the literature. *Computers, Informatics, Nursing, 35*(7), 338–343.

Rosseter, R. (2009). A new role for nurses: Making room for clinical leaders. *Joint Commission Perspectives, 9*(8), 5–7.

Sanderson, C. (2018). Ethical and bioethical issues in nursing and health care. In B. Cherry & S. Jacob (Eds.), *Contemporary nursing: Issues, leadership, and management* (7th ed.). St. Louis: Elsevier.

Schlariet, M. (2009). Bioethics mediation: The role and importance of nurse advocacy. *Nursing Outlook, 57*, 185–193.

Sensmeier, J. (2011). Information technology: Transforming nursing practice through technology and informatics. *Nursing Management, 42*(11), 20–23.

Southern Poverty Law Center. (2009). *Information on teaching tolerance and monitoring hate groups*. Retrieved from http://www.tolerance.org/.

Stop violence against women: A project by the advocates for human rights. (2010). Retrieved from http://www.stopvaw.org.

Substance Abuse and Mental Health Services Administration, Lipari, R., & Jean-Francosis, B. (2016). Center for Behavioral Health Statistics and Quality. Retrieved from https://www.samhsa.gov/data/sites/default/files/report_2361/ShortReport-2361.html.

Substance Abuse and Mental Health Services Administration. (2016). *Opioids*. Retrieved from https://www.samhsa.gov/atod/opioids.

The Joint Commission. (2016, February 24). *Sentinel Event Alert. Detecting suicide in all settings*. Issue 56. Retrieved from https://www.jointcommission.org/assets/1/18/SEA_56_Suicide.pdf.

Unver, V., Basak, T., Ayhan, H., et al. (2017, December 22). Integrating simulation based learning into nursing education programs: Hybrid simulation. *Technology and Health Care*. doi:10.3233/THC-170853.

U.S. Department of Health and Human Services. (2014). *Healthy People 2020, Diabetes: overview*. Retrieved from http://www.healthypeople.gov/2020/topicsobjectives2020/overview.aspx?topicid=8.

Veltri, L., & Barber, H. (2016). Forces and issues influencing curriculum development. In D. Billings, & J. Halstead (Eds.), *Teaching in nursing: A guide for faculty*. St. Louis: Elsevier.

Whitlow, M. L., Drake, E., Tullman, D., Hoke, G., & Barth, D. (2014). Bridging technology to the bedside using smartphones to improve interprofessional communication. *Computers, Informatics, Nursing, 32*(7), 305–311.

Whitty, K. K., & Burnett, M. F. (2009). Importance of instruction on mass casualty incidents in baccalaureate nursing programs: perceptions of nursing faculty. *Journal of Nursing Education, 48*(5), 291–295.

World Health Organization. (2016). *Nurse educator core competencies.* Retrieved from http://who.int/hrh/nursing_midwifery/nurse_educator050416.pdf.

World Health Organization. (2017). *Antimicrobial fact sheet.* Retrieved from http://www.who.int/mediacentre/fact sheets/fs194/en/

ZeroSuicide in Health and Behavioral Health. (2015–2017). Retrieved from http://zerosuicide.sprc.org/

Zurmehly, J. (2010). Personal digital assistants (PDAs): Review and evaluation. *Nursing Education Perspectives, 31*(3), 179–182.

4

Nursing Licensure and Certification

Susan R. Jacob, PhD, MSN, RN

Legal regulations and professional certification ensure safe, competent nursing care.

Ⓔ Additional resources are available online at: *http://evolve.elsevier.com/Cherry/*

LEARNING OUTCOMES

After studying this chapter, the reader will be able to:

1. Explain the development of licensure requirements in the United States.
2. Summarize current licensure requirements in the context of historical developments.
3. Analyze the various components of a nurse practice act.
4. Discuss the mutual recognition model and identify Nurse Licensure Compact states.
5. Describe the development of certification requirements for advanced practice.
6. Identify requirements for certification for advanced practice in different specialties.
7. Use appropriate resources to obtain current information on licensure and certification.

KEY TERMS

Accreditation Voluntary process by which schools of nursing are approved to conduct nursing education programs.

Advanced practice nurse (APN) Legal title for nurses prepared by education and competence to perform independent practice.

American Nurses Association (ANA) Professional organization that represents all registered nurses.

American Nurses Credentialing Center (ANCC) An independent agency of the American Nurses Association that conducts certification examinations and certifies advanced practice nurses.

Certification Process by which nurses are recognized for advanced education and competence.

Compact state A term of law. In the context of the Nurse Licensure Compact, a state that has established an agreement with other states allowing nurses to practice within the state without an additional license. The interstate compacts are enacted by the state legislatures.

Continued competency program A variety of initiatives to ensure nurses' knowledge, skills, and expertise beyond initial licensure.

Grandfathered In nursing, the statutory process by which previously licensed persons are included without further action in revisions or additions in nurse practice acts.

International Council of Nurses (ICN) Professional organization that represents nurses in countries around the world.

We thank Janet C. Scherubel, PhD, RN, for her contribution to this chapter in the fourth edition.

Licensure by endorsement The original program whereby nurses licensed in one state seek licensure in another state without repeat examinations. The requirements are included in state nurse practice acts or accompanying rules and regulations.

Mandatory continuing education Educational requirements imposed by individual states for renewal of a license.

Mutual recognition model Program developed by the National Council of State Boards of Nursing (2012). The Nurse Licensure Compact program establishes interstate compacts so that nurses licensed in one jurisdiction may practice in other compact states without obtaining duplicate licensure.

National Council of State Boards of Nursing (NCSBN) Organization whose membership consists of the board of nursing of each state or territory.

Nurse practice act Statute in each state and territory that regulates the practice of nursing.

State board of nursing Appointed board within each state charged with responsibility to administer the nurse practice act of that state.

Sunset legislation Statutes that provide for revocation of laws if not reviewed and renewed within a specified time.

PROFESSIONAL/ETHICAL ISSUE

Russell and Rudy were working PRN in a very busy comprehensive home health agency. The agency had recently experienced high RN turnover and numerous changes in administrative personnel. Mary, the efficient staff person with whom they had worked from the beginning of their employment, resigned 6 months ago, and temporary staff have been sporadically doing her job. Russell and Rudy discussed how they both missed Mary because she always reminded them of important things such as insurance enrollment periods, CPR certification expiration dates, and the date their nursing licenses were about to expire. Rudy stated, "I'm afraid critical things have been slipping through the cracks lately and going unnoticed since Mary resigned." Russell, who had told Rudy he was way over the limit on all of his credit cards and overdue on many of his bills, responded, "I know my RN license is about to expire, but I have no money to spend on that in the near future, so I am really hoping no one checks up on this detail. Then I might get away with not having a current license for a few months until I can get my financial issues worked out."

How should Rudy respond to Russell?

What are the implications for practicing as an RN without a current nursing license?

VIGNETTE

Three nurses are discussing their nursing practice licenses. Joe Branch, a senior nursing student, is preparing for initial licensure. Mary Stone's license is due for renewal.

Carmella Larkin has just moved into the state. As the three are talking about these changes in their practice, Giorgio Gonzales, a nurse practitioner, joins the group. Giorgio recently completed a certification examination and is interested in becoming certified for advanced practice. All the nurses have a general knowledge of the requirements for licensure and certification but lack the specific information needed to legally practice within the state.

Mary suggests contacting the state board of nursing. The nurses agree that this is a sensible idea, and Mary leaves to phone the board of nursing. On returning, Mary informs the group that the answers to all of their questions can be found in the state's nurse practice act and accompanying rules and regulations, which can be accessed online. She tells them that the state board of nursing office will also send free copies of both documents to individuals who request them.

The situation described here is not uncommon. Nurses need specific, current information on licensure and renewal of licensure. The most comprehensive sources for this information are the state nurse practice act and the state board of nursing. These resources provide accurate descriptions of the law governing nursing practice within each state and the U.S. territories.

Every nurse and nursing student will benefit from obtaining a copy of his or her state's nurse practice act and becoming familiar with its contents.

Questions to Consider While Reading This Chapter:

1. Who establishes the "rules" for nursing practice—the state or the employer?

2. Do graduates from different types of nursing education programs require different types of licenses?
3. If a nurse graduate passes the NCLEX-RN examination, does this person still need a license?
4. What happens if a nurse's license expires? Can the nurse still practice?
5. Must a nurse complete graduate school and take an examination to be an advanced practice nurse?
6. Are the regulations governing advanced practice the same in all states?

CHAPTER OVERVIEW

To practice nursing as a registered nurse (RN). That is the goal of every student nurse. A goal achieved through study, clinical practice, and successful completion of the National Council Licensure Examination–Registered Nurse (NCLEX-RN). This chapter discusses how and why nursing licensure developed, steps necessary to becoming licensed, licensure regulations, and the responsibilities of an RN.

After licensure as RNs, nurses must still maintain and increase their knowledge and skills. Many nurses may wish to specialize in a particular area of nursing and expand their practice. Nurses with these goals may seek certification in a specialty field. This chapter describes certification, the means to achieve certification, and the organizations that administer certifying examinations. Whether it is licensure or certification, the nursing profession is constantly progressing. Legal requirements to practice are continually being revised to ensure the protection of the public. Throughout history and in the current health care environment, nurses face complex issues and new challenges as they seek to increase their competence and ensure the delivery of excellent nursing services to patients. This chapter explores issues related to licensure and certification as well as some of the challenges nurses and students will face.

THE HISTORY OF NURSING LICENSURE

Recognition: Pins and Registries

The aim of caregivers throughout history has been to be recognized and acknowledged for one's skills and achievements. Early caregivers, particularly in the monasteries and convents of the medieval period, were identified by the habits they wore. Frequently, special insignias designated health personnel. During the Crusades, a large Maltese cross adorned the habits of the Knights Hospitalers of St. John of Jerusalem on the battlefield (Kalisch and Kalisch, 2003). These forms of identification allowed others to recognize their particular skills in caregiving and healing. More recently, nurses around the world wore a readily identifiable symbol of their school of nursing—the nursing cap.

Today, as in the past, the school of nursing pin identifies graduates from a particular school of nursing. Early in each school's history, the students and faculty crafted the pin. The pin's emblems and text symbolize the philosophy, beliefs, and aspirations of the nursing program. Students receive their own pins at graduation in a special pinning ceremony. Nurses wear their pins proudly as evidence of their achievement, learning, and skill. It is one way in which nurses distinguish themselves as distinct health care providers with a specialized body of knowledge and clinical skills.

Although White Coat Ceremonies have been an important rite of passage at medical schools for more than 20 years, it is now common to offer similar events at schools of nursing. In 2014, nursing schools in 43 states plus the District of Columbia were given financial support and guidance by The Arnold P. Gold Foundation and the American Association of Colleges of Nursing to offer a White Coat Ceremony. This ceremony usually consists of the recitation of an oath, cloaking of students in a white coat, an address by an eminent role model, and a reception for students and invited guests. Students typically also receive their nursing pins at the White Coat Ceremony.

Nursing programs also maintain a record of all graduates. Florence Nightingale started this practice in 1860, when she created a list of graduates of the St. Thomas's School of Nursing in England. This list became known as the "registry" of graduate nurses. The registry of nurses initiated by Nightingale provided institutions, as well as patients, with a system of identifying graduates of particular nursing programs. These lists proclaimed to all the skills and knowledge of graduates. These nurses could then be distinguished from lay practitioners and local citizens who provided care to the ill and infirm. Today nursing programs around the world continue the tradition started by Nightingale and maintain registries or listings of all of their graduates. In addition, state and international agencies maintain lists of nurses practicing in their jurisdictions.

Purpose of Licensure

As nursing programs proliferated, variations developed among the programs. Entry criteria differed, and many educational programs were structured to meet specific employer needs. A simple registry of nurse graduates was no longer sufficient to ensure minimal levels of competency in all nurses, regardless of the school in which the nurses were educated. Another system was necessary to distinguish those sufficiently trained to provide nursing care from untrained or lesser-trained individuals. Graduate nurses, physicians, and hospitals met to resolve this confusion. The outcome was criteria for the licensure of nurses in the United States. Then, as now, the primary purpose of licensure was protection of the public.

Early Licensure Activities

U.S. nursing programs developed in much the same manner as was the pattern in England. As early as 1867, Dr. Henry Wentworth Acland encouraged licensure of English nurses. However, it was not until 1896 that attempts were made to license nurses in the United States. Prior to the late 1800s, many hospitals established training programs to prepare nursing staff for their own institutions. The programs varied with the needs of the hospital, the availability of physicians and nurses for training students, and the resources devoted to the training. It became apparent to many nurses that consistent minimum standards to practice across settings were necessary. These standards would provide for safety of the public and improve the mobility of nurses among institutions. A key advocate for these standards was the Nurses Associated Alumnae of the United States and Canada. This organization later became the **American Nurses Association (ANA)**. However, the group met with resistance from hospitals, physicians, and even nurses. The early attempts at nursing licensure failed for lack of broad-based support (Joel, 2006).

Nurses worldwide mounted an extensive educational campaign explaining the purposes and safeguards inherent in licensure. Success was achieved, and in 1901 the International Council of Nurses (ICN) passed a resolution that each nation and state examine and license its nurses. Several U.S. states responded shortly thereafter. In 1903, North Carolina, New Jersey, New York, and Virginia were the first to institute permissive licensure. The licensure rules were voluntary. These permissive licenses permitted but did not require nurses to become registered.

Under permissive licensure, educational standards were set at a minimum of 2 years of training for nurses. State boards of nursing were established with rules for examinations as well as revocation of the license. Nurses not passing the examination could not use the title of RN. These early regulations served two purposes: first, to protect the public from unskilled practitioners; and, second, to provide legal sanctions to protect the title of RN. The New York State Board of Regents began a registry of nurses successfully completing all requirements. In 20 years, by 1923, all states had instituted examinations for permissive licensure. Each state's licensure examinations varied in content, length, and format and had written, oral, and practice components. The early work in examinations for licensure was the forerunner of today's licensure and certification requirements (Kalisch and Kalisch, 2003).

The early state efforts in licensing nurses were commendable. Nonetheless, there was considerable variability among states in the requirements for nursing education, the licensure examinations, and the **nurse practice acts** themselves. The widespread variability in nurse practice acts prompted the ANA (and later **the National Council of State Boards of Nursing [NCSBN]**) to design model nurse practice acts. The model acts provided a template for states to follow. The first was published in 1915. These model practice acts are revised and updated as nursing practice advances. For example, the NCSBN approved the most recent revision of the model practice act and administrative rules in 2011 (NCSBN, 2014). The NCSBN Model Act and Rules are exemplary legislation that can be adopted by a **state board of nursing (BON)**. The current Model Act & Rules were developed by an NCSBN committee, approved by the Delegate Assembly in 2012, and updated in 2014.

The model nurse practice act is composed of many sections, including a definition of nursing and the scope of practice for the RN, descriptions of advanced practice nursing, requirements for prescriptive authority of nurses, nursing education, compact guidelines, and processes for disciplinary actions against nurses who violate sections of the act. Separate sections of the model act provide guidelines for state boards of nursing and the necessary requirements for entry into practice. The latest model practice act is available online at the NCSBN website (https://www.ncsbn.org/3867.htm).

From these model acts, each state or jurisdiction developed a unique practice act. Although individual states, and territories' practice acts address the needs of the developing jurisdiction, every practice act includes the sections described in the model act. Students and practicing nurses may obtain the nurse practice act for any jurisdiction by contacting that state or territorial board of nursing.

Mandatory Licensure

Once each state had established permissive licensure, the next movement was toward a requirement that all nurses must be licensed. This practice is termed *mandatory licensure.* New York was the first state to require mandatory licensure, although this requirement was not in place until 1947. At the same time, nursing groups moved to standardize nursing licensure testing procedures.

After World War II, the ANA formed the NCSBN. The council was composed of a representative of each state and jurisdiction in the United States. As part of its original activities, the council advocated a standardized examination for licensure. These varied activities culminated in the National League for Nursing, which administered the first State Board Test Pool Examination in 1950. The written examination had separate sections on medical-surgical nursing, maternity nursing, nursing of children, and psychiatric nursing. This format for the examination continued for more than 30 years, and many of today's nurses took them.

The next major event in licensure efforts occurred in 1982 with the development of the first NCLEX-RN examination. The test was revised to include all nursing content within one section of the examination. In addition, the format was changed to present questions in a nursing process format. Just as with previous versions of licensing examinations, the NCLEX-RN examination has evolved over time. Paper-and-pencil testing was replaced with computerized adaptive testing in 1994. Extensive information on the NCLEX-RN examination may be found in Chapter 28 of this text.

COMPONENTS OF NURSE PRACTICE ACTS

Each state develops rules and regulations to govern the practice of nursing within that state. These rules are in the nurse practice acts or in its accompanying rules and regulations to administer the act. Many nurse practice acts are patterned after the ANA or NCSBN model practice act, and all contain comparable information.

Purpose of Act

Each act begins with a purpose. All nurse practice acts include two essential purposes. First, each act has statements that refer to protecting the health and safety of the citizens in the jurisdiction. The act describes the qualifications and responsibilities of those individuals covered by the regulations. Likewise, the act delineates those excluded from the practice of nursing. These provisions also serve to ensure protection of the public. The second purpose is to protect the title of RN. The legal title RN is reserved for those meeting the requirements to practice nursing. Only those licensed may use the designation RN. Thus, unlicensed personnel are prevented from using the title RN.

Definition of Nursing and Scope of Practice

In each state or jurisdictional nurse practice act, the practice of professional nursing is defined. The definition of nursing is of utmost importance because it delineates the scope of practice for nurses within the jurisdiction. That is, each act outlines the activities nurses may legally perform within the jurisdiction. Many states follow the guidelines incorporated in the model practice act, although each is specific and delineates practice within that state or jurisdiction. For example, some states describe nursing as a process that includes nursing diagnosis, whereas other states list broad areas of nursing activities. To avoid becoming outdated, the acts contain no lists of skills or procedures. As nursing knowledge and practices advance, new techniques are frequently allowable because of the comprehensive nature of the definition of nursing.

Many jurisdictions incorporate definitions of advanced practice nursing within one definition of nursing. In other states, the definitions of advanced practice nursing and the scope of practice for the **advance practice nurse** are separate.

Each state or jurisdiction establishes laws regulating practice within its borders. Therefore, it is imperative for the nurse to know and understand the definition of nursing in the states in which he or she practices. Further, each jurisdiction retains the right to govern practice within that jurisdiction. This right supersedes the presence of a mutual recognition agreement with other compact states. The retention of states' rights is an essential component in the mutual recognition model.

There are other important reasons for becoming familiar with the definition of nursing practice. Frequently, nurses are asked to perform in ways that are beyond the legal definition of nursing. This is illegal, and if the nurse complies, he or she could lose the privilege of practicing nursing. In other situations, labor laws or other statutes affect nurses. Definitions may include or exclude nurses on the basis of their legal definitions of nursing practice. As nursing practice becomes more complex and sophisticated, states may revise their nurse practice acts. Nurses are accountable for knowing the definition and scope of practice within their jurisdictions and practicing accordingly. In order to know and understand the laws regulating their practice, nurses should obtain copies of and become familiar with nurse practice acts for the states or jurisdictions in which they plan to practice.

Licensure Requirements

Entry into Practice Licensure. A section of each nurse practice act describes the requirements and procedures necessary for initial entry into nursing practice or nursing licensure. An initial requirement in all jurisdictions is graduation from both high school and an accredited nursing program. Candidates for licensure must submit evidence of graduation as defined by each state.

To verify an applicant's graduation from a nursing program, a transcript of coursework, a diploma, or a letter from the dean of the program is frequently necessary. Additional requirements for licensure may include a statement regarding the mental and physical health status of the applicant. Some jurisdictions conduct a review of prior legal convictions; this is especially important in reference to felony convictions. Some states also require declaration of misdemeanors, even those that have been expunged. Other states have appended provisions related to recreational drug abuse, and some states require declaration of termination and disciplinary action from a nursing or health care employer. Finally, most states require statements from the school of nursing attesting to the eligibility of the candidate for licensure. The requirements for licensure are detailed in each nurse practice act and the accompanying rules and regulations for practice.

In the past, it was customary for nurses to practice in only one state or territory. More than ever, nurses are practicing in more than one jurisdiction, either by their physical presence in that jurisdiction or through technological advances such as telephone and computer access to patients across state and territory lines. As laws are continually being revised to reflect the current practice of nursing, it is incumbent on the individual to be cognizant of the current licensure requirements in all states and territories in which he or she intends to practice.

Regardless of individual state requirements, all nurse practice acts require candidates to successfully complete the NCLEX-RN licensure examination before they can practice. In some states, it is possible to obtain a temporary permit to practice, pending receipt of success on the licensure examination. This arrangement was especially prevalent in past years because it took several months for results of the licensure examinations to be reported. Now, however, with computer testing and the prompt response from the testing services, the use of temporary permits to practice is becoming less frequent.

Temporary permits are still available for nurses moving from one jurisdiction to another. To obtain a license to practice in another state, the nurse applies for licensure by endorsement. Nurses licensed in one jurisdiction may apply for licensure in a second jurisdiction by submitting a letter to the second state board of nursing. Typically, evidence for the new license is similar to that for initial licensure. In addition, proof of the nurse's current license to practice, as well as any restrictions imposed on the license by the first state, is required. These procedures will continue for all states not participating in the Nurse Licensure Compact (NLC). For any state designated as a compact state, the nurse should contact the state board of nursing to determine the appropriate procedures for initiating nursing practice in that jurisdiction.

Advanced Practice Nursing Licensure. Advanced practice nurses must obtain separate nursing licensure in addition to licensure for entry into practice. State requirements vary; therefore, advanced practice nurses should contact the state board of nursing to determine the criteria and procedures.

Renewal of Licensure

In addition to outlining requirements for initial licensure, each nurse practice act includes the requirements and information necessary to renew one's nursing license. These regulations define the length of time a license is valid, generally from 2 to 3 years, as well as any specific requirements for renewal of licensure.

Mandatory Continuing Education

The nurse will find information on mandatory continuing education requirements for renewal of licensure in the section on license renewal. All nurses are expected to maintain continued competency to practice through various means of continuing education. In 1976, California was the first state to institute mandatory continuing education for renewal of licensure. Since that time, a number of states have instituted requirements of continuing education for renewal of licensure. The number of hours necessary varies depending on the jurisdiction, ranging from 20 to 40 hours over a 2- to 3-year period.

A few jurisdictions require specific continuing education coursework in the areas of health care ethics, the state nurse practice act, or other content specific to that jurisdiction. Clinical course content may be designated for specific health problems, such as sexually transmitted diseases, human immunodeficiency virus/acquired immunodeficiency syndrome, and family violence. In other states, the board of nursing allows the nurse wide latitude in meeting the requirements for renewal of licensure. Details of specific continuing education requirements are found in the nurse practice act and the accompanying rules and regulations.

ROLE OF REGULATORY BOARDS TO ENSURE SAFE PRACTICE

Membership of the Board of Nursing

An important section of every nurse practice act is the designation of a regulatory board of nurses and consumers to administer the act. Frequently, this responsibility is assigned to a state board of nursing. The practice act outlines guidelines for membership on the board. In addition, procedures by which members are appointed to the board of nursing are designated. In most cases, the members are appointed by the governor's office. Interested individuals or organizations, such as the state nurses' association, may submit names to the governor for consideration.

Duties of the Board of Nursing

The responsibilities and duties of the board of nursing are delineated in detail. Specific duties of the board may be outlined in the act itself or in the enabling laws. These enabling administrative statutes are frequently designated as rules and regulations for the practice of nursing. It is through the work of the board of nursing that nursing licenses are granted and renewed and disciplinary action is taken when provisions of the act are violated. Just as all nurses need to be cognizant of their nurse practice acts, nurses should also become familiar with the role of the state board of nursing.

A major responsibility of the board of nursing is addressing concerns about a nurse's practice. The review of a nurse's potential malfeasance or violation of the act or other state or federal laws is within the responsibilities of the board of nursing. The nurse practice act describes the due process and procedures for this review. The board of nursing then assigns appropriate disciplinary action. These activities are a key responsibility of the board of nursing. Actions may include restrictions on a nurse's license or its suspension or revocation. Just as all nurses need to be cognizant of their nurse practice acts, nurses should become familiar with the role of the state board of nursing.

SPECIAL CASES OF LICENSURE

Military and Government Nurses

There are many nurses whose practice takes them throughout the country on a regular basis. For example, many nurses are members of the military or join the military nursing services after graduation. The Veterans Administration and U.S. Public Health Service employ thousands of nurses who serve in many jurisdictions as well as outside U.S. boundaries. It is not necessary for these nursing personnel to obtain a nursing license in each jurisdiction in which they practice. The graduate takes the NCLEX-RN examination in one state. Upon successful completion, as an employee of the U.S. government, he or she may practice in other jurisdictions without additional licensure requirements. Nurses should obtain the current requirements for licensure because rules are updated to reflect current practices.

Internationally Educated Nurses

Internationally educated nurses (IENs) have become an integral part of the U.S. registered nurse workforce. Top countries represented by IENs passing the NCLEX-RN examination in 2010 include Philippines, South Korea, India, Canada, and Nigeria (Health Resources and Services Administration [HRSA], 2013).

Internationally educated nurses are another source of pipeline for the U.S. nursing workforce, especially in times of shortage in domestic supply. Health workforce migration, a critical issue for many years, has received increased attention as a result of the 2010 World Health Organization's Global Code of Practice on the International Recruitment of Health Personnel (Global Code). The Global Code represents an effort to promote ethical principles in the recruitment of international health personnel, with a particular focus on minimizing recruitment from countries experiencing critical shortages (HRSA, 2013).

Internationally educated nurses have met the requirements for practice in their own countries. When nurses move to the United States, they must show evidence of completing their original educational program and restrictions of their licenses. In addition, nurses need to demonstrate competency in English and the ability to take and pass the NCLEX-RN examination. Foreign nurses take a special examination administered by the Commission on Graduates of Foreign Nursing Schools. The examination is given in English and tests the knowledge required to practice in the United States. Upon successful completion, the foreign nurse graduate may apply for a license to practice in the United States. The intent of these regulations is not to be punitive or obstructive to the nurse. The regulations are yet another example of two key principles: first, the protection of the public and, second, the protection of the title of RN.

International Practice

In a similar manner, nurses licensed in the United States may want to practice in other countries. Nurses interested in these opportunities may contact either the International Council of Nurses (ICN) or the nursing regulatory board of the country in which they wish to practice. The ICN is composed of representatives of organized nursing worldwide. One of its functions is to assist nurses in obtaining licensure in other countries.

Each country has specific laws and regulations governing nursing practice that must guide the practice of the U.S. nurse. Just as a foreign nurse must demonstrate competency to practice in the United States, the U.S. nurse should be prepared to submit documentation on education, NCLEX-RN examination results, and proof of licensure and practice to officials in the foreign country. Advanced planning and contact with the appropriate regulatory agency will ease the transition for the nurse.

REVISION OF NURSE PRACTICE ACTS

Nurse practice acts, just as other sections of states' codes, are written and passed by legislators. As in any legislative endeavor, many governmental agencies, administrators, consumers, and special-interest groups seek to influence the legislation. These groups become actively involved in developing the accompanying rules and regulations. For example, physicians, dentists, pharmacists, licensed practical nurses, certified nursing assistants, emergency personnel, and physician assistants are just a few of the health care providers directly affected by the scope and definition of nursing practice. Likewise, organizations such as schools, hospitals, home health agencies, and extended care facilities are vitally concerned with the role of nurses today. Equally important, citizen groups are interested in determining nurses' roles and responsibilities. For this reason, the nurse practice act, as finally passed or amended by the state legislature, represents the aims and concerns not only of nurses but of many individuals and multiple-interest groups.

Review of a state's practice act reveals the influential parties involved in creating the act. Each group participates in defining the scope and practice of nursing and regulations affecting nursing practice within the jurisdiction. Because of these varied interests, it is essential for nurses to understand the practice act and the additional legislation that influences and controls their practice. Further, as proposals to amend the nurse practice act are promulgated at the state level, it is imperative for all nurses to be involved in the process. The resulting laws affect their profession, their practice, and their livelihood.

Sunset Legislation

One example of legislative activity affecting nurse practice acts is sunset legislation. Sunset laws, found in many states, are intended to ensure that legislation is current and reflects the needs of the public. When sunset provisions are included in a nurse practice act, the act must be reviewed by a specific date. If the act is not renewed, it is automatically rescinded. This review process allows for revisions to update practice acts to be consistent with current nursing practice. Many nurse practice acts contain sunset provisions. It is through these activities that the scope of nursing practice is updated and components, such as the diagnosis of nursing problems, have been incorporated into definitions of nursing. Other changes include changes in requirements for mandatory continuing education for licensure renewal. Equally important, sunset laws have provided the means to define advanced practice nursing and incorporate prescriptive authority for advanced practice nurses. Nurses should determine whether sunset regulations affect the nurse practice act in the state in which they practice. Likewise, nurses should be aware of, and involved in, activities to amend the nurse practice act.

DELEGATION OF AUTHORITY TO OTHERS

The rapid expansion of an array of health care providers, changes in health care delivery systems, and efforts to control health care costs have led to participation of many types of unlicensed personnel in the provision of health care. These personnel present a challenge to RNs working with them. Questions arise as to who can delegate what activities to which unlicensed provider groups. Guidelines for delegation have been developed by many nursing organizations, including the ANA and NCSBN (NCSBN, 2016). Although the professional organizations' guidelines are helpful, it is the nurse practice acts of individual states that establish the legal definitions of appropriate delegation practices. Because regulations differ among states, each nurse must identify and understand the regulations for the state in which he or she practices. Chapter 19 presents a detailed discussion of delegation and supervision.

CURRENT LICENSURE ACTIVITIES

Mutual Recognition Model

Efforts to provide common definitions of nursing practice, equivalent educational standards for practice, and uniform testing for entry into practice through the NCLEX-RN examination have been very successful. Nonetheless, most nurses are still required to apply for licensure in each state in which they practice. With the increased mobility of nurses, the telehealth movement, and the necessity of caring for patients across long distances, state boards of nursing have recognized the need to provide practicing nurses with more than procedures of endorsement of their initial licenses. This need has led to further changes in nursing licensure.

In 1997, the Delegate Assembly of the NCSBN moved to a new level of nursing regulation. The assembly endorsed a mutual recognition model of nursing regulation. Through this model, state boards of Nursing formed the Nurse Licensure Compact (NLC).

The original NLC allows nurses with a multistate license to practice physically, telephonically, or electronically in their home state and other original NLC states. In 2015, the NLC underwent revisions that led to new legislation known as the enhanced NLC (eNLC). At this time most NLC states and many non-compact states are moving forward with the process of joining the enhanced NLC. "Under the eNLC nurses are able to provide care to patients in other eNLC states, without having to obtain additional licenses. Nurses with an original NLC multistate license will be grandfathered into the eNLC" (NCSBN, 2018). Visit the NCSBN website for additional information.

The APRN Compact allows an advanced practice registered nurse to hold one multistate license with a privilege to practice in other compact states. The APRN Compact will be implemented when 10 states have enacted the legislation. NCSBN has developed a model for states to enact the Advanced Practice Nurse Compact (NCSBN, APRN, 2015). Visit the NCSBN website for key provisions of the new APRN contract (https://ncsbn.org/aprn-compact.htm).

"The newly enhanced compact or eNLC was approved by the BONs on May 4, 2015, as a licensure model of the future. It replaces the original NLC and adds extra protections. The original NLC states are currently enacting state legislation enabling them to transition into the eNLC. New states, not previously members of the original NLC, are also enacting state legislation to become members of the eNLC" (NCSBN, 2018).

A number of issues associated with mutual recognition concern nurses. On one hand, mutual recognition greatly facilitates interstate practice, telehealth programs, and movement of nurses to areas of shortage. In addition, a national nursing database provides information on individual nurses' practice and disciplinary actions taken against nurses. Nursys is "the first-ever comprehensive source of nursing licensure statistics for the U.S. and its territories" (NCSBN, Nursys, 2015). Compiled by NCSBN's database, Nursys "is an electronic information system where boards of nursing enter licensure data on a frequent basis. Of NCSBN's 58 (RN and PN) member boards, 56 share licensure data" (NCSBN, 2015, Nursys).

Nursys e-Notify is a free innovative nurse licensure notification system. The system helps nurses track their license and discipline status and provides license renewal reminders. The information is provided as it is entered into the Nursys database by participating boards of nursing. This database supports a key licensure goal—to protect the public health and safety. These advantages have resulted in support for the NLC by many nursing organizations.

On the other hand, concerns relate to monitoring nurses' practice in multiple jurisdictions, nurse privacy, and due process rights. Issues related to disciplinary action in home and distant states are still being resolved. In addition, differences in practice requirements in different states may cause nurses confusion as to their rights and responsibilities. The NLC is increasingly affecting all nurses. Nursing students and graduates must remain apprised of changing conditions. Because changes occur frequently in this area, the most comprehensive and current sources of information are the websites for the ANA, the NCSBN, and the state boards of nursing for individual jurisdictions.

Continued Competency

As discussed earlier in the chapter, the primary purpose of nurse licensure is protection of the public. Thus mandatory continuing education was instituted as a strategy to ensure that nurses were competent to remain in practice. These programs have continued for a number of years. However, a growing number of nurses believe that more is required than just attending seminars to demonstrate continued competency. Consortiums of nurses in a number of states are examining alternatives for renewal of licensure. These requirements may include designated numbers of clinical practice hours, portfolios of achievements in clinical practice, and other exemplars of practice. Nurses and students are encouraged to become aware of continued competency initiatives so that they may be prepared for changes in future licensure requirements.

There is increasing concern for patient safety and treatment in today's health care system. Models of continued competency are but one attempt by professional nurses to ensure that patients receive safe, effective nursing care. Another strategy in this quest is establishing programs for certification of advanced practice nurses.

CERTIFICATION
History of Certification

There are distinct differences between licensure and certification. At the most basic level, licensure establishes minimal levels of practice, whereas certification recognizes excellence in practice. Because of this difference, the background, requirements, and practice opportunities for licensure and certification differ markedly.

Just as with the development of nursing licensure, at its inception certification was not legally required; rather, it was voluntary. In an effort to recognize nurses who had completed additional education and demonstrated competency in clinical practice, a number of nursing graduate schools and nursing specialty organizations offered certification programs. In the 1970s and later, advanced clinical courses were designed for nurses as certificate programs. The programs varied in length and content and did not offer a full master's course of study in nursing.

A second distinct difference in licensure and certification pertains to the organizations that grant certification. Whereas licensure is granted and governed by legislation and administered through the state boards of nursing, certification is awarded by nongovernmental agencies. The first field of nursing practice to certify advanced practitioners was nurse anesthesia in 1946. Similarly, in 1961, the American College of Nurse-Midwives began certifying nurse-midwives. As certificate programs developed, it became apparent that program standardization was a necessity. In 1975, the ANA convened a national study group at the University of Wisconsin, Milwaukee, to explore the issue. This meeting was attended by 75 nursing specialty organizations. The report of the group recommended the formation of a central organization for certification of nurses. This report, in conjunction with efforts of many nurses, resulted in the formation of the American Nurses Credentialing Center (ANCC). More than a quarter million nurses in more than 40 areas of specialty practice (Box 4.1) have been certified by the ANCC since 1990. More than 80,000 advanced practice nurses are currently certified by the ANCC. Today, many of the ANCC's examinations are open to nurses with a variety of educational backgrounds.

In addition to the ANCC, other professional specialty nursing organizations (Box 4.2) offer certification examinations. These organizations have created certification

---

BOX 4.1   American Nurses Credentialing Center, Certifying Examinations 2012

Advanced Practice Certification
Acute Care NP
Adult NP
Adult Psychiatric and Mental Health NP
Diabetes Management—Advanced
Family NP
Family Psychiatric and Mental Health NP
Gerontologic NP
Pediatric NP
School NP

Clinical Nurse Specialists
Adult Gerontology CNS
Pediatric CNS
Public Community Health CNS

Specialties
Ambulatory Care Nursing
Cardiac Rehabilitation Nursing
Cardiac Vascular Nursing
Case Management Nursing
Certified Vascular Nursing

College Health Nursing
Community Health Nursing
Diabetes Management—Advanced
Genetics Nursing
General Nursing Practice
Gerontologic Nursing
Hemostasis Nursing
High-Risk Perinatal Nursing
Home Health Nursing
Informatics Nursing
Medical Surgical Nursing
Nursing Case Management
Nurse Executive—Advanced
Nursing Professional Development
Pain Management
Pediatric Nursing
Perinatal Nursing
Psychiatric Mental Health Nursing
Public Health Nurse—Advanced
Rheumatology
School Nursing

BOX 4.2   Other Nursing Certification Organizations

Advanced Practice Palliative Nurse—National Board for Certification of Hospice and Palliative Nurses (NBCHPN)
Clinical Nurse Leader—Commission on Nurse Certification
Comprehensive Care for DNPs—American Board of Comprehensive Care

---

boards that are separate from the parent organizations in order to maintain an independent role and to conform to department of education requirements. Nurses may contact these specialty nursing organizations directly for current guidelines and information.

All APRNs should be certified through a nationally recognized nursing certifying body and should understand that the examinations offered by these certification agencies will be used by state boards to grant APRNs the authority to practice. The lengths to which organized nursing has invested in certification of advanced practice in nursing are further indications of nurses' commitment to protection of the public and the patients they serve.

Certification began as a voluntary effort controlled by professional nursing organizations. State agencies were not involved in the credentialing process. This is still the case, although state nurse practice acts do include requirements for nurses to practice in advanced roles. Thus state practice acts first contained provisions requiring certification for nurse anesthetists and nurse-midwives. With the development of additional advanced practice roles, all states have included requirements for certification in their regulations for advanced practice nurses in all specialty roles.

Purpose of Certification

The purpose of advanced practice laws is, first and foremost, protection of the public. Within the acts are definitions of advanced practice nursing. A number of states further differentiate the advanced practice of nursing by including separate titles for nurse practitioners and clinical nurse specialists. The scope of practice of the advanced practice nurse is well defined. States describe supervisory or collaborative practice with physicians, with differences existing among states as to the regulations governing these relationships. Requirements for practice vary among states. Although many states require a master's degree in the specialty area for practice, this is not the case in all jurisdictions. All states require evidence of certification in the specialty area, and many require periods of practice in the specialty prior to awarding of certification status. All states incorporate specific provisions for prescribing medications.

Steps to Certification

The best strategy for a nurse wishing to practice in an expanded role is to become informed of specific requirements in the chosen field. The nurse should examine carefully the roles and responsibilities inherent in advanced practice nursing. First, the nurse should contact both the ANCC and the specialty organization in his or her area of practice to determine the education, experience, and examination requirements for certification. Concurrently, every nurse should contact the state boards of nursing in the state(s) in which he or she wishes to practice and should obtain information on legal requirements to practice in those jurisdictions. After gathering the requirements to practice, the nurse will be able to develop a plan of action to complete the necessary advanced coursework, clinical practice requirements, and examinations. Upon completion of the requirements of these agencies, the advanced practice nurse may practice in an expanded role. In addition to the certifying agencies, the nurse may wish to contact other advanced practice nurses, who will serve as valuable colleagues for the new advanced practice nurse.

Current Issues in Certification

Despite tremendous strides in less than 40 years, certification processes for the advanced practice nurse continue to evolve. As with any new endeavor, advances are made in small steps and great leaps.

Nurses in advanced practice face changing educational requirements for licensure and relicensure. Professional and legal issues regarding the scope of nursing practice and the independence of advanced practice nursing must change along with changes in the health care environment. Advanced practice nurses develop professional relationships with their physician colleagues, as do all nurses; however, the advanced practice nurses must define their legal relationships with physician practitioners and other caregivers. These issues are not uncommon to nurses in any practice setting; however, the advanced practice nurse is charting new territory.

A unique challenge to advanced practice nurses is reimbursement for nursing services. As advanced practice continues to expand, nurses have moved from secondary to independent billing for services. Federal regulations allow direct reimbursement for some nursing services, yet state and local practices vary. There are ongoing efforts at the state and national levels to resolve these issues. Advanced practice nurses are in constant communication with their peers and professional organizations. They look to all nurses to become involved in issues facing the advanced practice nurse.

Another issue in advanced practice nursing has emerged. Just as with the historical questions about which group will test and license nurses, a question is surfacing as to which organizations will credential and regulate advanced practice nursing. The NCSBN proposes that it is the appropriate agency to credential as well as license advanced practitioners in their vision for the future (2014). Nursing professional and specialty organizations are currently responding to the draft proposal. It is incumbent upon all nurses and potential nurses to become knowledgeable about this issue and to participate in the professional discussions. This issue clearly illustrates the changing practice and regulation of nursing.

Most recently, the ANCC Portfolio program for board certification, which was launched in 2012 as a strategy to certify nurses in specialty areas of practice where an examination was deemed not feasible to develop or did not currently exist, ended. Although the Portfolio program achieved some of its intended goals, applicant volumes did not reach a level whereby any of the programs achieved financial stability. In addition, persistent low applicant volumes precluded ANCC from applying for external accreditation (http://www.nursecredentialing.org/Certification/NurseSpecialties/FaithCommunity Nursing). Therefore, the Commission on Certification (COC), in collaboration with ANCC program leadership, decided to end the Portfolio program in the fall of 2017. Those who were certified by portfolio are able to maintain their certification by meeting ANCC's certification renewal requirements.

The Consensus Model for APRN Regulation, Licensure, Accreditation, Certification, and Education

"With approximately 300,000 advanced practice registered nurses (APRNs) in the United States, APRNs represent a powerful force in the health care system. The Consensus Model provides guidance for states to adopt uniformity in the regulation of APRN roles. . . . Today, many states have adopted portions of the Model elements but there still may be variation from state to state. APRNs moving from state to state need to ask themselves the following:

"Have I met the requirements to practice in this state?

Do I have the appropriate certification required to practice in this state?

Does my training/experience match within the scope of practice required to practice?

"As long as regulatory requirements differ from state to state, each state border represents an obstacle to portability—potentially preventing access to professionals and access to care. The *Consensus Model for APRN Regulation* has the potential to harness this power by outlining regulatory requirements in licensure, accreditation, certification, and education that should be adopted by every state.

"Visit the Consensus Model toolkit, a compendium of resources for understanding the Consensus Model at aprnconsensus@ncsbn.org" (NCSBN, APRN consensus model, 2018).

SUMMARY

Nurse practice acts provide protection for both the public and the title of RN. This is accomplished through the development of specific regulations regarding education and examination of competence to practice. Each act contains guidelines for disciplinary action to protect both the public and professional nursing. The nurse practice act of each jurisdiction addresses the needs of the state and the responsibilities of nurses practicing within that state. It is important for all nurses and students of nursing to become familiar with the regulations guiding their own practice.

As health care delivery evolves and nursing practice advances, new issues and initiatives arise. It is imperative to update nurse practice acts so that they remain responsive to the needs of all and allow nurses to practice to the full extent of their education and training. Nurses must be part of this process. Collaboration among professional nursing organizations, state boards of nursing, and individual nurses will enable nursing to continually meet the needs of patients.

REFERENCES

American Nurses Credentialing Center. (2018). Certifications available. Retrieved from http://www.nursecredentialing.org/certification.aspx.

Health Resources and Services Administration (HRSA). The registered nurse population: findings from the 2013 National Sample Survey of Registered Nurses. Retrieved from http://bhpr.hrsa.gov/healthworkforce/rnsurveys/rnsurveyfinal.pdf.

Joel, L. A. (2006). The nursing experience: trends, challenges, and transitions (5th ed.). New York: McGraw-Hill.

Kalisch, B. J., & Kalisch, P. A. (2003). The advance of American nursing (4th ed.). Philadelphia: Lippincott.

National Council of State Boards of Nursing. (2014). Advanced practice registered nurses. Retrieved from https://www.ncsbn.org/2632.htm.

National Council of State Boards of Nursing. (2015). APRN Compact. Retrieved from https://ncsbn.org/aprn-compact.htm.

National Council of State Boards of Nursing. (2016). National guidelines for nursing delegation. *Journal of Nursing Regulation*, 7(1), 5–14.

National Council of State Boards of Nursing. (2014). Model act. Retrieved from https://www.ncsbn.org/.

National Council of State Boards of Nursing. (2018). APRN consensus model; The consensus model for APRN Regulation, Licensure, adccreditation, certification, and education. Retrieved from https://www.ncsbn.org/aprn-consensus.

National Council of State Boards of Nursing. (2018). Enhanced Nurse Licensure Compact (eNLC) Implementation. Retrieved from https://www.ncsbn.org/enhanced-nlc-implementation.htm.

National Council of State Boards of Nursing. (2015). Nursys database. Retrieved from https://www.ncsbn.org/national-nursing-database.htm.

5

Nursing theory provides the direction for nursing practice and research.

Theories of Nursing Practice

Susan R. Jacob, PhD, MSN, RN

(e) Additional resources are available online at: *http://evolve.elsevier.com/Cherry/*

> *"Science is built up with facts, as a house is with stones. But a collection of facts is no more a science than a heap of stones a house."*
> **Jules Henri Poincaré, 1909, French scientist and mathematician**

LEARNING OUTCOMES

After studying this chapter, the reader will be able to:

1. Differentiate between a science and a theory.
2. Identify the criteria necessary for science.
3. Identify the criteria necessary for theory.
4. Explain a nursing theory and a nursing model.
5. Discuss two early and two contemporary nursing theorists and their theories.
6. Explain the effect of nursing theory on the profession of nursing.

KEY TERMS

Concept An idea or a general impression. Concepts are the basic ingredients of theory. Examples of nursing concepts include pain, quality of life, health, stress, and adaptation.

Conceptual model A group of concepts that are associated because of their relevance to a common theme.

Nursing science The collection and organization of data related to nursing and its associated components. The purpose of this data collection is to provide a body of scientific knowledge, which provides the basis for nursing practice.

Theory The compilation of data that define, describe, and logically relate information that will explain past nursing phenomena and predict future trends. Theories provide a foundation for developing models or frameworks for nursing practice development.

Proposition A statement that proposes the relationship between and among concepts.

Schematic model A diagram or visual representation of concepts, conceptual models, or theory.

We thank Margaret Soderstrom, PhD, RN, CS-P, APRN, and Linda C. Pugh, PhD, RNC, FAAN, for their contributions to this chapter in the fourth edition.

PROFESSIONAL/ETHICAL ISSUE

Bachelor of science in nursing (BSN) students Matt, Toni, and Britainy were studying together for their theory class when Matt spoke up and said, "I think all this theory is just a bunch of junk. Nurses in practice don't have time to learn about theories, and they sure don't use them to guide their practice."

Britainy spoke up and said, "My aunt is an RN on the cancer unit at Memorial Hospital and she has told me that on her unit they use Jean Watson's caring theory to guide their interactions with patients."

Toni said, "Really? Then maybe there is something to this theory stuff. I think we should take this class more seriously."

Britainy agreed and suggested that they divide the material among themselves and meet again the next day to prepare for the upcoming test.

Matt said, "You guys can do that if you want, but count me out. My plan is to skim the information and take my chances on the test. I am amazed you two really think we will ever need to know any of this stuff after we graduate. Nursing theory is never going to help me start an IV."

Is there a way for Britainy and Toni to show Matt he is wrong? If so, how?

How can Britainy and Toni persuade Matt to divide the theory material with them to prepare for the upcoming test?

VIGNETTE

When I was a nursing student, it was hard for me to understand why I needed to know anything about nursing theory, but now that I am in practice I see that theories provide a way for me to organize, deliver, and evaluate the care I provide. On our labor and delivery unit, we use Roy's adaptation model to guide our practice as we provide care to laboring moms. The use of this theory allows us to assess how well they are coping and provides guidance as we plan nursing interventions that promote their successful coping.

Questions to Consider While Reading this Chapter:
1. What is nursing theory?
2. How is nursing theory different from the theory of other disciplines?
3. How does theory relate to nursing practice?
4. Why is it important to understand nursing theory?
5. Why is it important for nurses to develop theory?

CHAPTER OVERVIEW

Explicit, detailed knowledge is the keystone, the foundation, and the carefully laid support that are critical to the classification of a discipline. In a seminal paper entitled "The Discipline of Nursing" (1978), Donaldson and Crowley note that a discipline "is characterized by a unique perspective, a distinct way of viewing all phenomena, which ultimately defines the limits and nature of its inquiry" (p. 113). Nursing, long ranked an art and a science, is actually quite young in its continuing struggle for professional and public recognition as a matchless, expert, and commanding profession. This notion is readily supported as one marks nursing's ongoing effort to define itself as a distinct discipline that is exclusive from other disciplines, particularly the medical practice model. Only when a substantial body of nursing knowledge is collected, organized, and developed will the profession be defined and its scope of practice differentiated. Key to this accomplishment is the development and practice of nursing theory.

It is important for nurses to study the development of nursing theory because without an idea of where you have been, how can you know how, why, when, or where to go? Nursing theory provides nurses with a focus for research and practice. You may consider using a theory as similar to using a map that provides direction while making available a variety of ways to get where you are going. As logical as this seems, the worth of studying nursing theorists, their theories, and the role of responsibility these theories contribute to the evolution of nursing science has been curiously under-appreciated. Even more surprising, many of the naysayers are nursing students. Nursing theory is not usually the favorite subject of undergraduates, who would rather learn technical, hands-on skills. Whether this is a maturation issue or an issue of knowledge and experience remains undetermined by nursing faculty and the profession itself.

This chapter in no way reflects the breadth and depth of nursing theorists and their theories. There are many scholarly works devoted to this topic. Instead it is a survey, a general overview; a smattering of nursing theories, with chosen segments intended to assist in providing the idea, the notion, and indeed, the semblance of what a theory is and how it is critical to the profession of nursing. Readers interested in examining the theoretic basis for nursing practice will find resources for further exploration at the end of the chapter.

SCIENCE AND THEORY

Science is a method of bringing together facts and giving them coherence and integrity. Science assists us in understanding how the unique yet related parts of a structure fit and become more than the sum of individual parts. In the opening metaphor, the stones represent the facts, the process of laying the stones represents the science, and the future ideas and new directions represent the theory.

Science is dynamic and static—dynamic in figuring out how a phenomenon happens, static in describing what happens. Scientific inquiry involves five steps: (1) hypothesis, (2) method, (3) data collection, (4) results, and (5) evaluation. These five steps are described in Box 5.1.

"Nursing theory is defined as an abstract generalization that presents a systematic explanation about the relationships among phenomena" (Polit and Beck, 2017, p. 746). Theory development functions in a parallel manner to scientific process, although theory generally applies to a more specific area of the larger scientific process. Even though Sigmund Freud and Carl Jung each had their individual theories about the psychology of humans, their theories were focused on specific ideas taken from the entire knowledge base surrounding psychology and psychotherapy and its scientific premise. Similarly, Albert Einstein's theory of relativity was but a fraction of the existing scientific knowledge base of mathematics at the time. Nevertheless, it is an undisputed fact that these theorists changed the thinking of their time and were responsible for the evolution of their philosophic and scientific interests (Anastasi, 1958). For a proposed theory to be accepted as a theory, it must meet the following six criteria: (1) inclusiveness, (2) consistency, (3) accuracy, (4) relevance, (5) fruitfulness, and (6) simplicity. These criteria are further explained in Box 5.2.

The importance of theories in the evolution of science is unquestioned. Nursing has evolved as a profession and a science in a similar manner. Nursing theories have explained, explored, defined, and delineated specific areas. They are foundational to nursing, helping to accumulate further knowledge and give indications of what direction nursing should take to develop the discipline. In practice, nursing theories help nurses by describing, explaining, and predicting everyday experiences. Theories can guide nurses in their assessments, interventions, and evaluations of nursing care.

Beginning with the work of Florence Nightingale in 1860, nursing theorists have taken the vast pool of

---

BOX 5.1 The Five Steps of the Scientific Process

Hypothesis: Ask the question that is to be the main focus. It usually includes independent and dependent variables.

Method: Decide what data will be collected to answer the question. Decide on and identify the step-by-step procedure that will be used to collect these data. Make sure this process can be easily replicated.

Data collection: Implement the step-by-step procedure that has been determined to answer the question.

Results: On the conclusion of the data collection, statistically identify the outcomes. Establish parameters (e.g., level of significance) that will determine whether the data are relevant.

Evaluation: Examine the results to determine the relevance of outcome data in answering the hypothesis. Determine the significance and identify the potential for future research.

BOX 5.2 Criteria for Theory Acceptance

Inclusiveness: Does the theory include all concepts related to the area of interest?

Consistency: Can the theory address new entities without having its founding assumptions changed?

Accuracy: Does the theory explain retrospective occurrences? Does the theory maintain its capacity to predict future outcomes?

Relevance: Does the theory relate to the scientific foundation from which it is derived? Is it reflective of the scientific base?

Fruitfulness: Does the theory generate new directions for future research?

Simplicity: Does the theory provide a road map for replication? Is it simple to follow? Does it make sense?

scientific information available and focused on precise target areas of interest. In so doing, theoretic models have been conceptualized to guide nursing actions, interventions, and implementation. Specific nursing theories are discussed later in the chapter.

Nursing Science

As might be expected, there are several definitions of nursing science (Abdellah, 1969; Jacox, 1974). Although these definitions differ, they generally support the premise that nursing science is a collection of data related to nursing that may be applied to the practice of nursing. These data encompass a vast array of knowledge that spans all of nursing and its diversity. This knowledge guides the practice of nursing to better serve patients through healing, prevention, education, and health maintenance.

Theories, Models, and Frameworks

Researchers use theories and conceptual models as their primary method to organize findings into a broader conceptual context (Reed and Shearer, 2012). Different terms are used in relation to conceptual contexts for research. These terms include *theories, models, frameworks, schemes,* and *maps.* Different writers often use terms differently, resulting in a blurring of distinct terms (Polit and Beck, 2017).

Theory. Theory is generally considered an abstract generalization that presents a systematic explanation about how phenomena are interrelated. Therefore, traditionally, a theory must have at least two related concepts that support it (Reed and Shearer, 2012).

Conceptual Model. A conceptual model deals with concepts that are assembled because of their relevance to a common theme. The term conceptual framework is used interchangeably with conceptual model. Conceptual models, or frameworks, also provide a conceptual perspective regarding interrelated phenomena, but they are more loosely structured than theories. There are many conceptual models of nursing that offer broad explanations of the nursing process. Four concepts basic to nursing that are included in these models are: (1) nursing, (2) person, (3) health, and (4) environment. The various nursing models define these concepts differently, link the concepts in various ways, and emphasize the relationships among the concepts

differently. For example, Roy's adaptation model emphasizes the patient's adaptation as a central phenomenon, whereas Martha Rogers emphasizes centrality of the individual as a unified whole. These models are used by nurse researchers to formulate research questions and hypotheses.

The terms *conceptual model* (or *framework*) and *nursing theory* are often used interchangeably. In this chapter, the nursing theories described may also be referred to as conceptual models. The term *model* is also used in reference to a diagram depicting the theory. In this chapter, *model* refers to a schematic model, which is a diagram or visual representation of the conceptual model or theory.

Nursing Theory

Theory and theoretic thinking guide research and practice. The basic ingredients of theory are concepts. Examples of nursing concepts include health, stress, and adaptation. **Propositions** are statements that propose the relationship between and among concepts (Polit and Beck, 2017). Theories provide us with a frame of reference, the ability to choose concepts to study, or ideas that are within one's practice. A theory helps guide research, and research helps validate theory.

In the research model, the researcher decides what to study and how and why the area of interest is important to the practice of nursing. In the practice model, the clinician decides what areas to directly assess, when to assess, and which intervention to implement. These decisions may or may not be knowingly based on a model or theory. Regardless, often the outcome supports the notion that behavior replicates a theoretic model, even though the nurse may be unaware that he or she is using a theoretic model in the practice process.

Just as in any other discipline, nursing theory has its own unique language. The words of this language identify linkages between the database of scientific nursing knowledge and the extracted information taken from this source for nursing theory. The interpretation of these words translates uniquely to the theory investigated. This application, or language of nursing theory, is the structure, or framework, from which one understands the theory. Table 5.1 presents the language of nursing theory along with definitions and examples.

TABLE 5.1	The Language of Nursing Theory	
Term	**Definition**	**Examples**
Concept	Labels given to ideas, objects, events; a summary of thoughts or a way to categorize thoughts or ideas	Comfort, fatigue, pain, depression, environment
Conceptual model	A structure to organize concepts (ideas)	Roy's adaptation model
Philosophy	Values and beliefs of the discipline	Watson's philosophy and science of caring
Theory	The organization of concepts or constructs that shows the relationship of the ideas with the intention of describing, explaining, or predicting. The purpose is to make scientific findings meaningful and generalizable. Our goal in science has been to explain, predict, and control.	Self-care, adaptation, caring, behavioral system, unitary man, hierarchy of needs, interpersonal relationships, humanistic, nurse-client transactions

Schematic Models

A schematic model is something that demonstrates concepts, usually with a picture. It is a visual representation of ideas. The model depicts concepts and shows how the concepts are related with the use of images, such as arrows and dotted lines (Polit and Beck, 2017). For example, a blueprint is a pictorial demonstration of a particular type of house someone might build. A model airplane is a detailed miniature replication of the original full-sized version. Diagramming a sentence outlines the specific parts (adverb, adjective, verb, subject, object, phrases) that make that particular sentence complete. Similarly, a nursing model gives a visual diagram or picture of concepts. Whether that is a critical pathway, decision tree, medication protocol, or other nursing-related practice, the model allows one to view the interrelated parts of the whole in picture form. A model of a nursing theory does the same thing. From the earliest model, offered by Florence Nightingale, nursing theory has been described and explained using this medium. Schematic models are used for clarifying complex concepts. The language of theory is translated into picture form, offering a comprehensive view, or model, of the theory. The schematic model shows how the concepts are related. A model, like a blueprint of a building, allows one to see the layout, including outlines of all features specific to the theory. Although it is not the same as understanding every little detail about the structure, its intent is to provide an overview, which at a glance is informative and descriptive.

Levels of Theory

Many people refer to the level of a nursing theory, which can range from broad in scope to a smaller, more specific scope. For example, grand theory is often broad in scope and may describe and explain large segments of human experience. Rogers's theory of unitary man describes the entire nursing process. Other levels include middle-range theory and practice theory, which are smaller in scope and may refer to a specific population, such as Jacob's theory of the grief process in older women whose husbands received hospice care (Jacob, 1996), or to a specific situation, such as Beck's (2012) theory of postpartum depression, or Pender's Health Promotion Model (Pender et al, 2015). Another example of a middle-range theory is the theory of unpleasant symptoms (Lenz and Pugh, 2003), which examines symptoms that are influenced by physiologic, psychologic, and situational factors as they relate to performance. The model of this theory is presented in Fig. 5.1. Nurses often use these middle-range theories, which are smaller in scope and simpler to understand, to guide their daily practice.

To better illustrate the application of theory to nursing practice, Case Study 5.1 presents a case example of middle-range theory application using Mishel's (1997) uncertainty in illness theory. In examining nursing theories, students may be surprised to discover that they are already using some of the concepts in their individual practices. Nursing theories assist with further defining and organizing these concepts into an underpinning that explains and details nursing practice and claims it as a unique discipline.

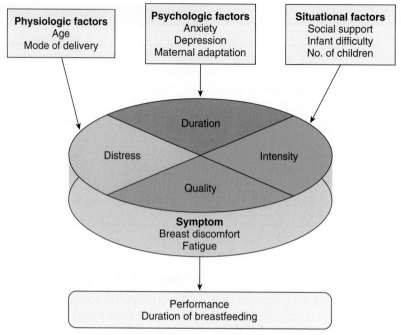

Fig. 5.1 Theory of unpleasant symptoms.

Mishel's Uncertainty in Illness Theory

A 9-year-old female client, Christine, is admitted to the pediatric unit for evaluation of a new onset of abdominal pain. The admission diagnosis is "intermittent abdominal pain, rule out appendicitis." It is her first time as a patient in a hospital. Her father, who is a surgeon, and her mother, who is a nurse, accompany Christine to the unit. Her mother will stay with her. After talking with the parents, you as the nurse are confident that Christine is well informed, well cared for, and well prepared for her admission. While her parents are speaking with Christine's attending physician in a nearby office, you talk with Christine, who goes from smiling and chatting to bursting into tears. You observe that she is quite upset as she expresses to you that she is afraid because her father told her that if she did need surgery she would not feel anything because she would be asleep. Christine tells you that when she sleeps she wakes up sometimes and that she is sure that if her appendix is "cut out" she will wake up during the operation and it "will hurt a lot." She tells you she has not told her parents she is afraid because they have told her how proud they are that she is so brave. You

realize Christine is terrified. Using Mishel's uncertainty in illness theory, you apply the four-stage framework:

1. *Stimuli frame:* Inadvertently, Christine, who concretely has understood the word "sleep" using her own filter for life experience, has misinterpreted the positive intention of the language used by her father. This misinterpretation has resulted in Christine's negative cognitive schema. Christine notably does not understand "sleep" and its use (or adult misuse, in this case) as a synonym for, or definition of, surgical anesthesia. This is the root cause of Christine's current uncertainty in illness.

   Nursing intervention: Listen carefully and caringly; explain in simple, understandable language, what "sleep" means in the context her father presented; initiate, seek, and clarify Christine's concerns and questions; use the term *anesthesia* to differentiate it from "sleep." Inform and involve her parents in the overall process.

2. *Appraisal stage:* As a result of Christine's concrete experiential interpretation of "sleep," she has applied a negative value to the environmental conditions

CASE STUDY 5.1   Application of Theory to Practice—cont'd

Mishel's Uncertainty in Illness Theory

surrounding her abdominal pain. This is particularly so as it relates to surgical anesthesia.

Nursing intervention: Follow up with Christine to make sure she comprehends the newly provided information. Elicit the support of Christine's parents and staff. If there are appropriate postsurgical patients on the unit, have them talk with Christine about their positive anesthesia experience.

3. *Initiation of coping mechanisms:* Christine is 9 years old. Her coping skills are limited to those used in her 9 years of life experience.

Nursing intervention: Check with Christine, and observe verbal and nonverbal cues. Have her verbalize any uncertainties she may be experiencing. Some of this process will be influenced by the progress of the illness.

4. *Adaptation:* Dependent on steps 1, 2, and 3

Nursing intervention: As Christine accepts the new information, new schema will follow. Although the

outcome of her abdominal pain may initially be uncertain, her acceptance of the new schema will hopefully result in an increased comfort zone and decreased fear.

Summary

A central tenet of Mishel's theory is the core position that uncertainty in illness must be addressed. If it is left unheeded, negative perceptions will escalate and clients will suffer. Their quality of life may be affected and positive outcomes may be compromised. Nursing's responsibility in applying Mishel's theory is to reframe the client's perceived loss of control, or uncertainty, and assist the client in developing new skills of assimilation and accommodation. The client will then be able to identify, develop, and master those targets capable of control.

FLORENCE NIGHTINGALE: THE FIRST NURSING THEORIST

If *theory* means to put concepts in a form in which relationships are described and predictions are made, then Florence Nightingale was the first nursing theorist. Nightingale did not deliberately set out to develop theory; rather her goal was to ease the suffering of soldiers and citizens of England. However, many important influences in her life directed her toward theory development:

- A classical education (philosophy [science], French, Italian, Greek, Latin, the arts, and history)
- Upper-class background, great wealth, and a prominent social life (operas, parties, balls)
- Religion and spirituality (spent much time daydreaming about how she could serve God and experienced four visions from God)
- Era of reform throughout England (Industrial Revolution and great divisions among the classes)

Despite her wealth and upper-class status, Nightingale was very dissatisfied with life. In 1852, she wrote a monograph titled "Cassandra," in which she pointed out the hopelessness inherent in being a woman in her day. "The family? It is too narrow a field for the development of an immortal spirit . . . The system dooms some minds to incurable infancy, others to silent misery. Marriage

is the only chance [and it is but a chance] offered to women for escape from this death; and how eagerly and how ignorantly it is embraced" (Nightingale, 1992, pp. 37-38). Her diary writings have been interpreted at times to be suicidal. Often depressed, Nightingale resorted to dreams as an escape from her unhappiness and discontent. Her personality and her lifestyle (dogmatic, practical, a critical observer who was fascinated by numbers and recorded everything she saw and experienced) set her apart. She was self-willed, unhappy, and dissatisfied at times in spite of having beauty, a brilliant social career, and an education of which few men of her day could boast.

She had enjoyed the best of music and art and the companionship of charming and important people. However, in refusing marriage and the round of social gaiety, she was revolting against the restrictions placed on women of her day, and she struggled to be allowed to work in a serious way.

Florence Nightingale eventually persuaded her family to allow her to attend nurses' training, and so began her distinguished career in the development of professional nursing. Nightingale is well remembered for her significant contributions to professional nursing in the areas of theory of practice, nursing education, scholarship, and statistics. Box 5.3 provides Nightingale's definitions of professional nursing.

BOX 5.3   Nightingale's Definition of Nursing

Nursing is an art—an art requiring an organized, practical, and scientific training.

Nursing is putting us in the best possible conditions for nature to preserve health—to prevent, restore, or cure disease or injury.

Nursing is, therefore, to help the patient live.

Nightingale's Theory of Practice

Nightingale's theory of practice, an environmental adaptation theory, was documented for nurses and laypersons alike and served as the foundation for the promotion of health. She referred to this theory as the canons of nursing that guided the practice of professional nursing. A description of these canons, or standards, follows.

Ventilation and warming: In the concept of ventilation and warming, Nightingale is very precise to "keep the air he breathes as pure as the external air without chilling him" (Nightingale, 1859, p. 8). She believed that good ventilation is necessary to carry off noxious elements from a sick person's lungs and skin.

Noise: "Unnecessary noise, or noise that creates an expectation in the mind is that which hurts a patient" (Nightingale, 1859, p. 25). The idea is that the nurse should guard against sudden noise, thoughtless chatter, and whispering in a patient's room, and believed that the effect of music may be beneficial.

Variety: Variety is another concept that helps alleviate suffering. Beautiful objects, brilliant colors, cut flowers, perhaps different things to do (e.g., handwork), and even pets may alleviate the boredom felt by those suffering.

Diet: The fourth concept is diet. "Sick cookery should half do the work of your poor patient's weak digestion" (Nightingale, 1859, p. 38). Nightingale reviews some of the common substances (gruel, arrowroot puddings, and egg flip) given to the sick.

Light: "It is the unqualified result of all my experience with the sick that second only to their need of fresh air is their need of light" (Nightingale, 1859, p. 47). Nightingale suggested taking the patient outside for direct sunlight, and keeping rooms well lighted with no bed curtains or dark windows.

Chattering hopes and advices: According to Nightingale, "chattering hopes and advices" are attempts by attendants and friends to cheer the patient. Nightingale warns against these attempts because she determines them to offer false hope and hollow advice. She clearly appeals, "Leave off this practice of attempting to cheer the sick by making light of their danger and by exaggerating their probabilities of recovery" (Nightingale, 1859, p. 54).

Cleanliness (health of houses): Nightingale's attention to cleanliness takes up a large portion of her book. She writes that health depends on this principle. Describing the care of bed, bedding, rooms, and walls, she states the exact steps needed to clean each. In addition, she details how to clean the sick person so as to prevent poisoning by the skin. She describes the patient's feeling of well-being after washing and drying. The nurse needs to wash her own hands with friction as well. Some believe that Nightingale's success was based primarily on cleaning up the hospitals.

Because of these significant contributions to nursing and to improving the health of soldiers and citizens alike, Nightingale was highly recognized. Her honors, decorations, medals, and citations may be seen in the United Services Museum in Whitehall, London. She was the first woman ever to receive the British Order of Merit, which was bestowed by King Edward VII. One of her biographers (Cook, 1942) said, "she was not only 'The Lady with a Lamp' throwing light into dark places but also a kind of galvanic battery stirring and sometimes shocking the dull and sluggish public to life and action."

SURVEY OF SELECTED NURSING THEORIES

A brief discussion of selected nursing theories follows. The date identified for each indicates the year in which the theory was first presented. However, most theories have continued to be refined and modified. A summary of the major nursing theorists with a brief description of their theory or conceptual model is presented in Table 5.2, which provides the reader with information to guide further exploration of nursing theory.

A useful nursing theory will make assumptions concerning health problems, environment, behaviors, and target populations that are logical, consistent, research supported, and similar to ones that have proved to be successful in previous programs.

TABLE 5.2 Summary of Major Nursing Theorists and Theory Description

Theorist and Date	Theory Description
Florence Nightingale, 1860	Investigates the effect of the environment on healing.
Hildegard E. Peplau, 1952	Interpersonal relations model explores the interpersonal relationship of the nurse and the client and identifies the client's feelings as a predictor of positive outcomes related to health and wellness.
Faye Abdellah, 1960	Twenty-one nursing problems. Client-centered interventions.
Ida Jean Orlando, 1961	Theory of the nursing process. Deliberate nursing approach that stresses the action of the individual client in determining the action of the nurse; focus is on the present or short-term outcome.
Virginia Henderson, 1966	Definition of nursing. Nursing assists patients with 14 essential functions toward independence.
Myra Estrin Levine, 1967	Conservation model. Four conservation principles of inpatient client resources (energy, structural integrity, personal integrity, and social integrity).
Martha E. Rogers, 1970	Science of unitary human beings: energy fields, openness, pattern, and organization; nurse promotes synchronicity between human beings and their universe or environment.
Betty Neuman, 1970	Systems model: wellness-illness continuum; promotes the nurse as the agent in assisting the client in adapting to and, therefore, reducing stressors; supports the notion of prevention through appropriate intervention.
Dorothea Orem, 1971	Self-care model. Nursing facilitates client self-care by measuring the client's deficit relative to self-care needs; the nurse implements appropriate measures to assist the client in meeting these needs by matching them with an appropriate supportive intervention.
Imogene King, 1971	Goal attainment theory. Goal attainment using nurse-client transactions; addresses client systems and includes society, groups, and the individual.
Sister Callista Roy, 1974	Adaptation model. Client's adaptation to condition using environmental stimuli to adjust perception.
Madeline Leininger, 1977	Theory of cultural care diversity and universality. Transcultural and caring nursing; concepts are aimed toward caring and the components of a culture care theory; diversity, universality, worldview, and ethnohistory are essential to the four concepts of care, caring, health, and nursing.
Jean Watson, 1978	Philosophy and science of caring and humanistic nursing; there are 10 "carative" factors that are core to nursing; this holistic outlook addresses the impact and importance of altruism, sensitivity, trust, and interpersonal skills.
Margaret Newman, 1979	Central components of this model are health and consciousness followed by concepts of movement, time, and space; all components are summative units, described in relationship to health and to each other.
Dorothy E. Johnson, 1980	Behavioral system model for nursing; separates the psychologic and physiologic aspects of illness; role of the nurse is to provide support and comfort to attain regulation of the client's behavior.
Rosemarie Rizzo Parse, 1981	Theory of human becoming proposes that quality of life from each person's individual perspective should be the goal of nursing practice. Parse first published the theory in 1981 as the "man-living-health" theory; however, the name was officially changed to "the human becoming theory" in 1992 to remove the term *man* after the change in the dictionary definition of the word from its former meaning of "humankind"; individual, by existing, actively participates in creating health according to environmental influences; individual is regarded as an open system wherein health is a process.

Betty Neuman (1970)—The System Model

The system model focuses on the response of the client system to actual or potential environmental stressors and on the use of several levels of nursing prevention intervention for attaining, retaining, and maintaining optimal client system wellness. Neuman defines the concern of nursing as preventing stress invasion. If stress is not prevented, then the nurse should protect the client's basic structure and obtain or maintain a maximum level of wellness. Nurses provide care through primary, secondary, and tertiary prevention modes.

Hildegard E. Peplau (1952)—Interpersonal Relations as a Nursing Process: Man as an Organism That Exists in an Unstable Equilibrium

When the client incurs an insult that renders her or him incapable of moving forward because of stressful environmental conditions, anxiety increases. This condition creates a situation wherein the option is to either move in a backward direction or remain on a plateau. Nursing intervention in Peplau's model focuses on reducing the related incapacitating stressors through therapeutic interpersonal interaction. Intervention involves the nurse's assisting the client with mutual goal setting. These goals may address exploration of the identified problem, identification of viable options, and implementation of available resources for resolution. The interpersonal nursing process is present and interactive, using associated and appropriate nursing intervention skills, which incorporate the roles of the nurse as resource person, educator, mentor, transfer agent, and counselor. Peplau's model requires that the nurse have self-awareness and insight regarding her or his own behaviors. This awareness may be applied in identifying and working through those behaviors unique to the client's schema. Fig. 5.2 presents Peplau's psychodynamic nursing model.

Martha E. Rogers (1970)—Science of Unitary Human Beings: Humans as Energy Fields That Interact Constantly with the Environment

According to Rogers's theory, when the client-human unit incurs an insult that renders him or her out of balance with the universe, nursing interventions must be geared toward helping the client-human unit attain an increasingly complex balance and synchronicity with the universe. Essential to Rogers's theory is the belief that each being is unique and consists of more than the collective sum of parts, and that each being is constantly evolving in a forward momentum as he or she interacts continually with the surrounding environmental field. Rogers's theory states that a brain integration is necessary to support the notion of human-environmental synergy, using the right side of the brain to recognize every human unit's capacity for imagery, sensation, and emotion and the left side of the brain for language, abstraction, and thought.

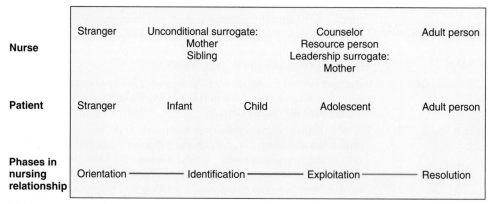

Fig. 5.2 Peplau's psychodynamic nursing model: Phases and changing roles in nurse-patient relationships. (From Peplau, H.E. [1952]. *Interpersonal relations in nursing* (p.54). New York: GP Putnam.)

Dorothea Orem (1971)—Self-Care Deficit Model: Self-Care, Self-Care Deficits, and Nursing Systems

When a client incurs an insult that renders him or her incapable of fully functioning, deficient self-care occurs, which makes nursing intervention necessary. The object of Orem's theory is to restore the client's self-care capability to enable him or her to sustain structural reliability, performance, and growth through purposeful nursing intervention. The aim of such intervention is to help the client cope with unmet care needs by acquiring the maximal level of function. This would be to either regain previous function or maximize available function present after the insult, hence restoring a sense of well-being.

Sister Callista Roy (1974)—Adaptation Model: Assistance with the Adaptation to Stressors to Facilitate the Integration Process of the Client

When the client incurs an insult that renders him or her in need of environmental modification, the nurse is the agent of change to assist the individual with this adaptation. Helping the "biopsychosocial" client to modify external stimuli allows adaptation to occur. In the case of illness, the outcome is a diminution or absence of integration of the constantly changing setting known as the *illness environment* with the constantly changing human, who is interacting with the existing outside surroundings. To attain wellness, adaptation must occur through this integration. The nurse's role is to promote this adaptation by modifying and regulating peripheral stimuli to enable the client's adaptation and integration with a supportive, healing environment. In so doing, the nurse is instrumental in assisting the client with the areas of health and well-being, life worth and value, and self-respect and dignity. Sister Callista Roy's adaptation model is depicted in Fig. 5.3.

Madeline Leininger (1977)—Theory of Cultural Care Diversity and Universality

Transcultural nursing and caring nursing concepts are aimed toward caring and the components of a culture care theory. In Leininger's theory, diversity, universality, worldview, and ethnohistory are essential to the four concepts of care, caring, health, and nursing.

Jean Watson (1978)—Theory of Human Caring: Transpersonal Caring as the Fulcrum; Philosophy and Science as the Core of Nursing

When the client incurs an insult that renders him or her in need, the transpersonal process between the client and the nurse is considered a healing nursing intervention. An assumption of Watson's theory is that everyone requires human caring to quell need. Hence, the transpersonal process of "caring," or the caring among nurse, environment, and client, is essential to healing. Caring promotes the notion that every human being strives for interconnectedness with other humans and with nature. The nurse who implements these "carative" factors is the facilitator in the goal of

Fig. 5.3 Roy's adaptation model: The person as an adaptive system. (From Roy, C. [1984]. *Introduction to nursing: an adaptation model* (2nd ed., p.30). Englewood Cliffs, NJ: Prentice-Hall.)

restoring congruence between the client's perceived self and the existent self through the promotion of health and equilibrium. The expectation is that the client will experience balance and harmony in mind, body, and soul. Harmony, or wellness, will prevail, whereas disharmony, or illness, will be altered, eliminated, or circumvented.

Margaret Newman (1979, Revised 1986)— Health as Expanding Consciousness

Margaret Newman's theory defines health as "expanding consciousness," or increasing complexity. The theory of health as expanding consciousness was stimulated by concern for those for whom health, defined as the absence of disease or disability, is not possible. Nurses often relate well to people facing the uncertainty, debilitation, loss, and eventual death associated with chronic illness. The theory has progressed to include the health of all persons regardless of the presence or absence of disease. The theory asserts that every person in every situation, no matter how disordered and hopeless it may seem, is part of the universal process of expanding consciousness—a process of becoming more of oneself, of finding greater meaning in life, and of reaching new dimensions of connectedness with other people and the world. (For more information, visit http://www.healthasexpandingconsciousness. org/home.)

Merle Mishel (1981, Revised 1990)— Uncertainty of Illness

Uncertainty in illness is frequently a stress-producing incident that is capable of contributing to negative physical and/or psychologic outcomes. Uncertainty exists when the client is unsure about a diagnosed illness. This uncertainty renders the client incapable of assigning a concrete value either to the illness itself or to a predictable outcome. Uncertainty can occur when a client misperceives a diagnosed illness because the information received is inadequate, the health care provider incorrectly presumes client knowledge, or the health care informant fails to recognize the client's individual unique filtering of provided illness information. Mishel's theory is used in chronic illness and other practice settings. Mishel's model outlines a four-step approach in defining her theory: (1) stimuli frame: antecedents generating client uncertainty; (2) appraisal stage: client assignment of a value (positive or negative) to the uncertainty; (3) initiation of coping mechanisms: client ability to develop, improvise, and implement skills to cope with uncertainty; and (4) adaptation: positive client assimilation and accommodation to uncertainty, resulting from effective coping. Mishel's theory establishes a framework that guides nursing practice by assisting nurses to work with clients in establishing interventions that promote positive outcomes.

FUTURE OF NURSING THEORIES AND THEORISTS

At no time in history have so many health care concerns been the primary focus of federal and state legislative agendas. New questions are being asked in the twenty-first century about how health care is being conducted and managed. It is imperative that nurses be on the front lines to provide testimony in response to these queries.

The current nursing shortage, scarce resources, patient safety and medical errors, managed care, Medicare, welfare-to-work plans, confidentiality issues, parity of reimbursement, advanced practice nurses and their scope of practice, mandatory overtime, whistle-blower protection, prescriptive authority, licensure, multistate compacts, telemedicine, and many other policy issues that directly affect nursing practice are coming before the U.S. Congress and individual state legislative bodies for practice-related decisions. The direct effect on nursing cannot be overemphasized.

As nursing continues to operate in an environment of ongoing change, outcome data will be analyzed in an effort to provide quality care and access to that care for all clients in need of health care services. Therefore, one may predict that established nursing theories will be reevaluated and modified accordingly. New theories will be created and developed that may help answer the health care questions of the twenty-first century. Simply put, nursing theories in the twenty-first century will embrace complex environmental changes that incorporate new technologies, such as genetics, computers, noninvasive surgery, robotics, decreasing energy sources, increasing pollutants under a thinning ozone layer, environmental hazards, new diseases, and antibiotic-resistant illness. These changes have already resulted in client needs that differ from those as recent as 5 years ago.

SUMMARY

Let the reader beware. As stated at the beginning of this chapter, the information provided here is in no manner a substitute for a comprehensive analysis of existing nursing theories and theorists. More theories exist than are presented here, and in fact, several comprehensive texts cover these theories in depth. Instead, this chapter offers an overview of theory in the attempt to familiarize readers with the idea of theory. Selected theories are described to that end. Readers should identify nursing theories as ideas that have shaped and continue to shape the nursing profession in practice and research. It is our intention to assist students with understanding that practice and theory are interdependent entities. In other words, practice and theory cannot efficiently or effectively exist one without the other. As in the metaphor at the beginning of this chapter, without the existence of the scientific data (stones), the organization of specific, concentrated yet related areas (house; theory) could not have happened.

REFERENCES

Abdellah, F. G. (1969). The nature of nursing science. *Nursing Research, 18*(5), 393.

Anastasi, A. (1958). Heredity, environment, and the question "how?" *Psychological Review, 65*(4), 197–208.

Beck, C. T. (2012). Exemplar: Teetering on the edge: A second grounded theory modification. In P. L. Munhall (Ed.), *Nursing research. A qualitative perspective* (5th ed., pp. 257–284). Sudbury, MA: Jones & Bartlett.

Cook, E. (1942). *The life of Florence Nightingale.* New York: Macmillan.

Donaldson, S. K., & Crowley, D. M. (1978). The discipline of nursing. *Nursing Outlook, 26*(2), 113–120.

Jacob, S. (1996). The grief process of older women whose husbands received hospice care. *Journal of Advanced Nursing, 24*(2), 280–286.

Jacox, A. K. (1974). Theory construction in nursing: an overview. *Nursing Research, 23*(1), 4.

Lenz, E. R., & Pugh, L. C. (2003). Theory of unpleasant symptoms. In M. J. Smith, P. Liehr (Ed.), *Middle range theory for nursing.* New York: Springer.

Mishel, M. H. (1981). The measurement of uncertainty in illness. *Nursing Research, 30*(5), 258–263.

Mishel, M. H. (1997). Uncertainty in acute illness. *Annual Review of Nursing Research, 15*, 57–80.

Nightingale, F. (1992). *Notes on nursing: What it is, and what it is not* (commemorative edition). Philadelphia: Lippincott.

Nightingale, F. (1859). *Notes on nursing: What it is, and what it is not.* London: Harrison and Sons.

Pender, N. J., Murdaugh, C. L., & Parsons, M. A. (2015). *Health promotion in nursing practice* (7th ed.). Upper Saddle River, NJ: Prentice Hall.

Polit, D., & Beck, C. (2017). *Nursing research* (10th ed.). Philadelphia: Wolters Kluwer Health/Lippincott.

Reed, P. G., Shearer, N. B. C. (2012). *Perspectives on nursing theory* (6th ed.). Philadelphia: Lippincott Williams & Wilkins.

6

Nursing Research and Evidence-Based Practice

Rosemary A. McLaughlin, PhD, CNE, RN-NIC,
Zoila V. Sanchez, PhD, FNP

Nursing research provides the foundation for evidence-based nursing practice.

ⓔ Additional resources are available online at: *http://evolve.elsevier.com/Cherry/*

LEARNING OUTCOMES

After studying this chapter, the reader will be able to:

1. Summarize major points in the evolution of nursing research in relation to contemporary nursing.
2. Evaluate the influence of nursing research on current nursing and health care practices.
3. Differentiate among nursing research methods.
4. Critically appraise the quality of research studies using established criteria.
5. Participate in the research process.
6. Use research findings to improve nursing practice.

KEY TERMS

Abstract A brief overview of a research study.

Clinical nurse specialist (CNS) An advanced practice nurse who provides direct care to clients and participates in health education and research.

Clinical practice guideline (CPG) An evidence-based guide to clinical practice developed by experts in a particular field for direct application in clinical environments.

Control group Subjects in an experiment who do not receive the experimental treatment and whose performance provides a baseline against which the effects of the treatment can be measured. When a true experimental design is not used, this group is called a comparison group.

Data collection The process of acquiring existing information or developing new information.

Empirical Having a foundation based on data gathered through the senses (e.g., observation or experience) rather than purely through theorizing or logic.

Ethnography A qualitative research method for the purpose of investigating cultures that involve data collection, description, and analysis of data to develop a theory of cultural behavior.

Evidence-based practice The process of systematically finding, appraising, and using research findings as the basis for clinical practice.

Experimental design A design that includes randomization, a control group, and manipulation between or among variables to examine probability and causality among selected variables for the purpose of predicting and controlling phenomena.

Generalizability The inference that findings can be generalized from the sample to the entire population.

Grant Proposal developed to seek research funding from private or public agencies.

Grounded theory A qualitative research design used to collect and analyze data aiming to develop theories grounded in real-world observations.

Integrative research review (IRR) Methodology that simultaneously synthesizes several experimental and non-experimental research findings to provide a comprehensive understanding of the phenomena of interest.

Meta-analysis Statistical method of quantitative synthesis of findings from several studies to determine what is known about a phenomenon.

Metasynthesis Interpretive translations produced from the integration or comparison of findings from qualitative studies.

Methodologic Research design used to develop the validity and reliability of instruments that measure research concepts and variables.

Naturalistic paradigm Holistic view of nature and the direction of science that guides qualitative research.

Needs assessment Study in which the researcher estimates the resource needs of a group.

Peer review A process by which a scholarly work (such as a paper or a research proposal) is checked by a group of experts in the same field to make sure it meets the necessary standards before it is published or accepted.

Practice guidelines Research-based recommendations stated as standards of practice, procedures, or decision algorithms.

Phenomenology Qualitative research design employing inductive descriptive methodology to describe the lived experiences of study participants.

Pilot study Conduct of a smaller version of a proposed study that develops or refines methodology prior to use in a larger study.

Qualitative research Systematic, subjective approach used to describe life experiences and give them meaning.

Quantitative research Formal, objective, systematic process used to describe and test relationships and examine cause-and-effect interactions among variables.

Quasi-experimental research A type of quantitative research study design that lacks one of the components of an experimental design (i.e., randomization, control group, manipulation of one or more variables).

Randomization The assignment of subjects to treatment conditions in a random manner (determined by chance alone).

Secondary analysis A research design in which data previously collected in another study are analyzed for different aims than the original study.

Survey A nonexperimental research design that focuses on obtaining information regarding the status quo of a situation, often through direct questioning of participants.

Triangulation The use of a variety of methods to collect data on the same concept.

PROFESSIONAL/ETHICAL ISSUES

Issue 1

Mary Smith is a 19-year-old female who comes to the health department women's center complaining about vaginal itching, foul-smelling discharge, and pain with sexual intercourse. She admits to being sexually active for the last 2 years with multiple partners and a prior history of trichomoniasis infections, twice within the last year. Ms. Smith has been on an oral contraceptive (OC) pill for the last 2 years and her last menstrual cycle was 4 days ago. Ms. Smith admits that there is family history of cervical cancer. Her mother was diagnosed and treated in 1992 for this condition. Ms. Smith has never had a Pap test. Ms. Smith stated, "The family planning center just did blood work to make sure I was not pregnant and gave me a prescription for oral contraceptive pills."

As a registered nurse you are aware that family history of cervical cancer needs further inquiry and follow-up. A vaginal examination is performed by a nurse practitioner, with findings of multiple fleshy, soft, pale-colored growths on the vagina and perianal area. As a nurse you are aware that most cervical cancers are caused by certain oncogenic (cancer-causing) strains of the human papillomavirus (HPV). Owing to the family history of cervical cancer, you anticipate that the nurse practitioner will follow up with a Pap test on this patient.

However, the current practice guidelines of the American Cancer Society and the American Society for Colposcopy and Cervical Pathology recommend that women younger than 21 should not be screened (Pap test) for cervical cancer or HPV, regardless of whether they are sexually active.

Issue 2

One of the latest epidemics in the United Sates involves the use and misuse of opioid analgesics. Although opioids can be safe and effective for certain pain conditions, such as postoperative acute pain and end-of-life pain, the long-term use of opioids to treat chronic pain is highly debatable. As a result, these conflicting reports have led to an increase in the misuse of opioids that has resulted in opioid hyperalgesia and an increase in opioid-related deaths.

Your friend in nursing school is getting her wisdom tooth removed and you have gone with her to drive her home. An opioid is offered for pain control. As a nurse, what would you do?

VIGNETTE

I did not understand why I had to take a research class when all I wanted to do was be a staff nurse in a critical care unit. Research? Evidence-based practice? Why are these topics in the nursing program? I have enough to do just learning all the content in my clinical courses. What do research and evidence have to do with developing my nursing abilities? I trust the faculty, the textbooks, and clinical experience to prepare me for nursing. I'm already getting what I need to know.

That was my earlier attitude. Now that I am practicing, I have a new appreciation for nursing research and the evidence it provides for application to practice. I have an entirely different way of addressing clinical questions. I'm starting to ask questions about how I can improve the care I give to patients and how I can be involved in my workplace's efforts to improve care for the patients it serves. I have discovered by purposeful reading in my practice area that research reports and research summaries contain many implications that apply to practice in the critical care unit.

Questions to Consider While Reading this Chapter

1. How can a desire to read research and evidence-based practice literature in students be facilitated?
2. How does research affect nursing practice?
3. How can nurses motivate colleagues to base their practice on research?

CHAPTER OVERVIEW

This chapter provides basic knowledge regarding the research process and the ultimate importance of evidence-based nursing practice. The intent is to inspire an appreciation for nursing research and to show both how it can improve nursing practice and how results can be translated into health policy. *Nursing research* is defined as a systematic approach used to examine phenomena important to nursing and nurses. A summary of major points in the evolution of nursing research in relation to contemporary nursing is presented. A description of private and public organizations that fund research is given, and their research priorities are listed. Major research designs are briefly described, and examples of each are given. Nurses of all educational levels are encouraged to participate in and promote nursing research at varying degrees. Evidence-based practice (EBP) is the use of the best scientific evidence, integrated with clinical experience and incorporating patients' values and preferences in the practice of professional nursing. Competencies have been developed to ensure that nurses are competent in providing EBP care and its uniformity in the application and generation of evidence. The process of locating research and evidence, including practice guidelines, is reviewed. Students are introduced to the research process and guided in the process of critically appraising published research and research syntheses. Ethical issues related to research are examined, and historical examples of unethical research are given. The functions of the institutional review board (IRB) and the use of informed consent in protecting the rights of human subjects are emphasized.

DEFINITION OF NURSING RESEARCH

Research is a process of systematic inquiry or study to build knowledge in a discipline. The purpose of research is to develop an empirical body of knowledge for a discipline or profession. Specifically, research validates and refines existing knowledge and develops new knowledge (Gray, Grove & Sutherland, 2017). The results of the research process provide a foundation on which practice decisions and behaviors are laid. Research results create a strong scientific base for nursing practice, especially when deliberately and carefully evaluated for application to specific clinical topics (Melnyk and Fineout-Overholt, 2015).

Nursing research is a systematic approach used to examine phenomena important to nursing and nurses. Because nursing is a practice profession, it is important that clinical practice be based on scientific knowledge. Evidence generated by nursing research provides support for the quality and cost-effectiveness of nursing interventions. Thus, recipients of health care— and particularly nursing care—reap benefits when nurses attend to research evidence and introduce change based on that evidence into nursing practice. The introduction of evidence-based change into the direct provision of nursing care may occur at the individual level, with a particular nurse, or at varied organizational or social levels. Research within the realms of nursing education, nursing administration, health services, characteristics of nurses, and nursing roles provide evidence for effectively changing these supporting areas of nursing knowledge (Gray, Grove & Sutherland, 2017).

EVOLUTION OF NURSING RESEARCH

Nursing research began with the work of Florence Nightingale during the Crimean War. After Florence Nightingale's work, the pattern that nursing research followed was closely related to the problems confronting nurses. For example, nursing education was the focus of most research studies between 1900 and 1940. As more nurses received their education in a university setting, studies regarding student characteristics and satisfactions were conducted. As more nurses pursued a college education, researchers became interested in studying nurses. Questions such as what type of person enters nursing and how are nurses perceived by other groups guided research investigations. Teaching, administration, and curriculum were topics that dominated nursing research until the 1970s. By the 1970s, more doctorally prepared nurses were conducting research, and there was a shift

to studies that focused on the improvement of patient care. The 1980s brought nursing research to a new stage of development. There were many more qualified nurse researchers, widespread availability of computers for collection and analysis of data, and a realization that research is a vital part of professional nursing (Polit and Beck, 2017). Nurse researchers began conducting studies based on the **naturalistic paradigm**. These studies were qualitative rather than quantitative. In addition, instead of conducting many small, unrelated research studies, teams of researchers, often interdisciplinary, began conducting programs of research to build bodies of knowledge related to specific topics, such as urinary incontinence, decubitus ulcers, pain, and quality of life. The 1990s brought increasing concern about health care reform, and now, in the twenty-first century, research studies focus on important health care delivery issues, such as cost, quality, and access. With the developing educational emphasis on the doctorate in nursing practice degree, research emphasis on patient care foci is gaining momentum, especially in view of the quality gaps highlighted by sentinel reports from the Institute of Medicine (IOM, 2001, 2011).

Increasingly, research findings are being used as the basis for clinical decisions. Evidence-based practice can be defined as the process of systematically finding, appraising, and using research findings as a basis for making decisions about patient care (Houser, 2015). The rise of technology and the worldwide access to and flow of information have transformed the decision-making processes of practitioners. No longer do nurses and other health care professionals simply compare outcomes of patient care between units in the same hospital; solutions, choices, and outcomes are sought on an international level. Hospitals must show improved outcomes and clinical practice based on current evidence. In recent decades, the nursing discipline is paying greater attention to the necessity of participating in research, as evidenced by the maintenance of magnet status for facilities (Wise, 2009).

RESEARCH PRIORITIES

Why set priorities for research in the nursing discipline? Can nurses do research in areas that match personal areas of interest? The answer to the second question is yes, certainly. But nursing exists to provide high-quality nursing care to individuals in need of health-promoting, health-sustaining, and health-restoring strategies. The main outcome of research activity for a nurse is to put the knowledge gained to work in health care delivery. Research priorities, often set by groups that fund research, encourage nurse researchers to invest effort and money into those areas of research likely to generate the most benefit to recipients of care.

Two major sources of funding for nursing research are the National Institute of Nursing Research (NINR) and the Agency for Healthcare Research and Quality (AHRQ), which are both funded by federal congressional appropriations. Private foundations and nursing organizations also provide funding for nursing research.

National Institute of Nursing Research

As part of the National Institutes of Health (NIH), NINR supports research on the biologic and behavioral aspects of critical health problems that confront the nation. The NINR's focus is designed to advance the "science of health" by encompassing four key themes: symptom science (promoting personalized health strategies); wellness (promoting health and preventing illness); self-management (improving quality of life for individuals with chronic illness); and end-of-life and palliative care (the science of compassion) (NINR, 2016).

The areas of research emphasis published by the NINR are useful guides for investigators developing proposals but are not considered prescriptive in nature. Investigators bring to bear their own unique expertise and creativity when proposing research in harmony with NINR priority research areas. Recently, the NINR Innovative Questions Initiative was launched to encourage new research questions, new thinking, and creativity in nursing to promote results-oriented innovations. This allowed for identification, discussion, and debate (Grady, 2014).

Agency for Healthcare Research and Quality

The AHRQ broadly defines its mission as improving "the quality, safety, efficiency, and effectiveness of health care for all Americans" (AHRQ, 2017a). As an agency of the U.S. Department of Health and Human Services, the AHRQ has health-related aims: to reduce the risk of harm by promoting delivery of the best possible health care, improve health care outcomes by encouraging the use of evidence to make informed health care decisions, transform research into practice to facilitate wider access to effective health care services, and reduce unnecessary costs (AHRQ, 2017a). Since the inception of the agency in 1989, strategic goals have centered on supporting improvements in health outcomes, strengthening measurement of health care quality indicators, and fostering access to and cost-effectiveness of health care. The 1999 reauthorizing legislation expanded the role of the agency by directing the AHRQ to:

- Improve the quality of health care through scientific inquiry, dissemination of findings, and facilitation of public access to information.
- Promote patient safety and reduce medical errors through scientific inquiry, building partnerships with health care providers, and establishing centers for education and research on therapeutics (CERTs).
- Advance the use of information technology for coordinating patient care and conducting quality and outcomes research.
- Establish an office on priority populations to ensure that the needs of low-income groups, minorities, women, children, older adults, and individuals with special health care needs are addressed by the agency's research efforts.

The research-related activities of the AHRQ are quite varied, but a recent shift emphasizes a more deliberate translation of research evidence into practice. In a process similar to that used by the NIH, investigators are invited to submit research proposals for possible funding through grant announcements. A listing of current areas of the agency's research interests can be found online at http://www.innovations.ahrq.gov.

The AHRQ actively promotes EBP, partially through the establishment of 14 EBP centers (EBPCs) in the United States and Canada. EBPCs conduct research on assigned clinical care topics and generate reports on the effectiveness of health care methodologies. Health care providers may then use the evidence in developing site-specific guidelines that direct clinical practice. AHRQ also actively maintains the National Guideline Clearinghouse (NGC) (http://www.guidelines.gov), a website that makes available to health care professionals a wide array of clinical practice guidelines that may be considered in health care decision making. Another addition to AHRQ's initiatives is the Healthcare Innovations Exchange (AHRQ, 2017b), which provides a public source of information about innovations taking place in health care delivery. Submitted innovations are reviewed for the quality of achieved outcomes, providing evidence as a foundation for decision making by others who may be searching for or considering similar innovations. Although most AHRQ activities are intended to support health care professionals and institutions, the agency supports health care recipients by designing some information specifically for dissemination to the lay public (AHRQ, 2017b).

Private Foundations

Obtaining money for research is becoming increasingly competitive, so voluntary foundations and private and community-based organizations should be investigated as possible funding sources. Many foundations and corporate direct-giving programs are interested in funding health care projects and research. Computer databases and guides to funding are available in local libraries. In addition, grant-seeking enterprises often purchase subscriptions that allow computer access to enhanced listings of funding foundations that include information about the types of projects those foundations typically fund. Although such subscriptions are expensive, costs are often balanced by the efficiency with which suitable funding prospects are identified. An example of such a service is Prospect Research Online (2015; http://www.iwave.com).

Private foundations, such as the Robert Wood Johnson Foundation (2017a, 2017b) and the W.K. Kellogg Foundation (https://www.wkkf.org/grantseekers), offer program funding for health-related research. Investigators are encouraged to pursue funding for small projects through local sources or private foundations until they establish a track record in research design and implementation, which will then lead to securing of funding from public sources.

Nursing Organizations

Sigma Theta Tau International (STTI), the American Nurses Association (ANA), and the Oncology Nurses Society (ONS) are a few of the nursing organizations that fund research studies. STTI makes research grant awards to increase scientific knowledge related to nursing practice. This organization supports creative interdisciplinary research and places importance on identifying best practices and benchmark innovations. Awards are made at the international and local chapter levels. The ANA awards small grants through the American Nurses Foundation. Specialty nursing organizations offer grants to support research related to their specialty. For example, the ONS awards grants that focus on issues related to oncology. A list of current nursing organizations offering funding opportunities can be found online at http://nursingworld.org/research-toolkit/Research-Funding.

Summary

Multiple potential sources of funding are available for research projects. The individual or group wishing to conduct research will need to carefully develop a proposal, search for a possible funding source, and submit the proposal. Libraries and the Internet provide ample information about the many foundations and organizations interested in funding research endeavors. Most research institutions establish offices that help in the search and procurement of funding that supports researchers in their work of knowledge building.

COMPONENTS OF THE RESEARCH PROCESS

The research process involves conceptualizing a research study, planning and implementing that study, and communicating the findings. The process involves a logical flow as each step builds on the previous steps. These steps should be included in published research reports so that the reader has a basis for understanding and critiquing the study (Box 6.1).

BOX 6.1 Components of the Research Process

Research is a process that takes place in a series of steps:
1. Formulating the research question or problem.
2. Defining the purpose of the study.
3. Reviewing related literature.
4. Formulating hypotheses and defining variables.
5. Selecting the research design.
6. Selecting the population, sample, and setting.
7. Conducting a **pilot study**.
8. Collecting the data.
9. Analyzing the data.
10. Communicating conclusions.

STUDY DESIGNS

Study designs are plans that tell a researcher how data are to be collected, from whom data are to be collected, and how data will be analyzed to answer specific research questions. Research studies are classified into two basic methods, quantitative and qualitative, two distinctly different approaches to conducting research. The researcher chooses the method on the basis of the research question and the current level of knowledge about the phenomena and the problem to be studied. Quantitative research is a formal, objective, systematic process in which numeric data are used. Qualitative research is a systematic approach used to describe and promote understanding of human experiences related to health in a nonnumeric fashion. The qualitative approach to research focuses on understanding the human experience as it is lived, thus complementing quantitative methodologies (Polit and Beck, 2017).

Quantitative Designs

Arising from early scientific models for doing research, the nursing discipline directly adopted the quantitative method of conducting research. Thus, quantitative design has traditionally been prevalent in nursing research studies. Deriving meaning from the statistical analysis of numerical data obtained from samples and populations has yielded significant contributions to nursing knowledge. The usual intent of quantitative study is to apply or generalize knowledge from a smaller sample of subjects to a larger population. The most common quantitative designs used in health care research are survey, needs assessment, experimental, quasi-experimental, methodologic, meta-analysis, and secondary analysis. A brief overview of these mostly quantitative study designs is given in Table 6.1. For in-depth understanding of particular methods and their suitability for studying

TABLE 6.1 A Sample of Quantitative Research Methodologies	
Method	**Description**
Survey	Survey research designs are popular in nursing research studies that are designed to obtain information regarding the prevalence, distribution, and interrelationships of variables within a population. This is a useful design for the collection of demographic information, social characteristics, behavioral patterns, and information bases.
Needs assessment	Needs assessments are used to determine what is most beneficial to a specific aggregate group. This design can be used by organizations, communities, or groups to establish priorities for their respective client groups (Polit and Beck, 2017).
Methodologic	Methodologic research focuses on the development of data collection instruments, such as surveys and questionnaires. The goal is to improve the reliability and validity of instruments. This work is time-consuming and tedious, but necessary for the implementation of research studies. However, when quality instruments are developed, they can be used in multiple studies.
Meta-analysis	Meta-analysis is an advanced process whereby multiple research studies on a specific topic are reviewed and the findings of these studies are statistically analyzed. Meta-analysis synthesizes quantitative data from multiple similar studies, thus enlarging the power of the results and allowing more confident generalizations than a single study.
Experimental study	Experimental studies, having several subtypes, include the manipulation of one or more independent variables, random assignment to either a control group or treatment group, and observation of the outcome or effect that presumably is a result of the independent variable. Rigor and control of extraneous variables allow researchers to establish cause-and-effect relationships, testing causal relationships (Polit and Beck, 2017).
Quasi-experimental design	A quasi-experimental design is lacking one of the required components of the experimental design. This is a useful design when randomization, a control group, or the manipulation of one or more variables is not possible. Several subtypes exist.
Secondary analysis	Secondary analysis involves asking new questions of data collected previously. The data may have been generated from previous formal research or may have resulted from any prior systematic collection of data. Examples of prior nonresearch data include the many inevitable records generated as a by-product of health care delivery systems.

particular phenomena, the reader should consult research methods texts.

Qualitative Designs

Qualitative research is designed for discovery rather than verification. It is used to explore little-understood or ambiguous phenomena rather than to verify a cause-and-effect issue. Qualitative methods can be important to the complex study of humans. Concepts that are important to health care professionals often are difficult to reduce in a quantitative way. Interviewing is the main technique used in qualitative methods to explore the meaning of certain experiences to individuals. This method is time-consuming and costly and uses small samples; therefore, generalizations cannot be made from findings. However, in an exploration of issues such as caregiver burden, it might be more appropriate to interview participants with open-ended questions to get their perspective than to send out a standard questionnaire, thereby broadening the data gathered. The main types of qualitative research designs include **phenomenology**, **ethnography**, and **grounded theory**. Table 6.2

TABLE 6.2   A Sample of Qualitative Research Methodologies

Method	Description
Phenomenology	Phenomenology is designed to provide understanding of the participants' "lived experience." This method is a valuable approach for studying intangible experiences, such as grief, hope, and risk taking.
Ethnography	Ethnography is a method used to study phenomena from a cultural perspective. Ethnographers spend time in the cultural setting with the research participants to observe and better understand their experience.
Grounded theory	Grounded theory is designed to explore and describe a social process. This method is used to explore a process that people use to deal with problematic areas of their lives, such as coping with a terminal illness or adjusting to bereavement.

provides brief descriptions of these methods. For a more complete understanding, the reader should refer to qualitative research texts.

Although there is a need for qualitative research studies in health care, qualitative one-on-one interviews take time; they must be recorded, typed, transcribed, and analyzed. Data analysis is conducted by the researcher, who then reviews each transcribed interview line by line to group common conceptual meanings. Concepts are combined to describe the experience for the particular group being studied. The researcher cannot assert that findings from a small unique sample would be the same in a large, diverse population. However, findings should be transferable. The researcher should give a thorough description of the sample and setting so that findings could be expected to occur in similar individuals in a similar setting. In addition, **triangulation** studies may provide the strength needed to increase **generalizability** of the findings.

Triangulation

Triangulation is the use of various research methods or different **data collection** techniques in the same study. *Triangulation* commonly refers to the use of qualitative and quantitative methods in the same study. This method can be useful when data from multiple sources and methods are necessary to provide a holistic understanding of the subject matter.

Pilot Studies

Pilot studies are small-scale studies used to identify the strengths and limitations of a planned larger-scale study. Pilot work is preliminary research that can be used to assess the design, methodology, and feasibility of a study, and typically includes participants who are similar to those who will be used in the larger research study. By performing each step, the researcher can evaluate the effectiveness of the proposed data collection methods to improve and assess the feasibility of the study (Polit and Beck, 2017). Pilot studies can serve to discover preliminary trends in outcomes for a particular agency, personnel, and clients.

EVIDENCE-BASED PRACTICE AND RESEARCH UTILIZATION

From the beginnings of the nursing research endeavor, nurses have been interested in using nursing research to effectively affect the care of individuals and aggregate groups. Despite other incentives for the conduct of research, none is more powerful for a nurse than the difference that might be made in the lives of individuals and aggregates for the betterment of health. Thus, early emphasis in the 1980s on research utilization has been expanded, with the increasing emphasis on EBP. Although the terms *research utilization* and *evidence-based practice* are related, research utilization has been described as a subset of EBP (LoBiondo-Wood and Haber, 2017). EBP encompasses multiple types of evidence, such as research findings, research reviews, and evidence-based theory, and the integration of that evidence with clinician's expertise and patient preferences and values (Melnyk and Fineout-Overholt, 2015) (Box 6.2).

In this second decade of the twenty-first century, EBP has become a major driving force in the disciplinary life of clinicians, students, educators, administrators, and policymakers. Discussion on barriers to research utilization and EBP has shifted to how to actively promote implementation of EBP. Extensive work is being done on the best ways to translate research into practice, spawning a new area of health care science called *translation science*. The promise of translation science is eventually to provide guidance on the best ways to incorporate best evidence into health care, including nursing. As an example of translation strategy, White (2011) describes "nurse champions" as key agents in the "timely integration of discovery" into daily practice. Nurse champions will take ownership of a practice project and personally oversee a practice innovation process from discovery to adoption and dissemination. Table 6.2 provides brief descriptions of the steps involved in the EBP process. Whole texts are available that explain the multiple aspects of EBP (Brown, 2014; Larrabee, 2009a; Malloch and Porter-O'Grady, 2010; Melnyk and Fineout-Overholt, 2015), and various models have been proposed that more carefully detail the process of incorporating evidence into practice (Larrabee, 2009b; Newhouse et al, 2007; Stetler, 1994).

Advancing Evidence-Based Practice

How does one get started with EBP? A list of strategies for encouraging a climate of EBP is likely to look somewhat different depending on the context of care—a clinic, a hospital, or a conglomerate. A short list of broad strategies suggested by Melnyk and Fineout-Overholt (2015) applies regardless of the setting:

- Assessment of barriers to EBP
- Correction of misperceptions about EBP goals and processes
- Questioning of current clinical practices

Assessment should be as comprehensive as possible in order to identify the knowledge, beliefs, and behaviors that are common in the existing system and to raise the awareness of a need for shifting decision making about clinical care toward a consideration of current best evidence. Raising questions about current clinical practices provides a strategy for getting the critical thinking juices flowing about particular clinical practices and problems. Individuals with common interests may form collaborative groups that further strengthen the EBP culture through bonding around specific patient problems and the discovery of evidence-based solutions. The specific tactics, processes, and events that undergird an EBP initiative require allocation of resources, creativity, and

---

BOX 6.2 Seven Steps of Evidence-Based Practice

The following is a brief overview of the multistep process involved in evidence-based practice (EBP):

1. Cultivating a spirit of inquiring.
2. Asking a clinical question in the PICOT format (P, population; I, intervention or interest area; C, comparison intervention or group; O, outcome; and T, time).
3. Searching for and collecting the most relevant best evidence to answer the question. Reliable sources include systematic reviews, pre-appraised literature and studies from **peer-reviewed** journals, and practice guidelines.
4. Critically evaluating the evidence. Making rapid critical appraisal of the findings (evidence) for validity, reliability and applicability, then synthesizing that evidence.
5. Integrating the best evidence with one's clinical expertise and patient preferences and values in making a practice decision regarding whether a practice change should be made.
6. Evaluating outcomes of the practice decision or change on the basis of the evidence. Outcomes should be measured to determine the positive or negative outcomes of the change.
7. Disseminating the outcomes of the EBP decision or change through presentations or publications so that others can benefit from the process.

dedication. Of particular significance to EBP initiatives is the availability of individuals in clinical environments who have the specific responsibility and expertise to understand and translate evidence into practice (Malloch and Porter-O'Grady, 2010).

In order to facilitate and advance the use of EBP by nurses, specific EBP competencies have been developed for the practicing registered nurses (RNs) and advance practice nurses (APNs) (Tables 6.3 and 6.4). The online Merriam-Webster Dictionary generally defines competency as the quality of being competent to perform or capable of performing a function. The ANA (2010) defines competency as "an expected and measurable level of nursing performance that integrates knowledge, skills, abilities, and judgement, based on scientific knowledge and expectations for nursing practice." Melnyk, Gallagher-Ford, & Fineout-Overholt (2016) outline 13 EBP competencies for RNs and APNs, and 11 EBP competencies specifically for APNs (Tables 6.3 and 6.4). The EBP competencies' goal is to ensure competency of nurses in providing EBP care and uniformity in the application and generation of EBP.

Nurse Researcher and Evidence-Based Practice Roles

Two nursing roles are specifically focused on research and EBP: the clinical nurse specialist and the clinical research nurse.

Clinical Nurse Specialist. The clinical nurse specialist (CNS) is a registered nurse with graduate preparation in a specialized area of nursing practice and an expert clinician with additional responsibility for education and research. A CNS is in an ideal position to link research to practice by assessing an agency's readiness for research utilization, consulting with staff to identify clinical problems, and helping staff to discover, implement, and evaluate findings that improve health care delivery (National Association of Clinical Nurse Specialists, 2004).

The CNS also may need to communicate results to legislators or other policymakers if the results potentially affect health policy. Research evidence is important to

Competency	Description
1	Questions clinical practices for the purpose of improving the quality of care
2	Describes clinical problems based on patient assessment date, outcomes management, and quality improvement data
3	Participates in the formulate clinical question using PICOT (P, population; I, intervention/area of interest; C, comparison/intervention group; O, outcome; T, time
4	Systemically searches current evidence (evidence generated from research) to address clinical question
5	Participates in critical appraisal of pre-appraised evidence (i.e., clinical practice guidelines, EB policies and procedures, evidence syntheses)
6	Participates in critical appraisal of published clinical research studies
7	Participates in the evaluation and synthesis of evidence retrieved
8	Systematically collects practice data (e.g., internal patient data, quality improvement, outcome data) for clinical decision making used in providing patient care
9	Integrates evidence gathered from internal and external sources in order to plan EBP changes
10	Implements practice changes based on evidence and clinical expertise and patient's preferences to improve care processes and patient outcomes
11	Evaluates outcomes of evidence-based decisions and practice changes to determine best practices
12	Disseminates best practices supported by evidence to improve quality care and patient outcomes
13	Participates in strategies to sustain an evidence-based practice culture

TABLE 6.3 Evidence-Based Practice (EBP) Competencies for Registered Nurses and Advanced Practice Nurses

From Melnyk, B.M, Gallagher-Ford, L., & Fineout-Overholt, E. (2016). *Implementing the evidence-based practice (EBP) competencies in healthcare: A practical guide for improving quality, safety, and outcomes.* Indianapolis, IN: Sigma Theta Tau International.

TABLE 6.4   Evidence-Based Practice Competencies for Advance Practice Nurses

Competency	Description
14	Systematically conducts an exhaustive search for external evidence* (clinical research studies) to address clinical questions
15	Critically appraises relevant pre-appraised evidence (i.e., clinical guidelines, summaries, synthesis of external evidence)
16	Integrates external evidence from nursing and related fields with internal evidence (i.e., patient data, outcomes management, and quality improvement data)
17	Leads transdisciplinary teams in applying synthesized evidence to initiate clinical decisions and practices changes to improve the health of individuals, groups, and populations
18	Generates internal evidence through outcome management and EBP implementation projects
19	Measures process and outcomes of evidence-based clinical decisions
20	Formulates evidence-based policies and procedures
21	Participates in generation of external evidence with other health care professionals
22	Mentors others in evidence-based decision-making and EBP process
23	Implements strategies to sustain an EBP culture
24	Communicates best evidence to individuals, groups, colleagues, and policymakers

*External evidence refers to evidence generated from research.
From Melnyk, B.M, Gallagher-Ford, L., & Fineout-Overholt, E. (2016). *Implementing the evidence-based practice (EBP) competencies in healthcare: A practical guide for improving quality, safety, and outcomes.* Indianapolis, IN: Sigma Theta Tau International.

policy making because it provides a logical foundation for policy change. The process of writing brief summaries of evidence or personally testifying about particular topics should be approached carefully. One should know the target audience, the exact policy issue, the background of the issue, and the full range of pertinent evidence (Melnyk and Fineout-Overholt, 2015).

If agencies do not have a CNS, they should be encouraged to develop relationships with researchers in university settings or other agencies. Professors in academic settings are expected to conduct research and often are interested in collaborating with health care agencies that might serve as a site. These agencies often have the patient population that can serve as a study sample. For example, a university professor interested in home health care issues might collaborate with an agency to examine the efficacy of various health care delivery models for patients with congestive heart failure. In today's care environment, it would be essential for the agency to offer care that is the most effective and efficient. Therefore, this collaborative relationship would reward the researcher and the health care agency.

Case Study 6.1 is an illustration of how a CNS led efforts to use research findings to improve practice.

Clinical Research Nurse. The Clinical research nursing role focuses on the care of research participants. In addition to providing and coordinating clinical care, clinical research nurses have a central role in assuring participant safety, ongoing maintenance of informed consent, integrity of protocol implementation, accuracy of data collection, data recording and follow up" (Hastings, 2009).

Emerging Roles. In addition to the CNS, there are emerging role definitions for the clinical nurse leader (CNL) and the doctor of nursing practice (DNP). Given the specified role definitions published by the American Association of Colleges of Nursing (AACN), the CNL and DNP are considered to be major contributors to the advancement of nursing research and EBP (AACN, 2014). CNLs use quality improvement methods in evaluating individual and aggregate client care and for self-improvement.

Nurses prepared at the DNP level provide leadership for EBP in nursing and translate evidence-based nursing research into their own practice. They are expected to disseminate and integrate new knowledge. Regardless of the official role definition, nurses at the point of care and

CASE STUDY 6.1

Mary, a CNS in a medical center, asks the staff nurses on a pediatric oncology unit to identify patient care problems that need to be investigated. The nurses identify pain control as a major problem for the children admitted to the unit. In talking with the nurses on the unit, Mary discovers that the nurses routinely use physiologic measures, such as heart rate and blood pressure, as indicators of pain. Occasionally, the nurses rely on parents' reports, but rarely do they consult the child.

Mary conducts a systematic review of the literature/evidence to determine proven ways to assess pain in children. In the *Western Journal of Nursing Research,* Mary discovers a meta-analysis of pediatric pain assessment techniques. Findings from this study indicate that self-report tools are appropriate for most children 4 years and older and provide the most accurate measure of children's pain. Mary discovers a pediatric pain interview tool in the literature that she thinks would be practical and feasible for use on the unit.

She then writes a utilization memo to the nurse manager citing the problem (inadequate pain control), the research findings documented in the literature, and a suggestion for change in practice (use of the self-report pain assessment) on the pediatric oncology unit. Next, Mary organizes a meeting with the nurses to discuss conducting a pilot study on the unit for the purpose of comparing the effectiveness of the pediatric pain assessment interview tool and their usual procedures for assessing pain in the pediatric oncology patients. Findings from this study are incorporated into practice through documentation of the preferred method of pain assessment in the unit's protocol.

The change instituted by the pediatric oncology unit is cited in the medical center's accreditation report as an example of how the medical center is meeting standards of care in pain management.

nursing division leaders increasingly may be called upon to lead and contribute to collaborative research and EBP initiatives at the health care agency level (Larrabee, 2009a).

About the Evidence

Practice decisions made from a foundation of evidence are more likely to be clear, rational, and motivational than those made from the foundation of mere authority. Although research evidence forms the backbone of EBP, other evidence types, such as patient values and preferences, expert opinion, theory-based information, evidence-based theories, and compiled database information, are also useful (Fawcett and Garity, 2009; Malloch and Porter-O'Grady, 2010; Melnyk and Fineout-Overholt, 2015). When care is being delivered to an individual, evidence regarding patient assessment and resource availability must also be considered (Melnyk and Fineout-Overholt, 2015).

Locating Published Research and Evidence Summaries for Evidence-Based Practice

The health care literature is continually and rapidly expanding; the task of keeping up with relevant health care information is daunting. Strategies to facilitate access to research evidence include formulating a clear and concise clinical question, identifying the research design that would best answer the question, and identifying the most appropriate place to look for studies that answer the question.

Many health care practitioners routinely read clinical practice journals but are unfamiliar with research or EBP journals. Computerized databases aid the process of locating research relevant to current practice. These databases list article information, provide a short summary, identify key words, and links to similar articles. *Cumulative Index to Nursing and Allied Health Literature* (CINAHL) (2017) is an index of selected journal articles about nursing, allied health, biomedicine, and health care. MEDLINE (Medical Literature Analysis and Retrieval System Online) is the most comprehensive online resource for national and international medical literature (U.S. National Library of Medicine, 2017). Multiple other useful databases may be available from academic and health care libraries. These databases consist largely of primary or original research studies as well as guidelines and best practices (National Guidelines Clearinghouse; http://www.guideline.org).

University and public libraries are the major access points to these databases and journals, which are available online directly from publishers. Because of online availability, novice users may be tempted to limit searches only to those articles that are available online as full text.

This is a serious mistake that any investigator of published literature should avoid.

The search for literature should be conducted with the intent of procuring all or most of the current articles appropriate to answer the clinical question. A truly comprehensive reading of the literature may include all articles of current and historical relevance to the topic.

Even though nurses may have access to computerized databases to assist with a literature search, they often are unaware of the journals that are entirely devoted to the publication of research studies. Box 6.3 contains a list of research journals and other health-related journals that publish research and evidence summaries.

BOX 6.3   Nursing and Health-Related Journals

Nursing
Advances in Nursing Science
Applied Nursing Research
Biological Research for Nursing
Clinical Nursing Research
Evidence-Based Nursing
International Journal of Nursing Studies
Journal of Nursing Scholarship
Journal of Advanced Nursing
Journal of Transcultural Nursing
Nursing Clinics of North America
Nursing Economics
Nursing Research
Nursing Science Quarterly
Qualitative Health Research
Research in Nursing and Health
Western Journal of Nursing Research
Worldviews on Evidence-Based Nursing

Health
American Journal of Public Health
Hastings Center Report
Health Affairs
Health Care Management Review
Health Services Research
Heart & Lung
Journal of Pain & Palliative Care Pharmacotherapy
International Journal of Evidence-Based Healthcare
Journal of Health Economics
Journal of the American Medical Association
New England Journal of Medicine
Oncology Nursing Forum
Social Science and Medicine

Other important sources for locating evidence are as follows:

- *Clinical practice guidelines* are systematically developed statements to assist practitioner and patient decisions about appropriate health care for specific clinical circumstances. In the United Kingdom, the Cochrane Collaboration (http://www.cochrane.org) is an electronic resource for locating high-quality information quickly. This resource has published hundreds of intervention guidelines based on meta-analyses and research reviews of health care practice areas. *Evidence-Based Nursing* (http://www.evidence-basednursing.com) selects original studies from more than 100 health care journals and presents critical appraisal and summary in brief abstracts.

- *The Internet* is a useful source of health care information for both health care professionals and consumers. However, the potential for harm from inaccurate information is substantial. As a result, it is important to evaluate the quality of web-based materials on the Internet.

Types and Levels of Evidence

Evidence exists in many forms. Perhaps the most obvious form is the journal article describing a single research study. Prior to the current disciplinary emphasis on EBP, it would have been the responsibility of the reader of these reports to critique each article and decide which, if any, of the research findings could be used in practice (research utilization). Though this technique continues to be somewhat useful, more systematic methods have been developed for synthesizing multiple research reports on a single topic. These systematic review methods include meta-analysis, integrative research reviews, and metasynthesis.

In a meta-analysis, the findings of multiple quantitative randomized controlled trials (RCTs), studies on a single topic, are statistically analyzed to produce a summary statistic. A metasynthesis takes the findings of multiple qualitative studies on a single topic and synthesizes and amplifies the narrative information contained in the reports. An integrated research review (IRR) takes the findings from experimental and non-experimental studies on a single topic and synthesizes them to provide a comprehensive understanding of the phenomena. The importance of such reviews is that they represent a meticulous integration of the best evidence available at the time the review was conducted and are considered to provide the highest possible evidence (Melnyk and Fineout-Overholt, 2015; Polit and Beck, 2017). Therefore, individuals or agencies with clinical questions are able to consult well-prepared knowledge syntheses for possible application in the practice arena. Fig. 6.1 illustrates an evidence hierarchy based on levels of evidence regarding the effectiveness of interventions and/or findings.

With such an array of evidence types, it is not surprising that evidence is viewed as requiring an assessment of just how strong it is. The terms *evidence hierarchy, levels of evidence,* and *strength of evidence* are used to refer to the categorical classifications that have been proposed to rate evidence along a continuum from best evidence to worst evidence. Most rating schemes rate meta-analyses of well-conducted RCTs as best evidence, with other

evidence types sitting lower in the hierarchy (Melnyk and Fineout-Overholt, 2015; Polit and Beck, 2017).

Clinical Practice Guidelines

A **clinical practice guideline (CPG)** is an evidence-based guide to clinical practice developed by experts in a particular field for direct application in clinical environments (Polit and Beck, 2017). Like systematic reviews, guidelines gather, appraise, and combine evidence. Guidelines, however, go beyond systematic reviews in attempting to address all the issues relevant to a clinical decision and all the values that could sway a clinical recommendation. Guidelines make explicit recommendations and, in some circumstances, may be used to define "standard of care." In this scenario a CPG *may* have legal ramifications. Several court cases have

Fig. 6.1 Quick guide to an evidence hierarchy of designs for cause-probing questions. RCT, randomized controlled trial. (From Polit, D.E., & Beck, T.C. [2017]. *Nursing research: Generating and assessing evidence for nursing practice,* Philadelphia: Lippincott Williams & Wilkins.)

addressed the use of CPGs, but there are no set judicial standards for how these documents may be used and interpreted in individual cases (Moffet and Moore, 2011). This is an evolving discussion because practice guidelines are playing important roles in guiding health care practices. In theory, any professional association, government agency, or health system can produce CPGs; however, practice guidelines are to be researched and driven by evidence. Practice guidelines are based on the consensus of a group of decision makers—ideally experts and front-line clinicians.

Critical Appraisal

Nurses at all levels of educational preparation should critically read research journal articles and research summary articles. These articles are accepted on a competitive basis and undergo a *blind review* because the reviewers are unaware of who wrote the article. Therefore, readers can assume that experts have scrutinized it for merit and relevance to nursing; however, the reader should critically appraise the findings for validity. This is accomplished through detailed analysis of study design and measurement strategies. The abstract gives an overview of the study, and the discussion or conclusion provides suggestions for nursing practice based on the findings of the research study.

Pre-appraised evidence such as systematic reviews also require appraisal, but the emphasis is on whether the review provides ample and trustworthy evidence for answering a particular clinical question. The appraisal of various types of research and research summary articles for application to practice is best approached by using defined appraisal guidelines that may be located on the Internet, such as those from the EQUATOR network (http://www.equator-network.org). Careful appraisal may or may not lead one to make a change in practice. If change is implemented, the health care provider has an ethical and moral responsibility to evaluate the quality of patient outcomes derived from the change.

Rather than being a simple process of implementing the practice suggestions found at the end of a research report, use of research requires careful and complex analysis, wise implementation, and patient outcome assessment. Clinical practice guidelines can be methodologically weak or strong and thus may yield either valid or invalid recommendations. When considering using a practice guideline as a basis for an agency protocol, or as a guide for providing patient care, health care providers need to critically assess the credibility, clinical significance, and applicability of the guideline's recommendations. To facilitate the review process there are instruments for appraising the quality of a clinical practice guideline. The Appraisal of Guidelines for Research and Evaluation (AGREE) Instrument is a reliable and valid instrument that evaluates the process of practice guideline development and quality of reporting (Brouwers et al, 2010). AGREE can be accessed at http://www.agree trust.org.

Evolution of Evidence-Based Practice: Some Examples

Though much work remains to be done, the potential effect of research on health care knowledge and practice can be demonstrated by two examples:

- The use of heparinized saline for flushing capped peripheral intravenous catheters was compared with saline only. Saline only was found to be clinically effective in maintaining patency of peripheral catheters (Goode et al, 1991, 1993) and in neonates (Cook et al, 2011; Shah et al, 2005). As a result of this research, many acute care facilities revised their institutional policies to recommend saline only as a flush for peripheral intravenous catheters.
- Pressure ulcers are a significant problem for multiple populations. It should not be surprising that many groups are interested in their prevention and treatment. An online search of the National Guideline Clearinghouse yielded multiple clinical guideline statements contributed by groups, public and private, nursing and medical. In the case of pressure ulcers, a significant amount of research evidence is available for implementing prevention and management strategies.

From these two examples, it can be seen that research evidence can play a significant role in health care practice. However, the process of spreading the "good news" about new or refined practice-related knowledge is a complex one. Researchers must make the knowledge they generate available and understandable. Practitioners must access, interpret, and carefully apply research evidence. The scientific process may take years to yield enough data to make clinical recommendations and more years to evaluate the effect of evidence-based changes through outcomes research. For instance, peptic ulcer disease was researched for many years before the discovery and acceptance of the presence of *Helicobacter pylori* in the stomach and duodenum (Marshall, 2002).

ETHICAL ISSUES RELATED TO RESEARCH

Institutional Review

In institutional review, a committee called an *institutional review board (IRB)* or human subjects committee examines research proposals to make sure that the ethical rights of those individuals participating in the research study are protected. Participants must sign an informed consent that explains the study and assures them of their rights, including their right to refuse to participate or to withdraw from the study. Institutions that receive federal funding or conduct drug or medical device research regulated by the U.S. Food and Drug Administration (FDA) are required by federal regulations to establish an IRB. Federally funded studies have to meet strict guidelines to ensure the protection of the human rights of subjects, such as self-determination, privacy, anonymity and confidentiality, fair treatment, and protection from discomfort and harm. The informed consent must include essential study information and statements about potential risks and benefits, protection of anonymity and confidentiality, voluntary participation, compensation, alternative treatment, and specific information on how to contact the investigator (Polit and Beck, 2017).

Historical Examples of Unethical Research

In addition to the institutional review process, a number of codes and regulations have been implemented to ensure ethical conduct in research. The two historical documents are the Nuremberg Code and the Declaration of Helsinki, which were developed in response to unethical acts such as the Nazi experiments. These experiments, which occurred in the 1930s and 1940s, used untested drugs, sterilization, and euthanasia on prisoners of war. The experiments were unethical because they caused grievous harm to the subjects and denied them the opportunity to refuse participation (Polit and Beck, 2017).

Another famous incident of unethical research that prompted the need to oversee the conduct of research is the famous Tuskegee syphilis study. This study, which was initiated by the U.S. Public Health Service, continued for 40 years. The study was conducted to determine the natural course of syphilis in African-American men. Many participants were not adequately informed about the purpose and procedures of the study. The subjects periodically were examined but did not receive treatment for syphilis, even after penicillin was determined to be effective. The study was not stopped until 1972, when published reports of it sparked public outrage (Centers for Disease Control and Prevention, 2017). *Bad Blood* a comprehensive documentary account of the Tuskegee syphilis study, clearly relates the study's adverse effects on research participation by African-Americans and on race relations in the United States (Jones, 1993).

As late as the 1960s, another famous study that violated human rights took place. The Jewish Chronic Disease Hospital in New York was the setting for a study to determine patients' rejection of liver cancer cells. Twenty-two patients were injected with liver cancer cells without being informed that they were taking part in the research. In addition, the physician directing the study did not have institutional approval for a study that had the potential to cause the subjects harm or even death (Murphy, 2004).

In institutions in which IRB approval is not required for non–federally funded programs, the researcher should seek external advice regarding ethical considerations. When IRB approval is an option, researchers should seek it because IRB approval demonstrates scientific rigor.

■ SUMMARY

Educators must prepare health care professionals to have an appreciation of research and to participate in research at the level of their preparation. Practicing nurses must seek, develop, and adopt EBP protocols while encouraging affiliated institutions to support this effort. Health care administrators must facilitate an environment that supports research efforts. Collaborative arrangements between health care agencies and universities must be developed for such activities as student projects, continuing education, development of clinical practice guidelines, and research endeavors. Consumers must be educated about the value of health care research, and policymakers must be informed of pertinent findings so that results can be translated into health policy.

REFERENCES

Agency for Healthcare Research and Quality. (2017a). *AHRQ vision*. Retrieved from http://integrationacademy.ahrq.gov.

Agency for Healthcare Research and Quality. (2017b). *Healthcare innovations exchange*. CDC. Retrieved from http://www.innovations.ahrq.gov.

Brouwers, M. C., Kho, M. E., Browman, G. P., Burgers, J. S., Cluzeau, F., Feder, G., et al. (2010). AGREE II: advancing guidelines development, reporting and evaluation in healthcare. *Canadian Medical Association Journal*, *182*, E839–E842.

Brown, S. (2014). *Evidence-based nursing: The research-practice connection* (3rd ed.). Sudbury, MA: Jones and Bartlett.

Centers for Disease Control and Prevention. (2017). *U.S. Public Health Service syphilis study at Tuskegee*. Retrieved from https://www.cdc.gov/tuskegee/timeline.htm.

CINAHL Information Systems. *Nursing resources from EBESCO*. Retrieved from https://www.ebscohost.com/nursing/products/cinahl-databases/cinahl-complete.

The Cochrane Collection. (2017). *Cochran reviews*. Retrieved from http:///www.cochrane.org/.

Cook, L., Bellini, S., & Cusson, R. M. (2011). Heparinized saline vs normal saline for maintenance of intravenous access in neonates: an evidence-based practice change. *Advances in Neonatal Care*, *11*(3), 208–215.

Department of Health and Human Services. (2017). *National Institutes of Health*. Retrieved from https://www.cc.nih.gov/nursing/crn/crn_2010.html.

Fawcett, J., & Garity, J. (2009). *Evaluating research for evidence-based nursing practice*. Philadelphia: FA Davis.

Goode, C. J., Titler, M., Rakel, B., Ones, D. S., Kleiber, C., Small, S., et al. (1991). A meta-analysis of effects of heparin flush and saline flush: quality and cost implications. *Nursing Research*, *40*(6), 324–330.

Goode, C. J., Kleiber, C., Titler, M., Small, S., Rakel, B., Steelman, V. M., et al. (1993). Improving practice through research: the case of heparin vs. saline for peripheral intermittent infusion devices. *Medsurg Nursing*, *2*(1), 23–27.

Grady, P. A. (2014). Charting future directions in nursing research: NINR's innovative questions initiative. *Journal of Nursing Scholarship*, *46*(3), 143.

Gray, JR, Grove, SK, & Sutherland, S. (2017). *Burns and Groves: Practice of nursing*, (8th ed.). Philadelphia, Elsevier/Saunders.

Hastings C. (2009). Nursing at the NIH Clinical center: clinical research nursing: background and overview. Retrieved from https://www.cc.nih.gov/nursing/crn/crn_2010.html.

Houser, J. (2015). *Nursing research: Reading, using, and creating evidence*. Burlington: Jones & Bartlett Learning.

Institute of Medicine. (2011). *The future of Nursing: Leading change, advancing health*. Washington, DC: The National Academies Press. Retrieved from https://www.nap.edu/catalog/12956/the-future-of-nursing-leading-change-advancing-health.

Institute of Medicine. (2001). *Report brief: crossing the quality chasm: a new health system for the 21st century*. Retrieved from https://www.iom.edu/~/media/Files/Report%20Files/2001/Crossing-the-Quality-Chasm/Quality%20Chasm%202001%20%20report%20brief.pdf.

Jones, J. (1993). *Bad blood: The Tuskegee syphilis experiment* (rev. ed.). New York: Free Press.

Larrabee, J. (2009a). *Nurse to nurse: Evidence-based practice*. New York: McGraw-Hill.

Larrabee, J. (2009b). *The model for evidence-based practice change, Nurse to nurse: Evidence-based practice*. New York: McGraw-Hill.

LoBiondo-Wood, G., & Haber, J. (2017). *Nursing research: methods and critical appraisal for evidence-based practice* (9th ed.). St. Louis: Elsevier.

Malloch, K., & Porter-O'Grady, T. (2010). *Introduction to evidence-based practice in nursing and health care* (2nd ed.). Sudbury, MA: Jones and Bartlett.

Marshall, B. (2002). The discovery that Heliobacter pylori, a spiral bacterium, caused peptic ulcer disease. In J. Barry, & B. Marshall (Eds.), *Helicobacter pioneers: Firsthand accounts from the scientists who discovered helicobacter, 1892–1982* (pp. 165–202). Oxford: Blackwell.

Melnyk, B. M., & Fineout-Overholt, E. (2015). *Evidence-based practice in nursing and healthcare: A guide to best practice* (3rd ed., pp. 3–23). Philadelphia: Lippincott Williams & Wilkins/Wolters Kluwer.

Melnyk, B. M., Gallagher-Ford, L., & Fineout-Overholt, E. (2016). *Implementing the evidence-based practice (EBP) competencies in healthcare: A practical guide for improving quality, safety, and outcomes*. Indianapolis, IN: Sigma Theta Tau International.

Moffett, P. & Moore, G. (2011). Standard of care: legal history and definitions: Bad and good news. *West J Emerg Med.*, *12*(1): 109–112.

Murphy, T. F. (2004). *Case studies in biomedical research ethics*. Cambridge, MA: MIT Press.

National Association of Clinical Nurse Specialists. (2004). *Statement on clinical nurse specialists practice and education* (2nd ed.). Retrieved from http://nacns.org/wp-content/uploads/2016/11/NACNS-Statement.pdf.

National Institute of Nursing Research. (2016). *NINR strategic plan*. Retrieved from https://www.ninr.nih.gov/aboutninr/-mission-and-strategic-plan.

Newhouse RP, Dearholt SL, Poe SS, et al. (2007). *Johns Hopkins nursing evidence-based practice model and guidelines*. Indianapolis: Sigma Theta Tau International.

Polit, D., Beck, C. (2017). *Nursing research: Generating and assessing evidence for nursing practice* (10th ed.). Philadelphia: Lippincott Williams & Wilkins.

Prospect Research Online. (2015). *Iwave information systems.* Retrieved from www.iwave.com/our-solutions/prospect-research-online.

Robert Wood Johnson Foundation. (2017a). *About RWJF.* Retrieved from https://www.rwjf.org/en/about-rwjf.html.

Robert Wood Johnson Foundation. (2017b). *Grants Explorer.* Retrieved from http://www.rwjf.org/en/grants.html#q/maptype/grants/II/37.91,-96.38/z/4.

Shah, P. S., Ng, E., & Sinha, A. K. (2006). *Heparin for prolonging peripheral intravenous catheter use in neonates.* The Cochrane Library, Issue 4. Chichester, UK: John Wiley & Sons, Ltd, Last updated June 1, 2005.

Stetler, C. B. (1994). Refinement of the Stetler/Marram model for the application of research findings to practice. *Nursing Outlook, 42*(1), 15–25.

Titler, M. G., Kleiber, C., Steelman V. J., Rakel, B. A., Budreau, G., Everett, L. Q., et al. (2001). The Iowa model of evidence-based practice to promote quality care, *Critical Care Nursing Clinics of North America, 13*(4), 497–509.

U.S. National Library of Medicine. (2017). *Fact sheet MEDLINE.* Retrieved from https://www.nlm.nih.gov/pubs/factsheets/medline.html.

White, C. L. (2011). Nurse champions: a key role in bridging the gap between research and practice. *Journal of Emergency Nursing, 37*(4), 386–387.

Wise, N. J. (2009). Maintaining magnet status: establishing an evidenced-based practice committee. *AORN Journal, 90*(2), 205–213. doi:10.1016/j.aorn.2009.02.016.

W. K. Kellogg Foundation. *Grantseekers.* Retrieved from https://www.wkkf.org/grantseekers.

7

Paying for Health Care in America: Rising Costs and Challenges

Barbara Cherry, DNSc, MBA, RN, NEA-BC

There is a tug of war for the shrinking health care dollar.

ⓔ Additional resources are available online at: *http://evolve.elsevier.com/Cherry/*

LEARNING OUTCOMES

After studying this chapter, the reader will be able to:

1. Analyze major factors that have influenced health care access and financing since the middle of the twentieth century.
2. Integrate knowledge of health care resources, access, and financing into managing professional nursing care.
3. Critique the relationship between contemporary economic issues and trends and professional nursing practice.
4. Discuss the implications of the Patient Protection and Affordable Care Act (PPACA) for nursing and health care.

KEY TERMS

Centers for Medicare & Medicaid Services (CMS) The federal government agency that administers Medicare and Medicaid.

DRGs (diagnosis-related groups) A common method of reimbursement for health care services based on a predetermined fixed price-per-diagnosis.

Effectiveness Production of a desired outcome; taking the right action to achieve the expected result.

Efficiency The extent to which resources, such as energy, time, and money, are used to produce the intended result.

GDP (gross domestic product) The measure of the total value of goods and services produced within a country; the most comprehensive overall measure of economic output; provides key insight into the driving forces of the economy.

Health Insurance Exchange Also known as the "Health Insurance Marketplace," an online marketplace for individuals to shop for and purchase health insurance at affordable rates and to identify whether they qualify for cost assistance subsidies to help pay the cost of the insurance; states

We would like to acknowledge Marylane Wade Koch, MSN, RN, for her contributions to this chapter in previous editions.

established health insurance exchanges as a component of the Patient Protection and Affordable Care Act to provide access to affordable health insurance options for American citizens and legal residents.

Marginal An economic term that refers to a small or insignificant change in some variable (e.g., the number of medical tests performed).

Medicaid A jointly sponsored state and federal program that pays for medical services for persons who are elderly, poor, blind, or disabled and for certain families with dependent children who meet specified income guidelines.

Medicare A federally funded health insurance program for the disabled, persons with end-stage renal disease, and persons 65 years of age and older who qualify for Social Security benefits.

Patient Protection and Affordable Care Act (PPACA) A federal statute enacted in 2010 that requires U.S. citizens and legal residents to have health insurance through comprehensive health care reform; expands health care coverage access to millions of people who were previously uninsured.

Private health insurance A method for individuals to maintain insurance coverage for health care costs through a contract with a health insurance company that agrees to pay all or a portion of the cost of a set of defined health care services such as routine, preventive, and emergency health care; hospitalizations; medical procedures; and/or prescription drugs. Typically, the private insurance is provided through an individual's employer with a portion of the cost paid by the employer and a portion paid by the employee. Private insurance policies can also be purchased by individuals but are generally much more expensive than when provided through an employer's group plan.

Prospective payment system A method of reimbursing health care providers (e.g., physicians, hospitals) in which the total amount of payment for care is predetermined on the basis of the patient's diagnosis; encourages increased efficiency in the use of health care services because providers are reimbursed at a predetermined level regardless of how many services are rendered or procedures performed to treat a particular diagnostic category; the most common method of payment in today's health care system.

Provider A licensed health care professional (e.g., physician or nurse practitioner) who or an organization (e.g., hospital) that receives reimbursement for providing health care services.

Retrospective payment system A method of reimbursing health care providers (e.g., physicians, hospitals) in which professional services are rendered and charges are billed based on the basis of the individual service provided; also known as the "fee-for-service" payment system. This system may encourage overuse of health care services because the more services rendered or procedures performed, the more revenue received by providers.

Single payer system A method of reimbursement in which one payer, usually the government, pays all health care expenses for citizens; funded by taxes; decisions about covered treatments, drugs, and services are made by the government. Though the terms universal health care and single payer system are sometimes used interchangeably, universal health care could be administered by many different payer groups; both offer all citizens health insurance coverage.

Third-party payer An organization other than the patient and the provider (e.g., hospital, physician, nurse practitioner), such as an insurance company, that assumes responsibility for payment of health care charges. An individual's health insurance plan provided by his or her employer is considered a third-party payer.

PROFESSIONAL/ETHICAL ISSUE

Susan and Matt Taylor have a 2-year-old daughter, Carmen. Susan worked full time as a nurse in a local clinic until Carmen was born. So far, the Taylors have been able to budget for Susan to work only one day a week so she can stay home and care for Carmen. They downsized to a smaller home and adjusted their spending to address the changes in the economy and rising costs of basic living such as food, gas, and utilities.

The Taylors have health insurance through Matt's employer, a small local business. The premiums and co-pays have increased over the past few years, stressing their tight budget. The Taylors believe that all people should have access to quality health care, and as a nurse, Susan has been an advocate for those who needed care, with or without insurance. However, the Taylors question why their insurance costs continue to increase and strain their already tight family budget. Matt and Susan did not anticipate the yearly increases in health insurance costs and are struggling with many questions. Is it fair that the Taylors' lifestyle should be negatively affected by the rising cost for health insurance, especially since they are a healthy family and practice good health behaviors? How are small businesses like Matt's employer affected by the cost of health insurance for their employees? Are there less expensive insurance alternatives available to the Taylors? What would happen if the Taylors chose not to carry health insurance?

VIGNETTE

As a home care nurse for many years, Callie Thompson primarily provided care to older adults. Knowledge of Medicare coverage guidelines for service was critical to the financial success of the home care agency she works for. Today, in the home care agency, she cares for patients of all ages with varying reimbursement guidelines. These guidelines, which affect the types of services she provides for her patients, differ among managed care organizations, government-provided coverage, and insurance companies. When she first took this job, understanding Medicare coverage guidelines was a new challenge. Now even more is required. Callie knows that today's nurse needs extensive knowledge of health care reimbursement guidelines and the economic influences on professional practice to provide quality patient care.

Questions To Consider While Reading this Chapter

1. What do health care economics and finance have to do with me as I provide patient care?
2. Why do I need to understand health care reimbursement and its implications for my practice? Is that not the role of the finance department or business office at my workplace?
3. With so many variations in health care insurance, I have a hard time understanding my own policy coverage. What role do I have in helping my patients understand their insurance or coverage options? Can being a more informed consumer add value to my practice?

CHAPTER OVERVIEW

In the past several decades, the costs of health care have continued to increase, with economic issues taking a central role in health care decision making. Hospital managers know that for most patients the hospital will receive a predetermined payment, regardless of length of stay and specific treatments. Physicians and nurse practitioners recognize that the prescribed course of treatment for their patients may be analyzed by a peer review committee; the costs their patients incur may be compared with those of other providers or against cost benchmarks. Businesses require employees to cover larger amounts of their health insurance premiums and/or pay larger deductibles and copayments. Health insurance companies "manage" care, sometimes placing limits on medical care coverage, on providers in the network, or on the site of care delivery. The **Patient Protection and Affordable Care Act (PPACA)** of 2010 added a new dimension to health care financing with various insurance options for universal coverage of American citizens and alternative models of reimbursement to promote quality and cost-effective health care.

The objective of this chapter is to provide an overview of the major economic issues and trends driving changes in health care delivery, how health care is paid for, and how these issues affect nursing practice. This chapter presents information about historical trends in health care finance, the problem of the uninsured and underinsured, methods of paying for health care, and the effect of health care finance on professional nursing practice.

HISTORY OF HEALTH CARE FINANCING

The high costs of health care did not occur overnight. To understand current health care financing, it is necessary to understand its history (Table 7.1). Historically, several underlying themes have driven health care financing in the United States. Among these are the following:

- The physician's role as being primarily responsible for health care decision making
- The broad objective of providing the "best" possible care to everyone
- The rapidly increasing sophistication and cost of medical technology
- Economic incentives and the fee-for-service payment method that encouraged overuse of health care services

For many years, physician domination in decision making and the fee-for-service payment method were intertwined and contributed to the lack of cost consciousness in health care. Physicians made all decisions about what health care services were needed; costs were rarely discussed between physician and patient, so the cost of care was not considered until bill-paying time. Medical tests or procedures were provided if the physician determined that they offered even marginal aid or diagnostic information.

Beginning in the 1960s, the attitude that "if it might help, do it" flourished as the rapid pace of sophisticated technologies enhanced providers' abilities to provide treatment. The more tests or procedures performed, the greater the earnings for providers (i.e., hospitals and physicians) because they were paid according to the number of procedures performed or services provided.

TABLE 7.1	Historical Highlights of Health Care Finance
1847	Massachusetts Health Insurance of Boston offers a group policy.
1861–1865	Insurance plans become available during the Civil War.
1890	Individual disability and/or illness policies become available.
1929	First group health coverage is offered for a monthly charge; teachers in Dallas, Texas, contract with Baylor Hospital. This is the beginning of Blue Cross/Blue Shield insurance.
1932	Blue Cross insurance forms.
1934	Hospitals receive payment through Blue Cross, a prepaid health insurance plan to protect hospitals during the Great Depression.
1945	Blue Cross captures 50% of the insurance market.
1946	California Physician Service ensures physician payment through Blue Shield plans.
1950s	Employee benefit packages are initiated to attract workers.
1954	Government disability program with Social Security coverage becomes available.
1965	Medicare and Medicaid programs are created, making comprehensive health care available to millions of Americans.
1977	Health Care Financing Administration (HCFA) is created to manage Medicare and Medicaid separately from the Social Security Administration.
1980–1990	Managed care plans emerge.
1983	Hospitals become answerable to the diagnosis-related group (DRG) system.
2001–2003	The Centers for Medicare & Medicaid Services is created, replacing the HCFA.
2003	Medicare Prescription Drug Improvement and Modernization Act of 2003, the most significant expansion of Medicare since its enactment, including a prescription drug benefit, is enacted.
2006	Blue Cross/Blue Shield plans cover more than 94 million (1 in 3) Americans. Pay-for-performance is introduced as a model of reimbursement for health care services.
2010	Patient Protection and Affordable Care Act, comprehensive health care reform for universal coverage of Americans, is enacted. Implementation is scheduled to occur over several years, from 2010–2018.

Instead of attempting to allocate medical resources to the highest medical need, the financial incentive was to provide as much care as possible using the most technically advanced methods of care. Overuse of health services and rapid cost inflation resulted.

Yet consumers of health care remained insulated from cost inflation. Most patients had some form of insurance or third-party payment and did not pay the full cost for their care or even for their health insurance premiums. The full cost of care remained hidden from consumers because costs were subsidized by employers or by taxpayers through such programs as Medicare and Medicaid. Providers had little incentive to contain costs, so the demand for medical care generated "perverse" economic incentives in which providers received more income for using more services with no financial risk for their use of additional resources.

These perverse economic incentives had a drastic effect on the Medicare program. Medicare was established by the U.S. Congress in 1965 to provide health insurance coverage for persons 65 years and older who are eligible for Social Security benefits, persons with end-stage renal disease, and the eligible disabled population. By the early 1980s, increased medical usage (increased intensity of care) and high inflation combined with a growing older adult population generated substantial increases in Medicare costs. The rapid growth of Medicare expenditures became a major factor in the federal budget deficit, causing the Centers for Medicare & Medicaid Services (CMS) to rethink the entire Medicare payment system. This process led to a revolution in how the government and private health insurance companies paid for health care.

Health Care Financing Revolution of the 1980s

The rising cost of health care over the last 50 years is a dangerous trend that poses a significant threat to the U.S. economy. In 1965, annual health care expenditures in the United States were $202 per person; in 2016, the national health expenditures had risen to $10,348 per person (CMS, 2017a). Total health care spending increased from $1.3 trillion in 2000 to $3.3 trillion in 2016; national health expenditures as a percentage of the gross domestic product (GDP) was 17.9% in 2016 and is projected to be 19.9% by 2025 (CMS, 2017a). This means that for every dollar a person spends buying products or services in the United States, almost 18 cents goes to pay for

health care. In contrast, health care spending in 2017 in neighboring Canada was expected to reach an all-time high of $6604 per person in 2017, with a health care GDP of 11.5% (Canadian Institute for Health Information, 2017).

To control rapidly rising health care costs, Medicare moved from a retrospective (fee-for-service) payment system to a prospective payment system (PPS) based on diagnosis-related groups (DRGs) in 1983. This shift was critical for hospitals because Medicare is the largest single payer of hospital charges. Under DRGs, each Medicare patient is assigned to a diagnostic grouping on the basis of his or her primary diagnosis at hospital admission. Medicare limits total payment to the hospital to the amount pre-established for that DRG, unlike with the previous approach, in which hospitals billed Medicare for any and all services provided to patients and Medicare reimbursed these charges with a generous payment schedule.

Since 1983, if hospital costs exceed the DRG payment for a patient's treatment, the hospital incurs a loss, but if costs are less than the DRG amount, the hospital makes a profit. Thus, hospitals face a strong financial incentive to reduce the patient's length of stay and minimize procedures and tests performed. Although DRGs originally applied only to hospital payments for Medicare patients, similar reimbursement arrangements were initiated by private insurance companies. Implementation of the DRG system created a new role for nurses as utilization review experts to review medical records and determine the most appropriate DRGs for patients.

The Development of Managed Care

With the shift to prospective payment under Medicare, private insurance companies followed Medicare's lead and developed managed care. Managed care organizations (MCOs) encompass several different approaches, such as health maintenance organizations (HMOs), preferred provider organizations (PPOs), and point-of-service (POS) plans (Table 7.2). The primary commonality among all of these health plans is that they use some method to review and approve (or deny) the use of health care services. In this review process, the patient's medical options are reviewed by a nurse or physician employed by the health insurance company, and a judgment is made as to the necessity of the service being considered. Coverage may be denied for unnecessary, excessive, or experimental procedures, in strong

TABLE 7.2	**Common Types of Health Insurance Plans in America**
Fee-for-service (FFS)/ indemnity plan	Member (covered individual) pays a premium for a fixed percentage of expenses covered Plan includes deductible and copayment Allows member to choose physician and specialists without restraint May cover only usual or reasonable and customary charges for treatment and services, with member responsible for charges above that payment Plan may or may not pay for preventive care
PPO (preferred provider organization)	Member (covered individual) pays a premium for a fixed percentage of expense covered Plan includes deductible and copayment Member may select physician, but pays less for physicians and facilities on the plan's preferred list Plan may or may not pay for preventive care
POS (point of service)	Offered by HMO or FFS Allows use of providers outside the plan's preferred list or network, but requires higher premiums and copayments for services
HMO (health maintenance organization)	Member (covered individual) pays a premium There is a a fixed copayment Member must select a primary care physician approved by the HMO Member must be referred for treatments, specialists, and services by the primary care physician Services outside of "network" must be preapproved for payment Plan may refuse to pay for services not recommended by primary care physician Plan encourages use of preventive care
Medicare	Federal health insurance plan for Americans 65 years of age and older and certain disabled persons Member must be eligible for Social Security or railroad retirement Part A covers hospital stays and care in skilled nursing facilities (does not cover long-term care) Part B requires payment of a premium and covers physician services and supplies Plan offers a prescription drug benefit
Medicaid	Health care coverage for low-income persons who are aged, blind, or disabled, and for certain families with dependent children Federal program is delivered and managed by each state for eligibility and scope of services offered Plan covers long-term care (i.e., nursing home care) for qualifying individuals
TRICARE: military health insurance (formerly CHAMPUS)	Civilian health and medical health insurance program for military, spouses, dependents, and beneficiaries Program offered through Military Health Services System

contrast to the previous "if it might help, do it" approach. The goal of managed care is to minimize payment of charges for inappropriate or excessive health care services.

As health care costs rise, the costs for businesses to provide health insurance for employees also rises; these increasing costs are then passed to consumers by increasing the price of the products or services produced by the business. However, health care costs have led to a situation in which U.S. businesses struggle to compete in an international market, in which health care costs are significantly lower. Large businesses, such as automobile manufacturers, pushed health insurance companies to decrease the rising costs of health insurance premiums, leading to a move from conventional insurance plans to MCOs. The overall goals of these types of managed care plans are to limit unnecessary health care services and to use the least expensive service when care is needed.

ACCESS TO HEALTH CARE—
THE PROBLEM OF THE UNINSURED
AND UNDERINSURED

As health care costs continue to rise dramatically in the United States, one major issue that must be addressed is access to health care for the uninsured or underinsured. Prior to the passage of the PPACA in 2010, lack of access to health care primarily reflected a lack of insurance coverage, so access was an issue of financial access. The uninsured and underinsured included the working poor employed by small businesses without insurance coverage, part-time workers, unemployed persons, and the homeless. The poor are more likely to lack a usual source of care, less likely to use preventive services, and more likely to be hospitalized for avoidable conditions than those who are not poor.

The uninsured and underinsured populations generate uncompensated or indigent care costs and bad debt for health care providers. Unpaid costs must be covered by those who do pay so the hospital can continue operating, a process known as *cost shifting*. Providers increase their charges against households and public and private insurers who pay for care to make a contribution for the care of the uninsured population. This practice raises insurance premiums, making it even more difficult for many households and businesses to afford coverage. The problem of uncompensated care and cost shifting was a major factor leading to health care reform and the passage of the PPACA.

In 2013, the percentage of the population without health insurance for the entire calendar year was 13.4%, or 42.0 million people (Barrett and Berchick, 2017). In 2016, the percentage of people without health insurance was down to 8.8% percent (Barrett and Berchick, 2017) as a direct result of the availability of more affordable health insurance options through the PPACA.

Despite these advances in providing health insurance through the PPACA, there are still about 28 million people in the United States without health insurance. People most likely to be uninsured are low-income adults and people of color; the major barrier to obtaining and maintaining health insurance is the cost of coverage (Foutz et al, 2017). Lack of health insurance is perhaps the greatest barrier to accessing health care services and has a tremendous negative effect on an individual's overall health status. Consider that people without health insurance (Foutz et al, 2017):

- Do not have a usual source for healthcare and are more likely to go without needed care due to cost;
- Have an increased risk of being diagnosed at the later stages of a disease leading to higher mortality rates;
- May not receive preventive care;
- Are less likely to receive care for chronic diseases; and
- May often seek treatment in emergency departments at a much higher cost to the health care system.

People without health insurance weigh their costs for daily living expenses, such as food, housing and transportation, against the cost of health insurance coverage and are simply not able to meet the financial demands for health insurance, even with assistance provided through the PPACA. The PPACA does not provide health insurance for every person for several reasons: A person's income may make him or her ineligible for financial assistance through the PPACA, yet he or she is still unable to afford the insurance premiums; the person is subject to immigrant eligibility restrictions; or the state in which the person lives did not expand Medicaid to his or her income level (Foutz et al, 2017).

Medicaid, a federal health insurance program administered by each state, is intended to improve access to health care for the poor, covering approximately 19.4% of the population in 2016 (Barrett and Berchick, 2017). The PPACA expanded federal Medicaid support to any state that accepted this assistance, allowing those states to increase the number of people who meet the qualifications for Medicaid. In 2017, 33 states expanded their Medicaid programs with federal support from the PPACA (Kaiser Family Foundation, 2017), increasing access to health insurance for a larger group of low-income families and individuals. The true impact of the PPACA on the percentage of the population that is uninsured remains to be seen and is certainly worth tracking over the next few years! The following section provides a more detailed discussion of the PPACA.

THE PATIENT PROTECTION
AND AFFORDABLE CARE ACT

On March 23, 2010, the Patient Protection and Affordable Care Act (Public Law 111-148) was signed into law. This comprehensive health care reform plan was designed to expand health insurance coverage to uninsured Americans while controlling costs and improving the quality of health care. In its broadest view, the PPACA is the plan for a comprehensive national health insurance program to provide funding for U.S. citizens and legal residents to secure health insurance beyond the current programs such as Medicare and Medicaid while also providing for provisions to improve the quality of health care and reduce costs.

Almost a decade after this legislation was signed into law, the PPACA continues to be debated in Congress, with various components of the law, or the entire law, being up for revisions or repeal. Thus it remains important for nurses to understand the following key components of the PPACA, which are still in effect in 2018 (Kaiser Family Foundation, 2013):

- U.S. citizens and legal residents must have qualifying health insurance coverage or else pay a penalty.
- Individuals and families at 133% to 400% of the federal poverty level receive financial assistance to help make health insurance more affordable.
- Employers with more than 200 employees must offer health insurance.
- State-based health insurance exchanges are offered whereby individuals and small businesses can purchase qualified coverage at more affordable rates.
- The health insurance plan must cover specified benefits to be deemed "qualifying health insurance coverage," including ambulatory patient services, emergency services, hospitalizations, maternity and newborn care, mental health and substance abuse treatment, prescription drugs, rehabilitative services, laboratory services, preventive and wellness services, chronic disease management, and pediatric services to include vision and oral care.
- Preexisting conditions and annual and lifetime caps to insurance plans are eliminated.
- Dependent coverage for children up to age 26 years must be included for all individual and group policies.
- Insurance companies must spend 80% of premiums on medical care, a requirement that forces them to reduce their administrative expenses.
- Medicare will no longer pay hospitals to treat hospital-acquired conditions (e.g., falls, decubitus ulcers, infections).
- The value-based purchasing program was established in which hospitals are paid on the basis of their performance on quality measures, including patient satisfaction.
- Medicare payments to hospitals for preventable hospital readmissions are reduced.

The PPACA represents the first major effort to reform the U.S. health care system by expanding health insurance coverage to uninsured populations and, just as important, slowing unsustainable health care costs, improving quality, and moving health care to a focus on prevention and population health rather than acute illness treatment. For a comprehensive summary of the PPACA, including updates and revisions to the law, visit the Kaiser Family Foundation website at http://www.kff.org and select "Health Reform."

HOW HEALTH CARE IS PAID FOR

A combination of private and public sources pays for health care services and supplies for individuals in the United States. Most individual health care is paid for either by households through direct out-of-pocket payments or by third-party public or private insurers (Table 7.3). Third-party payers include private insurance

TABLE 7.3 Health Insurance Coverage in America (2016)	
People with health insurance (for all or part of the year)	91.2% of the U.S. population
People without health insurance (for the entire year)	8.8% of the U.S. population
Children younger than 19 years without health insurance	5.4% of children
People covered by private health insurance plans (for all or part of the year)	67.5% of the U.S. population (55.7% employer-based)
People with government insurance (for all or part of the year)	37.3% of the U.S. population (19.4% Medicaid; 16.7% Medicare; 4.6% military)

From Barnett, J.C., & Berchick, E.R. (2017). *Health insurance coverage in the United States: 2016. Current population reports, P60-260.* Washington, DC: U.S. Government Printing Office.
Retrieved from https://www.census.gov/content/dam/Census/library/publications/2017/demo/p60-260.pdf.

companies and government health programs, such as Medicare, Medicaid, and the Veterans Administration health system.

Private Insurance

Private insurance accounts for the largest percentage of coverage for health care, with the cost of providing health insurance to employees passed on by the employer to the consumer in the pricing of goods and services. This means that everyone pays a part of the country's health care costs in every purchase made. Individuals still must pay a portion of their health care costs directly from their own pockets, through payments for insurance premiums, deductibles, and copayments.

With managed care products, such as HMOs, PPOs, and POS arrangements, the premium the consumer pays for coverage has continued to rise. In response to these concerns, some companies now offer their employees high-deductible health plans (HDHPs), health reimbursement accounts (HRAs), health savings accounts (HSAs), or a combination of these. These plans offer more flexibility and consumer discretion over their health care dollars and provide a tax-free way to save for future health care needs.

Public Insurance: Medicare and Medicaid

Government is the biggest influence in the health insurance market, generating half of hospital revenues and more than one fourth of physician incomes. The largest government health insurance program is Medicare. Medicare is an entitlement program based on age or disability criteria, rather than on need. Medicare Part A covers inpatient hospital services, skilled nursing facilities (SNFs), and home health benefits; Medicare does not cover long-term care. Hospital coverage has deductible and coinsurance requirements and some coverage limitations. Medicare Part B covers physician and outpatient services. In January 2006, Medicare added access to a prescription medication benefit, a noted and costly change from previous benefits.

Medicaid is a joint federal-state program to provide health insurance coverage for impoverished families, particularly those with children. Medicaid, along with the Children's Health Insurance Program (CHIP), offers health coverage to more than 62 million Americans. Those eligible for health care services include pregnant women, children and parents, persons with disabilities, and seniors who meet certain income criteria. Each state administers its own Medicaid program within minimal federal income guidelines, so some variances can occur from state to state. The PPACA expanded the minimum income levels for Medicaid eligibility for those less than 65 years of age, effective January 1, 2014. However, according to the 2012 Supreme Court ruling on the PPACA, states have the right to opt out of offering the expanded Medicaid coverage. Medicaid is a primary payer of long-term care nationwide. Medicaid represents the fastest-growing component in most states' budgets.

Effect of Payment Modes

Various methods of reimbursing providers for health care services have emerged because of rapid growth in health care costs combined with concerns about the safety and quality of health care and implementation of the PPACA. Hospitals and providers can now be rewarded for achieving improved health outcomes and are not paid for certain medical errors. Value-based payment models, "never events," value-based purchasing, and readmission reduction programs focus on aligning reimbursement with patient outcomes. Nurses are at the center of helping hospitals and other health care organizations successfully manage these new payment mechanisms by ensuring that errors are prevented, health outcomes are achieved, and financial rewards are realized.

Value-Based Payment Models

Medicare and private insurance companies have shown success with various methods of reimbursing providers (hospitals and physicians) based on quality measures that reflect the quality of care provided with an emphasis on providing evidence-based care, preventing complications, and coordinating care to reduce costs. Hospitals and other providers are rewarded through financial incentives for meeting standards of care for certain conditions such as diabetes, myocardial infarction, pneumonia, and heart failure.

To promote innovative models of care designed to improve care quality, reduce costs, support patient-centered practices, and keep people healthier, CMS established its Innovation Center, which allows for creating and testing of new care delivery models (CMS,

2017b). Such new models include Accountable Care Organizations, Medical Home Models, and Episode-based payment initiatives. Students are encouraged to visit the CMS Innovation Center at http://www.CMS.gov to learn more about these new models of care delivery.

Never Events. To save lives and millions of dollars, CMS adopted a policy that it will no longer pay hospitals for the extra costs of treating preventable errors. Medicare will no longer pay hospitals for the cost of treating *never events*—medical errors that are largely preventable and have serious consequences for patients. The purpose of the never events payment policy is to eliminate payments for certain medical errors and encourage hospitals to direct resources to preventing errors rather than being paid for them. Never events include hospital-acquired infections, injuries from falls, wrong-site surgery, and mismatched blood transfusions. Nurses have a highly visible and important role to play in preventing such complications and helping to control costs for hospitals.

Value-Based Purchasing. Value-based purchasing (VPB) is a CMS reimbursement model that rewards inpatient hospitals for providing quality care to include patient satisfaction. The incentives for VBP arise from two domains: (1) the patient experience of care and (2) clinical processes of care. The patient experience of care is based on the hospital's scores on the Hospital Consumer Assessment of Healthcare Providers and Systems (HCAHPS), which is essentially a standardized patient satisfaction survey (Box 7.1). Clinical process of care measures include such items as discharge

---

BOX 7.1 Components of the HCAHPS (Hospital Consumer Assessment of Healthcare Providers and Systems) Patient Experience

- Communication with nurses
- Communication with doctors
- Responsiveness of hospital staff
- Communication about medicines
- Cleanliness and quietness of hospital environment
- Discharge information
- Overall rating of hospital

---

instructions delivered to heart failure patients, receiving fibrinolytic therapy given within 30 minutes of hospital arrival to patients with acute myocardial infarction, and prophylactic antibiotic received within 1 hour prior to surgical incision. In addition to affecting hospital reimbursement, data from the VBP program is used to provide information to the public about hospital quality. Visit the CMS Hospital Compare website at http://www.medicare.gov/hospitalcompare to learn more about how quality measures are reported to the public. As the reader can easily see, nurses are at the center of addressing the clinical processes of care and the patient experience to enhance the hospital's VBP financial rewards and also its publicly available quality indicators.

Reducing Readmissions. A provision of the PPACA established the *Hospital Readmissions Reduction Program*, which reduces Medicare payments to hospitals with excessive readmissions. A *readmission* is defined as admission to a hospital within 30 days of a discharge from the same or another hospital (CMS, 2017c). The provision is currently focused on readmissions for acute myocardial infarction, heart failure, pneumonia, chronic obstructive pulmonary disease, total hip arthroplasty, total knee arthroplasty, and coronary artery bypass graft surgery. Nurses caring for patients with these conditions have a highly important role in ensuring effective discharge planning and education so the patient and family are fully prepared for recovery at home or in a transitional care setting. New roles for nurses as patient care navigators and transition care providers are rapidly emerging both in community settings and as part of the hospital's services to prevent readmissions. Just as with VBP models and never events, nurses are at the center of the efforts to prevent readmissions and avoid costly financial penalties to the hospital.

IMPLICATIONS FOR NURSES: MANAGING COST-EFFECTIVE, HIGH-QUALITY CARE

Nurses represent the largest health professional discipline in the United States and have an extremely important role in influencing the delivery of high-quality, lower-cost health care while also promoting health for individuals and communities. Never has there been a greater opportunity to advance the practice of

BOX 7.2 **Economic Issues and Trends**		
From		**To**
Illness treatment	$\longrightarrow$	Prevention and population health driven
Acute care	$\longrightarrow$	Preventive care, home care
Hospital or institution based	$\longrightarrow$	Noninstitution based (clinic or home)
Fee-for-service (cost based)	$\longrightarrow$	Value-driven payment models
If it might help, use it	$\longrightarrow$	Outcomes measurement and cost-effectiveness
Independent decisions (practice variation)	$\longrightarrow$	Protocols and guidelines (evidence-based practice)

professional nursing. Innovation and excellence in all nursing practices are needed to contain costs while attaining positive, measurable outcomes. As the reader can see from the various methods of reimbursement discussed earlier, nurses are at the center of ensuring positive patient outcomes, maximizing reimbursement, and decreasing financial penalties for errors and readmissions. Every setting in which professional nurses practice holds challenges in providing and managing care that is efficient, affordable, and of high quality. Box 7.2 summarizes the trends occurring in health care that affect professional nurses. These trends mandate that nurses have a clear understanding of the economic and financing issues underlying their continually evolving roles.

Care Coordination

One key to improving quality and reducing costs is to ensure that health care is coordinated in order to decrease duplication of services and reduce wasted resources. Effective care coordination requires the use of case management and other emerging practice models, such as patient care navigator and transition care coordinator, all with the same goal: to ensure care is delivered in the community through home care, outpatient clinics, and ambulatory care centers at less costly rates and to decrease more expensive hospital-based care. Nurses as care coordinators, case managers, patient care navigators, or transition care coordinators demonstrate cost-effectiveness by ensuring that patients have the resources they need to get effective treatment at the appropriate level of care across the continuum of care.

Expansion of Technology

Improved technology for diagnostic and therapeutic practice is under examination for cost-efficiency in comparison with outcome delivery. Leaders must balance the health contributions of the improved technology and the accompanying costs with issues of quality of life, access to care, risk-benefit analysis, and individual consumer choice.

U.S. consumers have had access to high levels of technology with little concern for costs. Nurses are key players in educating patients and their family members about the cost-to-benefit ratio of certain technologies and can assist in selecting alternative treatment options. One example is the increased use of pharmaceuticals; more advanced drugs are marketed although they have varying degrees of actual documented benefit in comparison with existing, less expensive drugs. Patients may not trust generic drugs, although they are less expensive. The nurse can be a key to educating patients and the public regarding the potential and implications of using a less expensive drug instead of a more expensive alternative.

The technology of the Internet offers promise for information and education that allows consumers (or patients) to access health care resources more effectively. Some health care plans offer subscribers free newsletters that highlight ways to prevent disease and to manage chronic illness for improved quality of life and lower costs.

Information technology provides the professional nurse the ability to gather and analyze health-related information and data for improved care. Health care information systems and electronic health records offer many opportunities for managing health care costs. Combining clinical skills with information technology skills can be a significant advantage in the success of professional nurses as they demonstrate their ability to provide cost-effective outcomes measurement. See Chapter 15 for a more detailed discussion of information technology in the clinical setting.

BOX 7.3 Ways Consumers Can Reduce Health Care Costs

- Practice good health behaviors—healthy eating, exercise, good sleep.
- Use the Internet to learn more about your health and preventing disease.
- Recognize early warning signs of disease and get prompt treatment.
- Practice preventive health with health screenings and routine self-examinations. Take advantage of free screenings offered at community sites, hospitals, or churches.
- Develop an active relationship with health care providers to improve communication. Ask providers to explain the purpose of all prescribed tests and medications. Become an informed consumer.
- Use emergency care only in emergencies. See your health care provider during office hours.
- Know health risks for lifestyle choices, such as alcohol and drug use, dietary habits, sedentary behaviors, and safety at home and while driving.
- Understand and use the health care benefits of your insurance plan to stay healthy. Take advantage of all preventive benefits offered.
- Determine whether the health care treatment is really necessary. Choose nonhospital alternatives for treatment whenever possible. Comparison shop for health care alternatives.
- Choose generic drugs whenever possible. Question expensive drugs or devices.
- Review your health care bills carefully, and notify the provider and/or facility of errors.

Consumer Empowerment

Health care customers demand quality health care services at affordable rates. Economic forces motivate the shift toward health promotion and preventive care to achieve cost-effectiveness. This relationship with the consumer emphasizes cost sharing through individual choices in health practices. For instance, the presence of unhealthy personal practices, such as smoking, illegal drug use, and a sedentary lifestyle, may lead to a higher insurance rate for an individual. Smokers may pay higher rates and have to be smoke-free for 1 year to qualify for lower rates. Being overweight may cost the subscriber more in premiums because this status poses additional health concerns and potential increased health costs. Box 7.3 shows ways consumers can reduce their health care costs.

■ SUMMARY

Changes in the U.S. health care system bring new challenges for professional nurses. Health care has moved from an emphasis on illness to an emphasis on wellness and prevention and is shifting from acute care services to preventive and community-based services, such as ambulatory care and home care. Financing of health care services has gone from retrospective, fee-for-service payment systems to prospective payment and managed care and continues to evolve through implementation of the PPACA to expand insurance coverage and new models of financial rewards and incentives (e.g., never events, value-based purchasing, readmission reduction programs) to improve quality and reduce costs. Today, technology is viewed as important to health care delivery, but its value is based on having the appropriate service at the right price.

U.S. leaders and legislators agree that health care costs are too high, but they differ in the best ways to stop the increased cost of health care. Most agree that when citizens practice healthy lifestyles, they require less health care and enjoy a better quality of life. However, what will motivate people to make healthier choices and practice disease prevention?

What do these changes in health care delivery mean to professional nursing? Nursing practice in a cost- and quality-conscious environment is here to stay. Nurses must constantly challenge current practice for quality improvement and cost-effectiveness. Accurate data must be collected to show cost containment and positive patient outcomes. Nurses need to be leaders and to have a voice in the ever-changing economic and political environment that determines payment for services. The PPACA has expanded the contributions of nursing in many ways. Roles on clinical teams, in administration, with insurance companies, and with the government hold promise for empowered change. Professional nurses can prepare for these evolving careers with a commitment to lifelong learning. Nurses can take the lead by being healthy role models, educating consumers, and encouraging personal responsibility for improved health practices. Managing care brings nurses back to the basics as society recognizes that healthy people are good business.

REFERENCES

Barnett, J.C., & Berchick, E.R. (2017). Health insurance coverage in the United States: 2016. Current Population Reports, P60-260. Washington, DC: U.S. Government Printing Office. Retrieved from https://www.census.gov/content/dam/Census/library/publications/2017/demo/p60-260.pdf.

Canadian Institute for Health Information. (2017). National health expenditure trends 1975 to 2017. Retrieved from https://www.cihi.ca/sites/default/files/document/nhex2017-trends-report-en.pdf.

Centers for Medicare and Medicaid Services. (2017a). National health expenditure fact sheet, 2016. Retrieved from https://www.cms.gov/research-statistics-data-and-systems/statistics-trends-and-reports/nationalhealthexpenddata/nhe-fact-sheet.html.

Centers for Medicare and Medicaid Services. (2017b). About the CMS Innovation Center. Retrieved from https://innovation.cms.gov/About/index.html.

Centers for Medicare and Medicaid Services. (2017c). Readmissions reduction program. Retrieved from https://www.cms.gov/medicare/medicare-fee-for-service-payment/acuteinpatientpps/readmissions-reduction-program.html.

Foutz, J., Damico, A., Squires, E., & Garfield, R. (2017). The uninsured: A primer - Key facts about health insurance and the uninsured under the Affordable Care Act. Kaiser Family Foundation. Retrieved from https://www.kff.org/report-section/the-uninsured-a-primer-key-facts-about-health-insurance-and-the-uninsured-under-the-affordable-care-act-executive-summary/#endnote_link_246155-3.

Kaiser Family Foundation. (2017). State Medicaid expansion approaches. Retrieved from https://www.kff.org/medicaid/fact-sheet/state-medicaid-expansion-approaches.

Kaiser Family Foundation. (2013). Summary of Affordable Care Act. Retrieved from http://files.kff.org/attachment/fact-sheet-summary-of-the-affordable-care-act.

8

Knowledge of the law enhances the nurse's ability to provide safe and effective care.

Legal Issues in Nursing and Health Care

Laura R. Mahlmeister, PhD, MSN, RN

 Additional resources are available online at: *http://evolve.elsevier.com/Cherry/*

LEARNING OUTCOMES

After studying this chapter, the reader will be able to:

1. Differentiate among the three major categories of law on which nursing practice is established and governed.
2. Analyze the relationship between accountability and liability for one's actions in professional nursing practice.
3. Outline the essential elements that must be proven to establish a claim of negligence or malpractice.
4. Distinguish between intentional and unintentional torts in relation to nursing practice.
5. Identify causes of nursing error and patient injury that have led to claims of criminal negligence.
6. Incorporate fundamental laws and statutory regulations that establish the patient's right to autonomy, self-determination, and informed decision making in the health care setting.
7. Incorporate laws and statutory regulations that establish the patient's right to privacy and privacy of health records.

KEY TERMS

Accountability Being responsible for one's actions; a sense of duty in performing nursing tasks and activities.

Advance directives Written or verbal instructions created by the patient that describe specific wishes about medical care in the event he or she becomes incapacitated or incompetent. Examples include living wills and durable powers of attorney.

Breach of duty Occurs when one person or company has a duty of care toward another person or company but fails to live up to that standard.

Case law Body of written opinions created by judges in federal and state appellate cases; also known as judge-made law and common law.

Civil law A category of law (tort law) that deals with conduct considered unacceptable. It is based on

societal expectations regarding interpersonal conduct. Common causes of civil litigation include professional malpractice, negligence, and assault and battery.

Common law Law that is created through the decisions of judges as opposed to laws enacted by legislative bodies (e.g., Congress).

Comparative negligence A type of liability in which damages may be apportioned among two or more defendants in a malpractice case. The extent of liability depends on the defendant's relative contribution to the patient's injury.

Criminal negligence Negligence that indicates "reckless and wanton" disregard for the safety, well-being, or life of an individual; behavior that demonstrates a complete disregard for another, such that death is likely.

Damages Monetary compensation the court orders paid to a person who has sustained a loss or injury to his or her person or property through the misconduct (intentional or unintentional) of another.

Defendant The individual who is named in a person's (plaintiff's) complaint as responsible for an injury; the person who the plaintiff claims committed a negligent act or malpractice.

Disclosure A process in which the patient's primary provider (physician or advanced practice nurse) gives the patient, and when applicable, family members, complete information about unanticipated adverse outcomes of treatment and care.

Durable power of attorney for health care An instrument that authorizes another person to act as one's agent in decisions regarding health care if one becomes incompetent to make one's own decisions.

Error A failure of a planned action to be completed as intended or the use of a wrong plan to achieve a specific aim.

Ethical issues A problem that requires a person or organization to choose between alternatives that must be evaluated as right (ethical) or wrong (unethical).

Gross negligence A legal concept that means extreme carelessness showing willful or reckless disregard for the consequences to a person (patient).

Health care law Federal, state, and local laws and associated rules and regulations applicable to the health care industry and health care workers.

Immunity Legal doctrine by which a person is protected from a lawsuit for negligent acts or an institution is protected from a suit for the negligent acts of its employees.

Legal liability Failure of a person or an entity to meet legally defined responsibilities and allows a lawsuit for resulting damages.

Liability Being legally responsible for harm caused to another person or property as a result of one's actions; compensation for harm is normally monetary.

Licensing laws Laws that establish the qualifications for obtaining and maintaining a license to perform particular services. Persons and institutions may be required to obtain licenses to provide particular health care services.

Malpractice Failure of a professional to meet the standard of conduct that a reasonable and prudent member of his or her profession would exercise in similar circumstances that results in harm. The professional's misconduct is unintentional.

Negligence Failure to act in a manner that an ordinary, prudent person (either a layperson or professional) would act in similar circumstances that results in harm. The failure to act in a reasonable and prudent manner is unintentional.

Nursing case law The body of written legal opinions developed by judges through court decisions that eventually contribute to the expected standard of nursing conduct.

Nursing malpractice An incident in which a nurse fails to competently perform his or her legal duty owed to a patient and that failure harms the patient.

Nursing Practice Act The body of state law that sets out the scope of practice and responsibilities of the registered nurse in order to protect the health and welfare of individuals or communities under the care of the registered nurse.

Plaintiff The complaining person in a lawsuit; the person who claims he or she was injured by the acts of another.

Preventable adverse event An injury caused by medical management rather than the patient's underlying condition. An adverse event attributable to error is a preventable adverse event.

Punitive damages Monetary compensation awarded to an injured person (patient) that goes beyond what is necessary to compensate for losses (e.g., the ability to function, death, income) and is intended to punish the wrongdoer.

Res ipsa loquitur Legal doctrine applicable to cases in which the provider (e.g., the physician) had exclusive control of events that resulted in the patient's injury; the injury would not have occurred ordinarily without a negligent act; a Latin phrase meaning "the thing speaks for itself."

Respondeat superior Legal doctrine that holds an employer indirectly responsible for the negligent acts of employees carried out within the scope of employment; a Latin phrase meaning "let the master answer."

Risk management Process of identifying, analyzing, and controlling risks posed to patients; involves human factor and incident analysis, changes in systems operations, and loss control and prevention.

Sentinel event As defined by The Joint Commission, an unintended adverse outcome that results in death, paralysis, coma, or other major permanent loss of function. Examples of sentinel events include patient suicide while in a licensed health care facility, surgical procedure on the wrong organ or body side, and a patient fall.

Standard of care In civil cases, the legal criteria against which the nurse's (and physician's) conduct is compared to determine whether a negligent act or malpractice occurred; commonly defined as the knowledge and skill that an ordinary, reasonably prudent person would possess and exercise in the same or similar circumstances.

Statute or statutory law Law enacted by a legislative body; separate from judge-made or common law.

Strict liability A legal doctrine, sometimes referred to as absolute liability, that can be imposed on a person or entity (e.g., a hospital) without proof of carelessness or negligence.

Vicarious liability Legal doctrine in which a person or institution is liable for the negligent acts of another because of a special relationship between the two parties; a substituted liability.

PROFESSIONAL/ETHICAL ISSUE

All health care systems are challenged to provide safe patient care when employees, physicians, or other providers report illness while at work. Although health care workers are advised to stay home if they are febrile and have signs of respiratory infection that may be spread to patients and coworkers, anecdotal evidence suggests that workers are in fact pressured to "tough it out" and come to work. The following is a scenario illustrating ethical issues and challenges related to working with sick colleagues.

A pregnant woman arrives in a labor and delivery unit at 6:45 AM for a scheduled repeat cesarean delivery. Her obstetrician, Dr. Mary Smith, is on call and planning to perform the surgical birth. The obstetrician is completing her preoperative documentation at the nurses' station. The charge nurse notes that Dr. Smith has obvious symptoms of a severe respiratory illness. She is coughing, sneezing, has copious nasal secretions, and looks quite ill. The patient's nurse observes Dr. Smith drinking about a third of a bottle of a liquid cold and flu remedy and pocketing the rest of the medication in her lab coat. The nurse knows that one of the side effects of the medication is significant drowsiness.

She approaches the physician and says, "Dr. Smith, you look quite ill. I am concerned about you and whether you are up to performing surgery this morning. Can we call your partner who is scheduled to start at 8:00 AM to come in and relieve you?"

Dr. Smith responds, "Look, it's just a bad cold. I've taken a large dose of a cold remedy. I will double-mask and use a splash shield. Let's get going. I'm off duty at 8:00 AM. If we move fast I'll be out of here before then. Call me when the patient's on the table." Dr. Smith then walks into the physician's lounge and reclines on a couch.

Questions

1. What is the nurse's ethical duty to the patient and coworkers at this time?
2. What danger does complying with Dr. Smith's plan to proceed with surgery pose to the patient and coworkers?
3. Does the nurse have an ethical duty to the physician?

PROFESSIONAL/LEGAL ISSUE

There are a broad range of health care laws underpinning nursing practice. The nurse must be familiar with these legal imperatives and how they affect professional nursing care. Ignorance of the law is not a defense against charges of negligence, malpractice, or criminal misconduct. An increasing number of cases have been filed alleging a violation of health care statutes by nurses.

VIGNETTE

On July 26, 2017, an unconscious man injured in a motor vehicle accident was conveyed to the University of Utah Hospital in Salt Lake City (Smart, 2017). A registered nurse was directed by a police officer, who had entered the Emergency Department (ED), to draw blood from the man who was still unresponsive. The blood sample would be tested for alcohol, drugs, and illicit substances that could alter mentation. A charge nurse explained to the officer that neither she nor the police were permitted to obtain the sample because the patient had not given consent. The police officer telephoned his supervisor, who supported the officer's directive to draw the blood sample. The nurse had alerted a hospital supervisor about the unresolved disagreement, but that person had not yet arrived in the ED.

A videotape captured the encounter between the nurse and officer. It was released in September of 2017 to the media (*The Salt Lake Tribune,* 2017). The nurse was able to contact a hospital representative to speak telephonically with the police officer. When the nurse continued to respectfully refuse the order, the officer arrested her, forcefully removed her from the ED, handcuffed her, and conveyed her to the police department.

Questions to Consider While Reading This Chapter:

1. What was the nurse's legal duty in this situation?
2. What legal principles underlie the nurse's obligations to the patient?
3. What laws, if any, would govern the nurse's decision-making process in this case?
4. In this situation, does the police officer's order to draw the blood supersede the nurse's right to refuse the order?
5. Could the patient sue the charge nurse if she had drawn the blood sample and given it to the police officer?
6. What would the likely claims of nursing negligence be if a lawsuit had been filed on behalf of the patient?

CHAPTER OVERVIEW

The preceding vignettes highlight growing clinical dilemmas that nurses and patients face in an ever-changing health care system. In an increasingly complex health care environment, the nurse's ability to make appropriate decisions about the provision of patient care services is assisted by a sound knowledge of ethical principles and the laws governing practice. In the case of the ED charge nurse, consent and diagnostic testing are regulated by a federal law known as the Emergency Medical Treatment and Active Labor Act (EMTALA) (CFR, 42 U.S.C. §1395dd). Furthermore, the Fourth Amendment to the U.S. Constitution, prohibiting unreasonable searches and seizures, underpins the patient's right to refuse drug testing under certain circumstances.

There also may be a specific state law regarding drug testing in the ED as well as other departments such as inpatient psychiatric units and obstetric departments. Additionally, sections of the state's nursing practice act or professional and business code often describe professional conduct of the RN. They would assist the nurse in

responding to a concern about possible physician impairment or a request by an officer of the law to obtain blood samples for drug testing. The role of the nurse as patient advocate also informs the nurse's actions when the patient's rights are jeopardized.

Each nurse must be able to describe his or her professional duty to the patient or client under the law and associated health care rules and regulations and to recognize legal risks in practice. Knowledge of the law enhances the nurse's ability to provide safe, effective, and humane care in all settings. This chapter examines the legal aspects of nursing practice. The concepts of law, professional accountability, legal liability, negligence, malpractice, and criminal offense are defined. Specific laws or statutes governing nursing practice are also reviewed. The reader is introduced to current, relevant information about case law, also known as common law or judge-made law, as it applies to professional nursing practice. Patients' rights are explored within the context of law and court opinions. Finally, the ongoing reports about medical errors published by organizations such as the Institute of Medicine (IOM), The Joint Commission (TJC), and the Agency for Healthcare Research and Quality (AHRQ) are discussed, and specific strategies to reduce errors and legal risk are detailed.

SOURCES OF LAW AND NURSING PRACTICE

The actions of all individuals are regulated through two systems of principles known as laws and ethics. *Laws* enforce a minimal level of conduct by imposing penalties for violations of acceptable behavior (Griffith and Tengnah, 2017). Laws are expressed in terms of "must" and "shall" and are based on a society's interest in prohibiting or controlling certain behaviors. *Ethics* are described in terms of "should" and "may" and address beliefs about appropriate behaviors within a societal context (Butts and Rich, 2016). Chapter 9 presents an in-depth discussion about nursing ethics. Along with ethics, professional nursing conduct is regulated by a variety of laws. The two major sources of law are statutory law and common law. The standards for professional nursing practice are in great part derived from statutory as well as common law. The following section deals with statutory law and describes how it governs and indirectly influences nursing practice.

STATUTORY LAW

The terms *law* and *statute* are used interchangeably in this chapter. Laws that are written by legislative bodies, such as Congress or state legislatures, are enacted as statutes. The previously mentioned law, EMTALA, is an example of a federal statute. Violation of law is a criminal offense against the general public and is prosecuted by government authorities. Crimes are punishable by fines or imprisonment. The list of federal and state statutes that govern nursing practice has multiplied over the past 25 years. Nurses at all levels of practice must develop a greater depth and breadth of knowledge about laws related to patient safety, professional practice, their specific practice setting (e.g., the ED in the case of EMTALA), and health care systems in general. Ignorance of the law is never a defense when a nurse violates a health care statute. A nurse who violates the law is subject to penalties, including monetary fines, suspension or revocation of his or her license, and even imprisonment in some instances (Brown, 2013).

Federal Statutes

Conditions of Participation for Hospitals in Medicare (42 CFR Part 482).

Federal laws, rules, and regulations have a major effect on nursing practice and hospital operations. In the *U.S. Code of Federal Regulations* (CFR), Title 42 is the principal set of rules and regulations issued by federal agencies regarding public health. Title 42, Part 482, contains the Conditions of Participation for Hospitals in Medicare (CoPs) and is abbreviated in references as "42 CFR Part 482." The CoPs delineate the minimal standards of care required in all health care settings that receive federal reimbursement for treatment of Medicare beneficiaries. Medicare is administered by the Centers for Medicare & Medicaid Services (CMS), which has the authority to establish new rules and regulations to enhance patient safety and quality and reduce the cost of care. For instance, the CoPs require nurses to develop an individualized written nursing care plan for each patient and to revise the plan as necessary. Other CoPs mandate that hospitals properly train nurses for their stated roles and responsibilities, provide adequate staff to meet patient needs, and begin discharge planning as soon as possible after the patient's admission to the hospital.

Hospitals that are not in compliance with the CoPs may lose their federal funding if the CMS determines the violations place a patient in "immediate jeopardy" of harm. The hospital or units within the hospital may be prohibited from accepting patients until corrective actions are taken to ensure the safety of all patients (Mahlmeister, 2015). Likewise, nurses engaged in unprofessional conduct that violate CoPs may be barred from employment in hospitals that participate in the Medicare program. Nurses can access information about the CoPs online and without cost at the CMS website: http://www.cms.gov/Regulations-and-Guidance/Legislation/CFCsAndCoPs/Hospitals.html. The CoPs can be downloaded from the site as a pdf file, *Appendix A of the State Operations Manual. The State Operations Manual* delineates each of the 23 CoPs pertaining to hospitals and provides Interpretive Guidelines for each of the requirements in language that can be easily understood by nurses and consumers of health care.

In 2008, the CMS issued new rules that halt payment to hospitals for treatment of preventable patient complications and injuries, often referred to as "never events." The CMS identified 10 categories of hospital-acquired conditions (HACs) that studies have demonstrated are "reasonably preventable" (CMS, 2008). Box 8.1 lists the 10 categories of adverse events that are subject to nonpayment. The new rules were enacted in 2015 and have already had a significant impact on hospital nursing care through the introduction of evidence-based practices to prevent complications such as falls, infections, and the development of stage III and stage IV pressure ulcers. The major revisions the CMS proposed in the CoPs took effect July 16, 2012. Under these rules, nurses are required to develop greater expertise in the provision of evidence-based patient care, case management, and discharge planning.

Legal concerns have been raised about a possible increase in malpractice claims related to hospital-acquired conditions. It may be more difficult for a hospital to defend a malpractice claim if "strict liability" is applied to these hospital-acquired events. In other words, if the federal government deems the HAC a cause for levying penalties or denying reimbursement, does the decision constitute negligence per se? Case law has yet to determine whether the courts will accept the "strict liability" claim. However, hospitals will still face serious financial losses when hospital-acquired events occur. Beginning in 2008, the Hospital-Acquired Condition (HAC) Reduction

BOX 8.1   Categories of Hospital-Acquired Conditions Subject to Nonpayment

1. Foreign object retained after surgery (e.g., instruments, surgical sponges)
2. Air embolism
3. Blood incompatibility (blood transfusion error)
4. Development of stage III or stage IV pressure ulcer
5. Falls and trauma:
   - Fractures
   - Joint dislocation
   - Intracranial injuries
   - Crushing injuries
   - Burns
   - Electric shock
6. Manifestations of poor glycemic control:
   - Diabetic ketoacidosis
   - Nonketotic hyperosmolar coma
   - Hypoglycemic coma
   - Secondary diabetes with ketoacidosis
   - Secondary diabetes with hyperosmolarity
7. Catheter-associated urinary tract infection (UTI)
8. Vascular catheter–associated infection
9. Surgical site infection following:
   - Coronary artery bypass graft—mediastinitis
   - Bariatric surgery
   - Orthopedic procedure
10. Deep vein thrombosis (DVT)/pulmonary embolism (PE)

Data from Centers for Medicare & Medicaid Services (CMS). (2016). *Medicare program; changes to the hospital inpatient prospective payment system and fiscal year 2017 rates*. 81 FR 56761. Retrieved from https://www.cms.gov/Medicare/Medicare-Fee-for-Service-Payment/HospitalAcqCond/Hospital-Acquired_Conditions.html: Accessed May, 2018.

Program, mandated by the Affordable Care Act, required the CMS to reduce hospital payments by 1% for hospitals that ranked among the lowest-performing 25% with regard to HACs. In addition, under the HAC Reduction Program, the CMS has the authority to penalize hospitals reporting HACs. The CMS announced a planned reduction in reimbursement to 758 hospitals across the United States in 2016, resulting in a $364 million savings for Medicare (California Healthline, 2015). Nurses will continue to play a central role in quality improvement activities that reduce the likelihood of revenue loss. Nursing homes are another highly regulated industry that must meet federal and state requirements to operate.

Federal laws have also established rules and regulations to ensure the confidentiality of patients' personal health information (Health Insurance Portability and Accountability Act [HIPAA]). Several federal laws protect the rights of patients who participate as subjects in research by mandating the creation of institutional review boards and an appropriate informed consent process. The Americans with Disabilities Act (ADA) requires health care entities to provide interpreter services and communication devices for patients who are unable to effectively communicate their needs or wishes. The Federal False Claims Act makes it an offense to submit a false claim to the government for payment of health care services. The U.S. Department of Justice recovered more than $4.7 billion in settlements and judgments from civil cases involving fraud and false claims against the government in fiscal year 2016 (U.S. Department of Justice, December 2016). Furthermore, the person who reports the false or fraudulent claim (often referred to as a "whistle-blower") is entitled to 15% to 25% of any monetary amount recovered by the federal government if the government wins the case in court. Nurses have been the recipients of these "bounties" in several recent false claim cases in which the federal government recovered several million dollars.

Three federal statutes that nurses must be familiar with and clearly understand are discussed in this section. The list is not comprehensive, but it includes examples of federal laws that directly affect nursing practice. Many federal laws are relevant to specific health care settings (e.g., mental health hospitals, nursing homes, EDs, maternity settings). When nurses are knowledgeable about the federal laws applicable to their area of practice, they are able to more effectively advocate for patients in that setting. Unfortunately, most nurses are unfamiliar with health care law and rely on authorities in their employment setting to know what is legal and therefore permissible. Automatically deferring to administrators or nurse managers about the legality of a particular issue is no longer acceptable behavior for the professional nurse. Each RN must take accountability for knowing the law and understanding how it relates to patient care and nursing practice.

Emergency Medical Treatment and Active Labor Law (CFR, 42 U.S.C. §1395dd). The federal statute known as EMTALA, often referred to as the "antidumping" law, was enacted in 1986 to prohibit the refusal of care for indigent and uninsured patients seeking medical assistance in an ED (Moy, 2016). This law also prohibits the transfer of unstable patients, including women in labor, from one facility to another. The law states: "All persons presenting for care must receive the same medical screening examination and be stabilized, regardless of their financial status or insurance coverage, before discharge or transfer."

EMTALA is applicable to people coming to non-ED settings, such as urgent care clinics. It even governs the transfer of a patient from an inpatient setting to a lower level of care in some parts of the United States (*Roberts v. Galen of Virginia, Inc.,* 1997). Significant penalties can be levied against a facility that violates EMTALA, including a $25,000 to $50,000 fine (not covered by liability insurance). The federal government also can revoke the facility's Medicare contract, an action that could result in a major loss of revenue for the institution, or even insolvency. Many legitimate concerns that nurses have about the discharge or transfer of patients could be promptly addressed if the nurses had a solid understanding of EMTALA. A 2006 case illustrates the importance of understanding EMTALA. In *Love v. Rancocas Hospital* (2006), a woman was transported by ambulance to the ED after losing consciousness at home. She had a history of hypertension and continued to have high blood pressure readings in the ED. The woman also fell off the bed twice while being monitored, but the ED nurse did not report these events to the physician. The nurse received a discharge order from the physician and sent the woman home in an unstable condition, thus violating the stabilization requirement of EMTALA. The woman returned 2 days later after experiencing a stroke. Understanding EMTALA is not a daunting task for nurses engaged in the triage and medical screening of patients presenting to the ED or obstetric triage department. Nursing journals have published many articles about EMTALA and the nurse's role in upholding this statute (Angelini & Howard, 2014; Brent, 2017).

Americans with Disabilities Act of 1990 (Public Law No. 101-336; 42 U.S.C. Section 12101).

The intent of the ADA is to end discrimination against qualified persons with disabilities by removing barriers that prevent them from enjoying the same opportunities available to persons without disabilities. Court cases have established that as a place of public accommodation, a health care facility must provide reasonable accommodation to

patients (and family members) with sensory disabilities, such as vision and hearing impairment (*Abernathy v. Valley Medical Center,* 2006; *Boyer v. Tift County Hospital,* 2008). In another case (*Parco v. Pacifica Hospital,* 2007), a nurse was caring for a ventilator-dependent quadriplegic patient who was unable to speak or use his call light. She requested a special pillow that activated the patient's call light when he turned his head but was told that all the pillows were in use. The patient subsequently experienced three episodes of respiratory distress that he was unable to alert the nurse about, and could only hope that someone would discover his problem before he suffered brain damage or death (Snyder, 2007). The patient sued for emotional distress and mental anguish. The court affirmed that the ADA requires hospitals to provide assistive devices to patients with communication problems related to a disability. The hospital settled the lawsuit for $295,000.

This statute has relevance for all nurses. As patient advocates, nurses have a legal and ethical duty to provide appropriate patient and family education and to support the process of informed consent. In *Parco v. Pacifica Hospital,* the court noted that it was a basic tenet of nursing practice that patients be given the ability to communicate with caregivers. The health care facility must have a policy that defines how it will meet the need for education and information of a client with a vision or hearing disability. The policy also describes how a nurse can obtain translators and special types of equipment needed to facilitate communication with clients who have physical disabilities or language barriers.

Patient Self-Determination Act of 1990; Omnibus Budget Reconciliation Act of 1990 (Public Law No. 101-508; Sections 4206 and 4751).

The Patient Self-Determination Act of 1990 is a Medicare and Medicaid amendment intended to support individuals in expressing their preferences about medical treatment and making decisions about end-of-life care. The law requires all federally funded hospitals to give patients written notice on admission to the health care facility of their decision-making rights and policies regarding advance health care directives in their state and in the institution to which they have been admitted. Under the Patient Self-Determination Act patients have the right to:
- Participate in their own health care decisions
- Accept or refuse medical treatment
- Make advance health care directives

These choices include collaborating with the physician in formulating "do not resuscitate" (DNR) orders. Facilities must inquire as to whether the patient already has an advance health care directive, and they must make note of this in the patient's medical record. The institution must also provide education to their staff about advance health care directives. The law provides guidance to nurses, who often are in the best position to discuss these issues with the patient (e.g., while completing a comprehensive admission assessment). (Legal considerations related to living wills, durable power of attorney, and DNR orders are discussed in "The Law and Patient Rights," the last section of this chapter.)

Health Insurance Portability and Accountability Act of 1996 (Public Law No. 104-191). The intent of HIPAA is to ensure confidentiality of the patient's health information. Legitimate concerns regarding the uses of and release of medical information, particularly to private entities such as insurance companies, led to the passage of this law. The introduction of electronic medical records provided additional impetus for introduction of this legislation. The statute sets guidelines for maintaining the privacy of health data. It provides explicit guidelines for nurses who are in a position to release health information. To maintain confidentiality of the patient's health information, all nurses must have a basic understanding of this federal law. Nurses should also take note that the HIPAA confers whistle-blower protection for individuals who report in good faith any illegal disclosure of patients' health. In 2005 a federal statute, the Patient Safety and Quality Improvement Act (Public Law No. 109-41), was enacted to allow certain disclosures of patient safety data. The law permits a provider to disclose *nonidentifiable* patient data to a qualified patient safety organization (PSO) for the purpose of analyzing medical errors. The law prohibits an accreditation body, such as TJC, from taking any action against a provider who reports patient safety data to an approved PSO (Public Law No. 109-41).

With the continued rise in the number of nurses using social media such as blogs, social networking sites, video sites, and online chat rooms and forums, a patient's right to privacy is threatened. In 2011, the ANA published the Principles of Social Networking Toolkit for Nurses (ANA, 2011) and the National Council of State Boards of Nursing (NCSBN) published a complimentary brochure, "A Nurse's Guide to the Use of Social Media" (NCSBN, 2011a). The publications review the benefits and risks of using social media in the workplace and bringing workplace issues to social media sites during free time. The release of private health data, either inadvertent or intentional, is a violation of HIPAA and is punishable by significant fines and a term of imprisonment. It may also result in suspension or revocation of the nurse's license. Civil actions may arise from a violation of patient confidentiality, alleging failure to maintain security and confidentiality of protected patient health data, unprofessional conduct, and violation of hospital policies and procedures that restrict access to patient information on a "need to know" basis. Posting photographs or videotapes of patients, or even ostensibly unidentifiable body parts, is expressly forbidden and also violates the ANA's Code of Ethics for Nurses (2015a). Discussing conflicts with managers or coworkers on social networking sites or posting unauthorized photos or videos of professional colleagues opens the nurse to claims of invasion of privacy, slander, intentional infliction of harm, and emotional distress, among other things. Further risks to livelihood and future employment as a nurse are presented when the nurse publicly airs dissatisfaction with his or her employer or discusses problems at work that make the employer vulnerable to ridicule or loss of reputation in the community or larger health care arena.

State Statutes

In addition to federal laws, nursing practice is governed by state laws that delineate the conduct of licensed nurses and define behaviors of all health care professionals in promoting public health and welfare.

State Nurse Practice Act and Board of Nursing Rules and Regulations. One of the most important state laws governing nursing practice is a nurse practice act (NPA), which defines the scope and limitations of professional nursing practice. The aim of regulating practice in this manner is to protect the public and make the individual nurse accountable for his or her actions. State legislatures authorize the nurses' licensing board to promulgate administrative rules and regulations necessary to implement the NPA. Once these administrative rules and regulations are formally adopted, they have the same force and effect as any other law.

Although NPAs vary from state to state, they usually contain the following information:

- Definition of the term *RN*
- Description of professional nursing functions
- Standards of competent performance
- Behaviors that represent misconduct or prohibited practices
- Grounds for disciplinary action
- Fines and penalties the licensing board may levy when an NPA is violated

For further exploration, excerpts from three separate state NPAs can be found on the Evolve site at http://evolve.elsevier.com/Cherry/ illustrating how an NPA defines the scope of practice for nurses.

Surprisingly, many nurses are not even aware that the NPA is a law, and they unknowingly violate aspects of this statute (Cronquist, 2013; NCSBN, 2011b). They are not familiar with the administrative rules and regulations enacted by the licensing board. This is an unfortunate lack because these administrative rules and regulations answer crucial questions that nurses have about the day-to-day aspects of practice and unusual occurrences. For example, the increasing complexity of health care requires effective communication, collaboration, and planning of care among many licensed health team members. Rules promulgated by the Ohio Board of Nursing Section 4723.03, which refer to the competent practice as an RN, direct the nurse in appropriate reporting and consultation, as follows:

"A registered nurse shall in a timely manner:
Implement any order for a client unless the registered nurse believes or should have reason to believe the order is:

1. Inaccurate
2. Not properly authorized
3. Not current or valid
4. Harmful, or potentially harmful to a client
5. Contraindicated by other documented information; and

Clarify any order for a client when the registered nurse believes or should have reason to believe the order is: [a through e as delineated in (1)]"

> **Ohio Administrative Code,**
> **Section 4723-4-03, E, 2014**

According to this section, an RN in Ohio who does not clarify a questionable order before administering a medication or carrying out the prescribed action is in violation of the law.

Each nurse should own a current copy of the NPA and the licensing board's administrative rules and regulations for the jurisdiction in which he or she practices. The nurse also must know how to access the licensing board online and by telephone in order to clarify issues related to nursing practice. The dramatic changes occurring in health care often lead to uncertainty among nurses about which functions constitute the exclusive practice of registered nursing and which patient care tasks may be lawfully delegated to a licensed practical nurse/licensed vocational nurse (LPN/LVN) or unlicensed assistive personnel. The NPA and licensing board rules and regulations provide essential information that clarifies these important questions. In 2008, the Texas Board of Nursing approved a new rule requiring all nurses to take and pass a Nursing Jurisprudence Exam prior to initial licensure. The examination tests knowledge regarding nursing board statutes, rules, position statements, disciplinary action, and other resource documents accessible on the Texas Board's website (http://bon.state.tx.us/index.html).

Nurses may also have questions and concerns regarding the legal aspects of floating to unfamiliar units. An NPA provides information regarding the scope of practice, the required competencies, and the responsibilities of a nurse who accepts an assignment or agrees to carry out any task or activity in the clinical setting. The NPA broadly defines the practice of registered nursing in accordance with nursing's rapidly evolving functions. In recent years, with the expansion of basic nursing functions and the development of advanced nursing practice, many states have revised their NPAs. Licensing boards also have been authorized in some states to provide guidelines for the development of "standardized procedures." Standardized procedures are a legal means by which RNs may expand their practice into areas traditionally considered to be within the realm of medicine. The standardized procedure is actually developed within the facility where the expanded nursing functions have been approved. It is developed in collaboration with nursing, medicine, and administration. An example of a standardized procedure is a written protocol authorizing a nurse to implement a peripherally inserted venous catheter for any patient in the neonatal intensive care unit. The NCSBN provides additional online resources for nurses covering diverse topics, including licensure and regulation (NCSBN, 2011b).

Violations of an NPA. State legislatures have given licensing boards the authority to hear and decide administrative cases against nurses when there is an alleged violation of an NPA or the nursing board's rules and regulations. Nurses who violate the NPA or board's administrative rules and regulations are subject to disciplinary action by the board. Table 8.1

contains a synopsis of the licensing board procedure for a complaint made about a nurse. Courts have consistently affirmed board of nursing decisions to restrict, suspend, or revoke the nurse's license when nurses have challenged the decision.

Box 8.2 presents the more common grounds for disciplinary action by state boards of nursing. Penalties that

TABLE 8.1   Licensing Board Procedure When a Complaint Is Filed

Action	Consequence
Complaint is made (initial complaint may be lodged by a telephone call or a letter mailed to the licensing board) by: • Consumer (patient) • Family member • Nurse or nurse manager or employer • Professional nursing organization • State board of nursing • Federal or state authority (i.e., CMS or Department of Health and Human Services)	Sworn complaints must be filed
Licensing board reviews complaint: • Examines evidence • Reviews reports	Insufficient evidence—no action; administrative review scheduled • Nurse notified
Board makes determination	Nurse summoned • Rules of proceeding explained • Witnesses called to testify • Further evidence examined
Licensing board makes decision	Nurse exonerated Nurse guilty of violating the NPA
Board takes disciplinary action	Possible actions • Board issues formal reprimand • Fines levied against nurse • Nurse placed on probation • License suspended or revoked • License not renewed
Nurse may challenge licensing board's actions	Nurse must file appeal in court
Court reviews case (court action depends on jurisdiction) • Reviews conduct of proceedings • Reviews board's decision	Licensing board ruling is reversed
Licensing board can appeal ruling	Court reviews case
Court renders a decision	Licensing board ruling is upheld
OR	OR
Court renders a decision	Licensing board ruling is overturned Licensing board can appeal to a higher court
Case scheduled for trial	Licensing board ruling is upheld OR Licensing board ruling is reversed

CMS, Centers for Medicare & Medicaid Services; *NPA,* nurse practice act.

BOX 8.2 Grounds for Disciplinary Action by State Boards of Nursing

- Practicing without a valid license
- Failure to use appropriate nursing judgment
- Guilty of a felony
- Falsification of records
- Failure to complete nursing documentation
- Incorrect nursing documentation
- Failure to practice in accordance with nursing standards
- Inappropriate behavior or occurrence at work
- Medicare fraud
- Misappropriation of personal items

licensing boards may impose for violations of an NPA include the following:

- Issuing a formal reprimand
- Establishing a period of probation
- Levying fines
- Limiting, suspending, or revoking a nurse's license.

It is estimated that 10% to 15% of RNs in the United States are chemically dependent (Cares et al, 2015; NCSBN, 2011c). The majority of disciplinary actions by licensing boards are related to misconduct resulting from chemical impairment, including the misappropriation of drugs for personal use and the sale of drugs and drug paraphernalia to support the nurse's addiction. For a nurse whose license is limited or suspended because of problems related to chemical impairment, the ability to practice in the future is often predicated on successful completion of a drug rehabilitation program and evidence of abstinence. An increasing number of state licensing boards have established programs to guide nurses through the process of rehabilitation to reestablish licensure.

Nurse-Patient Ratios and Mandatory Overtime Statutes

Inadequate and often unsafe nurse-patient ratios continue to plague nursing and result in missed nursing care (Carthon et al, 2015). A growing body of evidence confirms a strong association between nurse-patient ratios and patient outcomes (Konetzka et al, 2013; Silber et al, 2016; Simpson, 2016). The ANA launched its "Safe Staffing Saves Lives Campaign" in 2008, publishing the results of a poll conducted to examine nurses' perceptions of staffing problems (ANA, 2009). More than

50% of respondents were considering leaving their current nursing position, and 42% indicated that the reason for leaving was associated with inadequate staffing. Another study surveyed direct-care nurses about nursing errors of omission. More than 70% of respondents reported the inability at times to plan and implement required care and intervene in a timely manner. Forty-four percent of respondents missed essential assessments (Kalisch et al, 2012). Eighty-five percent of the nurses indicated that lack of human resources (nurse and support staff) was the primary reason for omissions in essential components of the nursing process. In 2015 the ANA responded to these findings, publishing a white paper to assist nurse leaders in developing effective staffing strategies.

Nurse staffing is influenced to some degree by federal law through the CoPs and, increasingly, by state laws. Hospitals risk losing federal Medicare and Medicaid funding for a confirmed pattern of understaffing that has not been properly addressed by managers and administrators and the hospital's Board of Directors. The CMS has fined hospitals for understaffing, in part owing to increased patient census. Hospital administrators and clinical leaders must prepare a corrective action plan and submit it to the CMS within a specified time when cited by the CMS for safety violations such as unsafe staffing levels. Nurses can positively affect nurse staffing levels when armed with knowledge regarding federal and state laws. When concerns about work-related issues arise (e.g., a reduction in RN staffing, mandatory overtime, or replacement of RNs with LVNs-LPNs or unlicensed assistive personnel), the first question the nurse asks and answers should be, "Is this legal?" (Brooke, 2009).

In 1999, California became the first state to enact a law (California Assembly Bill 394) that mandates the establishment of minimum nurse-patient ratios in acute care facilities (Tevington, 2011). The law, which took effect in January 2004, set minimum nurse-patient ratios in critical care units, step-down and medical-surgical units, and maternity departments. No other state has followed California's lead in establishing nurse-patient ratios, but by 2014, 14 states had enacted laws that regulate or restrict mandatory overtime for nurses, and two states have restrictions established by state regulations (ANA, n.d.). The ANA reintroduced the RN Safe Staffing Act (H.R. 2392/S.3401) in 2017 for the 2017-2018 session of Congress. It requires hospitals that participate in

Medicare to implement staffing plans, which are established by a committee composed of a majority of direct-care nurses for each nursing unit and shift.

An increasing number of lawsuits against health care facilities have set forth claims of corporate negligence for inadequate staffing or "understaffing" when adverse outcomes occur. A jury awarded a $1.7 million verdict against a nursing home for the death of a resident who fell from her wheelchair. Evidence revealed that there was a widespread pattern of understaffing at the nursing home (*Sunbridge Healthcare Corp. v. Penny,* 2005). In 2006, another jury awarded $240,000 in punitive damages (out of a total award of $400,000) against a nursing home because understaffing at the facility was considered an aggravating factor in a patient's death (*Miller v. Levering Regional Healthcare Center,* 2006). The patient was 91 years of age and suffered from Alzheimer's disease. The resident (patient) was left unattended and fell, hitting her head, and subsequently died of her injuries. The court records contained adequate evidence that the facility knew it had a chronic understaffing problem and that the problem directly led to the woman's death (Snyder, 2006). The director of nursing was also found negligent for failing to comply with Medicare guidelines that required the facility to provide sufficient staffing.

Reporting Statutes

The federal government and states seek to protect at-risk individuals (children and older adults) by requiring nurses and other health care providers to report specific types of suspected or actual patient-client injury, abuse, or neglect. Boards of nursing are created to protect the public from unethical, incompetent, or impaired nursing practice. Some states have enacted statutes that *mandate* nurses to report unsafe, illegal, or unethical practices by nursing colleagues or physicians (Starr, 2016) or by administrators of health care facilities that place patients in jeopardy. With these mandates and protections in mind, the following case illustrates the adverse consequences that nurses may still face when reporting and/or whistle-blowing.

A nurse practitioner was contracted to provide health care services to inmates at a county jail in the state of Nevada. During the course of her work, she collaborated with a physician who also treated those incarcerated in the jail. The nurse practitioner, as well as other health care workers providing services in the facility, objected when the physician did not at all times write progress notes as he evaluated and treated the inmates. The primary concern was one of patient well-being, because the nurse and other health care workers relied on the physician's notes to provide safe and effective care. Additionally, the nurse practitioner feared for the health and safety of patients because another physician, the prison's staff psychiatrist, failed to perform timely assessments of inmates with psychiatric disorders. The nurse practitioner lodged complaints about the two physicians through the facility's formal chain of command and was terminated by prison management. The nurse sued her employer, claiming wrongful termination under Nevada's whistle-blower protection statute. The nurse's former employer claimed she could not sue for wrongful termination because she did not comply with the state's "generic" whistle-blower law, requiring her to report patient safety concerns directly to a public agency (Nevada State Department of Health). However, the U.S. District Court for the District of Nevada ruled that the fired nurse practitioner had the right to sue her former employer for retaliating against her. The court based its opinion on the state of Nevada's "special" whistle-blower law for health care workers. That special law protected nurses from retaliation (including termination) for internally reporting a situation that could compromise patient safety (*Scott v. Corizon Health,* 2014). The outcome of the nurse's suit against her former employer has not yet been reported in the legal literature.

Nursing publications provide recommendations and guidelines to any nurse considering the duty to report and its consequences (Lachman, 2012; Philipsen and Soeken, 2011). Nurses should be extremely careful to clarify their state's whistle-blower protection law for health care workers before engaging in whistle-blower activities. States vary widely in the requirements that must be met in order for a nurse to claim protection against retaliation for whistle-blowing. A first step requires the nurse to contact the state's board of nursing to determine whistle-blowing requirements established by the licensing board and/or formalized in that state's whistle-blowing protection statute. An increasing number of legal experts advise the nurse to seek the services of an attorney who specializes in reporting and whistle-blowing activities for nurses before making a decision to report (Snyder, 2014).

The types of conduct that the boards of nursing require nurses to report vary from state to state. Nurses can access the specific requirements for reporting nurse coworkers at their board of nursing website. Some states require nurses and providers to report victims of domestic or interpersonal violence, whether or not the victim (patient) consents. Nurses can access current information from the state regarding reporting requirements under family or domestic violence statutes. For a list of family violence statutes compiled by the American Academy of Orthopedic Surgeons (2012), visit http://www.aaos.org/about/abuse/ststatut.asp. Certain specifiable communicable diseases must also be reported to the Centers for Disease Control and Prevention (CDC) such as bubonic plague, Ebola, anthrax, and botulism. (For the list of reportable diseases, visit http://www.cdc.gov/ncezid/.) State law may also require nurses to report injuries resulting from the use of weapons, attempts to harm the self, or impaired driving (Mathes, 2014). Nurse managers and administrators are responsible for ensuring that reports made by direct-care nurses are forwarded to the appropriate legal authorities. Nurse leaders who fail in this duty may face criminal charges, claims of negligence, and disciplinary action by the nursing board (Raper, 2008).

Child Abuse Reporting Statutes. In 1973, the U.S. Congress enacted the Child Abuse Prevention and Treatment Act, which mandates all states to meet specific uniform guidelines to qualify for federal funding of child abuse programs. All 50 states and the District of Columbia have created laws that require reporting of specific health problems and the *suspected* or confirmed abuse of infants or children. Nurses often are explicitly named within the context of these statutes as one of the groups of designated health professionals who must report the specified problems under penalty of fine or imprisonment. Nurses need not fear legal reprisal from individuals or families who are reported to authorities in suspected cases of abuse. Most legislatures have granted immunity from suit within the context of the mandatory reporting statute. There is also a long history of court decisions shielding the nurse from civil claims by parents or guardians when that report is made in good faith, and in compliance with federal and state laws. The case of *Heinrich v. Conemaugh Valley Memorial Hospital* (1994) upheld this doctrine of immunity. The family of an injured child initiated a lawsuit against a hospital that reported suspected child abuse after a state investigation found them innocent of the charge. The court ruled that the hospital and the physician who made the report in "good faith" were immune from litigation under the Pennsylvania Child Protective Service Law that required reports of suspected child abuse.

It is crucial that nurses understand the requirements of abuse reporting statutes as they apply to their practice setting. For example, ED and pediatric nurses must have in-depth knowledge regarding child abuse reporting laws. Agency policies and procedures in the work setting may provide guidance in regard to reporting duties. If in doubt, the nurse should immediately contact his or her supervisor, an administrator, or the agency's compliance officer (the individual responsible for understanding and ensuring adherence to federal and state statutes) for additional guidance in the matter. In rare situations, when information is not available within the institution, the nurse may consult with the state Department of Health and Human Services or the state nurses' licensing board for guidance and to obtain the reporting statutes. There are serious ramifications for failing to report as required by the state's specific statute, which could result in criminal charges and claims of negligence.

Institutional Licensing Laws

All facilities (e.g., hospitals, nursing homes, rehabilitation centers) providing health care services must comply with licensing laws promulgated by state legislatures. These laws are created to protect the public and ensure the safe and effective provision of health care services. Specific language usually is contained within health facility licensing statutes regarding the following issues:

- Minimal standards for the maintenance of the physical plant
- Basic operational aspects of major departments (nursing, dietary, clinical laboratories, and pharmacy)
- Essential aspects of patients' rights and the informed consent process

Many state licensing laws mandate minimal levels of education, experience, or credentialing for department administrators, such as nurses, anesthesia personnel, pediatricians, and obstetricians. Several states also require minimum nurse-patient ratios in critical care units and other specialty departments, such as the operating room, nursery, and ED.

Health care redesign and cost-reduction efforts have led to many changes in the way health care services are provided and the settings in which care is rendered.

Not all change has been positive, and some redesign schemes have resulted in adverse outcomes for patients (Mahlmeister, 2009a). Investigations by state authorities on reports of patient injuries or death have discovered that in some cases health care facilities have operated in violation of existing licensing laws. In the past, direct-care RNs generally could rely on their nurse managers to have a comprehensive knowledge of health facility licensing law and to create policies and procedures that implement and enforce applicable aspects of the law. The trend toward flattened management and reduction in role development for leaders has altered this picture. In an increasing number of settings, nurse managers have been replaced with non-nurse administrators, who may have minimal knowledge of the CoPs for Medicare and the state health facility licensing laws (Mahlmeister, 2015).

In light of these changes, direct-care nurses should have a working knowledge of current licensing laws as they relate to nursing care and patient care services. The nurse also is guided by the ANA's *Nursing: Scope and Standards of Practice,* which states: "The registered nurse systematically enhances the quality and effectiveness of nursing practice" (ANA, 2015c). In many instances, nurses who have serious questions regarding quality of care in their employment setting have been able to resolve these concerns once they have read applicable sections of the health facility licensing law relevant to their setting. Bringing the pertinent section of the law to the attention of managers, administrators, a compliance officer, or the risk management department is often the most effective strategy to resolve problems. In settings in which nurses are represented by union contracts, potential violations of health facility licensing laws may be most effectively addressed through union representatives.

Internet access has allowed nurses to obtain information about current institutional licensing laws easily. Information can be downloaded and printed quickly. Nurses also can obtain a copy of the health facility's licensing law for their employment setting through the state department or health division of licensing and certification. Other states provide the statute and address questions through the state department of health's divisions of facilities regulations, health facilities inspection, or health quality assurance. The telephone number for this agency can be found in the white pages of the local telephone directory under the heading "State of" (e.g.,

Michigan). Nurses can call their licensing board or the state nursing association for guidance in reaching the appropriate authority to obtain a copy of the licensing law and to speak to a consultant about concerns.

COMMON LAW

In addition to statutory law, nursing practice is guided by common law, also known as decisional or *judge-made law.* Common law is created through cases heard and decided in federal and state appellate courts. Throughout the years, judge-made law regarding nursing practice has accumulated in the form of written opinions. These opinions eventually contribute to the expected standard of nursing conduct (Mathes, 2014). The body of written opinions about nurses also is known as nursing case law. The importance of nursing case law in establishing the current standard of practice cannot be overstated.

One of the most important cases to establish the expected conduct of nurses was *Utter v. United Hospital Center, Inc.* (1977). This West Virginia case affirmed that nurses were required to exercise independent judgment to prevent harm when caring for patients. Before the 1970s, the issue of whether nurses were licensed professionals who made independent judgments was not clearly established. In the Utter case, a patient whose arm was casted had signs and symptoms of compartment syndrome. The affected limb became progressively more edematous and eventually turned black. The nurses failed to activate the chain of command when the primary providers did not respond to their reports and requests for medical re-evaluation. The patient's arm eventually had to be amputated. The court wrote:

> "*Nurses are specialists in hospital care who, in the final analysis, hold the well-being, in fact in some instances, the very lives of patients in their hands. In the dim hours of the night, as well as in the light of day, nurses are frequently charged with the duty to observe the condition of the ill and infirm in their care. If the patient, helpless and wholly dependent, shows signs of worsening, the nurse is charged with the obligation of taking some positive action . . . [T] here was evidence that certain nurses did not fulfill their obligation.*"

The duty to prevent harm, known as the nurse's "affirmative duty," has been supported in numerous court decisions. In *Rowe v. Sisters of Pallottine Missionary Society* (2001), a hospital and its ED nurses were found negligent for failing to question a physician's discharge order. A 17-year-old motorcyclist was admitted to the ED for an injury to his left leg. He complained of severe pain in his left knee and numbness in his left foot. The nurses were unable to find a pulse in the left leg or foot. The physician issued a discharge order and gave instructions that included the application of ice and elevation of the affected leg. The next day the man sought emergency care at another hospital for worsening pain and swelling of his leg. An examination revealed a lacerated popliteal artery and dislocated knee. He underwent extensive surgery and suffers permanent impairment of the affected limb. The physician settled the suit against him for $275,000. The jury returned a verdict for the patient in excess of $880,000 and found the nurses negligent for failing to question the discharge order and to invoke the chain of command to obtain additional medical consultation and advice.

Every nurse should understand the effect that nursing case law has on his or her current practice. Case law made in appellate court decisions has addressed a range of vital issues related to professional nursing, including the following:

- Nursing malpractice cases
- Questions concerning labor law and collective bargaining
- Lawsuits alleging wrongful termination
- Legal challenges to state board of nursing disciplinary action against a nurse's license
- Legal actions against the nurse instituted by medical licensing boards
- "Practicing medicine without a license" claims
- Lawsuits claiming violation of the nurse's civil rights, including free speech issues and reasonable accommodation for nurses with disabilities

Efforts should be made by professional nurses to review case law as it is published and discussed in nursing journals. There has been a trend to incorporate "legal advice" columns into many practice journals, and journals often include discussions about nursing case law. There also has been a proliferation of nursing journals dedicated solely to legal issues in nursing practice.

Nurse managers, in particular, should have knowledge regarding the disposition of cases in their jurisdiction. A risk manager or agency attorney may help any nurse understand how judge-made law in his or her state relates to expectations for nursing practice in the local community. Many medical libraries also subscribe to publications that review federal or appellate court decisions in health care law that are relevant to the local community. Although local jury verdicts do not contribute to common law, it is useful for managers and interested nurses to periodically review published reports of malpractice cases in the state and their immediate community. Medical libraries also often subscribe to a local "jury verdicts" publication. (More information on finding nursing case law is available on the Evolve site at http://evolve.elsevier.com/Cherry/.)

CIVIL LAW

Two major categories of law have been created to deal with conduct that is considered unacceptable—criminal law and civil law. Nurses generally are more familiar with civil law and, in particular, the branch of civil law that deals with torts. Tort law is discussed first, with a discussion of criminal law following.

A *tort* is a civil wrong or injury committed by one person against another person or a property. The wrong results from a breach in one's legal duty regarding interpersonal relationships between private persons. This duty is established through societal expectations regarding interpersonal conduct (Butts and Rich, 2016). Civil suits are almost always brought by one person against another and generally are based on the concept of "fault." The person who initiates the civil lawsuit, the plaintiff, seeks damages for the wrongful behavior from the offending person, known as the defendant. The determination whether wrongful behavior has occurred usually is made by a jury, although in certain cases the right to a trial by jury can be waived by the private parties in the suit; in that case, the judge considers the facts and determines the outcome. If the plaintiff succeeds in the civil lawsuit (plaintiff verdict), damages are generally awarded in the form of monetary compensation. Damages may include "hard" damages—financial reimbursement for treatment of injuries, loss of wages, rehabilitation services, or special equipment—and "soft" damages—monetary compensation for pain and suffering, loss of companionship, or mental anguish, among others (Griffith and Tengnah, 2017).

Negligence and Malpractice

There are two types of torts: an unintentional tort (or wrong) and an intentional tort. An unintentional tort is an unintended wrong against another person. The two most common unintentional torts are negligence and malpractice.

Negligence is defined as the failure to act in a reasonable and prudent manner. The claim of negligence is based on the accepted principle that everyone is expected to conduct themselves in a reasonable and prudent fashion. This is true of laypersons, student nurses, and licensed professionals. A more formal definition of negligence is the failure of a person to use the care that a reasonably prudent and careful person would use under similar circumstances (Griffith and Tengnah, 2017).

Malpractice is a special type of negligence (i.e., the failure of a professional, a person with specialized education and training, to act in a reasonable and prudent manner) (Mathes, 2014). As state NPAs have evolved to reflect the growing professionalism of RNs, courts have begun to recognize the negligent acts of nurses as malpractice. Evidence of this change in perceptions is apparent in the increasing use of RNs as expert witnesses in malpractice cases.

In general, expert testimony is not needed in cases of "simple negligence," if the actions of the defendant are so obviously careless that even a layperson would recognize the conduct as negligent. In contrast, if the jury does not possess the special knowledge and information that professionals ordinarily have, an expert witness is required to establish whether the person breached the expected standard of care. In this case, the breach of duty is not simple negligence but malpractice.

Elements Essential to Prove Negligence or Malpractice.

Although any patient (or surviving family member, in the case of a patient death) may sue the nurse and his or her employer, the following elements must be proved for the plaintiff to succeed in the case.

1. The nurse owed the patient or client a special duty of care based on the establishment of a nurse-patient relationship. The nurse's acceptance of a patient assignment establishes the relationship and requires the nurse to meet his or her duty to the patient. The duty of the nurse is to possess the knowledge and skill that a reasonable and prudent nurse would possess and exercise in the same or similar patient care situation. The duty of the nurse as described is the standard of care. A nurse-patient relationship also may be established through telephone communication in the case of a nurse who performs telephone triage and advice or via computer or audiovisual systems that are being introduced in some health care settings (American Academy of Ambulatory Care Nursing, 2011; American Telemedicine Association, 2014).

2. The nurse has breached his or her duty to the patient or client. Evidence is presented that proves the nurse breached the standard of care. The standard of care is derived from a multiplicity of sources; these are described in Box 8.3.

3. Actual harm or damage is suffered by the patient.

4. There is proximate cause or a causal connection between the breach in the standard of care by the nurse and the patient's injury:
   - No intervening event is responsible for the injury.
   - A direct cause and effect can be demonstrated.
   - In some jurisdictions, the nurse's breach of duty must only be proven to be a substantial cause of the patient's injury.

This last element merits further discussion. The relationship between the nurse's breach in the standard of care and the patient's injury must be established by the plaintiff. To prove proximate cause, there must be a direct causal link. For example, a patient reports that he has an allergy to penicillin and wears a MedicAlert bracelet to that effect. A physician orders penicillin to treat the patient's infection. The nurse fails to check or to ask the patient about allergies. The nurse administers the penicillin, and the patient suffers an anaphylactic reaction and dies. There is a direct connection between the nurse's actions and the patient's death. Proximate cause has been established.

One may ask what the physician's liability is in this case. The physician also owes a duty to the patient and may be found negligent for ordering penicillin, if he or she had knowledge of or should have had knowledge of the allergy. However, even in the case of a physician's negligence—"I knew about the penicillin allergy, but forgot"—the nurse has a separate and independent duty to the patient to prevent harm. The nurse must review the patient's medical record for information about allergies, ask the patient about allergies, and

---

BOX 8.3 Sources That Contribute to the Standard of Nursing Care

Federal Laws
Emergency Medical Treatment and Active Labor Law
Americans with Disabilities Act
Patient Self-Determination Act
Occupational Health and Safety Act
The Patient Safety and Quality Improvement Act

Federal Administrative Rules and Regulations
Rules and regulations for participation in Medicare

Federal Agencies
U.S. Food and Drug Administration
Agency for Healthcare Research and Quality clinical guidelines
National Institutes of Health publications
Centers for Disease Control and Prevention publications
(*Morbidity and Mortality Weekly Report*)

State Statutes
Nurse practice acts
State reporting statutes:
- Child abuse/elder abuse reporting statutes
- Domestic violence reporting statutes
- Health facility licensing laws

State Administrative Rules and Regulations
Licensing board rules

Board of Nursing
Position statements and advisories

Nursing Case Law
Appellate court decisions

Professional Organizations
Standards and guidelines for practice
Nursing journals
Position statements
Technical bulletins and practice resources
Code of Ethics

Manufacturer Guidelines
Durable medical equipment
Drugs and solutions
Disposable equipment and supplies

Agency Policies and Procedures
Job descriptions
Agency-specific documents
Nursing care plans
Care maps or critical pathways
Unit- or department-based standards of practice
Medical staff bylaws

---

check the patient's identification band before administering a drug.

In some jurisdictions, it is necessary only to prove that the nurse's actions were a substantial cause of the injury or harm to prove negligence. For example, in a large teaching hospital, a nurse notes a significant change in a patient's vital signs, suggesting deterioration in his condition. A first-year resident is called to the bedside and made aware of the patient's status. The resident orders the nurse to simply continue observing the patient. The first-year resident remains immediately available in the unit and receives repeated reports of a continued decline in the patient's condition. A clear chain-of-command policy is established in the hospital, which takes into account varying levels of skill and expertise of the residents in training. There is also a chain-of-command policy to deal with unresolved disagreements between health care professionals and nonresponsive providers. Despite the existence of these policies, the nurse does not activate the chain of command.

The patient suffers hypovolemic shock caused by internal bleeding, leading to permanent anoxic brain damage. In this case, the nurse's failure to obtain additional medical advice and consultation (a senior resident was physically present and available in the hospital) was a substantial cause of the patient's injury. These two examples illustrate that negligence may constitute a commission (inappropriate penicillin administration) or an omission (failure to activate the chain of command) in care.

Negligence and the Doctrine of *Res Ipsa Loquitur*. In the majority of cases, a plaintiff must retain a nurse expert witness because the jury does not ordinarily possess the scientific and technologic knowledge necessary to determine the required standard of care. When the negligent act clearly lies within the range of a jury's common knowledge and experience, the doctrine of *res ipsa loquitur* ("the thing speaks for itself") may be applied. For instance, studies have reported close to

5000 foreign objects (instruments, needles, surgical sponges) inadvertently left in patients' bodies following surgery each year. Retained foreign bodies were associated with a higher average cost of health services than uncomplicated postsurgical care ($26,678 vs. $12,648) (Al Qurayshi et al., 2015).

Leaving a surgical instrument in the patient's body after an operation is one case in which the doctrine of *res ipsa loquitur* may apply. It would be obvious to any layperson that failure to remove a surgical instrument is below the standard of care.

Dickerson v. Fatehi (1997) illustrates this point. A woman who underwent neck surgery experienced severe pain in her right arm, hand, and neck after the procedure. Approximately 20 months later, a second procedure was performed to determine the cause of the patient's continued pain. An 18-gauge hypodermic needle with a plastic attachment for a syringe was discovered in her neck and removed. The woman sued the surgeon and nurses involved in the original surgical procedure. The claims against the nurses included a failure to maintain a proper needle count and a failure to ensure the removal of the needle after surgery. The court hearing this case dismissed the suit. On appeal, the Supreme Court of Virginia reversed the lower court's decision and directed the case for trial. The Supreme Court held that in this particular case expert testimony was not necessary to establish the applicable standard of care and that the doctrine of *res ipsa loquitur* applied. A jury would be able to determine whether a reasonably prudent circulating nurse and scrub nurse should have made and reported an accurate needle count.

Gross Negligence. In some cases, the negligent act of the nurse is so reckless and reflects such a conscious disregard for the patient's welfare that it represents gross negligence. When the nurse acts with complete indifference to the consequences for his or her patient, the court may award special damages meant to punish the nurse for the outrageous conduct. These damages are referred to as *punitive damages*. Each state has established standards to determine when punitive damages may be awarded. In *Mobile Infirmary Medical Center v. Hodgen* (2003), the jury awarded $2.5 million in punitive damages (later reduced to $1.5 million) when a new graduate, not yet licensed, administered five times the ordered dose of digoxin. The jury found that the new graduate had been improperly supervised by the novice nurse assigned as her preceptor by the shift charge

nurse. The charge nurse was also found liable for failing to properly direct the preceptor in her role responsibilities. The Supreme Court of Alabama found that the nurses acted callously and wantonly, the legal threshold that must be crossed before punitive damages can be awarded (Snyder, 2003).

Claims of Negligence and Student Nurses

Claims of negligence may arise when student nurses provide care. The emphasis on patient safety and reporting preventable adverse outcomes has brought an increasing number of student errors to light (Mahlmeister, 2008; Reid-Searl et al, 2010; Wolf et al, 2009). Because the student is not yet a licensed professional, the faculty member or licensed nurse who is supervising the student is often named in the lawsuit (Brooke, 2009). The state board of nursing may have an advisory or position statement regarding the scope of practice of nursing students, and the duty of the supervising registered nurse supervising the student, to maintain the appropriate level of oversight. Such is the case in California, where the Board of Nursing has promulgated a position statement, "Clinical Learning Experiences: Nursing Students," to guide the supervising nurse in her duty (California Department of Consumer Affairs, 2008). The agency or hospital in which the student is practicing also may be named under the legal doctrine of vicarious liability. *Dimora v. Cleveland Clinic Foundation* (1996) is a case in point. A student nurse was assigned to care for a patient who had serious difficulty maintaining her balance and required close supervision when standing, walking, and transferring. The student nurse testified that she knew the patient had an unsteady gait but still left her unattended on a commode. The patient fell and was injured. The hospital was named in the lawsuit and appealed, claiming the student was not an employee. The Ohio Court of Appeals ruled that a hospital was held to the same legal standard of care for a student nurse's error as for the same error committed by a licensed professional nurse.

Several other cases reinforce the importance of informing the patient that a student is providing the care and of documenting that the patient agrees to the care. In *Lovett v. Lorain Community Hospital* (2004), a student nurse, under the direct supervision of an instructor, administered Demerol and Vistaril by the intramuscular route and punctured the patient's sciatic nerve. The patient sued the hospital for negligence. A lower court dismissed the initial lawsuit because the student and the instructor were not employees of the hospital. The Ohio Court of Appeals reversed the lower court's decision. The higher court affirmed that a patient may assume that the care he or she receives in a hospital is provided by that institution. The patient can assume that the student and instructor are agents of the hospital, unless the patient has been specifically informed and has agreed to receive care from the student (Snyder, 2004). Because a student nurse is not yet a licensed professional, if a lawsuit is filed the alleged claim is usually "ordinary negligence" rather than "professional malpractice."

Criminal Negligence

Criminal negligence applies when the negligent acts of the nurse (normally an unintentional civil wrong) also constitute a crime. In most states, a nurse can be prosecuted when the conduct is deemed so reckless that the action results in serious harm to or death of the patient. Nurses with criminal convictions accounted for approximately 10% of the disciplinary actions taken by state boards of nursing (BONs) between 2003 and 2013 (Zhong et al, 2016).

In 1997 two RNs and an advanced practice nurse licensed in Colorado were charged with criminal negligent homicide in the death of a newborn resulting from a medication error (Kowalski and Horner, 1998). In this case, an oil-based form of penicillin was erroneously administered to the infant. The drug was administered at 10 times the physician's prescribed dose. This case, first discussed in the nursing literature in 1998, describes medication dispensing and administration practices that still exist in many U.S. hospitals, placing patients in immediate jeopardy and exposing nurses to claims of criminal negligence. A case that occurred in Wisconsin in 2006 illustrates the ongoing risks for catastrophic medication errors. A labor and delivery nurse inadvertently administered a piggyback solution bag of epidural anesthesia through a peripheral intravenous line. The patient, a 16-year-old female, experienced cardiovascular collapse and died. The error was compounded by failures to place an identification band on the patient and to use the available point-of-care barcode system. In the root cause analysis of this sentinel event conducted at a later date, "multiple latent systems failures" were also identified (Smetzer et al, 2010). The Wisconsin Department of Justice charged the nurse with a felony criminal offense. The charge was eventually reduced to a misdemeanor count

of illegally administering prescription medications. The Wisconsin Department of Health and Human Services imposed restriction on the nurse's ability to participate in any capacity in a facility funded by Medicare and Medicare programs for 5 years. The Wisconsin Department of Regulation and Licensing suspended the nurse's license for 9 months, and the hospital terminated her employment. In response to the Wisconsin case, the ANA released a statement opposing charges of criminal misconduct against a registered nurse who did not intentionally mean to harm the patient (ANA, 2007). The American Association of Nurse Attorneys (TAANA) in collaboration with the American Association of Legal Nurse Consultants (AALNC) also published a Position Paper, "Criminal Prosecution of Health Care Providers for Unintentional Human Error" (TAANA, 2011). The organizations strongly oppose criminalization of negligence.

The Colorado and Wisconsin cases should be read by every student nurse and licensed nurse for full appreciation of the change in the legal climate in the United States. They reflect the changing perspective of our justice system when negligent acts of health care professionals result in patient death. Conservative estimates published by the Institute of Medicine (IOM) in 2000 suggested that as many as 98,000 patients die each year as a result of the negligence and malpractice of health care providers (IOM, 2000), and another 90,000 deaths per year are attributed to hospital-acquired infections (CMS, 2011). National data regarding hospital-acquired infections may be accessed at the Centers for Disease Control and Prevention's National Healthcare Safety Network (http://www.cdc.gov/nhsn/). Later data derived from surveillance activities conducted by the Institute for Healthcare Improvement (IHI) using a new tracking tool, the "Global Trigger Tool," found that the number of adverse events in hospitals may *be ten times greater than previously measured* (Classen et al, 2012). Medical error has risen from the fifth to the third leading cause of death in the United States (Makary and Daniel, 2016).

Other negative consequences that a nurse faces when criminal charges are filed include the loss of his or her job and disciplinary action by the state licensing board. Even when the criminal charges are not supported, the nurse's license can be suspended or revoked, and out-of-pocket fines may be levied by the board if there is evidence of violation of the NPA. An attorney may have to be retained to represent the nurse when criminal charges are filed, and the nurse's malpractice insurance generally does not cover the attorney's fees in this case. Neither is the nurse's employer obligated to pay the legal fees of a nurse charged with a felony. In the Colorado case, the nurse practitioner was immediately terminated. The two direct-care nurses were permitted to work in nonpatient care areas. The costs of the criminal defense of all three nurses were paid by the hospital.

Nursing care that is deemed "deplorable" by the courts may result in disqualification of the nurse's employer from participation in the federal government's Medicare or Medicaid programs. Essentially the facility will be without adequate funding to continue operating. A case in point is *Barbourville Nursing Home v. U.S. Department of Health and Human Services* (2006). During a compliance survey visit to the facility by the U.S. Department of Health and Human Services (USDHHS), major infractions of nursing home regulations were discovered. The federal government levied a fine in excess of $24,000 and, because the actions of the nurses placed the patients in immediate jeopardy (e.g., contaminating wounds with feces during dressing changes and inadequate skin care resulting in severe pressure sores), the nursing home was disqualified from participating in Medicare.

Defenses Against Claims of Negligence

In some cases, a nurse can use certain legal doctrines as a defense against a claim of negligence. These standard defenses are discussed in the next section. In no case may a nurse provide a defense of "only following the provider's orders" against allegations of negligence (ANA, 2015c; Greenberg, 2017; Snyder, 2007). The NPA, licensing board rules and regulations, and nursing case law have delineated the nurse's independent duty to evaluate all provider orders before implementing them. In doing so, the nurse must consider two points: (1) is the order lawful and (2) is the order in this particular patient's best interest?

Each nurse has an absolute duty to take some positive action to prevent harm when orders are inappropriate or incomplete or when the actions of another health care provider endanger the patient's well-being. This principle of affirmative duty is well recognized in law and in ethics. The ANA *Code of Ethics for Nurses* (2015a) and the American Medical Association's *Code of Medical Ethics* (2010–2011) recognize the central role of nurses in preventing patient harm. A second principle underlying the nurse's legal and professional obligation to address questionable physician's orders or plan of care is

patient advocacy (ANA, 2012a). The nurse's duty to "speak out" in order to support and protect patients has been reaffirmed by The Joint Commission in its "Speak Up" initiative (TJC, 2014).

In *Columbia Medical Center of Las Colinas v. Bush* (2003), a jury awarded $13.1 million to a patient who suffered permanent brain damage and had no independent motor function or capacity for speech after receiving the wrong medication for a cardiac dysrhythmia. After consulting with a cardiologist, the ED physician had ordered verapamil for treatment of the patient's ventricular tachycardia. The ED nurse, who was certified in advanced life support, and her nursing supervisor, who was present, knew the drug was contraindicated for ventricular tachycardia. The two nurses did not question the order and permitted an emergency medical technician (EMT) to give the drug. The patient suffered profound hypotension and cardiopulmonary arrest. The Texas Court of Appeals opined that the nurse and her supervisor had a duty, when they had serious questions about a medication involving extreme risk to the patient, to activate the chain of command to obtain additional medical consultation and advice (Tammelleo, 2003).

Emergency Situations

Nursing care rendered in a life-threatening emergency may breach the standard of care required under ordinary circumstances. For instance, a woman who is 8 months pregnant arrives in the labor and delivery suite. She is hemorrhaging because of a premature separation of the placenta (abruptio placentae). An emergency cesarean delivery is ordered by the physician. The woman is near death as a result of blood loss. There also are clear signs of fetal distress. To expedite the surgical delivery, the operating room team does not observe the strict aseptic technique normally required during insertion of a Foley catheter into the woman's bladder and forgoes the lengthy abdominal scrub normally performed with an iodine solution.

The mother and infant are brought through the crisis safely, although a skin infection develops at the site of the woman's abdominal incision, which causes noticeable scarring. She also must be treated for a bladder infection, which resolves by discharge on the fourth postpartum day. She sues the nurses and physician. In this case, the defense could argue that the methods used were reasonable and prudent to save the life of the mother and baby. Even a delay of seconds could have resulted in the death of the woman or her infant. Expert witnesses are produced to support the defense assertion that in this particular situation, following customary procedures in preparing this woman for surgery would have breached the standard of care.

Governmental Immunity

For nurses working in federal or state health care facilities, a defense of governmental immunity may be used. Laws have been enacted that shield individual health care workers employed in federal or (some) state facilities from personal responsibility for damages awarded in malpractice cases. Nurses employed by the Department of Veterans Affairs, the U.S. Public Health Service, the National Aeronautics and Space Administration, and the Department of Defense are shielded from civil suits when in the performance of professional duties. This immunity was granted through enactment of specific federal statutes, including the Federal Tort Claims Act of 1946 and the Federal Employees Liability Reform and Tort Compensation Act of 1988. The intent of these laws was to substitute the U.S. government as the defendant in a malpractice suit. The government has waived its sovereign immunity against suit and pays the damages for injuries caused by the negligent acts of health care professionals employed in the aforementioned federal agencies.

State immunity statutes vary. In some instances, individual states have not waived their sovereign immunity from lawsuits. In these cases, the state is *not* substituted for the individual health care provider in malpractice cases. Nurses and physicians are liable for their negligent acts in these states and are personally responsible for damages awarded. It may be imperative in this circumstance for the health care professional to have individual malpractice insurance. The nurse should seek the advice of an attorney to determine whether it would be prudent to purchase malpractice insurance. The state affiliate of the ANA may also be helpful in this regard.

Good Samaritan Immunity

Good Samaritan laws may limit a nurse's liability or shield the nurse from a malpractice claim if the nurse renders assistance in an emergency that occurs outside the employment setting. Although in most states the nurse owes no legal duty to an accident victim, once the nurse makes a decision to stop and render aid (an ethical decision), a nurse-patient relationship is established.

(Some states, including Vermont, Minnesota, and Wisconsin, have enacted "duty to rescue" or "compulsory assistance" laws.) Nurses should contact the state licensing board or the state association of the ANA to determine whether the state in which they are licensed has a "duty to rescue" law.

When the nurse renders care at the scene of an accident, he or she is required to render the standard of care that any reasonable and prudent nurse would render in a similar situation. To prevail in a malpractice suit under the Good Samaritan laws, the injured plaintiff must prove that the nurse intentionally caused the injury or was grossly negligent. Therefore, each nurse should be familiar with his or her state-specific Good Samaritan statute. Nurses also should be reassured by the fact that the preponderance of malpractice cases that invoke the Good Samaritan defense are settled in favor of the nurse.

Statutes of Limitation in Malpractice Cases

Each state has established a time limit in which a person may initiate a lawsuit. Although many states have established a time limit of 2 or 3 years from the date of the patient's injury or death in which the plaintiff must sue, statutes of limitation vary widely from state to state. In some jurisdictions, a "termination of treatment" rule exists. It is predicated on the assumption that some injuries result from a series of treatments over time. In this case, the statute of limitation does not begin to run until the treatment ends.

Other rules and regulations govern the "tolling" or running of the statutes of limitation. The court recognizes that an injured party cannot initiate a malpractice case until he or she discovers that some harm was done (discovery rule). This can occur when health care providers actually hide the facts in the case of an injury through fraud, deceit, or concealment, such as through:
- Fraudulent or misleading entries in the medical record
- Destruction of evidence
- Destruction of the medical record

An Iowa case provides an example of a situation in which the statute of limitations may be extended (*Hanssen v. Genesis Health*, 2011). An orthopedic nurse erroneously gave a patient twice the dose of narcotic pain medication ordered by the physician. The patient became lethargic, experienced breathing problems, and fell twice in the bathroom. After the patient was discharged from the hospital, the orthopedic unit nurse manager wrote a letter to him. In the letter, the manager falsely stated that upon review of his chart, it was discovered that he had not received an incorrect dose of medication, but that he had a sensitivity reaction to the drug. The patient subsequently requested a copy of his complete medical record and decided to file a lawsuit against the nurse and hospital. The suit was filed more than 2 years after the alleged malpractice, which exceeded Iowa's 2-year statute of limitations. The hospital petitioned the court to dismiss the case on the basis of the tolling of the statute. The court ruled that there were legal grounds for extending the statute because the patient was not aware of the medication error until he received a complete copy of the medical record, at which time he filed a claim.

The statute of limitation also is altered when a foreign object is left in the patient's body. Until the foreign object is discovered, the statute of limitation does not begin to run. States have rules that regulate the tolling of the statute of limitation in cases involving mentally incompetent adults and minors. In the case of an adult patient who is so severely injured that there is a loss of mental capacity, the statute of limitation may not begin to toll until the patient regains mental competence. The statute of limitation varies in the case of minors and may expire only when the child reaches the age of majority (18 or 21 years of age) (Griffith and Tengnah, 2017).

Each nurse should be familiar with the statute of limitation for his or her state. If the nurse suspects that some form of fraud or deceit has occurred relative to a patient's injury, the agency's risk manager or attorney should be contacted immediately. Major penalties and fines are applicable in cases in which health care providers deliberately deceive the patient or destroy evidence. These acts rise to the level of criminal misconduct and can result in loss of one's professional license and possible incarceration.

Transparency and Disclosure of Error. When errors occur in practice, studies repeatedly confirm that telling the patient (and family) about the mistake (voluntary disclosure) results in far less severe ramifications for the clinicians and health care facility (Hannawa et al, 2016). In 2001, TJC established a new patient safety care standard requiring that institutions have a process in place to disclose unanticipated outcomes to patients. Disclosure of errors and unanticipated adverse outcomes is a key element of the national patient safety movement. The process of disclosure has been delineated by the National Quality Forum (NQF) in its publication, "Safe Practices for Better Healthcare" (2011). Safe Practice Number 7 states,

> *Following serious unanticipated outcomes, including those that are clearly caused by systems failures, the patient, and as appropriate, the family should receive timely, transparent, and clear communication concerning what is known about the event (p. v).*

When an unanticipated outcome occurs, the provider is generally responsible for discussing the situation with the patient and/or family members. Other agency representatives may be involved in the disclosure process, including administrators, risk managers, and attorneys. The nurse should not assume responsibility for disclosure before speaking to the provider and agency leaders. It should be determined in advance who will speak with the patient (or family) and how questions and concerns about the patient's condition, subsequent treatment, and the cost of any required care will be addressed. Fear that disclosure will lead to a malpractice claim is a significant barrier to voluntary disclosure, despite research findings to the contrary (Hannawa et al, 2016). In fact, patients sue for many reasons, including withdrawal of health team members after the event, silence, mishandling of information about unanticipated outcomes, delayed communication about adverse events, and anger when they believe they have not been told the truth about events (Kachalia, 2009).

If a nurse believes that the patient has not received essential information, the nurse discusses such concerns first with the provider. If further clarification is required, the nurse refers to the facility's chain of command or unresolved dispute policy. Research conducted by Shannon and associates (2009) on nurses' perceptions regarding disclosure found that nurses conceived of disclosure as a team event rather than a physician-patient discussion. Nurses believed they were excluded from the disclosure process. Furthermore, nurses in the study focus groups admitted to routinely and independently disclosing nursing errors that did not involve serious injury, but believed that when systems flaws or team mistakes contributed to the error and injury, the physician should serve as the team leader in the disclosure discussion.

Nursing Malpractice Insurance

With more states recognizing nursing malpractice as a legitimate claim in a civil suit, the question of whether nurses should carry malpractice insurance has become increasingly important. Nursing journals have published a number of articles that either address this question or describe the types of malpractice coverage the nurse should consider (Pohlman, 2015); textbooks also discuss the issue of liability insurance. A growing consensus appears to recommend that because of changes in the health care system, civil law, and insurance company policies, all nurses purchase malpractice insurance. Legal writers also are quick to note the fallacy of the assumption that having malpractice insurance increases the risk that the nurse will be targeted in a malpractice case. Lack of coverage will not discourage a lawsuit when there is a legitimate claim. Reasons given for the purchase of malpractice insurance by RNs include the following:

- Expanding functions of RNs and advanced practice nurses
- Floating and cross-training mandates
- Increasing responsibility for supervising subordinate staff
- Failure of some employers to initiate an adequate defense for nurses
- Work liability (insurance) coverage limits that are lower than the actual judgment made against the nurse in a lawsuit

Other considerations that the nurse must take into account when considering malpractice insurance include whether he or she is employed by the federal government. In this case, the nurse may be shielded from personal liability by federal tort statutes, although some states still uphold the doctrine of "sovereign immunity," making it impossible to sue a state-run medical facility for negligence. In these states, it is a virtual necessity for nurses to purchase malpractice insurance because health care workers become the only available targets in a malpractice case.

Liability

Closely tied to the concepts of negligence and malpractice is that of liability. Liability asserts that every person is responsible for the wrong or injury done to another resulting from carelessness.

Personal Liability

Within the context of nursing practice, the nurse is always accountable for the outcomes of his or her actions in carrying out nursing duties. The rule of personal liability requires the professional nurse to assume responsibility for patient harm or injury that is a result of his or her negligent acts. The nurse cannot be relieved of personal liability by another professional, such as a provider or nurse manager, who asserts, "Don't worry; I'll take responsibility for the consequences."

The principle of personal liability is illustrated in a Connecticut case, *Osiecki v. Bridgeport Health Care Center, Inc.* (2005). A jury found that a nurse caring for a patient with a tracheostomy failed to provide proper tracheostomy care, assessment of breath sounds, and re-evaluation of the patient's pulmonary status at appropriate intervals. The patient died secondary to a pulmonary hemorrhage, and the breaches in the standard of nursing care were found to be a substantial factor contributing to the patient's death. Had the nurse properly assessed the patient and at frequent intervals, early identification of pulmonary congestion would have permitted timely treatment. The surviving spouse was awarded $827,000 for the nurse's negligent actions. In another case, *Janga v. Colombrito* (2011), the nurses caring for a patient receiving anticoagulants were sued individually for his death, which was due to complications of bleeding. The nurses were found negligent for failing to question the order for anticoagulants before a patient underwent a lumbar puncture. There was conflicting testimony about whether or not a physician had issued an order to discontinue the anticoagulants. However, even if the physician did not direct the nurses to stop the medications, the plaintiff's expert witness nurse asserted that they had a duty to recognize that anticoagulants should not be given prior to a lumbar puncture and to advise the physician that they had nevertheless been administered. The court directed the jury to weigh the extent to which the nurses' negligence contributed to the unfortunate outcome (comparative negligence). The jury directed the nurses to pay 15% of the monetary award.

In 1989, the ANA summarized the most frequent allegations of negligence leveled against nurses in malpractice cases (Box 8.4). These charges have not substantially changed in the ensuing decades (McGuire and Mroczek, 2014). As nurses assume more and more responsibility for the monitoring and care of patients with complex health problems, the claim of "failure to rescue" is made with increasing frequency (Garvey, 2015; Taenzer et al, 2011). Nurses may be educated to implement effective risk-control strategies that reduce these claims. These personal and system-wide strategies are discussed in the next section.

BOX 8.4   **Most Frequent Allegations of Nursing Negligence**

- Failure to communicate and report*
- Failure to monitor the patient and report significant findings
- Failure to ensure patient safety
- Failure to rescue
- Improper treatment or negligent performance of the treatment
- Medication errors
- Failure to follow the agency's policies and procedures
- Failure to invoke the chain of command/access the line of authority

*The Joint Commission found that communication failures (i.e., reporting, situation-background-assessment-recommendation [SBAR] communication, and shift handoffs) were the number-one contributing cause of medical error and preventable adverse outcomes.

The Joint Commission. (2005). *Joint Commission guide to improving staff communication.* Oakbrook Terrace, IL: TJC; and The Joint Commission. (2017). *Inadequate handoff communication.* Sentinel Event Alert Issue 58. Oakbrook Terrace, IL: TJC.
Adapted from McGuire, C., & Mroczek, J. M. (2014). *Nursing malpractice.* Course 125. Lakeway, TX: The National Center of Continuing Education. Retrieved from https://www.nursece.com/pdfs/125_NurseMalpractice.pdf.

Many nurses practice under the misconception that they are protected from personal liability when employed by a health care entity such as a hospital. I have heard nurses say, "Why would a patient sue me personally? I don't have the financial resources of this (hospital, nursing home, home health care agency)!" Nurses can and have been individually named in lawsuits and found negligent. Damages can be levied against the nurse's current assets and future earnings for negligent acts. Furthermore, as Snyder (2003) reports, hospitals have sued nurses to recoup financial losses suffered when they were required to pay damages for the alleged negligence of the nurses named in the malpractice case. Personal liability is illustrated in the case of *Siegel v. Long Island Jewish Medical Center* (2003).

Personal Liability with Floating and Cross-Training

New models of patient care often mandate floating and cross-training of patient care staff to enhance efficiency and reduce staffing costs. These models of care have increased the personal liability of nurses (Griffith and Tengnah, 2017). Professional nurses must be cognizant of state statutes and case law when asked to perform services outside of their usual area of practice. In no case is a nurse permitted to perform tasks or render services for which he or she lacks the requisite knowledge and skill to do so competently.

The NPA and the administrative rules and regulations of the licensing board provide explicit statutory language regarding a nurse's duty to provide safe and competent care. For example, the Administrative Rules of the Tennessee Board of Nursing (revised, 2011) state:

The Board believes that the individual nurse is responsible for maintaining and demonstrating competence in the practice role whether the recipient of the nursing intervention is the individual, family, community, nursing staff, nursing student body, or other.

Tennessee Rules and Regulations of Registered Nurses Rule 1000-01-14: Standards of Nursing Competence

In addition to the laws governing practice in floating and cross-training situations, an increasing body of nursing case law also defines the limitation of assignments. Appellate court decisions have addressed the issue of when a nurse may safely refuse an assignment to float without the risk of job termination. A landmark case, *Winkelman v. Beloit Memorial Hospital* (1992), addressed the legal issues surrounding floating. The Supreme Court of Wisconsin ruled in this case that under certain circumstances, a nurse had a right to refuse floating assignments without fear of reprisal.

Nurse Winkelman was a skilled maternity nurse who was employed for 16 years at Beloit Memorial Hospital, working exclusively in the nursery. In 1987, the hospital created a policy that required nurses in the maternity setting to float when the patient census was low in their unit. Nurse Winkelman was asked to float to an adult floor dedicated to the care of postoperative and geriatric patients. She notified her immediate supervisor that she did not feel qualified to float to that unit and that attempting to provide care in that setting would place the patients at risk. In her testimony, the nurse said that she was given three choices: float, find another nurse who would float in her place, or take an unexcused absence day. She subsequently went home, and her employer construed her actions as "voluntary resignation of her employment." Nurse Winkelman then filed a complaint for wrongful discharge and breach of contract. A jury verdict was rendered in favor of Nurse Winkelman on the charge of wrongful discharge. The case was appealed and affirmed by the Supreme Court of Wisconsin. The court found that the nurse had identified a fundamental and well-defined public policy in the Wisconsin Administrative Code, which stated that a nurse should not offer or perform services for which he or she is not qualified by education, training, or experience.

The nurse's right to refuse a floating assignment has not been supported in all cases. Courts have affirmed the right of a health care facility to redirect staff to meet the needs of patients. The New Mexico Supreme Court, in *Francis v. Memorial General Hospital* (1986), held that the hospital was not prohibited from discharging a nurse who refused to float when the employer had made a reasonable offer to train the nurse for new responsibilities. Nurse Francis, a critical care nurse, refused to float to an orthopedic unit, stating he did not feel qualified to care for orthopedic patients. The hospital then offered to provide him with an orientation to the floors where he might float in the future. When he refused the opportunity for orientation, he was terminated. The court upheld his discharge.

Although it is clear that nurses have a legal duty to refuse specific tasks that they cannot perform safely and competently, the prudent nurse should carefully consider the consequences of not floating. Careful negotiation with the nursing supervisor and the team leader making the actual assignment often results in a satisfactory compromise. The floated nurse should clarify which aspects of professional nursing care he or she can safely carry out and which tasks are beyond his or her current capabilities. A reasonable supervisor will not insist that a nurse attempt to perform a task that he or she has no education, training, or current expertise to implement.

Another important strategy that may reduce the nurse's personal liability is to request that the team leader appoint a resource nurse who is skilled in the care of the patients on the unit. The resource nurse can assist the floated nurse as needed. It also is prudent practice for the floated nurse to enter a note in the medical record naming the resource or support nurse who will be available and responsible to assist with planning and evaluating care. For instance:

> *Assumed care of Mrs. Jones after report completed. L. Doe, RN, will co-manage patient and assist with procedures, planning, and evaluation of care as needed.*
>
> *J. Smith, RN (Floater)*

An NPA affirms that an RN ultimately is responsible for the quality of care provided to each patient, regardless of who actually is delegated the responsibility of carrying out the task. A claim of negligence may be leveled against the team leader who does not assign a competent "backup" or resource nurse to assist the floater. Only a nurse who is competent in the care of the patients normally treated in the setting (hospital, clinic, or home) can properly supervise a lesser-skilled worker and evaluate the outcomes of care.

Furthermore, TJC requires accredited organizations to ensure that all staff providing patient care, including float staff and agency or registry nurses, are properly oriented to their jobs and the work environment before providing care (TJC, 2017). Chapter 13 provides additional information about floating and accepting assignments.

Personal Liability for Charge Nurses and Team Leaders and Managers

The concept of personal liability extends to nurses who function as team leaders, supervisors, and upper-level managers. Team leaders, charge nurses, and managers are held to the standard of care of the reasonably prudent nurse employed in that role (Mahlmeister, 2006). Claims of negligence leveled against charge nurses generally surround the following:

- Functioning as a first responder in emergencies
- Triage of patients and allocation of staff and equipment
- Delegation of patient care tasks
- Supervision of orientees, float staff, and subordinates
- Reporting performance deficits in team members
- Supporting or invoking the chain-of-command process when indicated

Nurse managers and administrators at the upper end of the management ladder also may be held liable for the following:

- Inadequate training
- Failure to periodically reevaluate staff competencies
- Failure to discipline or terminate unsafe workers

- Negligence in developing appropriate policies and procedures
- Failure to uphold institutional licensing laws and state and federal statutes

The critical role of the charge nurse in promoting positive patient outcomes and reducing error is reflected in an Ohio Nurses Association Nursing Practice Statement (NP 21) regarding charge nurse responsibilities. The Practice Statement identifies 18 essential duties of the charge nurse (ONA, 2016). The many and varied role responsibilities of the charge nurse or team leader increases the risk for claims of malpractice.

The implementation of new models of care that alter staffing patterns and mixes may place managers at the same risk for liability as the health care providers delivering the actual bedside care (Roussel, 2011). The ANA affirms this view in the *Code of Ethics for Nurses* (2015a): "Although nurses in administration, education, and research have relationships with patients that are less direct, in assuming the responsibilities of a particular role, they share responsibility for the care provided by those whom they supervise and instruct" (p. 17).

The appropriate standard of care is established in the case of team leaders, charge nurses, managers, and leaders by expert nurse witnesses who function in those positions. An increasing body of case law in malpractice suits also is contributing to expectations about team leader and manager conduct. Although nurse managers and administrators generally are well aware of their particular liability risks, direct-care nurses who are relatively unfamiliar with the expanding role of team leaders or charge nurses may be particularly vulnerable to claims of negligence. Health care redesign has resulted in considerable flattening of the chain of command for nursing departments.

In September 2003, the American Organization of Nurse Executives, the American Hospital Association, and other health-related organizations submitted an *amicus curiae* (friend of the court) brief in support of the unique role of the charge nurse (Oakwood Healthcare, Inc., 348 J.L.R.B.., No. 37, 2006). These associations responded to a National Labor Relations Board invitation to file briefs to provide guidance on the meaning of the term independent judgment and the scope of discretion required for independent judgment with respect to the charge nurse. The brief asserts: "The charge nurse's background in the hospital's organization and in nursing practice enables him or her to step in when there is crisis or conflict, quickly to assess the situation and identify needed resources. Charge nurses also direct other employees, sometimes making split-second decisions that can literally be a matter of life or death." (pp. 6-7)

Team leaders, regardless of their title or designation, have assumed greater responsibility for unit- or department-based functions.

Any RN functioning in the role of team leader or charge nurse should review the following documents from administration:

- Detailed job description for the role, including how responsibilities are limited when the nurse is asked to lead a team or serve as a charge nurse on an unfamiliar floor or department
- Job descriptions for the team members assigned delegated tasks
- Formal period of training and mentoring in the role
- Validated proof of competence before leading a team independently
- Guidelines regarding personal patient care assignment when also serving as team leader
- Chain-of-command model for the facility, department, or unit

Administrators and nurse managers should be aware of landmark case laws regarding incompetent charge nurses and team leaders. A jury directed a verdict in excess of $7 million against a hospital in a 1995 Illinois case, *Holston v. Sisters of the Third Order* (1995). A charge nurse repeatedly refused a direct-care nurse's requests to personally evaluate a patient whose vital signs were rapidly deteriorating after gastric bypass surgery. The charge nurse also refused to call the patient's physician until the patient experienced cardiopulmonary collapse. Emergency surgery revealed that a central venous pressure catheter had migrated and perforated the cardiac muscle. The patient experienced cardiac tamponade and died approximately 1 week after this critical incident.

This case illustrates the necessity of validating the strong clinical skill of all RNs who are being considered for a leadership role that includes clinical supervision and consultation. Effective risk management of an unresolved clinical problem requires direct-care nurses to consult early and frequently with team leaders or managers. Each consultation with the team leader or manager should be carefully documented in the patient's medical record to demonstrate that appropriate chain-of-command process has occurred. The employer will likely be named in any lawsuit under the rule of vicarious liability if the team leader or manager offers negligent advice. Vicarious liability is discussed later in this chapter.

Personal Liability in Delegation and Supervision of Team Members

Team leaders and charge nurses who are responsible for delegation and supervision of team members must be absolutely clear about the legality of patient care assignments. They must determine whether it is reasonable and prudent to delegate a particular task on the basis of their knowledge of the worker, the patient's status, and the current conditions in the work setting. The determination whether a team leader or charge nurse has been negligent in delegating any particular patient care task or supervising subordinates is based on these aforementioned considerations.

Mobile Infirmary Medical Center v. Hodgen (2003) is a case in point. A patient with cardiac problems sued after suffering catastrophic physical and mental disabilities when a graduate nurse, not yet licensed, administered five times the ordered dose of digoxin. The shift charge nurse assigned another nurse with only 7 months' experience to act as the graduate nurse's preceptor. The preceptor did not supervise the new graduate when she administered the drug. The jury found all three nurses negligent. The court criticized the shift charge nurse for assigning a novice nurse as a preceptor and for failing to give her explicit directions regarding the level of supervision required in the circumstances. The court also faulted the preceptor, who had never worked with the new graduate, for inadequate supervision. The jury awarded $2.5 million in punitive damages.

Criteria for lawful and safe delegation have been spelled out by state boards of nursing and professional organizations, including the ANA (2012a) and the National Council of State Boards of Nursing (NCSBN) (2016). These guidelines and a growing body of case law assist the nurse in making decisions about safe delegation of patient care.

In *Williams v. West Virginia Board of Examiners* (2004), the Supreme Court of Appeals of West Virginia upheld the Kentucky Board of Nursing's disciplinary action of an RN. The nurse was responsible for supervising the care of home health aides. Inspectors found numerous violations of the nurse's duty to delegate and supervise care given by the aides. Furthermore, there was evidence that the nurse falsified patients' records, indicating that home health aides were present when in fact they were absent from the home. The nursing board suspended the nurse's license for 1 year.

Employer Liability

Although a nurse is never relieved of personal liability, the doctrine of vicarious or substituted liability permits a person to also sue the employer for the negligent conduct of nurses within the scope of their employment. Vicarious liability is based on the legal principle of *respondeat superior,* a Latin term that means "let the master answer" (for the actions of subordinates or servants). Because the employer has some control over the worker, the courts have affirmed that the employer may be held responsible for the employee's negligent acts when injury occurs.

In a New York case, *Pedraza v. Wyckoff Heights Medical Center* (2002), a hospital was found liable for the negligence of its nurses when they failed to adhere to the explicit policy it had established that bedrails were to be raised at all times for a particular category of high-risk patients. An 86-year-old patient with Alzheimer's disease was admitted to the hospital for pulmonary problems. Because the woman had Alzheimer's disease, she was classified as high risk for falling, and a fall-injury prevention protocol was to be implemented per hospital policy. A safety alert sign was to be posted above the bed, the patient was to be checked every 2 hours, the bed was to be kept in the lowest position, and all bedrails were to be up at all times. This protocol was not followed. A nurse found the patient facedown on the floor in the hallway. One bedrail had been left down when the nurse put the patient to bed after ambulating her. The hospital argued, in its defense, that keeping all four bedrails raised amounted to physical restraints and that restraints could not be applied without a physician's order. The court ruled in favor of the injured patient. The court opined that express violation of the institution's own internal policy by a hospital employee is evidence of negligence. A further discussion about the legal aspects related to the use of restraints is presented later in this chapter.

Corporate Liability

Hospitals and other health care facilities have evolved into dynamic systems that coordinate the care provided by a range of health care professionals. As a consequence of these changes, the courts have expanded the concept of corporate negligence in verdicts rendered against health care giants. In *Brodowski v. Ryave* (2005), the Pennsylvania Superior Court ruled that there was sufficient evidence that a systematic breakdown in communication caused an improper diagnosis and led to the patient's admission to a psychiatric unit before a stroke had been ruled out (Passarella, 2005). The patient was not properly treated, is now partially paralyzed, and has brain damage. The "standard of care" required of a health care corporation has been established through these cases but varies from state to state. Some jurisdictions have permitted TJC standards or state department of health licensing laws to define the "corporate standard of care." An agency's own medical bylaws or policies and procedures have been admitted as evidence of the appropriate corporate standard of care. In an earlier case, *Thompson v. Nason Hospital* (1991), the court elaborated four duties of a health care corporation:

1. Maintain safe and adequate physical facilities and equipment.
2. Select and retain competent physicians.
3. Oversee the acts of all persons who practice medicine within the facility as they relate to patient care.
4. Formulate, adopt, and enforce rules and policies to ensure quality of care.

The court in the *Brodowski* case based its ruling on the doctrine of corporate liability outlined in the *Thompson* case.

Health care facilities also have been found corporately liable for failing to have adequate numbers of qualified nursing staff assigned on each shift to meet the needs of patients. In a landmark case, *HCA Health Services v. National Bank* (1988), an unattended infant experienced respiratory arrest and suffered permanent anoxic brain damage. The jury rendered a verdict for the plaintiff and awarded $2 million in compensatory damages (for the cost of ongoing care) and $2 million in punitive damages for failing to provide an adequate number of qualified staff.

Nurses must develop a clear understanding of the principles of safe staffing and must advocate for appropriate staffing levels. Guidelines published by the ANA (2012a and 2013) can assist nurses to ensure the efficient use of human resources. Nurses should review position statements published by the Board of Nursing as well as their specialty nursing organizations (e.g., Association of PeriOperative Registered Nurses [AORN] or the Association of Women's Health, Obstetric and Neonatal Nurses [AWHONN]). Staffing guidelines promulgated by these organizations may assist the nurse in articulating concerns and formulating recommendations for improved staffing levels.

As more nurses become independent contractors working for temporary staffing agencies, courts have been asked to determine whether a hospital using temporary nursing staff is liable for the acts of an agency nurse. In *Ruelas v. Staff Builders Personnel Services, Inc.* (2001), an agency nurse was alleged to have abused a patient during administration of an enema. (The precise nature of the abuse was not delineated.) The court affirmed that as a general rule, the employer (in this case, Staff Builders) is legally liable for an employee's wrongful conduct. However, in this case, the agency had no practical or even theoretical right to control how its nurses carried out their clinical responsibilities in a particular setting. Although the agency is responsible for ensuring that the nurse has the requisite license, education, experience, and certifications, the hospital has direct control and supervision of the nurse's actions. Staff Builders was dismissed from the lawsuit.

TJC has developed detailed standards related to the orientation, training, and education of agency (contracted) staff (TJC, 2017). Courts have affirmed that facilities have a duty to provide a targeted orientation for agency nurses. A job-based or unit-based handout, if readily available, can be a useful reference for the agency nurse. A mentor or resource nurse should be provided during the targeted orientation and thereafter as needed when a new task or problem is encountered. Team members should have an opportunity to evaluate the agency nurse and provide written feedback about performance.

REDUCING LEGAL LIABILITY

Risk Management Systems

One of the most powerful allies the nurse has in any health care setting to facilitate positive change and reduce personal and corporate liability is the risk manager. The risk manager is a professional who tracks accidents and injuries that occur in the facility. The job of the risk manager is to establish and strengthen systems within the agency to reduce preventable patient injuries or deaths and to eliminate the loss of revenues as fines or the payment of damages through the insurance carrier. The risk manager may assist nurse managers in the development of effective policies and procedures to improve practice. The risk manager also is knowledgeable about federal and state administrative rules and regulations affecting health care systems, health care licensing laws, and health care case law. This knowledge is essential to prevent inadvertent violation of health care laws and to reduce claims of negligence and malpractice within the institution.

The IOM report *To Err Is Human: Building a Safer Health System* (2000) recommends a proactive approach to risk management. Nurses are encouraged to anticipate the potential for errors, report "near misses," and work closely with the risk manager to reduce preventable adverse events. All health care providers are urged to develop high-reliability operating systems. This concept is derived from the airline and nuclear energy industries. Both have established excellent safety records despite the highly complex and dangerous nature of their operations. The IOM report recommends creation of a nationwide mandatory reporting system for collection of information about adverse events and the development of performance standards that focus on patient safety.

Incident Reports or Unusual Occurrence Reports

Nurses are legally bound to report critical incidents to their nurse managers, agency administration, and the risk manager through a formal intra-agency document titled the "Unusual Occurrence Report" or "Incident Report." Emphasis on patient safety and quality has resulted in renaming of the Incident Report in many health care settings. The document is frequently referred to as the "Unusual Occurrence Form" but is also known by other titles, such as the "Quality Variance Report." This form often is directed to the risk management department through the nurse's immediate manager. The nurse manager has an opportunity to review the written report and begin the process of collecting information and mitigating any identified systems flaws in a timely fashion, depending on the nature of the incident. The report then is forwarded (usually within 24 hours) to the risk manager. If an ongoing problem does not appear to be any closer to resolution as the nurse works through the formal chain of command, beginning with the immediate nurse manager, the nurse may speak directly to the risk manager for guidance and advice.

Unfortunately, studies indicate that the rate of incident reporting still remains relatively low, particularly among physician providers (Polisena et al, 2013; USDHHS, 2012). As a condition of participation in the Medicare program, federal regulations require that hospitals develop and maintain Quality Assessment and Performance Improvement (QAPI) programs. To satisfy these requirements, hospitals must "track medical errors and adverse patient events, analyze their causes, and implement preventive actions and mechanisms that include feedback and learning throughout the hospital" (USDHHS, 2012). Unfortunately, a report released by the Office of Inspector General (OIG) found that hospital incident reporting systems captured only an estimated 14% of the patient harm events experienced by Medicare beneficiaries. Hospital risk managers, clinical managers, and administrators investigated only those reported events that they considered most likely to lead to quality and safety improvements. Few policy or practice changes were implemented as a result of reported events. Hospital administrators classified the remaining events (86% of all incident reports) as either events that staff did not perceive as reportable (61%) or as events that staff commonly report but did not report in this case (25%). The OIG recommended that (1) the CMS and AHRQ collaborate to create and promote a list of potentially reportable events for hospitals to use and (2) the CMS provide guidance to accreditors regarding their assessments of hospital efforts to track and analyze events.

Critical incidents that result in patient injury or death eventually may lead to a malpractice claim. Because state laws vary as to whether the incident report may be "discovered" by the plaintiff's attorney in a lawsuit, it is essential that the nurse follow appropriate procedures when completing and filing this document:

1. The nurse should describe all events objectively and should avoid subjective comments, personal opinions about why the incident occurred, and assumptions about events that were not witnessed. For example, if a patient was found lying on the floor at the foot of the bed, the nurse should avoid the statement, "Patient fell out of bed—found on floor." That the patient fell out of bed is an unfounded assumption. The nurse should instead state, "Entered room. Patient discovered lying prone at the foot of the bed. Both upper and lower side rails were raised."

2. The nurse should never note in the patient's medical record that an incident report has been completed and filed. This notation might alter the protection from discovery normally provided the document in some states. The jury also would be made aware that an incident report has been filed because they have access to nurses' notes submitted in evidence during the trial.

3. The nurse should never photocopy the incident report for his or her personal files. Photocopying an incident report generally is prohibited by agency policy and may be expressly prohibited in writing on

the incident report itself. Photocopying the incident report and taking it out of the agency violates patient confidentiality. It may fall into the hands of individuals who are not authorized to read any information about the patient. It may fall into the hands of the plaintiff's attorney, should a lawsuit be filed, with damaging effects on the agency's ability to defend against the claims of negligence.

4. Physicians and advanced practice nurses should not write an order for an incident report to be filed. Doing so would bring the existence of an incident report to the attention of the plaintiff's attorney.

5. The nurse should report every unusual occurrence or incident. He or she should not assume that "everyone knows about the problem or event." Box 8.5 lists circumstances under which an incident report should be filed.

BOX 8.5   Circumstances Under Which an Incident Report Should Be Filed*

- Patient or client injury
- Unanticipated patient death
- Malfunction or failure of durable medical equipment
- Significant or unanticipated adverse reactions to ordered therapy or care
- Inability to meet a patient's need(s), ordered therapy, medications, or treatments after consultation with appropriate nurse mangers or providers. This may be related to:
  - System problems (e.g., pharmacy closed, drug not available)
  - Unresolved problem with order (e.g., incomplete or illegible order)
  - Lack of qualified staff to implement order to provide needed care (e.g., registered nurse [RN] not available to perform task that law stipulates only an RN may perform)
  - Patient or family refusal of care (e.g., request for do-not-resuscitate [DNR] orders)
- Unresolved problems with physical plant that jeopardize patient well-being (e.g., electrical hazard, loose carpet section, delay in repair of essential equipment)
- Unethical, illegal, or incompetent practice that is witnessed or reported
- Patient complaint about provider or health care worker
- Toxic spills, fires, other environmental emergencies
- Violent behavior on the part of family or patient

*This list is not comprehensive but is a representative list of occurrences that should be reported.

INTENTIONAL TORTS IN NURSING PRACTICE

Ordinarily, in the course of carrying out one's nursing duties, breaches in the applicable standard of care are assumed to be unintentional acts. In other words, the nurse did not intend to harm the patient. As noted, this civil wrong is referred to as an *unintentional tort*. An intentional tort is a second category of civil wrong. It involves the direct violation of a person's legal rights. In this case, the nurse intends to perform the offensive act, although normally most nurses do not mean to harm the patient. The following acts are intentional torts:

- Assault
- Battery
- Defamation of character
- False imprisonment
- Invasion of privacy
- Intentional infliction of emotional distress

In the case of intentional torts, the plaintiff does not have to prove that the nurse breached a special duty or was negligent. The duty is implied in law (e.g., the duty to respect a patient's right to privacy). In general, legal remedies for intentional torts include fines and punitive damages, although some intentional torts rise to the level of a criminal act (such as battery) and may result in a jail sentence. Some states, such as California, also have enacted penalties that include a term of imprisonment for willful and malicious breach of confidentiality in releasing information about a patient's human immunodeficiency virus (HIV) status.

Assault and Battery

Patients who agree to treatment or nursing care do not surrender their rights to determine who touches them. Assault is causing the person to fear that he or she will be touched without consent. Battery is the unauthorized or the actual harmful or offensive touching of a person. It is important to note that a charge of battery does not require proof of harm or injury. Nurses engaged in drawing blood samples or in therapeutic procedures may face charges of battery if they touch a patient without consent. In *O'Brien v Synnott* (2013), a man was admitted to a hospital for surgery. He had suffered a gunshot wound after ramming a police cruiser. A police officer attempted to obtain a blood sample from the patient in the post-anesthesia care unit (PACU) for the purposes of alcohol screening. The patient, who objected to the blood draw, was uncooperative and resisted the officer's efforts. After the police officer was unsuccessful, a PACU nurse drew the blood sample, "implicitly leading the patient to believe that she was acting" in her capacity as a care provider. The patient believed the nurse was obtaining the sample for medical purposes, not for drug testing. The Supreme Court of Vermont ruled that the patient could sue the nurse and her employer for medical battery.

It is essential that the nurse ask the patient's permission to proceed before drawing blood samples or initiating any procedure, particularly those of an invasive nature. The nurse must be truthful regarding the reason for performing the procedure. Nurses also should document that the patient has given permission for the treatment or procedure. Consider the following situation:

A woman in active labor cries out through each contraction. The nurse has a standing order from the obstetrician for administration of an intravenous narcotic should the woman request pain relief. However, the woman refuses, being determined to experience a medication-free birth. As labor progresses, the woman's cries become so loud that other laboring women and visitors in the unit express concern and anxiety. Repeated efforts to assist the woman with breathing and relaxation exercises to reduce her vocalization have failed.

The nurse finally says to the patient, "Look, if you don't stop screaming and making those horrible noises, I'm going to give you the pain medication your doctor has ordered, whether you want it or not. You're frightening the other patients!" She repeats this threat several times and in the presence of the woman's family.

Although the woman continues to cry out, the nurse does not give the medication. The delivery of the infant is uneventful and without problems.

After discharge from the hospital, the patient retains a lawyer, claiming she was threatened with being sedated against her will. She further asserts that the nurse's repeated threats to inject her with a narcotic created an unbearable level of anxiety that interfered with her ability to cooperate with other necessary procedures during the birth. This assertion could result in a charge of negligence or intentional infliction of emotional distress.

In this case, the nurse is charged with assault (i.e., threatening the patient with unauthorized touching). Had the nurse actually carried out her threat of giving the medication, the charge could be expanded to assault and battery. Consequences for the nurse charged with assault may include the following:

- Imposition of fines and punitive damages
- State board of nursing disciplinary action
- Termination by the employer

When battery occurs, the nature of the touching may raise the offense to the level of a crime. In the aforementioned scenario, assume that the nurse decides to give the narcotic against the woman's will. She engages the assistance of a scrub technician to physically restrain the woman so that she can access a vein for the injection.

The technician, becoming frustrated with the woman's resistance to the procedure, says, "You're going to be sorry if you don't stop struggling." The technician purposefully hyperextends the woman's arm and says, "There, maybe if it hurts enough, you'll stop this nonsense."

A loud snapping sound is heard, and tests indicate that the technician has fractured the woman's arm. The charge of battery in this case may result in more serious ramifications, including punitive damages and a term of imprisonment.

Defamation of Character

A person has a right to be free from attacks on his or her reputation (defamation of character). *Libel* is a form of defamation caused by written work. *Slander* refers to an injury to one's reputation caused by the spoken word. Nurses may be subject to a charge of libel for subjective comments meant to denigrate the patient that are placed in the medical record or in other written materials read by others.

For example, a patient suffering from extreme pain who requests narcotics frequently is labeled as a "whiner," a "liar," and a "drug seeker" with an "addictive personality." These comments are noted on the medical record, on the nursing Kardex, and in the nurses' notes attached to a clipboard, which is kept on a wall peg outside the patient's room. The patient subsequently is found to have a severe intra-abdominal infection that accounts for the intense pain he experiences.

The patient sues for failure of the medical staff to identify and treat the infection. In the process of discovery, the patient, his family, and the attorney he has retained read the defamatory comments about his character. It is a distinct possibility that other family members, coworkers, and the patient's employer who visited may have read these subjective comments on the clipboard. A charge of libel is leveled against the nursing staff.

Nurses also may face charges of slander when they repeat similar types of subjective comments about patients in public places, such as elevators and hospital cafeterias. All patient care staff must be extremely cautious about discussing a patient or their opinions about a patient in public places. Even in report rooms or conference rooms, nurses should consider who in the immediate vicinity could inadvertently overhear the conversation. In all circumstances, only objective, professional language should be used in discussing patients.

False Imprisonment

False imprisonment is defined as the unlawful restraint or detention of another person against his or her wishes. Actual force is not necessary to support a charge of false imprisonment. An adult of sound mind (mentally competent) has a right to refuse any treatment that has previously been agreed to (Mathes, 2014). If he or she refuses, the person may leave the facility (e.g., hospital, rehabilitation center, long-term care facility) whenever he or she chooses. The nurse has no authority to detain the patient, even if discontinuing therapy may result in harm or injury.

The nurse has a duty to immediately notify the provider and appropriate nursing supervisors when a competent patient intends to leave "against medical advice" (AMA) but may not in any way prevent the individual from leaving the facility. Many agencies request that a patient sign an AMA form when they intend to leave in contradiction to the plan of care and despite the absence of a discharge order. The form may provide the facility with a reasonable defense against a malpractice claim if the patient's condition worsens or an injury is sustained and a malpractice claim is filed.

Intentional Infliction of Emotional Distress

When the nurse's behavior is so outrageous that it leads to emotional shock in a patient, the court can compensate the patient for emotional distress. A case in the area of maternity nursing illustrates the potential for a claim of intentional infliction of emotional distress.

In *Roddy v. Tanner Medical Center* (2003), a woman brought suit against the hospital after she was treated in the ED for a miscarriage at approximately 10 weeks' gestation. While en route to the hospital, Ms. Roddy felt something large extrude from her vagina, and she bled heavily. She reported to the ED nurse that whatever she had passed was still in her underpants with a great deal of blood. Ms. Roddy indicated that the nurse told her she would take whatever she could out of her clothes, and then the nurse placed the soiled clothes in a plastic bag.

Ms. Roddy was subsequently discharged home in stable condition after a gynecologic examination confirmed that she had passed the products of conception. When she returned home and began to remove her clothes from the plastic bag to launder them, the intact fetus dropped to the floor. Ms. Roddy claimed intentional infliction of emotional distress. The court permitted the case to go forward, indicating that there was evidence of "reckless disregard" of the rights of the patient.

Invasion of Privacy

Another basic right is to be free from interference with one's personal life. An invasion of privacy occurs when a person's private affairs (including health history and status) are made public without consent. The nurse has a legal and ethical duty to maintain patient confidentiality, and there may be serious repercussions when the nurse breaches this duty and violates this fundamental patient right.

With the growing use of electronic information systems, issues related to patient confidentiality and invasion of privacy are now being addressed by federal and state legislatures. Statutes, including the HIPAA, have been enacted to control access to electronic health data. Nurses are given passwords to access patients' electronic medical records. Nurses should never share passwords with colleagues because doing so increases the risk of unauthorized access to patients' records. Discussion of patients on social media Internet sites and taking unauthorized pictures of patients with personal electronic devices is a growing area for claims of HIPAA violation and invasion of privacy. The ANA (2011a and 2013) and the NCSBN (2011a) have both published guidelines to use of social media for nurses, along with precautionary advice.

In certain circumstances, the law permits divulging information contained in a patient's medical record. These situations include reporting certain communicable diseases, child abuse, and gunshot wounds to the proper authorities. If a nurse is asked to provide information to any sources, the matter should immediately be referred to the agency's administrator or risk manager. In no case should the nurse personally divulge the information or provide copies of the patient's record to another person or agency. Another fact-based case known to this author illustrates the intentional torts of invasion of privacy and intentional infliction of emotional distress. Consider the following situation:

A nurse works in a physician's office in a small, semirural community. The majority of the town's residents know one another. A patient being treated for several opportunistic infections is tested for HIV. The nurse also is aware that the patient has been questioned by the physician about his sexual activities and that he has divulged that he is gay and has had unprotected sex with several male partners. When the test results are reported as positive, the nurse calls several close friends (who also know the patient) and reports the finding and information about the patient's sexual conduct. Before the physician informs the patient about his diagnosis, he encounters two of the people who have been told about the HIV test result. They tell him that they know he is gay and infected with the HIV virus. He then discovers that the nurse has informed them about his condition. Suffering from intense shock and emotional pain, the man unsuccessfully attempts suicide.

In this case, the nurse's actions rose to the level of willful, malicious, and intentional infliction of emotional distress. The nurse faces serious charges and, in some states with HIV confidentiality laws, could face a prison sentence for intentionally violating the patient's confidentiality in a manner meant to harm the patient. It is likely that the nurse's license also will be revoked for her actions, and the board may impose a significant fine.

The Nurse and Criminal Law

A crime is an offense against society, defined through written criminal statutes or codes. A criminal act is deemed to be conduct so offensive that the state is responsible for prosecuting the offending individual on behalf of society. Legal remedies for crimes include fines, imprisonment, and, in some states, execution (death penalty). Criminal acts are classified as either minor offenses (misdemeanors) or major offenses (felonies). Misdemeanors that nurses are commonly charged with include the following:

- Illegal practice of medicine
- Failing to report child or elder abuse
- Falsification of a patient's medical record
- Assault and battery and physical abuse of patients

Felony acts may be committed against the federal government and generally involve drug trafficking offenses and, increasingly, fraud in billing for services of Medicare patients. Other serious criminal acts include theft, rape, and murder. A nurse found guilty of a felony generally serves time in prison and usually suffers the permanent revocation of his or her nursing license. For example, in the death of a 97-year-old nursing home patient, five RNs were indicted on 21 counts, including falsification of records, alteration of forms filed with the state department of health, and tampering with physical evidence (Kelley, 2000). The patient died after being fed through a stomach tube attached to an enema bag. The nurses used the enema bag in lieu of the appropriate feeding equipment, which was not available. The nursing director was found guilty on three counts and also surrendered her nursing license.

THE LAW AND PATIENT RIGHTS

Advance Directives

Society now recognizes the individual's right to die with dignity rather than be kept alive indefinitely by artificial life support. As a consequence, the majority of states have enacted "right-to-die" laws. These statutes grant competent adults the right to refuse extraordinary medical treatment when there is no hope of recovery. The term **advance directive** refers to an individual's desires regarding end-of-life care. These wishes generally are made through the execution of a formal document known as a living will. Right-to-die statutes vary from state to state; therefore, the nurse must become familiar with the state-specific statute. Agency policies and procedures in the nurse's employment setting also guide the nurse in an understanding of the patient's rights in this matter.

Living Wills

A living will is a legal document, a type of advance directive, in which a competent adult makes known his or her wishes regarding care that will be provided in the final stages of a terminal illness. A living will generally contains the following:

- Designation of the individual (proxy or surrogate) who is permitted to make decisions once the patient is incapacitated and no longer able to make decisions (often referred to as "decisionally incompetent" or "decisionally incapacitated")

- Specific stipulations regarding what care is acceptable and which procedures or treatments are not to be implemented
- Authorization of the patient's physician to withhold or discontinue certain life-sustaining procedures under specific conditions

Although living wills are legal in every state, they may not be legally binding. In some cases, a proxy is not recognized or sanctioned by the state statute. Living wills have been overturned, particularly if disputes arise among family members or significant others when the terminally ill patient is no longer able to make decisions. A living will may be revoked under any of the following conditions:

- There is evidence that the patient was not competent when the living will was executed.
- The patient's condition is not terminal.
- A state-imposed time for enforcement of the will has expired, and a new living will must be executed.
- The patient's condition has changed substantially, and the stipulations of the will no longer apply.

A living will must be written (in some cases, using a state-specific document), dated, signed, and witnessed. If asked to witness a patient's living will, the nurse should refer the matter to the agency's risk manager. It may not be lawful in a particular state for the nurse to witness this document.

Medical or Physician Directives and DNR Orders.

A more specific type of living will that the patient may execute is known as the medical or physician directive. This document lists the desire of the patient in a particular scenario, such as whether he or she would want to be resuscitated if cardiopulmonary arrest occurs. The physician writes DNR orders on the basis of written medical directives dictated by the patient. This medical directive, when properly executed, provides the physician with immunity from claims of negligence or intentional wrongdoing in the patient's death. The physician must also follow any state-specific statute and the agency's policies and procedures before writing a DNR order. Research has discovered a serious lack of uniformity among and within health care facilities in making certain that direct-care nurses and providers are aware of a patient's DNR status. The lack of awareness can result in a significant risk for confusion and error and contribute to claims of negligence.

The nurse has an absolute duty to respect the patient's wishes in the case of DNR orders. A lawfully executed DNR order must be followed. Nurses have been sued for failure to observe DNR orders. Claims against the nurse include battery, negligent infliction of pain and suffering, and "wrongful life" (*Anderson v. St. Francis– St. George Hospital,* 1992). Three problems may arise regarding a DNR order: A physician refuses to comply with the patient's wishes and initiates resuscitation; the patient revokes consent to the DNR order; and a family member demands that the DNR order be rescinded despite the patient's continued objection to resuscitation (Teno, 2008). If one of these issues arises, the nurse must act promptly to enlist the assistance of the nursing supervisor or a hospital administrator. One must remember that a patient may revoke a living will, including a DNR order, at any time. The ANA has published a Position Statement "Nursing Care and Do Not Resuscitate (DNR) and Allow Natural Death (AND) Decisions" to clarify the nurse's roles and responsibilities related to DNR and AND issues (ANA, 2012b).

Durable Power of Attorney for Health Care.

In 1993, the Uniform Health-Care Decisions Act was approved. The Act recognizes an individual's right to make decisions about health care and enables a patient to accept or refuse treatment. The act is also designed to give the patient autonomy to make end-of-life decisions. Durable power of attorney is a legal document that authorizes the patient to name the person (the health care proxy) who will make the day-to-day and final end-of-life decisions once he or she is decisionally incompetent. Naming a proxy who is intimately knowledgeable about the person's true wishes is important to ensure that the patient's desires will be carried out when he or she is no longer able to make decisions. Health care law experts recommend that individuals interested in naming a proxy seek legal assistance with executing a **durable power of attorney** for health care.

Nurses may be asked questions about living wills and durable power of attorney for health care by patients and their families. An important aspect of speaking to the patient about these issues is to provide the written materials about **advance directives** that are required under the federal statute the Patient Self-Determination Act, which was passed in 1990.

Informed Consent

For any patient to make meaningful choices about a particular procedure or treatment, the provider must convey certain material information. Under the doctrine of informed consent, the physician or advanced practice nurse has a duty to disclose information so that the patient can make intelligent decisions (Grady, 2015). This duty is mandated by federal statute (in the case of Medicare and Medicaid patients) and state law and is grounded as well in common law. In the case of routine as well as specialized care, the primary provider must disclose the following:

- Nature of the therapy or procedure
- Expected benefits and outcomes of the therapy or procedure
- Potential risks of the therapy or procedure
- Alternative therapies to the intended procedure and their risks and benefits
- Risks of not having the procedure

This duty to disclose rests with the provider and cannot be delegated to the RN. When the nurse has reason to believe that the patient has not given informed consent for a procedure, the provider should be immediately notified. In no case should the nurse proceed with initiating any part of the therapy that he or she is responsible for implementing. The patient's questions or concerns should be documented in the medical record to indicate why there has been a delay in carrying out the procedure (Mahlmeister, 2009b). If the nurse is responsible for witnessing the patient's signature on a consent form for the specified procedure, this process also should be deferred until the provider has had an opportunity to clarify the patient's questions.

A variety of negligence claims arise out of the informed consent process. The provider may be alleged negligent for failure to obtain informed consent. With adoption in some states of the corporate negligence doctrine, an increasing number of appellate courts have ruled that hospitals and nurses may be liable for failure to ensure that informed consent was given to the provider (Doctors Hospital of Augusta v. Alicea, 2016 Ga. LEXIS 448 (2016); *William McDougald et al. v. St.* Francis North Hospital Inc. 2014). Nurses have a duty to discuss concerns about informed consent with the primary provider. Should the nurse be unable to resolve the issue, the chain of command should be invoked to clarify questions or concerns.

In some cases, timely notification of a nursing manager may be essential to prevent violation of the patient's right to give consent. The following scenario provides a case in point. An RN is circulating in a surgical procedure intended to clean a severe leg wound. The consent form signed by the patient explicitly lists "wound debridement" as the procedure to be performed. On beginning the procedure, the surgeon asks for additional instruments, indicating that the wound is so infected that the leg will have to be amputated below the knee. Because the patient has received general anesthesia and is unable to give consent, and the consent form itself does not authorize an amputation procedure, the nurse must question the surgeon's intention to remove the leg. If the surgeon refuses to discuss the matter, or again requests the instruments necessary for the procedure, the nurse must obtain immediate assistant from her supervisor and if possible, the medical administrator (chief of surgery). The instruments for surgical amputation should not be placed on the sterile table, and in compliance with intraoperative communication standards, all other team members should be alerted that there is an unresolved question about the procedure and that a manager or administrator is on the way to evaluate the surgical plan.

Communication Barriers and Informed Consent. Health care organizations that receive federal funds are required to meet the language access provision of the Culturally and Linguistically Appropriate Services (CLAS) Standards for Health. The standards were issued in 2001 by USDHHS and were substantially enhanced in 2011 through a collaboration of the USDHHS Office of Minority Health (OMH) (2011) and the National Partnership for Action to End Health Disparities.

The standards require that the hospital or health facility must:

- Offer and provide free and timely language assistance services, including bilingual staff and interpreter services, at all points of contact at all hours of operation.
- Provide verbal and written notices (in the individual's preferred language) of the right to receive language assistance services.
- Ensure competence of language assistance provided by interpreters and bilingual staff.

Family and friends should *not* be used as interpreters except at the care recipient's request (USDHHSOMH, 2011). The duty to ensure appropriate communication is also established by the ADA (discussed previously). When an interpreter is used to facilitate communication, the nurse should document this process. The medical record should contain the name of the interpreter, the topic of the educational session or substance of the informed consent discussion, and the patient's questions and consent, if given.

TJC's *Comprehensive Accreditation Manual for Hospitals* requires the facility to respect a patient's right to and need for effective communication (TJC, 2017). Written materials, including consent forms and discharge instructions, should be available in the patient's preferred language. Educational materials should be culturally sensitive, and at a reading level that recognizes literacy limitations. TJC provides detailed information and guidance for development of a central office to coordinate all communication services, including the availability of interpreters fluent in medical terminology, for informed consent discussions between the provider and patient (TJC, 2008). Language access also includes access to interpreters skilled in signing for hearing-impaired patients and materials in Braille for vision-impaired individuals.

A New Jersey case (*Borngesser v. Jersey Shore Medical Center* [2001]) illustrates the duty to provide an interpreter before informed consent is given for an invasive procedure. A female patient was admitted to the hospital with severe cardiac disease. She was also completely deaf and mute. Notes in the medical record stated, "Patient deaf and dumb and difficult to assess." The nurses established a diagnosis of "Sensory deficit: hearing impaired" and recorded that it was difficult to communicate with the patient. Providers and nurses documented continued difficulty with assessments, patient education, and obtaining informed consent. The patient's 17-year-old daughter was not deaf and could sign but was not a trained medical interpreter. Ms. Borngesser subsequently died from severe cardiac disease and associated complications. Her daughter sued the hospital, claiming that the facility failed to make reasonable accommodation for her deaf and mute mother. *There were no claims of medical or nursing negligence.* The Superior Appellate Court of New Jersey affirmed that the case against the hospital could go forward. The court stated, among other things, that when a hearing-impaired patient is asked to give informed consent, the hospital has a duty to ensure that communication is effective by providing an interpreter fluent in American Sign Language (ASL).

The unique legal requirements related to informed consent in minors is a complex issue. The American Academy of Pediatrics (AAP) published a *Technical Report,* delineating important aspects of informed consent for pediatric patients (AAP, 2016.) All 50 states and the District of Columbia explicitly allow a minor to consent to testing and treatments for sexually transmitted diseases, except HIV testing and treatment. All other statutes regarding informed consent in adolescents vary widely from state to state. As noted earlier, when dealing with minors, the nurse must use agency resources, including social workers, managers, administrators, and risk managers, when facilitating an appropriate informed consent process between the provider and adolescent or older child.

The Right to Refuse Diagnostic Testing, Treatment, and Care

As noted, an adult of sound mind has a right to refuse any treatment that has previously been agreed to (Colwell, 2016; Selde, 2015). A Connecticut Supreme Court decision affirmed the fundamental right of adults to refuse medical treatment. In the case of *Stamford Hospital v. Vega* (1996), a woman who hemorrhaged after the birth of her infant refused blood on the grounds that it violated her beliefs as a Jehovah's Witness. The hospital obtained an emergency court order authorizing the facility to administer blood. The woman survived and was discharged in good health. Although it was a moot point (the blood already had been given), the family appealed the initial court decision authorizing the blood transfusion. The Supreme Court decided to hear the case and reversed the lower court's decision, stating the hospital did not have a right to substitute its decision for that of the patient.

If a patient who is under the nurse's care refuses treatment, the nurse has a duty to notify the primary provider. The same principles pertaining to the informed consent process apply to situations in which the patient refuses care. The physician or advanced practice nurse should provide the patient with information about the consequences, risks, and benefits of refusing therapy. The provider also must explore any alternative treatments that may be available to the patient.

Leaving Against Medical Advice

A common allegation made when a patient self-discharges against medical advice and is subsequently injured is that the patient was not fully apprised of the risks inherent in leaving the facility. If a patient intends to leave the facility without a written order, the nurse must act promptly to notify the provider. When circumstances suggest that the person may suffer immediate physical harm, the nurse must clearly articulate the dangers inherent in leaving (Levy et al, 2012). This precautionary statement is reserved for situations in which the life and limb of the patient are at risk and the appropriate providers (physicians or advanced practice nurses) are not available to address the direct and indirect consequences with the patient. The nurse should document all of these actions and any communication with the aforementioned parties.

If the primary provider has not arrived before the patient leaves, the nurses' notes should reflect the specific advice given the patient, which should include the fact that leaving the facility could:

- Aggravate the current condition and complicate future care.
- Result in permanent physical or mental impairment or disability.
- Result in complications leading to death.

In the case of a competent elder, prompt notification of the immediate family would also be a reasonable and prudent action.

Lyons v. Walker Regional Medical Center (2000) is a case in point. An ED nurse was found negligent for failing to warn a patient who was leaving AMA that his laboratory results indicated a state of diabetic keto-acidosis, a condition that could be lethal. When the "panic" value laboratory findings were displayed on the computer, the nurse did not bring the results to the physician's or patient's attention. Instead, she directed the unit secretary to complete the patient's discharge paperwork. The patient left, and he died 3 days later.

A study of patient characteristics associated with discharge AMA has found that low socioeconomic status, substance abuse, sickness within the family, underlying (and often untreated) psychiatric disorders, anger and anxiety about the admission diagnosis, and lack of effective communication with team members correlate with self-discharge (Alfandre, 2009). Nurses and providers should collaborate to address immediate patient concerns, communicate a time-limited plan of care, and advocate for appropriate consultations (e.g., psychiatry, social work, pastoral services, pain management) to reduce the likelihood of patient self-discharge.

Almost all health care facilities have an AMA form that patients are asked to sign when they decide to refuse or discontinue ordered therapy or intend to leave the facility. The value of the document in countering a claim of negligence should the patient or family later sue will depend in great part on the quality of the nurse's charting.

Nurses have also been charged with a variety of offenses when unlawfully detaining patients, including assault, battery, and false imprisonment (Snyder, 2001). These charges generally arise when well-meaning nurses try to prevent the patient from carrying out his or her intent. Actions that lead to a claim of false imprisonment include applying restraints, refusing to give the patient his or her clothes or access to a telephone, intimidating the patient by assigning a security person to guard his or her room, and sedating the patient against his or her will.

Use of Physical Restraints

One last but equally important area of patient rights to be discussed is the right of a competent adult to be free of restraint. Even patients with mental illness cannot be incarcerated or restrained without due process, and the institution must have the treatment and rehabilitation services necessary to reintegrate the individual into society (Bellenger et al, 2017). Restraint of any kind is a form of imprisonment, and the reasonable and prudent nurse will closely adhere to all laws, rules, and policies pertaining to the use of restraints. The goal when restraints are clinically indicated is to use the least restrictive restraint and only when all other strategies to ensure patient safety have been exhausted. Patients may never be restrained physically or chemically because there is not enough staff to properly monitor them. Nurses have a legal and ethical duty to report institutions or individuals who violate patient rights through unlawful restraint.

As noted, one of the most common allegations leveled against nurses is a failure to ensure patient safety. Nurses in many practice settings must balance the right of patients to unrestricted control of their bodies and movements against the need to keep vulnerable patients safe from harm. The use of seclusion, chemical restraints, and physical restraints, including vests, mittens, belts, and wrist restraints, is governed by federal and state statutes and accrediting bodies, such as TJC. Many nurses do not realize that even bedrails and chair trays fall under the category of physical restraints; these articles may not be used indiscriminately.

Violation of restraint statutes and the administrative rules and regulations promulgated to enact these laws can result in stiff penalties. The institution can lose its Medicare contract (decertification) and TJC accreditation, effectively putting it out of business. Patients and family members may initiate civil suits for unlawful restraints, resulting in monetary damages if the plaintiff succeeds in the suit. Charges of assault, battery, and/or false imprisonment may be leveled against nurses who use restraints improperly. Claims of negligence may arise from improper monitoring of the patient who has been appropriately placed in restraints in compliance with applicable laws and hospital policy.

Careful nursing documentation is essential when restraints are applied. The patient's mental and physical status must be assessed at regular and frequent intervals as prescribed by law and the agency's policies. The chart must reflect these assessments and the frequency with which restraints are removed. Neurovascular and skin assessments of limbs or other body parts covered by the restraints also must be entered in the medical record. Written physician orders for restraints must be timed and dated, and renewal of orders must be accompanied by evidence of medical evaluations and nursing reassessments.

On the basis of the aforementioned information, some nurses are under the misconception that current law prohibits restraining patients until a written order is obtained. Nurses may lawfully apply restraints in an emergency, when in their independent judgment no other strategies are effective in protecting the patient from harm. The physician must be contacted promptly to discuss the patient's condition and the need to restrain and to obtain an order for temporary continuance of restraints. The nurse is guided in the decision to restrain by knowledge of the laws, the agency's policies and procedures, qualifications of the staff, and conditions on the unit or in the department.

■ SUMMARY

Professional nursing practice is governed by an ever-widening circle of federal and state statutes and is constantly evolving in great part because of an accumulating body of nursing case law. The law provides guidance for every aspect of practice and can assist the nurse in managing the complexities of practice in a rapidly changing health care system. Knowledge is power, and the nurse who possesses a sound understanding of the law as it pertains to professional practice is empowered.

This chapter has reviewed the major sources and categories of law influencing nursing practice. The reader has been introduced to the doctrines of civil and criminal law that affect all nurses. The chapter has explored issues related to the legal rights of patients who are served by professional nurses. As patient advocates, all nurses should keep these fundamental rights uppermost in their minds as they attempt to provide safe, effective, quality care in all settings.

REFERENCES

Abernathy v. Valley Medical Center, WL 3754792 (W.D. Wash., 2006).

Alfandre, D. J. (2009). "I'm going home": discharges against medical advice. *Mayo Clinic Proceedings, 84*(3), 255–260.

Al-Qurayshi, Z. H., Hauch, A. T., Slakey, D. P., & Kandil, E. (2015). Retained foreign bodies: risks and outcomes at the national level. *Journal of the American College of Surgeons, 220*(4), 749–759.

American Academy of Ambulatory Care Nursing. (2011). *Scope and standards of practice for professional telehealth nursing* (5th ed.). Pitman, NJ: American Academy of Ambulatory Care Nursing.

American Academy of Pediatrics. (2016). Informed consent in decision-making in pediatric practice. Technical Report. *Pediatrics, 138*(2), e1-e16. Retrieved from http://pediatrics.aappublications.org/content/pediatrics/early/2016/07/21/peds.2016-1485.full.pdf.

American Association of Critical-Care Nurses. (2004). *AACN delegation handbook* (2nd ed.). Aliso Viejo, CA: American Association of Critical-Care Nurses.

American Medical Association. (2010–2011). *Code of medical ethics.* Chicago: American Medical Association.

American Nurses Association. (n.d.). *Mandatory Overtime. Policy and Advocacy.* Washington, DC: ANA. Retrieved from http://www.nursingworld.org/MainMenuCategories/Policy-Advocacy/State/Legislative-Agenda-Reports/MandatoryOvertime.

American Nurses Association. (2015a). *Code of ethics for nurses.* Washington, DC: ANA.

American Nurses Association. (2015b). *Optimal Nurse Staffing to Improve Quality of Care and Patient Outcomes.* Washington, DC: ANA.

American Nurses Association. (2011a). *Social networking principles toolkit.* Washington, DC: ANA. Retrieved from http://www.nursingworld.org/socialnetworkingtoolkit.

American Nurses Association. (2013). *Nurse Staffing 101: A decision-making guide for the RN.* Washington, DC: ANA. Retrieved from http://www.nursesbooks.org/Main-Menu/eBooks/General/eBook-Nurse-Staffing-101.aspx.

American Nurses Association. (2012a). *Principles of delegation.* Washington, DC: ANA. Retrieved from http://www.nursingworld.org/MainMenuCategories/ThePracticeof

ProfessionalNursing/workplace/PrinciplesofDelegation.
aspx.

American Nurses Association. (2007). *The American Nurses
Association comments on the Wisconsin Department of Justice
decision to pursue criminal charges against an RN in Wisconsin.*
Retrieved from http://ana.nursingworld.org/FunctionalMenu
Categories/MediaResources/PressReleases/2006/Criminal
ChargesAgainstanRNinWisconsin.aspx.

American Nurses Association. (2009a). *Safe staffing saves
lives.* Washington, DC: ANA. Retrieved from http://
www.safestaffingsaveslives.org/WhatIsANADoing/
StateLegislation/StaffingPlansandRatios.GM5Editor.html.

American Nurses Association. (2015c). *Nursing: Scope and
standards of practice* (3rd ed.). Washington, DC: American
Nurses Association.

American Nurses Association. (2012b). *Nursing Care and Do
Not Resuscitate (DNR) and Allow Natural Death (AND)
Decisions. ANA Position Statement.* Washington, DC:
ANA. Retrieved from http://www.nursingworld.org/
MainMenuCategories/EthicsStandards/Ethics-Position-
Statements/Nursing-Care-and-Do-Not-Resuscitate-DNR-
and-Allow-Natural-Death-Decisions.pdf.

American Telemedicine Association. (2014). *Telehealth nursing.* Retrieved from http://www.americantelemed.org/
docs/default-document-library/fact_sheet_final.pdf?
sfvrsn=2.

Anderson v. St Francis–St George Hospital, 614 NE 2d 841
(OH, 1992).

Angelini, D., & Howard, E. (2014). Obstetric triage: A systematic review over the past 15 years: 1998-2013. *MCN.
The American Journal of Maternal Child Nursing, 39*(5),
284–297.

Barbourville Nursing Home v. USDHHS, No 05-3421, 6 Cir
04/06/2006 (F3d-KY).

Bellenger, E. N., Ibrahim, J. E., Lovell, J. J., & Bugeja, L. (2017,
May 7). The nature and extent of physical restraint-related
deaths in nursing homes: a systematic review. *Journal of
Aging and Health.* http://doi.org/10.1177/0898264317704541.

Borngesser v. Jersey Shore Medical Center, 774 A. 2d 615 (N.J.
App. Ct., 2001).

Boyer v. Tift County Hospital, WL 2986283 (M.D. Ga.,
2008).

Brent, N. (2017). Nurse.com on Course Learning. *Court case
highlights nurses' duty to follow EMTALA.* Retrieved from
https://www.nurse.com/blog/.../court-case-highlights-
nurses-duty-to-follow-emtala/.

Brief *amici curiae* American Hospital Association. American
Organization of Nurse Executives, American Society for
Healthcare Human Resources Administration, Michigan
Health and Hospital Association in response to the
National Labor Relations Board's July 24, 2003 Notice
and Invitation to File Briefs, Filed Sept 22, 2003, United
States of America before the National Labor Relations
Board.

Brodowski v. Ryave, 885 A.2d 1045 (PA Supr Ct. 2005).

Brooke, P. (2009). When can you say no? *Nursing, 39*(7),
43–47.

Brown, A. (2013). Nurses and noncompliance, *Nurse Leader,
11,* 46–47.

Butts, J., & Rich, K. (2016). *Nursing Ethics.* Burlington, MA:
Jones & Bartlett Learning.

California Department of Consumer Affairs. (2008, November).
Clinical learning experiences of nursing students. California
Board of Registered Nursing. Retrieved from http://www.
rn.ca.gov/pdfs/regulations/npr-b-66.pdf.

California Healthline. (2015, December 11). *CMS penalizes
758 hospitals over hospital-acquired-conditions.* Retrieved
from https://californiahealthline.org/morning-breakout/
cms-penalizes-758-hospitals-over-hospital-acquired-
conditions/.

Cares, A., Pace, E., Denious, J., Crane, L. A. (2015). Substance
use and mental illness among nurses: workplace warning
signs and barriers to seeking assistance. *Substance Abuse,
36,* 59–66.

Carthon, J. M., Lasater, K. B., Sloane, D. M., Kutney-Lee, A.
(2015). The quality of hospital work environments and
missed nursing care is linked to heart failure readmissions:
a cross-sectional study of US hospitals. *BMJ Quality &
Safety, 24,* 255–263.

Centers for Medicare & Medicaid Services. (2008). *Hospital-
acquired conditions.* Retrieved from http://www.cms.gov/
Medicare/Medicare-Fee-for-Service-Payment/Hospital
AcqCond/index.html?redirect=/HospitalAcqCond/06_
Hospital-Acquired_Conditions.asp.

Classen D. C., Resar, R., Griffin, F., Federico, F., Frankel, T.,
Kimmel, N., et al. (2011). 'Global Trigger Tool' shows that
adverse events in hospitals may be ten times greater than
previously measured. *Health Affairs, 30*(4), 581–589.

Colwell, C. (2016). Know when uncooperative patients can
refuse care and transport. *Journal of Emergency Medical
Services, 41*(8), 45–47.

Columbia Medical Center of Las Colinas v. Bush, WL 22725001
WW3d (Tex., 2003).

Cronquist, R. (2013). Management of complaints against
nurses: Review, investigation, action, resolution. *Journal of
Nursing Regulation, 4*(1), 25–33.

Dickerson v. Fatehi, 84 SE 2d 880 (Va., 1997).

Dimora v. Cleveland Clinic Foundation, 683 NE 2d 1175
(Ohio App, 1996).

Doctors Hospital of Augusta v. Alicea (Administrator), 2016
Ga. LEXIS 448 (2016).

Francis v. Memorial General Hospital, 726 P 2d 852 (N.M., 1986).

Garvey, P. K. (2015). Failure to rescue: The nurse's impact.
Medsurg Nursing, 24(3), 145–149.

Grady, C. (2015). Enduring and emerging challenges of informed consent. *The New England Journal of Medicine, 372*: 855–862.

Greenberg, P. (2017). *Medication-related malpractice claims.* CRICO 2016 CBS Benchmarking Report. CRICO Strategies, Boston.

Griffith, R., & Tengnah, C. (2017). *Law and professional issues in nursing* (4th ed.). Los Angeles: Sage Publishers.

Hannawa, A. F., Shigemoto, Y., & Little, T. D. (2016). Medical errors: disclosure styles, interpersonal forgiveness, and outcomes. *Social Science and Medicine, 156*, 29–38.

Hanssen v. Genesis Health, WL 665318 (Iowa Appel. Ct., 2011).

HCA Health Services v. National Bank, 745 SW 2d 120 (Ark., 1988).

Heinrich v. Conemaugh Valley Memorial Hospital, 648 A 2d 53 (Pa., 1994).

Holston v. Sisters of the Third Order, 650 NE 2d 985 (Ill., 1995).

Institute of Medicine. (2000). *To err is human: Building a safer health system.* Washington, DC: National Academies Press.

Janga v. Colombrito, S.W, 3d WL6146197 (Tx. Appel. Ct. 2011).

Kachalia, A. (2009, January). *Disclosure of medical error.* Agency for Healthcare Research and Quality. Retrieved from http://www.webmm.ahrq.gov/perspective.aspx?perspectiveID=70.

Kalisch, B., Lee K. (2012). Missed nursing care: magnet versus non-magnet hospitals. *Nursing Outlook, 60*(5), 32–39.

Kelley, T. (2000, November 7). *Death at a nursing home leads to indictment of five* (p. B–1). *New York Times.*

Konetzka, R. T., Park, J., Ellis, R., & Abbo, E. (2013). Malpractice litigation and nursing home quality of care. *Health Services Research, 48*(6 Pt 1), 1920–1938.

Kowalski, K., & Horner, M. D. (1998). A legal nightmare: Denver nurses indicted. *MCN. The American Journal of Maternal Child Nursing, 23*(3), 125–129.

Lachman, V. D., Murray, J. S., Iseminger, K., & Ganske, K. (2012). Doing the right thing: Pathways to moral courage. *The American Nurse, 7*(5), 1–3.

Levy, F., Mareiniss D. P., & Iacovelli, C. (2012). The importance of a proper Against-Medical-Advice discharge: How signing out AMA may create significant liability protection for providers. *The Journal of Emergency Medicine, 43*(3), 516–520.

Love v. Rancocas Hospital, WL1541052 (Distr Ct New Jersey, 2006).

Lovett v. Lorain Community Hospital, WL239927 N.E. 2d. (Ohio, 2004).

Lyons v. Walker Regional Medical Center, 791 So. 2d 937 (Ala., 2000).

Mahlmeister, L. (2015). Crosswalk: the joint commission and centers for medicare and medicaid services pathways to patient safety and quality. *The Journal of Perinatal & Neonatal Nursing, 29*(2), 107–115.

Mahlmeister, L. R. (2006). Best practices in perinatal nursing: professional role development for charge nurses. *The Journal of Perinatal & Neonatal Nursing, 20*(2), 122–124.

Mahlmeister, L. R. (2008). Best practices in perinatal nursing: collaborating with student nurses to ensure high-reliability. *The Journal of Perinatal & Neonatal Nursing, 22*(1), 8–11.

Mahlmeister, L. R. (2009a). Best practices in perinatal care: maintaining safe and cost-effective staffing models during the current economic downturn. *The Journal of Perinatal & Neonatal Nursing, 23*(2), 111–114.

Mahlmeister, L. R. (2009b). Best practices in perinatal nursing: partnering with patients to enhance informed decision-making. *The Journal of Perinatal & Neonatal Nursing, 23*(3), 213–216.

Makary, M. A., & Daniel, M. (2016). Medical error – the third leading cause of death in the U.S. *BMJ, 353*, 2139.

Mathes, M. (2014). *Nurse's Law*. Indianapolis: Sigma Theta Tau International.

McGuire, C., & Mroczek, J. M. (2014). *Nursing malpractice.* Course 125. Lakeway, TX: The National Center of Continuing Education. Retrieved from https://www.nursece.com/pdfs/125_NurseMalpractice.pdf.

Miller v. Levering Regional Healthcare Center, S.W. 3d. WL1889883 (Mo. App. Ct., 2006).

Mobile Infirmary Medical Center v. Hodgen, So 2d, WL 22463340 (Ala., 2003).

Moy, M. (2016). *The EMTALA answer book.* Gaithersburg, Md: Aspen.

National Council of State Boards of Nursing. (2016). National guidelines for nursing delegation. *Journal of Nursing Regulation, 7*(1), 5–13.

National Council of State Boards of Nursing. (2011a). *A nurse's guide to the use of social media.* Chicago. Retrieved from http://www.ncsbn.org/NCSBNSocialMedia.pdf.

National Council of State Boards of Nursing. (2011b). *What you need to know about nursing licensure and boards of nursing.* Chicago. Retrieved from https://www.ncsbn.org/Nursing License.pdf.

National Council of State Boards of Nursing. (2011c). *Substance use disorder in nursing.* Chicago. Retrieved from https://www.ncsbn.org/Working_with_Others.pdf.

National Quality Forum. (2011). *Safe practices for better healthcare—2010 update.* Executive summary. Washington, DC: National Quality Forum. Retrieved from http://www.qualityforum.org/Publications/2010/04/Safe_Practices_for_Better_Healthcare_%E2.

Oakwood Healthcare, Inc., 348 J.L.R.B.., No. 37, September 29, 2006.

O'Brien v. Synnott, ___A 3d___2012 WL 2124161 (Vt. May 17, 2013).

Ohio Nurses Association. (2016). *The role of the registered nurse as charge nurse. Nursing Practice Statement 21, 2016.* Columbus, Ohio: ONA.

Osiecki v. Bridgeport Health Care Center, Inc., 2005 WL 1331225 (Conn. Super, May 12, 2005).

Parco v. Pacifica Hospital, WL 2491516 (Supr Ct. Los Angeles County, Calif., 2007).

Passarella, G. (2005, October 31). *Hospital faces trial on corporate negligence claim.* Legal Intelligencer. Retrieved from http://thelegalintelligencer.typepad.com/tli/gina-passarella/.

Pedraza v. Wyckoff Heights Medical Center, NYS2d, 2002 NY Slip Op 22094, 2002 WL 1364153 (N.Y. Sup, June 4, 2002).

Philipsen, N. C., & Soeken, D. (2011). Preparing to blow the whistle: a survival guide for nurses. *Journal of Nurse Practitioner, 7*(9), 740–746.

Pohlman, K. (2015, November). Why you need your own malpractice insurance. *American Nurse Today, 10*(1). Retrieved at: https://www.americannursetoday.com/need-malpractice-insurance/.

Raper, J.L., Hudspeth, R. (2008). Why board of nursing disciplinary actions do not always yield the expected results. *Nursing Administration Quarterly, 32*(4), 338–345.

Reid-Searl, K., Moxham, L., & Happell, B. (2010). Enhancing patient safety: The importance of direct supervision for avoiding medication errors and near misses by undergraduate nursing students. *International Journal of Nursing Practice, 16*(3): 225–232.

Roberts v. Galen of Virginia, Inc, 111 F 3d 405 (6 Cir, 1997).

Roddy v. Tanner Medical Center, 585 SE 2d 175 (Ga., 2003).

Roussel, L. (2011). *Management and leadership for nurse administration.* Boston: Jones & Bartlett.

Rowe v. Sisters of Pallottine Missionary Society, WL 1585453 SE 2d (W.Va., 2001).

Ruelas v. Staff Builders Personnel Services, Inc., 18 P 3d 138 (Ariz. App, 2001).

Saucedo A, Dall Oro, C et al. (2017 Aug 31). What impact does nursing care left undone have on patient outcomes? Review of the literature. *J Clinical Nursing*, Doi: 10.1111/jocn.14058.

Scott v. Corizon Health, 2014 WL 1877431 (D. Nevada, May 9, 2014).

Selde, W. (2015). Know when and how your patient can legally refuse care. *Journal of Emergency Medical Services, 40*(3), 3.

Shannon, S. E., Foglia, M. B., Hardy, M., & Gallagher T. H. (2009). Disclosing errors to patients: perspectives of registered nurses. *Joint Commission Journal on Quality and Patient Safety, 35*(1), 5–12.

Siegel v. Long Island Jewish Medical Center, NYS 2d NY Slip Op 17790 WL 22439814 (N.Y., NY)

Silber, J. H., Rosenbaum, P. R., McHugh, M. D., Ludwig, J. M., Smith, H. L., Niknam, B. A., et al. (2016). Comparison of the value of nursing work environments in hospitals across different levels of patient risk. *JAMA Surgery, 151*, 527–536.

Simpson, K. R. (2016). Nurse staffing and failure to rescue. *MCN. The American Journal of Maternal Child Nursing. 41*(2), 132.

Smart, C. (2017, September 4). University Hospital boss talks changes after nurse arrest, says 'this will not happen again.' Retrieved from http://www.sltrib.com/news/health/2017/09/04/live-university-hospital-officials-discuss-arrest-of-nurse-who-refused-to-draw-blood.

Singleton v. AAA Home Health, Inc., WL 1693814, So 2d (La., 2000).

Smetzer, J., Baker, C., Byrne, F. D., Cohen, M. R. (2010). Shaping systems for better behavioral choices: Lessons learned from a fatal medication error. *Joint Commission Journal on Quality and Patient safety, 36*(4), 152–163.

Snyder, E. (2001). Automatic blood pressure cuff: nurses ignored the patient, committed battery. *Legal Eagle Eye Newsletter for the Nursing Profession, 9*(4), 1.

Snyder, E. (2003). Digoxin overdose: $1.5 million punitive damages. *Legal Eagle Eye Newsletter for the Nursing Profession, 11*(12), 1, 4–5.

Snyder, E. (2004). Student nurse/instructor: court discusses host hospital's legal liability. *Legal Eagle Eye Newsletter for the Nursing Profession, 14*(3), 4.

Snyder, E. (2006). Understaffing, fall, no neuro assessment, epidural hemorrhage, death: nurses faulted. *Legal Eagle Eye Newsletter for the Nursing Profession, 14*(8), 6.

Snyder, E. (2007). Disability discrimination: Quad on ventilator could not communicate with his caregivers. *Legal Eagle Eye Newsletter for the Nursing Profession, 15*(10), 1.

Snyder, E. (2014). Whistleblower: Court upholds nurse's rights. *Legal Eagle Eye Newsletter for the Nursing Profession, 23*(2), 6.

Stamford Hospital v. Vega, 674 A 2d 821 (Conn., 1996).

Starr, K. T. (2016). Reporting a physician colleague for unsafe practice: What's the law? *Nursing, 46*(2), 14.

Sunbridge Healthcare Corp. v. Penny, SW3d, 2005 WL 562763 (Tex. App, March 11, 2005).

Taenzer, A. H., Pyke, J. B., McGrath, S. P. (2011). A review of current and emerging approaches to address failure to rescue. *Anesthesiology, 115*(2), 421–431.

Tammelleo, D. 2003. Failure to act when you know error on meds risk lives. *Nursing Law's Regan Report, 44*(11), 1.

Teno, J. *The wrongful resuscitation. April, 2008). Patient Safety Network. Agency for Healthcare Research and Quality.* Retrieved from https://psnet.ahrq.gov/webmm/case/175/the-wrongful-resuscitation.

Tevington, P. (2011). Mandatory nurse-patient ratios. *Medsurg Nursing, 20*(5), 265–267.

The American Association of Nurse Attorneys and the American Association of Legal Nurse Consultants. (2011, August). Criminal Prosecution of Health Care Providers for Unintentional Human Error. TAANA – AALNC Position Paper. August, 2011. Retrieved from http://www.taana.org/position_papers#cphcpuhe.

The Joint Commission. (2008). Promoting effective communication—language access services in health care. *Joint Commission Perspectives, 26*(2), 8–11.

The Joint Commission. (2017). *Comprehensive accreditation manual for hospitals.* Oakbrook Terrace, IL: The Joint Commission.

The Joint Commission. (2014). *Speak up initiatives.* Oakbrook Terrace, Il: The Joint Commission. Retrieved from http://www.jointcommission.org/speakup.aspx.

The Salt Lake Tribune. (2017, August 31). Arrest of university hospital nurse Wubbels. Retrieved from https://youtu.be/ihQ1-LQOkns.

Thompson v. Nason Hospital, 591 A 2d 703, 707 (Pa., 1991).

U.S. Department of Health and Human Services Office of Minority Health. (2011). National Partnership for Action to End Health Disparities. U.S. Office of Inspector General (OIG). Retrieved from http://minorityhealth.hhs.gov/npa.

U.S. Department of Health and Human Services, Office of Inspector General. (2012). Hospital incident reporting systems do not capture most patient harm: Summary. Report OEI-06-09-00091. Retrieved from http://oig.hhs.gov/oei/reports/oei-06-09-00091.pdf.

U.S. Department of Justice Office of Public Affairs (December 14, 2016). *Justice Department recovers over $4.7 billion from False Claims Act cases in Fiscal Year 2016.* Retrieved from https://www.justice.gov/oa/pr/justice-department-recoversover-47-billion-false-claims-act-cases-fiscal-year-2016.

Utter v. United Hospital Center, Inc., 236 SE 2d 213 (W.Va, 1977).

William McDougald et al. v. St. Francis North Hospital Inc. No. 48,955 (L. App. 2nd Cir. April 9, 2014).

Williams v. West Virginia Board of Examiners, S.E. 2d WL1432298 (W.Va., 2004).

Winkelman v. Beloit Memorial Hospital, 483 NW 2d 211 (Wis., 1992).

Wolf, Z. R., Hicks, R. W., Altmiller, G., Bicknell, P. (2009). Nursing student medication errors involving tubing and catheters: a descriptive study. *Nurse Education Today, 29*(8), 681–688.

Zhong, E., McCarthy, C., Alexander, M. (2016). A Review of Criminal Convictions Among Nurses 2012–2013. *Journal of Nursing Regulation, 7*(1), 27–33.

Ethical dilemmas are the puzzles of life.

Ethical and Bioethical Issues in Nursing and Health Care

Carla D. Sanderson, PhD, RN

ⓔ Additional resources are available online at: *http://evolve.elsevier.com/Cherry/*

LEARNING OUTCOMES

After studying this chapter, the reader will be able to:

1. Integrate basic concepts of human values that are essential for ethical decision making.
2. Analyze selected ethical theories and principles as a basis for ethical decision making.
3. Analyze the relationship between ethics and morality in relation to nursing practice.
4. Use an ethical decision-making framework for resolving ethical problems in health care.
5. Apply the ethical decision-making process to specific ethical issues encountered in clinical practice.

KEY TERMS

Accountability An ethical duty stating that one should be answerable legally, morally, ethically, or socially for one's activities.

Autonomy Personal freedom and the right of competent people to make choices.

Beneficence An ethical principle of compassion and patient advocacy, stating that one should do good and prevent or avoid doing harm.

Bioethics The study of ethical problems resulting from scientific advances.

Code of ethics A set of statements encompassing rules that apply to people in professional roles.

Deontology An ethical theory stating that moral rule is binding.

Ethics Science or study of moral values.

Ethics acculturation The didactic and experiential process of developing ethical reasoning abilities as a part of ongoing professional preparation.

Fidelity The agreement to keep promises and commitments, based on the virtue of caring.

Justice The equal and fair distribution of resources, regardless of other factors.

Nonmaleficence An ethical principle stating the duty to not inflict harm.

Paternalism On the basis of the health care provider's belief about what is in the best interest of the patient, he/she chooses to reveal or withhold patient information such as diagnosis, treatment, or prognosis.

Rights of conscience The civil right that protects conscientious health care providers against discrimination, allowing them the right to act according to the dictates of their consciences.

Utilitarianism An ethical theory stating that the best decision is one that brings about the greatest good for the most people.

Values Customs, ideas of life, and ways of behaving that society regards as desirable.

Veracity An ethical duty to tell the truth.

PROFESSIONAL/ETHICAL ISSUE

Nursing students are introduced to the ethical and legal implications of the profession of nursing during the foundational nursing course offered early in their nursing program.

The most dreaded course in the entire nursing curriculum is now Adult Health Nursing. For the first time in your nursing program, your grade point average in the course is only two points above passing. There is so much to learn, so many concepts to put together, so many possible ways to think through test questions, and, in fact, your professor has told you that you are overthinking the answers.

The last unit test is in 5 days: the Unit 4 examination. So much is riding on your ability to do well. You need to score higher than you have on any Adult Health unit examination to date, yet the Unit 4 examination has the reputation for being the hardest of all, with the lowest scores of the semester.

As you begin to organize your study plan for the test, a friend sends a text to tell you that his friend has a copy of an old Adult Health–Unit 4 examination. He invites you to his apartment that evening, where a group of six to eight students will be reviewing for the examination with the copy in hand.

Your nursing program has made it very clear that no copies of prior exams are available or appropriate for use. You know how important it is to be competent in Unit 4 materials, to possess the independent reasoning ability to pass the examination unaided. In fact, you know that knowing the Unit 4 material could easily be a matter of life and death for a patient who will someday soon be in your care.

And what about those six to eight other nursing students? What if they are able to pass the test without developing the knowledge needed to give safe, competent care?

What are you to do? Do you attend the review with your classmates? Do you determine that it is more important to pass this test and get through nursing school, thinking you can worry about truly learning the material later? Do you have any responsibility over the actions of your classmates? What is your moral and ethical responsibility for the wrongdoing of others?

VIGNETTE

Joe Smith has accepted a position as the nurse manager in a very busy urban emergency department, which serves patients from diverse cultures. Among Joe's many responsibilities is developing the 24-hour, 7-day–week work schedules of the department's nursing workforce in which he has 10 unfilled positions. Another responsibility is implementing the hospital's policy of offering all patients, regardless of cultural beliefs, the right to an advance directive for end-of-life care. At the same time, Joe must ensure that each patient who enters the emergency department receives appropriate high-quality care from competent professional care providers who respect and respond to patients' individual needs and desires. With these responsibilities come challenges, sometimes so significant that the nurse manager is faced with an ethical dilemma.

Questions to Consider While Reading This Chapter:

1. How will ethical and bioethical issues in nursing and health care affect my professional nursing practice?
2. What ethical theories and principles serve as a basis for nursing practice?
3. How am I to think about ethical dilemmas with moral integrity and consistency with my belief system?
4. What goals can I establish to move me toward excellence in moral and ethical reasoning?
5. How can I assist patients and families who face difficult ethical decisions?

CHAPTER OVERVIEW

In a nursing education program, nursing students begin to embrace the complexities and profound opportunities that are characteristic of the profession of nursing. Prelicensure nursing education is only an introduction to a discipline in which there are no knowledge boundaries. The abundance of nursing practice information is evident from a quick glance across the nursing textbook selections in the campus or online bookstore.

Most of that information addresses the "how-to" aspects of nursing care. The scientific aspects of nursing care are rapidly evolving as a host of nurse researchers delve into questions about the safe, competent, and therapeutic aspects of professional nursing care. As quickly as nursing science produces new knowledge, "how-to" information is shared through journals, textbooks, and Internet resources. The scientific aspects of care evolve constantly through "how-to" research.

A myriad of potential questions surpass the "how-to" body of knowledge that is inherent in the profession of nursing. Everywhere in today's health care delivery system are potential questions of another nature—the "how should" questions, which are challenging and sometimes evolve into ethical dilemmas. The "how should" questions that the emergency department nurse manager faces may sound something like the following:

- How should I determine the competency of an acutely ill 80-year-old patient who comes to the emergency department without an advance directive? Is her competency intact? How should I determine whether she is capable of giving an informed advance directive?
- How should I act if her decision for her own end-of-life care is not consistent with what her family wants for her? Or how should I respond if the family, because of cultural beliefs, will not even allow information about end-of-life care to be shared with their loved one?
- How should I view the care of this 80-year-old patient? Is an emergency resuscitation effort for such a patient considered ordinary and routine, or is it considered extraordinary and heroic?
- How should I respond to her if, in the course of efforts to stabilize her, she calls me in to ask me whether she is dying?
- How much of the truth is warranted?
- How should I decide when the availability of one-on-one trauma care beds becomes threatened and the decision must be made to move someone out of one bed to make room for this 80-year-old woman whose condition is rapidly deteriorating?
- Is the life of this 80-year-old woman any less significant than that of the 40-year-old father of four who has just been admitted after a tragic car accident?
- How should I react when another health care provider on duty devalues the significance of this patient's life?
- How should I feel when this 80-year-old patient is entered into a research study designed to test a new drug for flash pulmonary edema from congestive heart failure that has previously been tested only on a younger population?
- How should I make staffing assignments when the number of nurses on a given shift is insufficient to provide effective and adequate emergency department care to all?

- How should I respond when one of the few nurses reporting to work on a given day refuses to accept the care of patients because of inadequate staffing?
- How should I react when presented with situations that test my own sense of conscience and moral integrity?

This chapter introduces the nursing student to a different aspect of nursing care—the "how should" aspect or, as it is more appropriately called, the ethical aspect. Ethics is a system for deciding, on the basis of principles, how one should think and what one should do. With the goal of developing excellence in moral and reasoning ability, the nursing student begins a career-long process of ethics acculturation. This process allows the professional nurse to practice with an increasing level of understanding that goes beyond the scientific and moves toward a more complete and whole understanding of human existence.

NURSING ETHICS

Nursing ethics is a system of principles concerning the actions of the nurse in his or her relationships with patients, patients' family members, other health care providers, policymakers, and society as a whole. A profession is characterized by its relationship to society. The results of a 2016 Gallup poll on professional honesty and ethics indicate that the public ranks nursing as the most ethical of all professions and has for almost two decades (Gallop News, 2017). Codes of ethics provide implicit standards and values for the professions. A nursing code of ethics was first introduced in the late nineteenth century and has evolved through the years as the profession has evolved and as changes in society and health care have come about. Current dynamics, such as the Patient Protection and Affordable Care Act, the emerging genetic interventions associated with therapeutic and reproductive cloning, debates about securing stem cells for research and treatment, ongoing questions about euthanasia and assisted suicide, and escalating threats to the effective delivery of health care as a result of significant nursing shortages, now being called "the ethical climate in the workplace," bring nursing's code of ethics to the forefront (Boxes 9.1 and 9.2).

BIOETHICS

Nursing ethics is part of a broader system known as bioethics. Bioethics is an interdisciplinary field within the

BOX 9.1   American Nurses Association Code of Ethics for Nurses

- The nurse practices with compassion and respect for the inherent dignity, worth, and unique attributes of every person.
- The nurse's primary commitment is to the patient, whether an individual, family, group, community, or population.
- The nurse promotes, advocates for, and protects the rights, health, and safety of the patient.
- The nurse has authority, accountability, and responsibility for nursing practice; makes decisions; and takes action consistent with the obligation to promote health and to provide optimal care.
- The nurse owes the same duties to self as to others, including the responsibility to promote health and safety, preserve wholeness of character and integrity, maintain competence, and continue personal and professional growth.

- The nurse, through individual and collective effort, establishes, maintains, and improves the ethical environment of the work setting and conditions of employment that are conducive to safe, quality health care.
- The nurse, in all roles and settings, advances the profession through research and scholarly inquiry, professional standards development, and the generation of both nursing and health policy.
- The nurse collaborates with other health professionals and the public to protect human rights, promote health diplomacy, and reduce health disparities.
- The profession of nursing, collectively through its professional organizations, must articulate nursing values, maintain the integrity of the profession, and integrate principles of social justice into nursing and health policy.

Reprinted with permission from American Nurses Association. (2015). *Code of ethics for nurses with interpretive statements,* Silver Spring, MD: Nursesbooks.org, American Nurses Association. Available online at http://www.nursesbooks.org/Main-Menu/Ethics/Code-of-Ethics.aspx.

BOX 9.2   International Council of Nurses Code of Ethics for Nurses

1. Nurses and people

The nurse's primary professional responsibility is to people requiring nursing care.

In providing care, the nurse promotes an environment in which the human rights, values, customs and spiritual beliefs of the individual, family and community are respected.

The nurse ensures that the individual receives accurate, sufficient and timely information in a culturally appropriate manner on which to base consent for care and related treatment.

The nurse holds in confidence personal information and uses judgement in sharing this information.

The nurse shares with society the responsibility for initiating and supporting action to meet the health and social needs of the public, in particular those of vulnerable populations.

The nurse advocates for equity and social justice in resource allocation, access to health care and other social and economic services.

The nurse demonstrates professional values such as respectfulness, responsiveness, compassion, trustworthiness and integrity.

2. Nurses and practice

The nurse carries personal responsibility and accountability for nursing practice, and for maintaining competence by continual learning.

The nurse maintains a standard of personal health such that the ability to provide care is not compromised.

The nurse uses judgement regarding individual competence when accepting and delegating responsibility.

The nurse at all times maintains standards of personal conduct which reflect well on the profession and enhance its image and public confidence.

The nurse, in providing care, ensures that use of technology and scientific advances are compatible with the safety, dignity and rights of people.

The nurse strives to foster and maintain a practice culture promoting ethical behaviour and open dialogue.

3. Nurses and the profession

The nurse assumes the major role in determining and implementing acceptable standards of clinical nursing practice, management, research and education.

The nurse is active in developing a core of research-based professional knowledge that supports evidence-based practice.

The nurse is active in developing and sustaining a core of professional values.

The nurse, acting through the professional organisation, participates in creating a positive practice environment and maintaining safe, equitable social and economic working conditions in nursing.

The nurse practices to sustain and protect the natural environment and is aware of its consequences on health.

The nurse contributes to an ethical organisational environment and challenges unethical practices and settings.

4. Nurses and co-workers

The nurse sustains a collaborative and respectful relationship with co-workers in nursing and other fields.

The nurse takes appropriate action to safeguard individuals, families and communities when their health is endangered by a co-worker or any other person.

The nurse takes appropriate action to support and guide co-workers to advance ethical conduct.

From International Council of Nurses. (2012). *ICN code of ethics for nurses*. Geneva: ICN.

health care organization that has developed only in the past 50 years. Whereas ethics has been discussed since there was written language, bioethics has developed with the age of modern medicine, specifically with the development of hemodialysis and organ transplantation. New questions surface as science and technology produce new ways of knowing. Think of the questions that come from stem cell research, sexual reassignment, organ transplantation, funding for end-of-life care, and reproductive-assisting technologies such as donor insemination, in vitro fertilization, removal of unused zygotes, and surrogate parenting. Bioethics is a response to these and other contemporary advances and challenges in health care. It is difficult to imagine a time when answers will be more plentiful than bioethical questions.

Dilemmas for Health Professionals

Physicians, nurses, social workers, psychiatrists, epidemiologists, clergy, philosophers, theologians, researchers, and policymakers are joining through interprofessional initiatives to address ethical questions, difficult right-versus-wrong questions. As they seek to deliver quality health care, these professionals debate situations that pose dilemmas. They are confronting situations for which there are no clear right or wrong answers. Because of the diverse society in which health care is practiced, there are at least two sides to almost every issue faced.

Every specialization in health care has its own set of questions. Life and death, the margin of viability, quality of life, design of life, one life offering cure for another, right to decide, informed consent, medical confidentiality, and alternative treatment issues prevail in every field of health care. Questions about the economics of nursing care and the use of technologies in the diagnosis and treatment of illness abound. In every aspect of the nursing profession lie the more subtle and

intricate questions of how this care should be delivered and how one should decide when choices are in conflict.

Many nursing students do not consider health care and the practice of nursing in terms of the personal, truthful, faithful (i.e., keeping promises to patients), qualitative, and subjective side; rather, they look at it only in terms of the technical, quantitative, and objective side. Yet there are distinctively subjective factors that influence the way patients are actually treated, or at least the way they perceive their treatment, that go beyond the data-driven aspect. In many ways, advanced technology has changed the face of health care and created the troubling questions that have become central in the delivery of care.

Dilemmas Created by Technology

Advances in health care through technology have created new situations for health care professionals and their patients. For the young, the old, and generations in between, illnesses once leading to death have become manageable and are classified as high-risk or chronic illnesses. Although people can now be saved, they are not being saved readily or inexpensively. Care of the acutely or chronically ill person sometimes creates hard questions for which there are no easy or apparent answers. Mortality for most will be a long, drawn-out phenomenon, laced with a lifetime of potential conflicts about what ought to be done.

Even the nature of life itself and the technical manipulation of DNA are under investigation. Health care professionals who adhere to an exclusively scientific or technologic approach to care will be seen as insensitive and will fail to meet the genuine needs of the patient—needs that include assistance with these more subjective concerns, such as how to think about the many advanced care choices laid before the patient.

THE ETHICS OF CARE

The very nature of the profession of nursing is the obligation and responsibility to care (Beauchamp and Childress, 2009). The ethic of care involves the nurse fulfilling the caring task by seeking the best way to care for each patient, one patient at a time, thus fulfilling a moral imperative to alleviate suffering by taking action. Caring defines nursing, as curing often defines medicine (Lachman, 2012).

Toward this end, nursing's Code of Ethics, first written in 1950 with ongoing revisions across the years, was updated in 2015 to provide a "definitive framework for ethical analysis and decision-making for RNs across all practice levels, roles and settings" (American Nurses Association [ANA], 2015). The new Code is made up of nine provisions, which are elaborated on through interpretive statements. Each provision establishes nursing's values and commitments, its boundaries, and its duties beyond direct patient care to duties to society. ANA describes the Code as "the promise that nurses are doing their best to provide care for their patients and their communities and are supporting each other in the process so that all nurses can fulfill their ethical and professional obligations" (ANA, 2015).

Today's professional nurse will be deemed competent only if he or she can promote well-being through the scientific and technologic aspects of care *and* uphold his or her ethical and professional obligations. A competent nurse is an ethically sensitive nurse (Weaver et al, 2008) who can deal with the human dimensions of care that include a search for what is good and right as well as for what is accurate and efficient. The previously listed "how should" questions are just as important as the "how-to" questions surrounding day-to-day decision making in the emergency department or the care of the 80-year-old patient introduced previously. As the nurse seeks to understand the "how-to" aspects of nurse management and patient care, he or she also must seek to understand more about respecting the rights of patients.

Answering Difficult Questions

Care that combines human dimensions with scientific and technical dimensions forces some basic questions:
- What is safe care?
- What effect might a patient's cultural preferences have on safe care?

- When staffing is inadequate, what care should be accepted or refused?
- What are other barriers to ethical practice brought about by the workplace environment?
- What does it mean to be ill or well?
- What is the proper balance between science and technology and the good of humans?
- Where do we find balance when science will allow us to experiment with the basic origins of life?
- What happens when the proper balance is in tension?
- What happens when tension exists between personal beliefs and values and institutional policy or patient desires?

No tension is created in the effort to save the life of a dying healthy adolescent or set the broken leg of a healthy older adult. Science and the human good are not in conflict here. No conflict exists when there is a competent nursing staff, sufficient in number to provide quality care. However, what is the answer when modern medicine can save or prolong the life of an 8-year-old child but the child's parents refuse treatment for religious reasons? Or what is the answer when modern medicine has life to offer a 30-year-old mother in need of a transplanted organ but the woman is without the financial means to cover the cost of the treatment? What is the answer when a family refuses to allow the physician to share news of a terminal illness with their grandmother? What is the answer when new discoveries allow some would-be parents to choose biologic characteristics of children not yet conceived? What is the answer when the emergency department is full of acutely ill patients and there too few nurses expected for the next shift? At one end of the spectrum lies the obvious; at the other there is uncertainty. Health care professionals in everyday practice often find themselves somewhere between the two.

Balancing Science and Morality

If nursing care is to be competent, the right balance between science and morality must be sought and understood. Nurses must first attempt to understand not just what they are to do for their patients but who their patients are. They must examine life and its origins, in addition to its worth, usefulness, and importance. Nurses must determine their own values and seek to understand the values of others.

Health care decisions are seldom made independently of other people. Decisions are made with the patient, the family, other nurses, and other health care providers. Nurses must make a deliberate effort to recognize their own values and learn to consider and respect the values of others.

The nurse has an obligation to present himself or herself to the patient as competent. The dependent patient enters a mutual relationship with the nurse. This exchange places a patient who is vulnerable and wounded with a nurse who is educated, licensed, and knowledgeable. The patient expects nursing actions to be thorough because total caring is the defining characteristic of the patient-nurse relationship. The nurse promises to deliver holistic care to the best of his or her ability. The patient's expectations and the nurse's promises require a commitment to develop a reasoned thought process and sound judgment in all situations that take place within this important relationship. The more personal, subjective, and value-laden situations are deemed to be among the most difficult situations for which the nurse must prepare.

VALUES FORMATION AND MORAL DEVELOPMENT

A value is a personal belief about worth that acts as a standard to guide behavior; a value system is an entire framework on which actions are based and is the backbone to how one thinks, feels, and takes action. Perhaps many nursing students come to their education with a strong backbone and an intact value system. No doubt anyone living in these times has faced many situations in which important choices had to be made. The challenges faced in this generation are too numerous to avoid difficult choices. Values have been applied to those decisions. Yet often people do not take time to seriously contemplate their value system, the forces that shaped those values, and the life and worldview decisions that have been made on the basis of such values.

Examining Value Systems

To become a competent professional in every dimension of nursing care, nurses must examine their own system of values and commit themselves to a virtuous value system. A clear understanding of what is right and wrong is a necessary first step to a process sometimes referred to as *values clarification,* in which people attempt to examine the values they hold and how each of those values functions as part of a whole. Nurses must acknowledge their own values by considering how they would act in a particular situation.

Diane Uustal was one of nursing's first leaders to describe the role of values clarification in the decision-making process of the nurse. A values clarification process is an important learning tool for nursing students preparing themselves to become competent professionals (Uustal, 1992). The deliberate refinement of one's own value system leads to a clearer lens through which the nurse can view ethical questions in the practice of the profession. A refined value system and worldview can serve the professional as he or she deals with the meaning of life and its many choices. A worldview provides a cohesive model for life; it encourages personal responsibility for the living of that life, and it prepares one for making ethical choices encountered throughout life. Tools to assist the reader in values clarification can be found online (http://evolve.elsevier.com/Cherry/).

Forming a worldview and a value system is an evolving, continuous, dynamic process that moves along a continuum of development often referred to as *moral development.* Just as there is an orderly sequence of physical and psychologic development, there is an orderly sequence of right and wrong conduct development. Consider an adult of strong physical strength and moral character. With each biologic developmental milestone there is a more mature, more expanded physical being; likewise with each life experience that has choices between right and wrong, there is a more mature, more virtuous person.

Learning Right and Wrong

The process of learning to distinguish right and wrong is often described in pediatric textbooks. Donna Wong describes such development in children (Hockenberry and Wilson, 2010). Infants have no concept of right or wrong. Infants hold no beliefs and no convictions, although it is known that moral development begins in infancy. If the need for basic trust is met in infancy, children can begin to develop the foundation for secure moral thought. Toddlers begin to display behavior in response to the world around them. They will imitate behavior seen in others, even though they do not comprehend the meaning of the behavior that they are imitating. Furthermore, even though toddlers may not know what they are doing or why they are doing it, they incorporate the values and beliefs of those around them into their own behavioral code.

By the time children reach school age, they have learned that behavior has consequences and that good behavior is associated with rewards and bad behavior with punishment. Through their experiences and social interactions outside their home or immediate surroundings, school-age children begin to make choices about how they will act on the basis of an understanding of good and bad. Their conscience is developing, and it begins to govern the choices they make (Hockenberry and Wilson, 2010).

The adolescent questions existing moral values and his or her relevance to society. Adolescents understand duty and obligation, but they sometimes seriously question the moral codes on which society operates as they become more aware of the contradictions they see in the value systems of adults.

Adults strive to make sense of the contradictions and learn to develop their own set of morals and values as autonomous people, sometimes referred to as *developing a moral compass*. They begin to make choices based on an internalized set of principles that provides them with the resources they need to evaluate situations in which they find themselves (Hockenberry and Wilson, 2010).

Understanding Moral Development Theory

Perhaps the most widely accepted theory on moral development is the now classic theory developed by Lawrence Kohlberg (1971). He theorizes a cognitive developmental process that is sequential in nature with progression through levels and stages that vary dramatically within society. At first, morality is all about rules imposed by some source of authority. Moral decisions made at this level (preconventional) are simply in response to some threat of punishment. The good-bad, right-wrong labels have meaning, but they are defined only in reference to a self-centered reward-and-punishment system. A person who is in the preconventional level has no concept of the underlying moral code informing the decision of good or bad or right or wrong.

At some point, people begin to internalize their view of themselves in response to something more meaningful and interpersonal (conventional level). A desire to be viewed as a good boy or nice girl develops when the person wants to find approval from others. He or she may want to please, help others, be dutiful, and show respect for authority. Conformity to expected social and religious mores and a sense of loyalty may emerge.

Not all people develop beyond the conventional level of moral development. A morally mature individual (postconventional level), one of the few to reach moral completeness, is an autonomous thinker who strives for a moral code beyond issues of authority and reverence. Integrative thinking is required to move toward having the critical components necessary to make moral judgments. The morally mature individual's actions are based on principles of justice and respect for the dignity of all humankind and not just on principles of responsibility, duty, or self-edification (Kohlberg, 1971).

Moving Toward Moral Maturity

The rightness or wrongness of the complex and confounding health care decisions being made today depends on the level of moral development of those professionals entrusted with the tough decisions. Moving toward the level of moral maturity required for sound ethical decision making requires strong commitment. Nurses must commit themselves to such learning, to a process called ethics acculturation across the span of their career. The issues will only get more complex and confounding as new advances are introduced. The desired outcomes of ethics acculturation are integrity, personal growth, practical wisdom, and effective problem solving on behalf of patients and their families (Weaver et al, 2008). These are the qualities characteristic of an ethically sensitive and morally mature person.

As a matter of the civil rights afforded to all members of U.S. society, health care professionals have been afforded rights of conscience to practice their own convictions about what is right and ethical care. Rights of conscience are relevant in the debate on abortion and euthanasia. Historically much liberty has been given to professionals in choosing to participate in care they believe in and refusing to participate in care they may find ethically unsound. The current debate on health care reform has sparked discussion on threats to continued rights of conscience for practitioners as federal funding for abortion has been allocated. Professional nurses must be ready to take up the challenge of debating the matter of whether or not the right to act according to conscience should continue to be a part of one's civil rights. Doing so will require careful examination of right and wrong, the principles and motivations that govern actions and thoughts, and accountability for actions taken.

The development of value-based behavior is essential for professional nursing. The American Association of Colleges of Nursing (AACN) has delineated five essential values, described in Table 9.1. Students who seek to become morally mature health care providers will appraise nursing's values and strive to find a comfortable union of those values with their own.

The complexity of today's healthcare environment may lead to value conflicts and the potential for moral distress that comes from knowing the morally right thing to do but not being able to do it because of constraints outside one's control. *Moral courage* refers to being able to stand up for what is right, taking action based on ethical principles and protecting ethical values such as honesty, integrity, fairness, respect, responsibility, empathy, compassion, and courage, regardless of the possible consequences taking such action might present (Murray, 2010). Moral courage

can be developed by simulating ethical dilemmas that students and nurses can process together. The study of ethical theory and ethical principles can guide the dialogue for processing dilemmas and give one a basis for moving forward as a morally courageous professional nurse.

ETHICAL THEORY

Ethical theory is a system of principles by which a person can determine what should and should not be done. Although there are others, utilitarianism and deontology are the theories most frequently cited in the Western world as foundational for processing ethical dilemmas.

Utilitarianism

Utilitarianism is an approach that supports what is best for most people, rooted in the assumption that an action or practice is right if it leads to the greatest possible balance of good consequences or to

---

TABLE 9.1 Essential Nursing Values and Behaviors

Essential Values	Attitudes and Personal Qualities	Professional Behaviors
Altruism—concern for the welfare of others	Caring, commitment, compassion, generosity, perseverance	Gives full attention to the client when giving care; assists other personnel in providing care when they are unable to do so; expresses concern about social trends and issues that have implications for health care
Autonomy—right to self-determination	Respectfulness, trust, objectivity	Provides nursing care based on respect of patients' rights to make decisions about their health care; honors individual's right to refuse treatment
Human dignity—respect for inherent worth and uniqueness of individuals and populations	Consideration, empathy, humaneness, kindness, respectfulness	Values and respects all patients and colleagues, regardless of background
Integrity—acting in accordance with an appropriate code of ethics	Moral, ethical, and legal professional behavior	The nurse is honest and provides care based on an ethical framework that is accepted in the profession
Social justice—acting in accordance with fair treatment regardless of economic status, race, ethnicity, age, citizenship, disability, or sexual orientation	Courage, integrity, morality, objectivity	Acts as a health care advocate; allocates resources fairly; reports incompetent, unethical, and illegal practices objectively and factually

From American Association of Colleges of Nursing. (2008). *Essentials of baccalaureate education for professional nursing.* Washington, DC: American Association of Colleges of Nursing.

the least possible balance of bad consequences. For instance, the utilitarian approach would be at work if the government made a decision to forgo Medicare funding treatment for a particular population with terminal disease and to redistribute funding to other Medicare-eligible individuals with a greater likelihood for longevity or quality of life. Utilitarian ethics are noted to be the strongest approach used in bioethical decision making. An attempt is made to determine which actions will lead to the highest ratio of benefit to harm for all persons involved in the dilemma.

Deontology

Deontology is an approach that is rooted in the assumption that humans are rational and act out of principles that are consistent and objective and compel them to do what is right. Ethics are based on a sense of a universal principle to consistently act one way. For instance, the deontological approach would be at work if a decision is made to resuscitate and provide mechanical ventilation to a 23-week, otherwise viable fetus, despite ability to pay for care and availability of newborn intensive care beds. In bioethical decision making, moral rightness is the act that is determined not by the consequences of the actions it produces but by the intentions and moral qualities intrinsic to the act itself. Deontological theory claims that a decision is right only if it conforms to an overriding moral duty and wrong only if it violates that moral duty. All decisions must be made in such a way that the decision could become universal law. Persons are to be treated as ends in themselves and never as means to the ends of others.

ETHICAL PRINCIPLES

Perhaps the most useful tool for the morally mature professional nurse is a set of principles, standards, or truths on which to base ethical actions. Common ground must be established between the nurse and the patient and family, between fellow nurses, between the nurse and other health care providers, and between the nurse and other members of society. Such common ground can be established by adhering to a set of principles that can move everyone involved toward understanding and agreement.

The practice of ethics involves applying principles to the two ethical theories described—utilitarianism and deontology—or to other theories that are described elsewhere. Principles can permit people to take a consistent position on specific or related issues. If the principles, when applied to a particular act, make the act right or wrong in one situation, it seems reasonable to assume that the same principle, when applied to a new situation, can have the same result.

Three principles have proven to be highly relevant in bioethics: (1) autonomy, (2) beneficence and nonmaleficence, and (3) veracity. These principles do not form a complete moral framework. One principle may be relevant to a particular situation but the others are not. Yet these principles are sufficiently comprehensive to provide an analytic framework by which moral problems can be evaluated.

Autonomy

Autonomy, the principle of respect for a person, is sometimes called the primary moral principle. This concept holds that humans have incalculable worth or moral dignity not possessed by other objects or creatures. There is unconditional intrinsic value for everyone. People are free to form their own judgments and whatever actions they choose. They are self-determining agents, entitled to determine their own destiny.

If an autonomous person's actions do not infringe on the autonomous actions of others, that person should be free to decide whatever he or she wishes. This freedom should be applied even if the decision creates risk to his or her health and even if the decision seems unwise to others. Concepts of freedom and informed consent are grounded in the principle of autonomy.

Although the principle of autonomy may seem basic and universal, there are times when this principle may be in conflict with other principles, such a familial ones. For instance, in some male-dominated or patriarchal cultures, the family leader's rights may override the individual and autonomous rights of a family member. In this situation, action based on the moral principle of autonomy may perpetuate conflict.

Beneficence and Nonmaleficence

In general terms, to be *beneficent* is to promote goodness, kindness, and charity. A different yet related principle is *nonmaleficence,* which is a duty not to inflict harm. In ethical terms nonmaleficence is abstaining from injuring others and helping others further their own well-being by removing harm and eliminating threats, whereas *beneficence* is to provide benefits to others by promoting their good. The beneficence-nonmaleficence principle is largely a balance of risk and benefit. At times, the risk for harm must be weighed against the possible benefits. The risk should never be greater than the importance of the problem to be solved.

Although it may seem natural to promote good at all times, the most common bioethical conflicts result from an imbalance between the demands of beneficence and those acts and decisions within the health care delivery system that might pose threats. For instance, it is not always clearly evident what is good and what is harmful. Is the resuscitation effort for the 90-year-old woman good or harmful to her overall sense of well-being? How much beneficence is there in supporting someone toward a peaceful death? What is the balance between beneficence and nonmaleficence in an understaffed emergency department? Is it better to do as much good as you can with the limited resources you have or to refuse to assume care in an effort to prevent harm that can come from being understaffed?

Veracity

Most contemporary professionals believe that telling the truth in personal communication is a moral and ethical requirement. If there is the belief in health care that truth telling is always right, then the principle of veracity can itself pose some interesting challenges.

In the past, truth telling was sometimes viewed as inconvenient, distressing, or even harmful to patients and families. In fact, the first American Medical Association Code of Ethics in 1847 contained such a message: "The life of a sick person can be shortened not only by the acts, but also by the words or the manner of a physician. It is, therefore, a sacred duty to guard himself carefully in this respect, and to avoid all things that have a tendency to discourage the patient and to depress his spirits."

The belief that the truth could at times be harmful was held for many years. Only recently, with the shift from a provider-driven system to a consumer-driven system, has the adherence to silence begun to break down. With this shift have come interesting questions. Is the provider-patient relationship generally understood by both parties to include the right of the provider to control the truth by withholding some or all of the relevant information until an appropriate time for disclosure? How much deception of patients is morally acceptable in the communication of a poor or terminal prognosis?

Difficult questions surface, but at the heart of the principle of veracity is trust. Health care consumers today expect accurate and precise information that is revealed in an honest and respectful manner. A few generations ago, the trust factor may have been such that it was acceptable for providers to share parts of truth or to distort the truth in the name of beneficence. Today, however, for trust to develop between providers and patients there must be truthful interaction and meaningful communication. The moral conflict that results from being less than truthful to patients is too troublesome for today's practitioner. The deontologic theory that the health care provider has a duty to tell the patient the truth has taken precedence over the fear of harm that might result if the truth is revealed.

The challenge today is to mesh the need for truthful communication with the need to protect. Health care providers must lay aside fears that the truth will be harmful to patients and come to the realization that more often than not, the truth can alleviate anxiety, increase pain tolerance, facilitate recovery, and enhance cooperation with treatment. With a pledge to human decency, health care providers must commit themselves to truth telling in all interactions and relationships.

ETHICAL DECISION-MAKING MODEL

Theories provide a cognitive plan for considering ethical issues; principles offer guiding truths on which to base ethical decisions. With the use of these theories and principles, it seems appropriate to consider a system for moving beyond a specific ethical dilemma toward a morally mature and reasoned ethical action.

Many ethical decision-making models exist for the purpose of defining a process by which a nurse or another health care provider actually can move through an ethical dilemma toward an informed decision. Box 9.3 depicts one ethical decision-making model.

Situation Assessment Procedure

Identify the ethical issues and problems. In the first step of assessment, there is an attempt to find out the technical and scientific facts and the human dimension of the situation—the feelings, emotions, attitudes, and opinions. A nurse must make an attempt to understand what values are inherent in the situation. Finally, the

---

BOX 9.3   Situation Assessment Procedure

- Identify the ethical issues and problems.
- Identify and analyze available alternatives for action.
- Select one alternative.
- Justify the selection.

From Wright, R.A. (1987). *The practice of ethics: Human values in health care.* New York: McGraw-Hill.

---

nurse must deliberately state the nature of the ethical dilemma. This first step is important because the issues and problems to be addressed are often complex. Trying to understand the full picture of a situation is time-consuming and requires examination from many different perspectives, but it is worth the time and effort to understand an issue fully before moving forward in the assessment procedure. Wright (1987) poses some important questions that must be addressed in this first step:

- What is the issue here?
- What are the hidden issues?
- What exactly are the complexities of this situation?
- Is anything being overlooked?

Identify and Analyze Available Alternatives for Action.

In the second step, a set of alternatives for action is established. The second step is an important step to follow. Because actions are based most commonly on a nurse's personal value system, it is important to list all possible actions for a given situation, even actions that seem highly unlikely. Without a deliberate listing of possible alternatives, it is doubtful that the full consideration of all possible actions will take place. Wright's (1987) questions for the second step are as follows:

- What are the reasonable possibilities for action, and how do the different affected parties (patient, family, physician, nurse) want to resolve the problem?
- What ethical principles are required for each alternative?
- What assumptions are required for each alternative, and what are their implications for future action?
- What, if any, are the additional ethical problems that the alternatives raise?

Select One Alternative. Multiple factors come together in the third step. After identifying the issues and analyzing all possible alternatives, the skillful decision maker

steps back to consider the situation again. There is an attempt to reflect on ethical theory and to mesh that thinking with the identified ethical principles for each alternative. The decision maker's value system is applied, along with an appraisal of the profession's values for the care of others. A reasoned and purposeful decision results from the blending of all of these factors.

Justify the Selection. The rational discourse on which the decision is based must be shared in an effort to justify the decision. The decision maker must be prepared to communicate his or her thoughts through an explanation of the reasoning process used. According to Wright (1987), the justification for a resolution to an ethical issue is an argument wherein relevant and sufficient reasons for the correctness of that resolution are presented. Defending an argument is not an easy task, but it is a necessary step to communicate the reasons or premises on which the decision is based. A systematic and logical argument will show why the particular resolution chosen is the correct one. This final step is important to allow the nurse to advance ethical thought and to express sound judgment. Wright's formula for the justification process is as follows:

1. Specify reasons for the action.
2. Clearly present the ethical basis for these reasons.
3. Understand the shortcomings of the justification.
4. Anticipate objections to the justification.

Usefulness and Application of the Situation Assessment Procedure

A procedure or model for ethical decision making is useful for individuals and groups alike. The more subtle and tenuous issues that arise in health care often are resolved within the context of the patient-provider relationship that exists between two people. Dilemmas resulting from questions about truth telling, acknowledging uncertainty, paternalism, privacy, and fidelity are examples of issues that may be resolved between as few as two people.

Questions that are more encompassing are often addressed in group settings. Institutional ethics committees are now common within health care agencies. The purpose of the committee is to provide ethics education, aid in ethical policy development, and serve as a consultative body when resolution of an ethical dilemma cannot be reached otherwise. Although institutional ethics committees do not make legal decisions that are the province of the patient, the family, or the health care provider, a model such as the situation assessment procedure can be a useful procedure to guide the thinking of a group that has been asked to provide counsel.

More and more nurses are finding themselves facing ethical dilemmas as members of hospital administration teams or policymaking bodies within professional organizations or governmental bodies. Nurses contribute a highly relevant perspective to discussions and decisions about safe and effective care in these times of change. The situation assessment procedure can be applied to the decision-making process when procedures and policies are being developed to address conflicting variables.

Thus application of the situation assessment procedure can occur on two levels. The procedure is applicable to the daily practice level of ethical decision making as patients and providers make choices between right and wrong actions. The procedure is equally applicable to the policymaking level, where professionals come together to consider right and wrong choices that affect society as a whole. Professional organizations including the ANA have established committees, such as the Ethics and Human Rights Committee, which allow nurses to meet to set policy for the practice of nursing. Inherent in the policy formation are questions that affect patient care. The situation assessment procedure can be applied to difficult questions that arise in any setting in which the nurse is responsible for or contributes to ethical decision making.

BIOETHICAL DILEMMAS: LIFE, DEATH, AND DILEMMAS IN BETWEEN

Bioethical dilemmas are situations that pose a choice between perplexing alternatives in the delivery of health care because of the lack of a clear sense of right or wrong. It is imperative that every nursing student consider the potential dilemmas that might arise in a given practice setting. Concepts of life and death are central to nursing's body of knowledge, but a discussion of these concepts is incomplete unless the threats of conflict also are explored. A nursing student must not assume that conflict is rare or that it is to be dealt with primarily by other professionals on the health care team. Conflict must be addressed as the concepts of life and its origins, birth, death, and dying are addressed.

Life

Entire textbooks are written to address the potential conflict that surrounds questions about the beginning of life. The most significant conflict that will be recorded in the historical accounts of the twentieth century is the debate about when life begins. The abortion conflict became central in 1973 when the Roe v. Wade decision was made by the U.S. Supreme Court. Although the legal aspects of abortion have been resolved in courtrooms in the United States, the bioethical concerns continue to be debated 45 years later. The bioethical abortion conflict has been debated through the use of ethical theories and principles, value systems, rights issues, questions regarding the nature of choice, and so on. Answers acceptable to society as a whole have not materialized; thus, the right or wrong of abortion continues to rest with each person. Nurses serving in health settings for women and children must be prepared to face this morally laden issue.

Closely akin to the abortion question are newer questions about reproduction. Genetic screening, genetic engineering, stem cell therapy, and cloning are newer, highly advanced, and sophisticated techniques that bring with them the most ethically entangled questions ever encountered; the entire Human Genome Project with its rapidly developing advances represents the greatest challenge to date. Definitions of family, surrogacy, and other related issues also bring ethically entangled questions. Moving beyond the question about when life begins, health care providers must now address their patients' questions about the right or wrong of designing life itself through the manipulation and engineering of DNA or the right and wrong of new parenting models. Twenty-first-century science has created a whole new dimension of bioethics.

Genomic applications in health care, and the ethical implications surrounding them, are becoming increasingly relevant to the day-to-day delivery of care to patients. The National Institutes of Health provide a resource for understanding the ethical implications of genomics, the Genetics/Genomics Competency Center (G2C2), which can be accessed online (www.g-2-c-2.org). Nurses can use this center to learn how to apply ethical principles when deliberating genetic/genomic issues related to decision making, privacy, confidentiality, and informed consent, as well as to process situations when patients' beliefs and values influence genomic care choices, and can find resources for resolving ethical dilemmas.

The End of Life

The second most debated conflict in health care involves the issue of death and dying. Since the development of lifesaving procedures and mechanical ventilation, questions about quality of life and the definition of death have escalated. With advances in health care, it has become unclear what is usual and what is heroic care. The purpose and quality of life of a person in a vegetative state continue to be debated. Health care providers regularly contend with questions of cerebral versus biologic death in their dealings with patients and families.

The United States is now experiencing the aging of its largest segment of the population and is facing ethical dilemmas related to the limited resources available to care for them. There is growing concern in the public arena about the expenses associated with prolongation of the dying process, which often also prolongs suffering. Euthanasia and assisted suicide present the newest ethical questions surrounding the dying process, although the ANA has an official statement in opposition to these activities (ANA Center for Ethics and Human Rights, 2013). The morally courageous nurse must be prepared to recognize his or her own attitudes, values, and expectations about death in order to take ethical action for the good of the dying patient.

Dilemmas In Between

Life and death dilemmas receive the most attention through the media and in real-life drama played out in the news and on television and theater screens. However, a host of other questions make up most ethical decision-making activities for the professional nurse in the practice of today's health care. Between questions of life and death are questions of existence, reality, individual rights, responsibility, informed consent, cultural competence, equality, justice, ability to pay, and fairness. Added to these are an unlimited number of other questions that arise from the human dimension of caring.

It is in these ordinary day-to-day situations that many professionals find significant and troublesome ethical questions. Basic notions of individual and social justice are viewed in terms of fairness and what is deserved. A person has been treated justly when he or she has been given what is due or owed. Any denial of something to which a person has a right or entitlement is an act of injustice.

The Right to Health Care. Handling injustice has been a part of nursing since the days of Florence Nightingale and has been at the forefront of the implementation of the Patient Protection and Affordable Care Act as individuals, businesses, and the legislature debate providing quality health care for the many without sacrificing the basic rights of the few. What basic right to health care do people have? Is each person entitled to the same health care package? Should ability to pay affect the specific level of entitlement? Resolutions to such questions have been based largely on the doctrine of justice, which states that like cases should be treated alike and equals ought to be treated equally. Such issues grip at the core of nursing practice, wherein access to health care and a respect for human dignity are paramount. Justice becomes a bioethical issue at the point that it affects whether, when, where, and how a patient will receive health care. Americans have different values, beliefs, and priorities about how to surmount the injustices. Nurses must consider how their practice relates to injustice in health care and must address factors that work against individual well-being and societal health (Sorrell, 2012). The opportunity for true health care reform will challenge nurses and the entire nation to consider the important ethical issues of justice.

Allocation of Scarce Resources. The issues of organ transplantation and the allocation of scarce resources flow from the doctrine of justice. The problem of scarce medical resources is becoming more common. Which people in need of transplantation should receive organs when available organs are in shorter supply than the number of people who could benefit from them? The justice question is applicable to this situation. The utilitarian view argues that the allocation decision should be framed so as to serve the greatest good for the greatest number of people affected. Should the selected recipient be the man with the largest, most loving family who does the greatest work for society? Or should a more universal law be applied? Should the people in need of organ transplantation be placed on a first-come, first-served list, or should they be entered into a lottery? Distributive justice, or taking into consideration the needs, interests, and wishes of each patient, cannot alone answer allocation dilemmas. Who has the more meaningful life? Who has the best prognosis? Who can pay? As unjust as it may seem to some, these are the kinds of questions responsible parties must answer regarding the allocation of scarce resources. And what about the fact that nurses themselves are scarce resources? What about the challenge of the nurse's autonomous right to refuse to work in understaffed settings? Whose rights come first?

Ethical Challenges

What about the doctrines of justice and freedom and the need for human experimentation and biomedical research? What about animal experimentation? It is accepted that human and animal experimentation is necessary for the progression of health care knowledge, but what about the risk for harm and the moral imperative that providers should, above all, do no harm? What about specifically problematic aspects of research, such as the use in research of institutionalized or imprisoned subjects or the practice of research on a viable fetus? Memories of harmful medical research and human experimentation, such as the Nazi atrocities and the Tuskegee syphilis study, have resulted in governmental regulations involving the use of human subjects in medical research. The Nuremberg Code is a set of provisions that researchers must follow so their research is approved by the federal government. Institutional review boards are established within research institutions for the purpose of ensuring that the degree of risk to the subject is minimized, if not eliminated. Human experimentation tests the principles of autonomy and respect for personhood.

The Challenge of Veracity

Everyday issues that test the principle of veracity are the concepts of alternative treatment and acknowledging uncertainty. It is the nature of health science that new knowledge must come forth to abolish less effective dogma. However, new ignorance comes along with these new discoveries. Which treatment of two or more is best for a patient in a specific situation? Which of the new drugs should be used? Should every patient be subjected to every possible form of diagnostic evaluation? Should a particular patient be treated with surgery, medication, or both? How do the economics of treatment costs factor into the decision? And most important, should the patient be made aware of all of

these questions and various options for his or her care? Can patients comprehend medicine's esoteric knowledge, in general, and its accompanying certainties and uncertainties, in particular? Is disclosure of uncertainty ultimately beneficial or detrimental?

Acknowledging uncertainty is difficult for today's health care provider. As never before, it seems that providers need to present themselves as confident, knowledgeable, and sensitive to patients who may see them as arrogant, dogmatic, and insensitive. Acknowledging uncertainty may be worth the effort. For the diagnostician, it may lighten the burden by absolving him or her of the responsibility for implicitly making decisions for which there may be conflicting answers. For the patient, knowing about the uncertainty may give him or her a greater voice in decision making and, in the event of treatment failure, may leave him or her better informed and more trustful of the caregiver. It seems that disclosure of uncertainty is ultimately beneficial to both parties. In fact, full disclosure and open communication through a commitment to veracity could prevent many everyday ethical situations. Optimal health care results from an exchange between patient and provider with open communication about the patient's wants and needs and the provider's judgment and advice. All too often, time is not taken for open communication, and the exchange becomes one in which the patient listens to what the all-knowing and wise provider says about the patient's needs. In this scenario, it is easy for the provider to assume a paternalistic attitude in the delivery of health care.

The Challenge of Paternalism

Paternalism is an action and an attitude wherein the provider tries to act on behalf of the patient with the belief that his or her actions are justified because of a commitment to act in the best interest of the patient. Paternalism is a reflection of the "father knows best" way of thinking. The phenomenon of paternalism presumes, in the name of beneficence, to overlook the patient's right to autonomy. Thus, in the process of attempting to act in the best interest of the patient, paternalism involves actions not based on the patient's choices, wishes, and desires. Paternalism interferes with a patient's right to self-determination and occurs when the provider believes that he or she can make a better decision than the patient.

Whereas it must be recognized that some cultures are highly paternalistic, the most common belief and value system in North America views paternalism as a threat to the patient-provider relationship. Every provider must guard against actions and attitudes that are paternalistic. Perhaps in the past, paternalism was associated with the image of the white-coated physician as a sovereign god. Today paternalistic actions and attitudes can be found among nurses, pharmacists, physical therapists, occupational therapists, social workers, clergy, or anyone who assumes the image of the all-knowing in the delivery of care. A current threat to a healthy patient-provider relationship is the emergence of entrepreneurship in medicine, in which health care providers are called on to be business managers. The bottom-line financial realities can be threats to safe care.

The healthy patient-provider relationship is based on the open communication described previously, wherein patient choice and respect for personhood are deemed just as important as scientific knowledge and sound health care advice. In paternalistic cultures when the patient is denied knowing "the truth" about his diagnosis or choices for care, it is a challenge for health care providers to know when to give the patient information or have discussions with the patient in spite of the family's wishes. The provider-patient relationship is built on trust when the right to confidentiality and privacy become ethical and legal obligations.

The Challenge of Autonomy

The provider-patient relationship makes way for the crucial legal concept of informed consent, which stipulates that the patient has the right to know and make decisions about his or her health. These decisions take the form of consent or refusal of treatment. Based on the principle of autonomy, the consent process must be voluntary and without coercion; the fully informed patient must clearly understand the choices being offered.

Informed consent dilemmas evolve from questions about whether patients are competent to make informed decisions and whether there are family members or surrogates to make these decisions by proxy. Difficult questions are posed for health care providers by the need for informed consent from minors, confused older adults, persons in emergency situations, and persons who are mentally compromised, imprisoned, inebriated, or unconscious. The burden of informed consent lies with the physician in most circumstances, although the nurse frequently is responsible for aspects of informing and obtaining consent.

In the latter part of the twentieth century, another crucial concept of consent was introduced. Advances in technology and the potential to keep people alive for extended periods have brought about legislation aimed at giving people choices about end-of-life decisions while they are still healthy and well enough to make informed decisions. The opportunity for people to make advance directives is now common and is even a requirement for admission to hospitals and other health care agencies that receive federal dollars. People are not required to decide, but must be given an opportunity to do so. Ideally the health care community will provide such an opportunity while the patient is well, perhaps in a community setting, such as a public library or community center. Health care professionals, such as nurses and other health care educators, have an ethical obligation to educate the public about the use of advance directives. These opportunities can serve as excellent means of educating patients not only about advance directives but also about their rights in general, changes in health care delivery and managed care, and the role of the various health care providers. These are excellent opportunities to educate the public about the scope of practice of today's professional nurse.

The Challenge of Accountability

A host of specific ethical issues exists within the practice of nursing itself. Professional nursing is a complex profession that is unlike most others. The accountability factor in the practice of nursing is such that a keen sense of responsibility and personal integrity are necessary qualities for every practicing nurse. It is the nurse's ethical obligation to uphold the highest standards of practice and care, to assume full personal and professional responsibility for every action, and to commit to maintaining quality in the skill and knowledge base of the profession. Failure to meet such obligations places the patient-nurse relationship at risk.

Failure to be accountable for one's own actions damages the health care team, causing rifts, blame, and potentially shifting work/responsibilities and patient care between shifts. In other words, lack of accountability can negatively affect quality patient care and team building. In health professions in which the safety and health of society are at stake, the obligation of professionals to police the practice of their colleagues is important.

There are public and legal official policing bodies, such as the state board of nursing, for matters of public record and formal conviction. However, there are countless situations in which the official policing body will never be involved, and the obligation to denounce a harmful action or potentially threatening situation falls to a fellow member of the profession. Sometimes known as *whistle-blowing,* the obligation to denounce is based on the fact that to remain silent is to consent to the action or threatening situation. Whether denouncing a chemical impairment, negligence, abusiveness,

incompetence, or cruelty, the obligation is a moral one based at least in part on the principle of beneficence.

Every person bearing the title of nurse must aspire to maintain himself or herself as a professional of integrity who is willing to blow the whistle on those whose actions are irresponsible and harmful. If this is not the case, the wrong will continue, and the harm to others will escalate. In the end, the profession as a whole will suffer, and the well-being of society will be diminished.

▇ SUMMARY

Professional nurses must take up the ethic of caring and be prepared to face any number of potential ethical conflicts in the day-to-day practice of their profession. They must realize that each situation is different and that recognizing this uniqueness demands that responsible parties seek a loving and humane solution to every situation that poses an ethical dilemma. When the answer remains clouded, the decision maker must choose the most appropriate action, given the situation, on the basis of a variety of potentially applicable principles.

To think that dilemmas such as the ones described here are unlikely or far removed is to think that the surgery patient will not be troubled by pain or the trauma patient by anxiety or the cancer patient by fear. Ethical conflict is inherent in the practice of nursing and is played out in every practice setting every day. The challenge is not to escape the conflict but to meet it with expectancy and preparedness.

If the profession of nursing is the discipline of human caring, relationships are the foundation of safe, ethical practice. Those seeking a career in nursing must realize the multifaceted aspects of the profession. They also should appreciate the rich and diverse opportunities that will be afforded them. Braced with scientific knowledge and the resources for critical examination of health and illness, the professional nurse is provided access to life's most intimate and precious encounters. Perhaps more than any other health care provider, a sensitive and caring nurse is invited to join patients who are experiencing the most intense moments of their lives. Nurses are given the opportunity to embrace patients in their joy over the birth of a child or the good news of the success of surgery or chemotherapy treatment. They also are privileged to support patients and their families during the trials of waiting for the outcome of a tragic head injury

or the last breath in a life devastated by terminal illness. To all of this, nurses are invited.

With such privilege comes responsibility. The purpose of this chapter is to introduce nursing students to the idea that ethical conflict in health care abounds and to increase students' awareness of their role in resolving conflict. It is important for professional nurses to have a basic knowledge of the ethical thinking enterprise described in this chapter and to realize that there are other resources for committed professionals to draw on in an effort to stay abreast of the issues they are likely to face in their practice. Resources include the National Science Foundation's Hastings Center; the Center for Health and Human Dignity; the Institute of Society, Ethics, and the Life Sciences; the Kennedy Institute Center for Bioethics; and the ANA Committee on Ethics and Human Rights. These groups prepare position statements and write papers on specific ethical dilemmas arising from today's health care practice. Learning centers, libraries, and websites generally provide access to these resources.

Bioethics and ethical decision making are philosophic enterprises. Many activities in nursing practice require an actual skill that involves training, practice, and technique development. For example, nursing students are introduced to the principles of intravenous line insertion while in a campus laboratory setting. They may have an opportunity to practice starting an intravenous line in a simulated setting before actually assuming the responsibility for starting one on a patient. The first few times that students insert an intravenous line, their effort is based on a deliberate thinking through of each step and each principle of asepsis, circulation and blood flow, and positioning. In time, the principles of starting an intravenous line become a well-developed technique and skill activity. The same process can be used to develop one's capacity for a critical thinking activity.

This chapter has presented a vignette describing a nursing management situation laden with potential for ethical conflict within patient care. As nursing students move through their educational experience, they will be assigned to care for many different kinds of patients. Every nursing management and patient care situation has the potential of presenting an ethical dilemma. As students are faced with ethical decisions, they refine their decision-making skills. Each time they reflect on ethical theories or consider ethical principles, they develop critical thinking ability. In time, the professional nurse is able to incorporate what he or she has learned into a morally mature personal code of ethics. At this point, there is a liberating joy that comes from knowing that competence in professional nursing practice goes beyond technique and skill to include the ability to reason life's most difficult and challenging questions, and all for the benefit of another human being. Although it is not as easy as it may sound, it is well worth the effort.

Girded with truth, nurses must commit themselves to take a bold stance for what is right and against what is wrong. Nurses should feel empowered through their roles as primary patient advocates to voice their morality in the face of a new century that promises sweeping changes in health care delivery. Nurses must speak in support of patient choice and self-determination in the era of managed care. They must speak against the moral wrong of understaffed practice trends wherein patient safety is jeopardized. Nurses must monitor legislation that affects health care and must study current issues, such as assisted suicide and cloning. Professional nursing embodies a commitment to not just think and act wisely in the administration of therapeutic nursing interventions but also to think and act in accordance with specified values and basic principles of right and wrong. Nursing is making a commitment to all of these principles.

REFERENCES

American Nurses Association Center for Ethics and Human Rights. (2013, April). *Position Statement–Euthanasia Assisted Suicide and Aid in Dying.* Retrieved from http://www.nursingworld.org.

American Nurses Association, Code of Ethics for Nurses with Interpretive Statements, Silver Spring, MD: *American Nurses Association*, April 2015.

Beauchamp, T. L., & Childress, J. F. (2009). *Principles of biomedical ethics* (6th ed.). Oxford, England: Oxford University Press.

Gallop News. Americans Rate Nurses Highest on Honesty, Ethical Standards. news.gallup.com/poll/180260/americans-rate-nurses.

Hockenberry, M. J., & Wilson, D. (2010). *Wong's nursing care of infants and children* (9th ed.). St Louis: Mosby.

Kohlberg, L. (1971). *Stages of moral development as a basis for moral education* (pp. 42–53, 86–88). Center for Moral education, Harvard University. Cambridge: Harvard University Press.

Lachman, V. D. (2012). Applying the ethics of care to your nursing practice. *Medsurg Nursing, 21*(2), 112–116.

Murray, J. S. (2010). Moral courage in healthcare: acting ethically even in the presence of risk. *OJIN: The Online Journal of Issues in Nursing, 15*(3), 2. Retrieved from http://www.gallup.com/poll/180260/americans-rate-nurses-highest-honesty- ethical-standards.aspx.

Sorrell, J. M. (2012, November 9). Ethics: The Patient Protection and Affordable Care Act: ethical perspectives in 21st century health care. *OJIN: The Online Journal of Issues in Nursing, 18*(1). doi:10.3912/OJIN.Vol18No02 EthCol01.

Uustal, D. (1992). *Values and ethics in nursing: From theory to practice* (4th ed.). Greenwich, RI: Educational Resources in Nursing and Holistic Health.

Weaver, K., Morse, J., & Mitcham, C. (2008). Ethical sensitivity in professional practice: concept analysis. *Journal of Advanced Nursing, 62*(5), 607–618.

Wright, R. A. (1987). *The practice of ethics: Human values in health care.* New York: McGraw-Hill.

10

Cultural Competency and Social Issues in Nursing and Health Care

Susan R. Jacob, PhD, MSN, RN

Clients deserve culturally competent care.

ⓔ Additional resources are available online at: *http://evolve.elsevier.com/Cherry/*

LEARNING OUTCOMES

After studying this chapter, the reader will be able to:

1. Integrate knowledge of demographic and sociocultural variations into culturally competent professional nursing care.
2. Provide culturally competent care to diverse client groups that incorporates variations in biologic characteristics, social organization, environmental control, communication, and other phenomena.
3. Critique education, practice, and research issues that influence culturally competent care.
4. Integrate respect for differences in beliefs and values of others as a critical component of nursing practice.

KEY TERMS

Cultural humility Incorporates a lifelong commitment to self-evaluation and self-critique, to redressing the power imbalances in the patient-clinician dynamic, and to developing mutually beneficial and advocacy partnerships with communities on behalf of individuals and defined populations (Tervalon and Murray-Garcia, 1998).

Cultural sensitivity Experienced when neutral language, both verbal and nonverbal, is used in a way that reflects sensitivity and appreciation for the diversity of another (American Academy of Nursing Expert Panel on Cultural Competence, 2007).

Culture Shared values, beliefs, and practices of a particular group of people that are transmitted from one generation to the next and are identified as patterns that guide thinking and action.

Ethnicity Affiliation resulting from a shared linguistic, racial, or cultural background.

Ethnocentric Believing that one's own ethnic group, culture, or nation is best.

Minority An ethnic group smaller than the majority group.

Prejudice Preconceived, deeply held, usually negative, judgment formed about other groups.

Stereotyping Assigning certain beliefs and behaviors to groups without recognizing individuality.

Transcultural Being grounded in one's own culture, but having the skills to be able to work in a multicultural environment.

PROFESSIONAL/ETHICAL ISSUE

Yei Wu, a 64-year-old Chinese female, was admitted to the emergency room (ER) with a temperature of 103°F, severe nausea and vomiting, and uterine bleeding. She was brought to the ER by her 36-year-old son, who had found her lying on the floor in her home when he went to visit her earlier in the afternoon. Because Yei speaks no English, her son provided the necessary information for her admission to the hospital. When the attending physician heard the charge nurse, Chandra, request an interpreter, he interrupted her by saying that an interpreter would not be needed because the bilingual son could provide interpretation. Chandra remembered learning in her cultural competence training that family members should be used for interpretation only as a last resort.

What avenues should Chandra explore for interpretation services? What are the potential risks of having family members interpret for the patient?

VIGNETTE

When my instructor taught the session on cultural differences, she stressed the high alcoholism rates of American Indians. I began to fear that my instructor and fellow classmates would stereotype me because of my American Indian background. However, no one in my family drinks alcohol because we belong to the Mormon Church, where drinking is not accepted. I wish the instructor had stressed the importance of not stereotyping.

Questions to Consider While Reading This Chapter:

1. What preconceived ideas do you have about the following cultural groups: Hispanic, Appalachian, Moroccan, black/African-American, South African, and Chinese?
2. What strategies can you implement to overcome prejudice?
3. How can nurses provide effective care to different cultural groups who each have a unique set of beliefs about illness?
4. How can nursing research affect the attitudes and beliefs of health professionals in regard to minority populations?

CHAPTER OVERVIEW

The United States has always been represented by a culturally diverse society. However, the volume of cultural groups entering our country is increasing rapidly. Professional nurses must provide care to persons of various cultures who have different values, beliefs, and perceptions about health and illness. This chapter explores cultural phenomena, including environmental control, biologic variations, social organization, communication, space, and time in relation to major cultural groups. It also examines different views about health, illness, and cure. Federally defined minority groups, which include African-Americans or Blacks, Asians, Hispanics, and American Indians, are emphasized. The need for diversity in the health care force is explored, and strategies for recruiting and retaining minorities in nursing are suggested. Strategies that nurses can use to improve their own cultural competence also are given.

POPULATION TRENDS

The demographic and ethnic composition of the U.S. population has experienced a marked change in the past 100 years. Minority groups have grown faster than the population as a whole. In some U.S. cities, the number of persons from diverse cultural groups is increasing at such a rapid pace that minorities constitute more than half the population. The nation will be more racially and ethnically diverse, as well as much older, by midcentury, according to 2013 projections released by the U.S. Census Bureau. Minorities, now roughly one third of the U.S. population, are expected to become the majority in 2044, with the nation projected to be 54% minority in 2050. By 2023, minorities will account for more than half of all children.

Two factors—longer lifespans and aging baby boomers—will combine to double the population of Americans aged 65 years or older during the next 25 years to about 72 million. By 2030, older adults will account for roughly 20% of the U.S. population (Centers for Disease Control [CDC], 2013).

Along with the dramatic aging of the U.S. population during the next several decades will become significant increases in racial and ethnic diversity. The older population is becoming more racially and ethnically diverse. Between 2014 and 2060 the share of the older population that is non-Hispanic white is projected to drop by 24 percentage points, from 78.3% to 54.6% (Mather, 2016).

Language barriers, reduced access to health care, low socioeconomic status, and differing cultural norms can be major challenges to promoting health in an increasingly diverse older population (CDC, 2013). This demographic change introduces many interrelated social, economic, political, educational, and health problems. The fact that people are living longer allows more opportunity for the development of chronic illness. Social isolation and depression that result from losses of friends and family will present a challenge for mental health care providers. Primary care providers will be faced with identifying risks to independence and health for the aging population (Stanhope and Lancaster, 2016). Health care providers must guard against issues of *ageism,* that is, assuming that health issues and levels of cognition are the same for every senior adult.

Federally Defined Minority Groups

Federally defined minority groups are as follows:
- Asian American
- Black or African-American
- Hispanic or Latino
- Native Hawaiian and other Pacific Islander
- American Indian and Alaska Native

The populations within the federally defined minority groups have grown faster than the population as a whole. In 1970, minority groups accounted for 16% of the population. As previously mentioned, if current trends, continue by the time the 2020 census is conducted, more than half of the nation's children are expected to be part of a minority race or ethnic group. (Visit https://www.census.gov/newsroom/press-releases/2015/cb15-tps16.html for more information.)

ECONOMIC AND SOCIAL CHANGES

Changing world economics have had profound consequences, such as increased joblessness, homelessness, poverty, and limited access to health insurance and health care. Anxiety, hopelessness, depression, and despair commonly affect the individuals in our society who find themselves suddenly without jobs and sometimes even without homes as a result of economic downsizing. These conditions are often associated with increased stress-related symptoms, substance abuse, violence, and crime (Lenburg et al, 1995). Dramatic

changes in technology and specialization in the health care field have made health care costs skyrocket. Therefore, not everyone can afford health care services. A higher percentage of minorities lack health insurance than that of the general population (Nies and McEwen, 2015). Higher costs of living and lower wages for minority groups make it difficult to rise out of poverty (Stanhope and Lancaster, 2016).

Poverty

Most families with racially or ethnically diverse backgrounds have a lower socioeconomic status than does the population at large. Blacks, Hispanics, and American Indians have much higher rates of poverty than non-Hispanic whites and Asians. The median family income of Asians is slightly higher than that of non-Hispanic whites and is consistent with Asians' high levels of education and the higher percentage of families with two wage earners. However, opportunities for education, occupation, income earning, and property ownership that are available to upper- and middle-class Americans often are not available to members of minority groups (Stanhope and Lancaster, 2016).

Poverty rates are important indicators of community well-being and are used by government agencies and organizations to allocate need-based resources. The American Community Survey (ACS) 5-year data allow for the analysis of poverty rates by race and Hispanic origin for many levels of geography. Poverty rates are also presented for selected detailed race and origin groups in the cities and towns with the largest populations of these groups. For the nation and selected places, poverty rates are summarized for detailed Asian groups with populations of 750,000 or more, detailed Native Hawaiian and other Pacific Islander groups with populations of 25,000 or more, and detailed Hispanic groups with populations of 1 million or more (Macartney et al, 2013).

- *The official poverty rate in 2016 was 12.7 percent, down 0.8 percentage points from 13.5 percent in 2015. This is the second consecutive annual decline in poverty. Since 2014, the poverty rate has fallen 2.1 percentage points from 14.8 percent to 12.7 percent.*
- *In 2016 there were 40.6 million people in poverty, 2.5 million fewer than in 2015 and 6 million fewer than in 2014 (Semega et al, 2017).*

By race, the highest national poverty rates were for American Indians and Alaska Natives (26.2.0%), the only group in which the poverty rate did not decline, and blacks or African-Americans (22%). Native Hawaiians and other Pacific Islanders had a national poverty rate of 17.6%. For the Asian population, poverty rates were 10.1% For Hispanics, national poverty rates were 19.4% (https://www.census.gov/library/publications/2017/demo/p60-259.html).

The poor also suffer more than the population as a whole for nearly every measure of health. Substantial disparities remain in health insurance coverage for certain populations. In 2016, non-Hispanic whites had the lowest uninsured rate. Around the time the 2020 census is conducted, more than half of the nation's children are expected to be part of a minority race or ethnic group. The uninsured rates for blacks and Asians were higher than for non-Hispanic whites, at 10.5% and 7.6%, respectively. Hispanics had the highest uninsured rate, at 16.0%. Lack of health care coverage has major implications for health (Barnett and Berchick, 2017). For more information, see the U.S. Census Bureau's web page on health insurance coverage (Barnett and Berchick, 2017).

Minority members of society often live in poverty. This social stratification leads to social inequality. For instance, it is widely known that school systems and recreational facilities vary significantly between the inner city and the suburbs (Nies and McEwen, 2015). Residential segregation, substandard housing, unemployment, poor physical and mental health, and poor self-image are part of the cycle of poverty. This inequality is especially disturbing as it relates to health care. The United States has a history of providing the highest quality health care to those with the highest socioeconomic status and the worst health care to those with the lowest socioeconomic status. Social, economic, and health problems have led to heated debates about the philosophy, scope and costs, and sources of funding for health care and insurance programs. "It is important to enable seldom heard, hard to reach populations and facilitate their participation in research (through the use of interpreters, increased sensitivity, and a detailed consideration of ethical issues) in order to understand how vectors of disadvantage intersect" (Floyd and Sakellarious, 2017).

VIOLENCE

Changing economic and social conditions have contributed to the rising level of violence in our society. Statistics indicate that homicide is the second leading cause of death among Americans 15 to 24 years of age (Nies and McEwen, 2015). Businesses, schools, restaurants, playgrounds, and churches have become common settings for random acts of violence. Although the increasing incidence of violence affects all segments of society, women, children, older adults, and culturally vulnerable groups are especially at risk. Unemployment rates among young minority men in the United States are consistently high (Stanhope and Lancaster, 2016). This group also has the highest rate of violence, with homicide being a major problem for young black males. The differing rates of violence among races are more likely a result of poverty than of race (Stanhope and Lancaster, 2016).

Intimate partner violence (IPV), formerly known as *domestic violence,* is the single greatest cause of injury to women 15 to 24 years of age. IPV crosses all ethnic, racial, socioeconomic, and educational lines. It includes battering, resulting in physical injury, psychologic abuse, and sexual assault (Nies and McEwen, 2015).

ATTITUDES TOWARD CULTURALLY DIVERSE GROUPS

The range of attitudes toward culturally diverse groups can be viewed along a continuum of intensity, as illustrated in Figure 10.1 (Lenburg et al, 1995).

Fig. 10.1 A continuum of intensity of the range of attitudes toward culturally diverse groups. (From Lenburg et al., American Academy of Nursing. [1995]. *Promoting cultural competence in and through nursing education: a critical review and comprehensive plan for action.* Washington, DC.)

The extreme negative manifestation of prejudice is hate in its many violent and nonviolent forms. Contempt is somewhat less intense but is problematic because it is so widespread and undermines many aspects of society. Tolerance reflects a more neutral attitude that accepts differences without attempting to convert them; it is the minimal-level attitude essential in democratic societies. Respect for diversity is manifested in behaviors that integrate differences into positive interactions and relationships. Respect is a demonstration of the inherent worth of the individual, regardless of differences. The most positive attitude is portrayed as a celebration (or affirmation) of the positive merits of cultural differences (e.g., the value added to life experiences by multiple perspectives, traditions, rituals, foods, and art forms). The combination of ignorance of other cultures and arrogance about one's own culture fosters disrespect and hate. The deliberate attempt to discover and apply the positive benefits of cultural variation promotes respect and a celebration of the value of diversity, whereas perpetuating prejudice fosters narrow-mindedness and contempt. By integrating these perspectives as part of professional role behavior, educators can help students prepare for culturally competent practice in communities of diversity.

DIVERSITY IN THE HEALTH CARE WORKFORCE

Need for Diversity in the Health Care Workforce

Members of some cultural groups are demanding culturally relevant health care that incorporates their beliefs and practices (Nies and McEwen, 2015). Consumers are becoming much more aware of what constitutes culturally sensitive and competent care and are less willing to accept incompetent care (Douglas et al, 2011). There is a lack of diversity and ethnic representation among health care professionals, as well as limited knowledge about values, beliefs, experiences, and health care needs of certain populations, such as immigrants, older adults, and gays and lesbians. Each of these groups has a unique set of responses to health and illness.

Nurses make up the largest segment of the workforce in health care delivery. Therefore, they have an opportunity to be proactive in changing health care

Stereotypes should be trashed.

inequities and access to health care (Douglas et al, 2011). The changing health care system must reflect the community, and as health care moves into the community, it is vital that partnerships be formed between health care providers and the community. For these partnerships to become a reality, minority representation in all health professions is essential. Some factors inhibiting minority members from attaining a career in nursing include inadequate academic preparation, especially in the sciences; financial costs; inadequate career counseling; lack of valuing the role of nursing by some cultures; and better recruitment efforts by other disciplines (Loftin et al, 2012).

Current Status of Diversity in the Health Care Workforce

According to the U.S. Census Bureau, individuals from ethnic and racial minority groups accounted for more than 24% of the U.S. population in 2017. With projections that minority populations will become the majority by 2044, professional nurses must demonstrate a sensitivity to and understanding of a variety of cultures to provide high-quality care across settings.

Diversity within the nursing workforce—in terms of race/ethnicity and sex—is desirable because it can improve both access to and quality of care for minorities and medically underserved populations. The nursing workforce does not mirror the U. S population seeking care, matching for gender, ethnicity, or age (Buerhaus et al, 2017). Nursing has historically been dominated by white females, and as Figure 10.2 shows, the nursing workforce is still predominantly white, out of proportion to the general population, with some

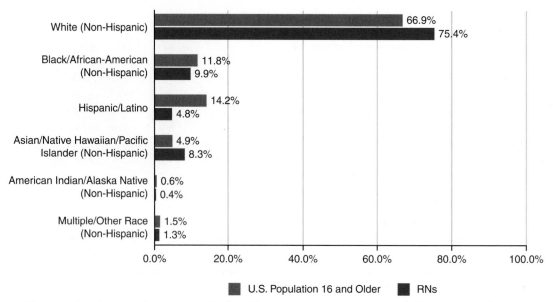

Fig. 10.2 Distribution of RNs, by Race/Ethnicity, relative to the Working-Age Population. (From U.S. Department of Health and Human Services, Health Resources and Services Administration, National Center for Health Workforce Analysis. [2013]. *The U.S. Health workforce chartbook: part I: clinicians.* Rockville, MD. Retrieved from https://bhw.hrsa.gov/sites/default/files/bhw/nchwa/chartbookpart1.pdf; data Source: HRSA analysis of the /American Community Survey Public Use Microdata Sample, 2008-2010.)

minorities being more under-represented than others. According to a 2013 survey conducted by the National Council of State Boards of Nursing (NCSBN) and the Forum of Nursing Workforce Centers, nurses from minority backgrounds represent 19% of the registered nurse (RN) workforce. In terms of racial/ethnic backgrounds, the RN population is 83% white/Caucasian; 6% black/African-American; 6% Asian; 3% Hispanic; 1% American Indian/Alaska Native; 1% Native Hawaiian/Pacific Islander; and 1% other (NCSBN, 2013).

A 2017 analysis of the Current Population Survey (CPS) found that men have steadily composed 11% of all RNs for the past 5 years (Center for Interdisciplinary Health Workforce Studies [CIHWS], 2017). There are increasing numbers of men in the nursing workforce, who are younger than female RNs and continue to earn higher wages. Since 1994, the CPS data indicate, full-time equivalent (FTE) male RNs continue to earn, on average, $2 more per hour than their female counterparts (CIHWS, 2017).

According to the report by the American Association of Colleges of Nursing (AACN) on Enrollment and Graduations in Baccalaureate and Graduate Programs in Nursing (2016-2017), nursing students from minority backgrounds represented 29.7% of students in entry-level baccalaureate programs, 31.8% of master's students, 30.2% of students in research-focused doctoral programs, and 26.8% in practice-focused doctoral programs (Fang et al, 2017). In terms of gender breakdown, men made up 13.3% of students in baccalaureate programs, 11.7% of master's students, 10.5% of research-focused doctoral students, and 12.7% of practice-focused doctoral students. Although nursing schools have made strides in recruiting and graduating nurses who reflect the patient population, more must be done before equal representation is realized. The need to attract diverse nursing students is paralleled by the need to recruit more faculty from minority populations. Few nurses from racial/ethnic minority groups with advanced nursing degrees pursue faculty careers. According to 2017 data from AACN's annual survey, only 15.8% of full-time nursing school faculty come from minority backgrounds, and only 6% are male (Fang et al, 2017).

Recruitment and Retention of Minorities in Nursing

It is clear that we have been slow in preparing nurses to be reflective of our population, just as we have been unaware of the need for culturally sensitive patient care and sometimes less than welcoming to students different from the preponderant population (Loftin et al, 2012). Recruitment and retention of students from minority populations must not be separated. In other words, recruitment programs must have retention as their primary focus because there is no point in recruiting minorities into nursing programs and then not helping them succeed.

Before World War II, the only known effort to recruit minority students into nursing on a national scale was made by the National Association of Colored Graduate Nurses (NACGN), which had had recruitment of blacks into nursing as one of its objectives since its inception in 1908. During the Second World War, the federal government set into motion a mechanism to produce additional nursing personnel by financing basic nursing education. This was done through the Cadet Nurse Corps. The corps had a number of recruiters, two of whom were black. These two nurses confined their recruiting to 82 black/African-American colleges and universities. By the end of the war, 21 black/African-American nursing schools had participated in the corps and more than 2000 black nurses had acquired their basic nursing education through this mechanism.

After the war, national recruitment efforts for black nurses reverted to the NACGN, an organization that voted itself out of existence in 1949 and was dissolved in 1951. However, individual black/African-American schools in the North and South continued to recruit. In the South law segregated the nursing schools, and in the North custom did so. In 1954, the unanimous Supreme Court decision *Brown v. Board of Education* asserted that "separate educational facilities were inherently unequal," making racial segregation in public schools unconstitutional. This decision was interpreted to mean that all kinds of educational discrimination would be considered, including nursing.

It was around the time of the Brown decision that schools of nursing were being accredited by national standards, and many schools, both black/African-American and white, just did not measure up to the standards. As a result, many schools closed. With integration permitting black students to be admitted to formerly all-white schools, quality black/African-American schools had difficulty attracting enough students, and many of the schools closed. However, the white schools that began admitting black students did not admit the number that would have been admitted by the black/African-American schools. For example, many white schools admitted only one or two black students per class.

In the late 1960s, many efforts were made to help the economically disadvantaged in this country. Although not all people of minority groups are economically disadvantaged, the vast majority of disadvantaged people are members of ethnic minority groups. Nursing, too, became concerned about the disadvantaged and began concerted efforts to recruit more members of minority groups into nursing schools. The Sealantic Fund, one of the Rockefeller Brothers' funds, was one of the first foundations that helped minorities enter nursing school. Sealantic funded projects in 10 universities in different parts of the country to recruit students from minority groups and help them achieve success. The best example of an ongoing project, funded by the division of nursing since 1971, is the National Student Nurses Association's Breakthrough to Nursing, intended to accelerate the recruitment of minorities, including men.

In 1997, the American Nurses Foundation published a report of a project it had funded, titled *Strategies for Recruitment, Retention and Graduation of Minority Nurses in Colleges of Nursing*. Through survey and interview analysis, Hattie Bessent and a cadre of knowledgeable leaders investigated the most effective approach to increasing the nursing profession's representation of minority nurses (Bessent, 1997). Members of Chi Eta Phi, a national black/African-American nursing society with chapters throughout the country, serve as mentors to minority nursing students. As mentors, sorority members provide intellectual and inspirational stimulation along with counseling.

In 1997, the AACN published its first position statement affirming that diversity and inclusion had emerged as central issues for organizations and institutions. The AACN encouraged leadership in nursing to respond to these issues by finding ways to accelerate the inclusion of groups, cultures, and ideas that traditionally had been underrepresented in higher education.

As the demographics of the population rapidly change in the twenty-first century, there have been numerous strategies to recruit and retain minority nursing faculty, students, and practicing nurses in the profession to better reflect the population demographics. Just as contributions of diverse cultural groups are increasingly valued, the profession has begun to value the need for diversity in their students and faculty and to view this diversity as strength.

Strategies for Recruitment and Retention of Minorities in the Nursing Workforce

All national nursing organizations, the federal Division of Nursing, hospital associations, nursing philanthropies, and other stakeholders within the health care community agree that recruitment of underrepresented groups into nursing is a priority for the nursing profession in the United States. For more information, visit AACN's web page on resources in enhancing workforce diversity (http://www.aacnnursing.org/News-Information/Fact-Sheets/Enhancing-Diversity).

Nursing shortage reports, including those produced by the American Hospital Association, the Robert Wood Johnson Foundation (RWJF), The Joint Commission, and the Association of Academic Health Centers, point to minority student recruitment as a necessary step to addressing the nursing shortage. For more information on these reports, visit http://www.aacnnursing.org/News-Information/Fact-Sheets/Enhancing-Diversityin Nursing Workforce.

A lack of minority nurse educators may send a signal to potential students that nursing does not value diversity or offer career ladder opportunities to advance through the profession. Students looking for academic role models to encourage and enrich their learning may be frustrated in their attempts to find mentors and a community of support. Academic leaders are addressing this need by working to identify minority faculty recruitment strategies, encouraging minority leadership development, and advocating for programs that remove barriers to faculty careers.

There also is a need to increase the number of nurse educators and researchers from diverse, marginalized, and vulnerable populations. Raising consciousness involves increasing the level of awareness of nurses and other health care professionals about the issues surrounding diversity. This can be accomplished by encouraging participation in forums related to different aspects of various cultural phenomena, such as environmental control, communication, and health beliefs. Such forums might be offered by state and local professional nurses' organizations and health care facilities.

Another successful strategy for recruiting and retaining minorities in education and clinical practice is matched mentoring, which involves matching same-culture mentors in either the same institution or different institutions. A different mentoring strategy involves teaching and modeling by nurses who have been trained in cross-cultural care. Cross-cultural nursing consultants in the care of specific groups are available to agencies, professional groups, licensing bodies, and individual nurses. (Organizations should contact the Transcultural Nursing Society, at http://www.tcns.org, to obtain the names of consultants in the field of transcultural nursing.)

Audiovisual media should be used to teach the importance of human health conditions cross-culturally. Video conferencing can provide international links for students and faculty who cannot travel. Students from various cultures can share their clinical experiences. One of the greatest benefits is the discovery that thinking, values, and decision making differ in various cultures. Collaborative arrangements should be encouraged between colleges and universities so that exchange programs can be offered to students. Such exchanges can give students firsthand in-depth experience with cultures that are different from their own. Interactive media can be used to gain a clearer perspective than can be obtained through the print medium on particular cultures.

Strategies such as mentoring by the same-culture professional are effective in recruiting and retaining minorities in nursing. In addition, the value of workshops, continuing education programs, and use of consultants to promote culturally competent care should not be overlooked.

CULTURAL COMPETENCE

Health professionals, educators, and health care systems must all respond to the consequences of increasing cultural diversity for the future well-being of all populations. The worldwide shortage of nurses and the global immigration of both nurses and populations have heightened the need to educate nurses to deliver culturally competent care for increasingly diverse populations regardless of geographic location. *The Standards of Practice for Culturally Competent Nursing Care: 2011 Update* provides universally applicable guidelines for use by nurses around the globe to guide clinical practice, research, education, and administration. The recipient of the nursing care described in these standards is assumed to be an individual, a family, a community, or a population (Douglas et al, 2011). These 12 standards (Table 10.1)

TABLE 10.1   Standards of Practice for Culturally Competent Nursing Care: 2011 Update

Standard	Description
Standard 1: Social justice	Professional nurses shall promote social justice for all. The applied principles of social justice guide nurses' decisions related to the patient, family, community, and other health care professionals. Nurses will develop leadership skills to advocate for socially just policies.
Standard 2: Critical reflection	Nurses shall engage in critical reflection of their own values, beliefs, and cultural heritage to have an awareness of how these qualities and issues can affect culturally congruent nursing care.
Standard 3: Knowledge of cultures	Nurses shall gain an understanding of the perspectives, traditions, values, practices, and family systems of culturally diverse individuals, families, communities, and populations they care for, as well as a knowledge of the complex variables that affect the achievement of health and well-being.
Standard 4: Culturally competent practice	Nurses shall use cross-cultural knowledge and culturally sensitive skills in implementing culturally congruent nursing care.
Standard 5: Cultural competence in health care systems and organizations	Health care organizations should provide the structure and resources necessary to evaluate and meet the cultural and language needs of their diverse clients.
Standard 6: Patient advocacy and empowerment	Nurses shall recognize the effect of health care policies, delivery systems, and resources on their patient populations and shall empower and advocate for their patients as indicated. Nurses shall advocate for the inclusion of their patients' cultural beliefs and practices in all dimensions of their health care.
Standard 7: Multicultural workforce	Nurses shall actively engage in the effort to ensure a multicultural workforce in health care settings. One measure to achieve a multicultural workforce is through strengthening of recruitment and retention effort in the hospital and academic setting.
Standard 8: Education and training in culturally competent care	Nurses shall be educationally prepared to promote and provide culturally congruent health care. Knowledge and skills necessary for assuring that nursing care is culturally congruent shall be included in global health care agendas that mandate formal education and clinical training, as well as required ongoing, continuing education for all practicing nurses.
Standard 9: Cross-cultural communication	Nurses shall use culturally competent verbal and nonverbal communication skills to identify clients' values, beliefs, practices, perceptions, and unique health care needs.
Standard 10: Cross-cultural leadership	Nurses shall have the ability to influence individuals, groups, and systems to achieve outcomes of culturally competent care for diverse populations.
Standard 11: Policy development	Nurses shall have the knowledge and skills to work with public and private organizations, professional associations, and communities to establish policies and standards for comprehensive implementation and evaluation of culturally competent care.
Standard 12: Evidence-based practice and research	Nurses shall base their practice on interventions that have been systematically tested and shown to be the most effective for the culturally diverse populations that they serve. In areas where there is a lack of evidence of efficacy, nurse researchers shall investigate and test interventions that may be the most effective in reducing the disparities in health outcomes.

Douglas, M., Pierce, J., & Rosenkoetter, M. (2011). Standards of practice for culturally competent nursing care: 2011 update. *Journal of Transcultural Nursing, 22*(4), 317–333.

can serve as a guide and resource by emphasizing cultural competence as a priority.

Lenberg and colleagues (1995) suggest that it is essential that nurses take responsibility to:

- Be sensitive to and show respect for the differences in beliefs and values of others.
- Take responsibility to inquire, learn about, and integrate beliefs and values of others in professional encounters.
- Take responsibility to try to change negative and prejudicial behaviors in themselves and others.

In light of societal changes, responsible persons at all levels in education and health care delivery systems acknowledge the need to reassess the influence of culture on achieving expected health outcomes. There is a significant need for nurse educators, administrators, students, and others to promote sensitivity to, acceptance of, and respect for the rights of all individuals within the context of their cultural orientation and society as a whole. Nurses must be culturally competent because:

- The nurse's culture often is different from the client's culture.
- Care that is not culturally competent may be costlier.
- Care that is not culturally competent may be ineffective.
- Specific objectives for persons in different cultures need to be met as outlined in the federal government's *Healthy People 2020* initiative.
- Racial and minority groups experience profound disparities in health and health care.
- Nursing is committed to social justice, providing safe quality care to all.
- Nurses are expected to respond to global infectious disease epidemics.

Achieving cultural competence should be our goal, although it may take most of us a lifetime to attain. However, we can all aspire to achieve cultural humility, which incorporates a lifelong commitment to self-evaluation and self-critique, to redressing the power imbalances in the patient-clinician dynamic, and to developing mutually beneficial and advocacy partnerships with communities on behalf of individuals and defined populations (Tervalon and Murray-Garcia, 1998). If we acquire cultural humility, we should also demonstrate cultural sensitivity, which shows appreciation of the diversity of others.

CULTURAL COMPETENCE IN NURSING EDUCATION

Since the 1960s, there has been a united effort to include concepts sensitive to cultural diversity in nursing education. The National League for Nursing (NLN) and the AACN have made this effort mandatory for accreditation of nursing programs. In 2008, the AACN developed five end-of-program competencies for graduates of baccalaureate nursing programs as well as a faculty toolkit for integrating these competencies into undergraduate education (AACN, 2008a). *The Essentials of Baccalaureate Education for Professional Nursing Practice* (2008) mandates the inclusion of culturally diverse nursing care concepts in the curriculum with attention to cultural, spiritual, ethnic, gender, and sexual orientation diversity. The AACN (2008b) developed the following five competencies to serve as a framework for integrating cultural content into existing curricula:

1. Apply knowledge of social and cultural factors that affect nursing and health care across multiple contexts.
2. Use relevant data sources and best evidence in providing culturally competent care.
3. Promote achievement of safe and quality outcomes of care for diverse populations.
4. Advocate for social justice, including commitment to the health of vulnerable populations and the elimination of health disparities.
5. Participate in continuous cultural competence development.

Also, in collaboration with leading foundations and stakeholders, the AACN took the following steps to enhance diversity in nursing education:

New Careers in Nursing (NCIN) *was a national scholarship program of the Robert Wood Johnson Foundation (RWJF) and the American Association of Colleges of Nursing (AACN). Founded in 2008 to help alleviate the nursing shortage and increase the diversity of nursing professionals, NCIN awarded its final grants in 2015 to schools with accelerated baccalaureate and master's degree nursing programs. In total, grants have provided scholarships to 3517 students at 130 unique schools of nursing (http:// www.newcareersinnursing.org/).*

The Future of Nursing Scholars program, another effort supported by RWJF, created "a diverse cadre of PhD prepared nurses who are committed to a long-term leadership career; advancing science and discovery through research; strengthening nursing education; and furthering transformational change in nursing and health care" (Future of Nursing Scholars, 2018). In December 2017 the RWJF "announced the 31 schools of nursing selected to receive grants to support up to 58 nurses as they pursue their PhDs. These 31 schools comprise the fifth and final cohort of grantees of the *Future of Nursing Scholars* program" (Future of Nursing Scholars, 2018).

In 2013, AACN and the RWJF initiated the Doctoral Advancement in Nursing (DAN) Project to enhance the number of minority nurses completing PhD and Doctor of Nursing Practice (DNP) degrees. DAN's expert committee has developed a white paper featuring student recruitment and retention strategies that can be used by schools of nursing; comprehensive approaches to leadership and scholarship development for students; suggestions for model doctoral curriculum; and more. For more information, see DAN's web page (http://www.newcareersinnursing.org/doctoral-advancement-nursing.html).

In April 2008, the RWJF joined with the AACN to launch funding for Nursing Workforce Development Programs, including funding for Nursing Workforce Diversity Grants. This program provides funding for projects to increase nursing education opportunities for individuals from disadvantaged backgrounds, including racial and ethnic minorities underrepresented among RNs.

CULTURAL BELIEF SYSTEMS

A value is a standard that people use to assess themselves and others. It is a belief about what is worthwhile or important for well-being. There is a tendency for people to be "culture bound" (i.e., to assume that their own values are superior to, more sensible than, or more correct than that of others). Cross-cultural health promotion requires the nurse to work with clients without making judgments as to the superiority of one set of values over another.

Each culture has a value system that dictates behavior directly or indirectly by setting norms and teaching that those norms are right. Health beliefs and practices tend to reflect a culture's value system. Nurses must understand each patient's value system to foster health promotion.

CULTURAL PHENOMENA

Giger and Davidhizar (2008) have identified six cultural phenomena that vary among cultural groups and affect health care. These phenomena are environmental control, biologic variations, social organization, communication, space, and time orientation.

Environmental Control

Environmental control is the ability of members of a particular culture to control nature or other environmental factors. Some groups perceive humans as having mastery over nature; others perceive humans to be dominated by nature; and still other groups see humans as having a harmonious relationship with nature (Stanhope and Lancaster, 2016). People who perceive that they have mastery over nature believe that they can overcome the natural forces of nature. Such individuals would expect positive results from medications, surgery, and other treatment modalities. Persons who believe that they are subject to the forces of nature or that they have little control over what happens to them may not be compliant with treatments because they believe that whatever happens to them is part of their destiny. Included in this concept are the traditional health and illness beliefs, the practice of folk medicine, and the use of traditional and nontraditional healers. Environmental control plays an important role in the way clients respond to health-related experiences and use health resources (Stanhope and Lancaster, 2016).

Biologic Variations

Biologic variations, such as body build and structure, genetic variations, skin characteristics, susceptibility to disease, and nutritional variations, exist among different cultures. For example, babies who are born in Western culture weigh more than non-Western babies. Other common variations include skin color, eye shape, hair texture, adipose tissue deposits, shape of earlobes, and body configuration (Stanhope and Lancaster, 2016).

Social Organization

Social organization refers to the family unit (nuclear, single-parent, or extended family) and the religious or ethnic groups with which families identify. *Family* is defined differently among cultures. Families depend on the extended family for emotional and financial support in times of crisis.

Communication

Communication differences include language differences, verbal and nonverbal behaviors, and silence. Language can be the greatest obstacle to providing multicultural care. If the client does not speak the same language as the nurse, a skilled interpreter is mandatory (Douglas et al, 2011). Comfort with direct eye contact during communication is an area that varies among cultures. Although some cultures value direct eye contact as a sign of attention, other cultures may view direct eye contact as rude behavior.

Health professionals should not assume that a first-name basis is appropriate for client relationships. With any client, terms of endearment such as "honey" and "dear" are unacceptable and can be interpreted as disrespectful, derogatory, or condescending. The best solution to the challenge of different communication styles and preferences is always to ask the client how he or she prefers to be addressed.

If the nurse and the client do not speak the same language, an interpreter should be consulted. An interpreter can help the nurse establish rapport with the client and explain concepts to the patient that are foreign to the nurse. When interpreters are needed, they should be selected carefully. Friends are possible choices, as are bilingual staff and community volunteers. Nurses should be aware that some ethnic groups consider it a breach of confidentiality to have a stranger interpret, whereas certain individuals may not want other family members or friends to know the specifics of their medical condition.

The nurse also should be careful to consider the different dialects spoken in the same country and the culture's view of women and children. Children should not be used as interpreters because of the subject matter and because of certain cultural views of authority. Many cultures view adults as having more authority than children. In many cultures, women would not be acceptable interpreters because of the cultural view of women.

Nurses should be aware of the possibilities for interpreter services. A language line can be accessed 24 hours a day, 7 days a week by calling 1-800-528-5888 and asking for the language wanted. A live translator comes on the line to serve in any of 77 languages. The nurse can conference call, use two phones on the same line, or simply pass the phone back and forth to the person with whom he or she wishes to converse. For more information, visit http://www.languageline.com.

Health care facilities may get a reasonable subscription rate that is less costly than the individual rate for these services.

Space

Space refers to people's attitudes and comfort level regarding the personal space around them. There are vast cultural differences in the comfort level associated with the distance between persons. Most nurses tend to feel comfortable with an intimate zone of 0 to 18 inches. This usually is the distance between the nurse and the patient when the nurse performs certain parts of a physical assessment, such as an eye or ear examination. Entering this zone could be uncomfortable for clients and nurses who have not had time to establish a trusting relationship. This discomfort would be greater for persons whose culture is not comfortable at all with such a limited space (Stanhope and Lancaster, 2016).

Time

Time orientation is the view of time in the present, past, or future. Present-oriented persons enjoy what they are experiencing at the moment and move on to the next event or activity only "when the time is right." Punctuality and "watching the clock" are definitely part of Western culture, but many cultural groups do not view time in the same way. This difference in time orientation can have implications for the present-oriented professional in the work setting, who may always be late for work without thinking it is an important issue. In addition, there are implications for health teaching. For example, when teaching medication schedules to a patient, it would be important to consider how that individual views time.

Clients who view the past as more important than the present or the future may focus on memories of the past. For instance, some ethnic groups may take actions that they believe are consistent with the views of their ancestors and look to them for guidance (Giger and Davidhizar, 2008). In some cultures, time is viewed as being more flexible than in Western culture, and being on time for appointments is not a priority (Stanhope and Lancaster, 2016).

People who are future oriented are concerned with long-range goals and health care measures that can be taken in the present to prevent illness in the future. These persons plan ahead in scheduling appointments and organizing activities. They may be seen as having "distant" or "cold" personalities because they are not always engaged in communication at the moment, commonly because they may be thinking about their plans for the future. Persons who are oriented more to the present may be late for appointments because they are less concerned with planning ahead.

PRACTICE ISSUES RELATED TO CULTURAL COMPETENCE

Health Information and Education

According to the Task Force on Black and Minority Health of the U.S. Department of Health and Human Services (DHHS), some minority populations are less knowledgeable about specific health problems than are whites. Successful programs to increase public awareness about health problems are being offered to minority groups, but efforts must be continued to reach more of the population. Families, churches, employers, and community organizations need to be involved in facilitating behavior changes that will result in healthier lifestyles. Education programs have the greatest effect on diseases that are affected by lifestyle, such as hypertension, obesity, and diabetes. For example, if patients with diabetes could improve their self-management skills, complications could be prevented, saving human suffering and health care dollars (Nies and McEwen, 2015).

Education and Certification

Increasingly more universities and colleges offer graduate programs in transcultural, cross-cultural, and international nursing. Many nurses have not been exposed to transcultural nursing in their basic education program. Therefore, the availability of graduate study in this area often is an unrecognized possibility.

Transcultural nursing is the study of differences and similarities of various cultural health values and beliefs among different ethnic and minority groups. The Transcultural Nursing Society has been certifying nurses in transcultural nursing since 1988. Certification as a transcultural nurse is based on oral and written examinations and evaluation of the nurse's educational and experiential background. Certification has increased recognition of transcultural nursing as a legitimate nursing specialty. Transcultural nurses are interested in finding universal care for clients that will improve, maintain, and restore health and improve client satisfaction.

International Marketplace

Nurses trained in the United States work, teach, and consult in hundreds of foreign countries on every continent. They often are recognized as international pacesetters and are viewed as "commodities for import" by both the more developed countries and the less developed third- or fourth-world nations. Nurses can make a difference in the health outcomes of people all over the world. Technology has enhanced global communication and facilitated travel. As nurses help solve emerging health problems in countries throughout the world, they are the most valuable assets of the health care system. They will be called on to design, implement, and evaluate international projects, educational endeavors, and research with an intercultural focus. Therefore, it is important that nurses understand the intercultural issues related to our global society (Nies and McEwen, 2015).

Nursing Literature

The number of journal articles about culturally diverse clients, transcultural nursing research, international nursing, and the inclusion of transcultural concepts in nursing curricula has increased considerably since the 1950s. The *Journal of Transcultural Nursing* is a refereed journal that was first published in 1989. This journal was created to advance transcultural nursing knowledge and practices. It focuses on theory, research, and practice dimensions of transcultural nursing and provides a forum for researchers. Other journals that address cultural issues include the *Western Journal of Medicine:*

Cross Cultural Issues, the *Journal of Cultural Diversity,* the *Journal of Multicultural Nursing,* the *International Journal of Nursing Studies,* the *International Nursing Review,* and the *Journal of Holistic Nursing.* Nurse writers also need to be encouraged to publish articles related to clients' cultural views and health care needs in nursing specialty and practice journals that are more widely read by nurses who actually are providing care on a daily basis to clients from diverse cultures.

Although research articles on transcultural issues are becoming a common feature in health care journals, there is a need for additional research that examines individual behavioral responses to normal life processes, such as pregnancy, birth, death, and human growth and development. There also is a need for well-designed studies that explore the biologic, psychologic, sociologic, and spiritual differences within, between, and among cultural groups (Douglas et al, 2011). Dr. Madeline Leininger created the theory of culture care diversity and universality to guide transcultural research. Even though numerous research studies have been conducted on cultural diversity issues, a significant time gap often exists between the identification of findings and the publication of results. The limited dissemination of research findings inhibits widespread acceptance of new interventions that could improve health care practices of culturally diverse populations. Computer information technology and online networks help narrow this gap and distribute research findings in a timely manner (Douglas et al, 2011).

Responsibility of Health Care Facilities for Cultural Care

Nursing policies should reflect openness to including extended family members and folk healers in the nursing care plan, provided that their presence is not harmful to the client's well-being. Most hospital chaplaincy programs have access to religious representatives available for patients of various religions.

Clients may need to consult with their support persons and folk healers before making medical decisions. Nurses must respect the client's right to privacy and allow time for the client to interact with his or her spiritual or cultural healers. Nurses must respect unconventional beliefs and health practices, and must work with clients to develop a plan of care that builds on their beliefs and incorporates nontraditional health practices that are not harmful. These nontraditional

healers should be received with respect and provided privacy to enable the healers to interact with their patients (Nies and McEwen, 2015).

Health care facilities should provide resources for nurses and other health care professionals to assist with the culture-specific needs of clients. Health care facilities should have a list of interpreters fluent in the major languages spoken by persons typically using the organization. Translators who have knowledge of health related terminology are more effective than those who do not. Gender, birth origin, and socioeconomic class need to be considered in the selection of a translator. Gender is an important consideration because many cultures prohibit discussion of intimate matters between women and men. Birth origin of the client and translator should be determined because often many dialects are spoken within the same country, depending on the particular region (Stanhope and Lancaster, 2016). Differences in socioeconomic class between client and interpreter can lead to problems of interpretation.

Clinical nurse specialists (CNSs) in transcultural nursing should be added to the staff of institutions serving large numbers of culturally diverse individuals. The transcultural CNS could be a role model to the staff in delivery of culturally sensitive and competent care, provide in-service education to staff related to cultural differences, and conduct research related to cultural and social issues. In addition, consultants should be used to deal with specific cultural issues.

Continuing education programs for nurses should be offered by health care institutions. Programs should focus on promoting awareness of the nurses' own culturally based values, beliefs, and attitudes, cultural assessment, biologic variations of cultural groups, cross-cultural communication, and culture-specific beliefs and practices related to childbearing and childrearing, death and dying, issues of mental health, and cultural aspects of aging.

Recommended Standards for Culturally and Linguistically Appropriate Services (CLAS)

Culture and language have a considerable effect on how patients access and respond to health care services. To ensure equal access to quality health care by diverse populations, the Office of Minority Health in the DHHS developed guidelines for health care organizations. In its report *Assuring Cultural Competence in Health*

Care: Recommendations for National Standards and an Outcomes Focused Research Agenda, the following standards are recommended (Fortier et al, 1999):

- Promote and support the attitudes, behaviors, knowledge, and skills necessary for staff to work respectfully and effectively with patients and each other in a culturally diverse work environment.
- Have a comprehensive management strategy to address culturally and linguistically appropriate services, including strategic goals, plans, policies, procedures, and designated staff responsible for implementation.
- Utilize formal mechanisms for community and consumer involvement in the design and execution of service delivery, including planning, policymaking, operations, evaluation, training, and, as appropriate, treatment planning.
- Develop and implement a strategy to recruit, retain, and promote qualified, diverse, and culturally competent administrative, clinical, and support staff members that are trained and qualified to address the needs of the racial and ethnic communities being served.
- Require and arrange for ongoing education and training for administrative, clinical, and support staff in culturally and linguistically competent service delivery.
- Provide all clients with limited English proficiency (LEP) access to bilingual staff or interpretation services.
- Provide oral and written notices, including translated signage at key points of contact, to clients in their primary language informing them of their right to receive interpreter services free of charge.
- Translate and make available signage and commonly used written patient educational material and other materials for members of the dominant language groups in service areas.
- Ensure that interpreters and bilingual staff can demonstrate bilingual proficiency and receive training that includes the skills and ethics of interpreting as well as knowledge in both languages of the terms and concepts relevant to clinical or nonclinical encounters. Family or friends are not considered adequate substitutes because they usually lack these abilities.
- Ensure that the clients' primary spoken language and self-identified race or ethnicity are included in the health care organization's management information system as well as any patient records used by provider staff.
- Utilize a variety of methods to collect and use accurate demographic, cultural, epidemiologic, and clinical outcome data for racial and ethnic groups in the service area. Become informed about the ethnic and cultural needs, resources, and assets of the surrounding community.
- Undertake ongoing organizational self-assessments of cultural and linguistic competence; integrate measures of access, satisfaction, quality, and outcomes for CLAS into other organizational internal audits and performance-improvement programs.
- Develop structures and procedures to address cross-cultural ethical and legal conflicts in health care delivery and complaints or grievances by patients and staff about unfair, culturally insensitive, or discriminatory treatment; difficulty in accessing services; or denial of services.
- Prepare an annual progress report documenting the organizations' progress with implementing CLAS standards, including information on programs, staffing, and resources.

CULTURAL ASSESSMENT

Cultural Self-Assessment

The first step to becoming a culturally sensitive and competent health care provider is to conduct a cultural self-assessment. The nurse should engage in a cultural self-assessment to identify individual culturally based attitudes about clients who are from a different culture. Cultural self-assessment requires self-honesty and sincerity as well as reflection on attitudes of parents, grandparents, and close friends toward different cultures. Through identification of health-related attitudes, values, beliefs, and practices, the nurse can better understand the cultural aspects of health care from the client's perspective. Everyone has ethnocentric tendencies that must be brought to a level of consciousness so that efforts can be made to temper the feeling that one's own culture is best.

Cultural Client Assessment

After the nurse performs a cultural self-assessment, he or she should obtain a cultural assessment of the client. Nursing assessments in institutional and community settings should include the gathering of data pertinent to cultural beliefs and practices. Cultural assessments lead to culturally relevant nursing diagnoses and give direction to effective nursing intervention. Basic cultural data include ethnic affiliation, religious preference, family patterns, food patterns, and ethnic health care practices. Cultural assessments should be used as an adjunct to other patient assessments. These data will give the nurse sufficient information to determine whether a more in-depth assessment of cultural factors is needed. A major reason that cultural assessments are performed is to identify patterns that may assist or interfere with a nursing intervention or treatment regimen (Douglas et al, 2011). The nurse needs to find out whether the client's beliefs, customs, values, and self-care practices are adaptive (beneficial), neutral, or maladaptive (harmful) in relation to nursing interventions. For example, if a client who is diagnosed with hypertension insists on taking garlic instead of an antihypertensive, this practice could be harmful. If the client agrees to take the garlic in addition to the antihypertensive, this practice would be neutral. An adaptive or beneficial practice would include daily exercise in addition to the garlic and antihypertensive.

In some cultures, dermal methods are perceived as ways to relieve headaches, muscle pains, sinusitis, colds, sore throats, diarrhea, or fever. Cupping involves placing a heated cup on the skin; as it cools, it contracts, drawing what is believed to be toxicity into the cup. A circular ecchymosis is left on the skin. Pinching may be done at the base of the nose or between the eyes. Bruises or welts are left at the site of treatment. Rubbing or "coining" involves rubbing lubricated skin with a spoon or a coin to bring toxic "wind" to the body surface. A similar practice is burning, which involves touching a burning cigarette or piece of cotton to the skin, usually the abdomen, to compensate for "heat" lost through diarrhea (Nies and McEwen, 2011). These practices nurture the client's sense of well-being and security in being able to do something to correct disturbing symptoms. In most cases, the practice would be considered adaptive (beneficial) or neutral. However, if the client had a clotting disorder, the practices would pose a threat to physical integrity and therefore would be considered maladaptive (harmful) (Nies and McEwen, 2011).

Cultural Client Nutrition Assessment

A cultural nutrition assessment should be obtained for clients who are minorities. It is necessary to assess the client's cultural definition of food. For example, certain cultures do not consider greens to be food. Therefore, when asked to keep a food diary, individuals would not list greens, which are an important source of vitamins and iron. Frequency and number of meals, amount and types of food eaten, and regularity of food consumption are other important factors to consider.

In cultures in which obesity is a problem, it is helpful for the nurse to have an idea of food preferences to help the client select low-calorie, low-fat foods. Asians tend to prefer spicy foods, which may lead to their high incidence of stomach cancer, ulcers, and gastrointestinal bleeding (Purnell and Paulanka, 2009).

Nurses should avoid cultural stereotyping as it relates to food because not all Italians necessarily like spaghetti, nor do all Chinese like rice. However, knowing the clients' food preferences makes it possible to develop therapeutic interventions that do not conflict with their cultural food practices (Stanhope and Lancaster, 2016).

Cultural Beliefs About Sickness and Cures

It also is important for the nurse to consider the nontraditional beliefs of sickness and cure of various cultures. For example, there are diseases that are not classified as Western culture diseases. For different cultural groups, they are real diseases for which the group has medicines and treatments. Examples of such diseases are mal ojo, susto, bilis, and empacho.

It is important to determine how culturally diverse clients define health and illness and whether their health beliefs and practices differ from the norm in the Western health care delivery system (Spector, 2016).

Health represents a balance within the body, mind, and spirit. It is strongly affected by the family and the community (Box 10.1). Spector (2016) has developed a guide that can be used to assess clients' personal methods for maintaining, protecting (preventing illness), and restoring health (Table 10.2).

BOX 10.1   Health Traditions Assessment Model

Maintaining Health

Physical	Are there special clothes one must wear; foods one must eat or not eat, or combinations to avoid; exercises one must do?
Mental	Are there special sources of entertainment; games or other ways of concentrating; traditional "rules of behavior"?
Spiritual	Are there special religious customs; prayers; meditations?

Protecting Health and Preventing Illness

Physical	Are there special foods that must be eaten after certain life events, such as childbirth; dietary taboos that must be adhered to; symbolic clothes that must be worn?
Mental	Are there special sources of entertainment, games or other ways of concentrating; traditional "rules of behavior"?
Spiritual	Are there special religious customs, superstitions, amulets, oils, or waters?

Restoring Health

Physical	Are there special folk remedies; liniments; procedures, such as cupping, acupuncture, and moxibustion?
Mental	Are there special healers, such as curanderos, rituals, folk medicines?
Spiritual	Are there special rituals and prayers, meditations, healers?

From Spector, R.E. (2016). *Cultural diversity in health and illness* (9th ed.). Upper Saddle River, NJ: Prentice-Hall.

TABLE 10.2   Assessment Guide for Personal Methods to Maintain, Protect (Prevent Illness), and Restore Health

	Physical	Mental	Spiritual
Maintain health	Are there special clothes you must wear at certain times of the day, week, or year? Are there special foods you must eat at certain times? Do you have any dietary restrictions? Are there any foods that you cannot eat?	What do you do for activities, such as reading, sports, or games? Do you have hobbies? Do you visit family often? Do you visit friends often?	Do you practice your religion and attend church or other communal activities? Do you pray or meditate? Do you observe religious customs? Do you belong to fraternal organizations?
Protect health or prevent illness	Are there foods that you cannot eat together? Are there special foods that you must eat? Are there any types of clothing that you are not allowed to wear?	Are there people or situations that you have been taught to avoid? Do you take extraordinary precautions under certain circumstances? Do you take time for yourself?	Do you observe religious customs? Do you wear any amulets or hang them in your house? Do you have any practices, such as always opening the window when you sleep? Do you have any other practices to protect yourself from "harm"?
Restore health	What kinds of medicines do you take before you see a doctor or nurse? Are there herbs that you take? Are there special treatments that you use?	Do you know of any specific practices your mother or grandmother may use to relax? Do you know how big problems can be cared for in your community? Do you drink special teas to help you unwind or relax?	Do you know any healers? Do you know of any religious rituals that help to restore health? Do you meditate? Do you ever go to a healing service? Do you know about exorcism?

From Spector, R.E. (2016). *Cultural diversity in health and illness* (9th ed.). Upper Saddle River, NJ: Prentice-Hall.

SUMMARY

In a society as diverse as the United States, health care cannot come in one form to fit the needs of everyone. Culture has a powerful influence on one's interpretation of health and illness and response to health care. All clients have the right to be understood and respected, despite their differences. They have the right to expect health care providers to acknowledge that their perspectives on and interpretations of health are legitimate. Health care professionals must make a commitment to increase their knowledge, sensitivity, and competence in cultural concepts and care. Perhaps no other group in the health profession has recognized the effect of cultural diversity on outcomes of health care more than nurses. Nurses always have supported the concept of holistic care. By understanding the client's perspective, the nurse can be a better advocate for the client. With increased knowledge, sensitivity, respect, and understanding, therapeutic interventions can be maximized to promote the highest quality of health for clients in our multicultural society.

REFERENCES

American Academy of Nursing. (1995). *Diversity, marginalization, and culturally competent health care issues in knowledge development*. Washington, DC: American Academy of Nursing.

American Association of Colleges of Nursing. (2008a). *The Essentials of baccalaureate education for professional nursing practice*. Washington, DC: American Association of Colleges of Nursing.

American Association of Colleges of Nursing. (2008b). Cultural competency in baccalaureate nursing education. Available at http://www.aacnnursing.org/Portals/42/AcademicNursing/CurriculumGuidelines/Cultural-Competency-Bacc-Edu.pdf?ver=2017-05-18-143551-883.

American Association of Colleges of Nursing. (2015). *Enhancing Diversity in the Workforce*. Retrieved from http://www.aacnnursing.org/News-Information/Fact-Sheets/Enhancing-Diversity.

American Academy of Nursing Expert Panel on Cultural Competence. (2007). *American Academy of Nursing standards of cultural competence*. Washington, DC: American Academy of Nursing Expert Panel on Cultural Competence.

American Academy of Nursing Expert Panel on Culturally Competent Health Care: culturally competent health care. *Nursing Outlook*, 40(6), 277–283, 1992.

American Association of Colleges of Nursing. *Policy Brief: The Changing Landscape: Nursing Student Diversity on the Rise*. Retrieved from http://www.aacn.nche.edu/government-affairs/. Student-Diversity-FS.pdf. Ethnic Minorities.

Barnett, J. C., & Berchick, E. R. (2017). *Health insurance coverage in the United States: 2016: Highlights. U.S. Census Bureau. Current Population Reports P60-260*. Washington, DC: U.S. Government Printing Office. Retrieved from https://www.census.gov/library/publications/2017/demo/p60-260.html.

Bessent, H. (1997). *Strategies for recruitment, retention and graduation of minority nurses in colleges of nursing*. Washington, DC: American Nurses Foundation.

Budden, J. S., Zhong, E. H., & Moulton, P. (2013). Highlights of the national workforce survey of registered nurses. *Journal of Nursing Regulation*, 4(2), 5–14.

Buerhaus, P. I., Skinner, L. E., Auerbach, D. I., & Staiger, D. O. (2017). Four challenges facing the nursing workforce in the United States. *Journal of Nursing Regulation*, 8(2), 40–46.

Center for Interdisciplinary Health Workforce Studies. 2017 Data Brief Update: Current Trends of Men in Nursing. Retrieved from http://healthworkforcestudies.com/publications-data/data_brief_update_current_trends_of_men_in_nursing.html.

Centers for Disease Control and Prevention. (2017). *Healthy Aging*. Atlanta, GA: Centers for Disease Control and Prevention, US Department of Health and Human Services. Retrieved from http://www.cdc.gov/aging.

Douglas, M., Pierce, J., & Rosenkoetter, M. (2011). Standards of practice for culturally competent nursing care: 2011 update. *Journal of Transcultural Nursing*, 22(4), 317–333.

Fang, D., Li, Y., & Kennedy, K.A. (2017). *Enrollment and graduations in baccalaureate and graduate programs in nursing (2016-17)*. Washington, DC: American Association of Colleges of Nursing.

Floyd, A., & Sakellarious, D. (2017). Healthcare access for refugee women with limited literacy: layers of disadvantage. *International Journal for Equity in Health*, 16:195

Fortier, J. P., Convissor, R., & Pacheco, G. (1999). *Assuring Cultural Competence in Health Care: Recommendations for National Standards and an Outcomes-Focused Research*

Agenda. Rockville, MD: U.S. Department of Health and Human Services, Office of Minority Health.

Future of Nursing Scholars. (2018). *About the program*. Retrieved from http://futureofnursingscholars.org.

Giger, J. N., Davidhizar, R. E. (2008). *Transcultural nursing: assessment and intervention*. (5th ed.). St. Louis: Elsevier.

Health Resources and Services Administration. (2013). *The U.S. nursing workforce: Trends in supply and education*. Retrieved from http://bhprhrsa.gov/healthworkforce/ reports/nursingworkforce/. Washington, DC: U.S. Department of Health and Human Services.

Lenburg, C. B., Lipson, J. G., Demi, A., et al. (1995). *Promoting cultural competence in and through nursing education: a critical review and comprehensive plan for action*. Washington, DC: American Academy of Nursing.

Loftin, C., Newman, S. D., Dumas, B. P., Gilden G., & Bond, M. L. (2012). Perceived barriers to success for minority nursing students: An integrative review, *International Scholarly Research Notices*, doi:10.5402/2012/806543.

Macartney, S., Bishaw, A., & Fontenot, K., U.S. Census Bureau. (2013, February). *Poverty rates for selected detailed race and Hispanic groups by state and place, 2007–2011*. Report Number: ACSBR/11-17. Retrieved from http://www. census.gov/library/publications/2013/acs/acsbr11-17.html.

Mather, M. (2016). The Population Reference Bureau report, Fact sheet: aging in the United States. Retrieved from http://www.prb.org/Publications/Media-Guides/2016/ aging-unitedstates-fact-sheet.aspx.

Meleis, A., Isenberg, M., Koerner, J., et al. (1995). *Diversity, marginalization, and culturally competent healthcare issues in knowledge development*. Washington, DC: American Academy of Nursing.

National Center for Health Statistics. (2017). *Health, United States, 2016: With Chartbook on Long-term Trends in Health*. Hyattsville, MD. Retrieved from https://www.cdc. gov/nchs/hus/index.htm.

National Council of State Boards of Nursing. (2013). The National Council of State Boards of Nursing and The Forum of State Nursing Workforce Centers, National Workforce Survey of RNs. *Journal of Nursing Regulation, 4*(2), S1–S72.

Nies, M., & McEwen, M. (2011). *Community/public health nursing: Promoting the health of populations* (5th ed.). St Louis: Elsevier.

Nies, M., & McEwen, M. (2015). *Community/public health nursing: Promoting the health of populations* (6th ed.). St Louis: Elsevier.

Purnell, L., & Paulanka, B. (2009). *Guide to culturally competent healthcare* (2nd ed.). Philadelphia: FA Davis.

Semega, J. L., Fontenot, K. R., & Kollar, M. A. (2017.) *Income and poverty in the United States: 2016: Highlights*. U.S. Census Bureau, Current Population Reports P60-259. Washington, DC: U.S. Government Printing Office. Retrieved from https://www.census.gov/library/publications/ 2017/demo/p60-259.html.

Spector, R. (2016). *Cultural diversity in health and illness/ culture care: Guide to heritage assessment health*. In R. Spector (Ed.), Cultural diversity in health and illness (9th ed.). Upper Saddle River, NJ: Prentice-Hall.

Stanhope, M., & Lancaster, J. (2016). *Public health nursing: Population-centered health care in the community* (9th ed.). St Louis: Mosby.

Tervalon, M., & Murray-Garcia, J. (1998). Cultural humility versus cultural competence: a critical distinction in defining physician training outcomes in multicultural education. *Journal of Health Care for the Poor and Underserved, 9*(2), 117.

U.S. Census Bureau. Health Insurance Coverage in the United States: 2016. Retrieved from https://www.census. gov/library/publications/2017/demo/p60-260.html.

U.S. Department of Health and Human Services. (2010). *Public Health Service: Healthy People 2020*, Washington, DC: U.S. Government Printing Office.

11

Complementary and Alternative Healing

Charlotte Eliopoulos, PhD, RN, MPH, ND

Consumers are increasingly seeking natural remedies for health promotion and disease management; nurses have a responsibility to be aware of the potential effects.

ⓔ Additional resources are available online at: *http://evolve.elsevier.com/Cherry/*

LEARNING OUTCOMES

After studying this chapter, the reader will be able to:

1. Describe various complementary and alternative healing practices.
2. Identify how to effectively incorporate effective complementary and alternative therapies into care.
3. Provide patient education regarding uses, limitations, and precautions associated with selected complementary and alternative healing practices and products.

KEY TERMS

Complementary and alternative medicine (CAM) Healing philosophies, practices, and products that are outside of what Western society considers mainstream medicine and are not typically taught in the educational programs of physicians, nurses, and other health professionals.

Conventional medicine Western style of medicine practiced in the United States; also called allopathic medicine.

Energy therapies Qi gong, Reiki, therapeutic touch, healing touch, magnet therapy.

Manipulative and body-based methods Chiropractic, massage, and related techniques (e.g., manual lymph drainage, Alexander technique, Feldenkrais method, pressure point therapies, Trager psychophysical integration), osteopathy.

Mind-body interventions Aromatherapy, art therapy, biofeedback, dance therapy, hypnosis, imagery, meditation, music therapy, prayer, qi gong, progressive relaxation, self-help support groups, tai chi, yoga.

Movement therapies Alexander technique, Feldenkrais method, Rolfing, Trager psychophysical integration.

Natural products Herbal therapies, individual and orthomolecular biologic therapies, special diets.

PROFESSIONAL/ETHICAL ISSUE

Mr. Jensen is a 50-year-old man who has been diagnosed with a rare liver cancer that is typically fatal within 1 year. His oncologist has recommended a form of chemotherapy that cannot offer a cure but could possibly slow the cancer's spread and offer a few added months of life to Mr. Jensen.

Mr. Jensen, accompanied by his wife, are meeting with the oncologist, who is your employer and whom you are assisting. Mr. Jensen informs the oncologist that after giving it thought, he has decided against the chemotherapy. "I saw what my brother went through with his chemo for lung cancer and I don't want to do the same," Mr. Jensen states. "My wife found this natural health practitioner who offers some kind of touch therapy and uses herbal blends. I've seen him a couple of times now and have to tell you, I feel great so I'm going that route," he adds.

The oncologist is noticeably annoyed and responds, "You are wasting your time and money on that foolishness. If anything is going to help you it is what medicine has to offer, so I'd think about scheduling your next chemotherapy. The nurse will help you with that." He then exits the room.

Mr. and Mrs. Jensen appear upset and somewhat confused. You heard what the oncologist recommended and understand that there is no evidence supporting the effectiveness of the natural healing methods, yet you also know that the chemotherapy offers no cure and does carry risks and side effects. What do you do?

VIGNETTE

Ruth Jeffers is a registered nurse (RN) who works in a rehabilitation unit in which many clients suffer from chronic musculoskeletal pain. Ms. Jeffers has noted that a growing number of clients have a history of independently using acupuncture, nutritional supplements, and other alternative and complementary healing therapies to improve their symptoms. Although they report beneficial results, most do not tell their physicians that they are using these therapies.

Last year, Ms. Jeffers completed a course in the use of therapeutic touch and has used this therapy to promote relaxation and pain control with friends and family with considerable success. She is aware of many positive reports on the benefits of these unconventional approaches. She believes therapeutic touch and some other complementary healing therapies could benefit clients on the rehabilitation unit and informally introduces the topic to the team with whom she works. With the exception of one nurse who states that she believes these therapies are associated with the occult and wants no part of them, the nursing staff is enthusiastic and eager to implement complementary therapies. The physical and occupational therapists believe that complementary therapies could prove helpful to clients but that only therapists within their departments, not nursing, should provide them. The physician on the team opposes the use of all alternative and complementary therapies, stating, "I'm not about to put my license on the line for these unproven ideas."

Questions to Consider While Reading this Chapter:

1. What is the best course of action for Ruth Jeffers, RN, if she really believes that complementary and alternative therapies could benefit clients on the unit?
2. What would a hospital need to do to prepare for the inclusion of complementary and alternative therapies in its existing services?
3. What are some of the potential obstacles to introducing complementary and alternative therapies into a conventional setting?
4. What discipline(s) should be responsible for providing and/or coordinating or supervising the practitioners who provide complementary and alternative therapies in the hospital?

CHAPTER OVERVIEW

This chapter presents an overview of complementary and alternative medicine (CAM) therapies and products, which have gained popularity in Western society and are being integrated into health care. As increasing numbers of consumers and clinical settings become interested in and actually use CAM therapies, nurses must become knowledgeable about the uses, limitations, and precautions associated with these new practices and products. Professional nurses have an obligation to understand such practices and products so as to advise patients and effectively incorporate pertinent therapies into patients' care. Nurses who have knowledge and skills in this area are in key positions to empower patients for self-care that complements conventional medicine.

USE OF COMPLEMENTARY AND ALTERNATIVE HEALING METHODS

Complementary and alternative healing methods include healing philosophies, practices, and products that fall outside what Western society considers mainstream (conventional) medicine and that are not typically taught in the educational programs of physicians, nurses, pharmacists, and other health professionals.

The past few decades have seen CAM progress from a fringe movement to highly popular, widely used therapies that are being integrated into conventional care. According to a nationwide government survey, more than 38% of U.S. adults 18 years and older and approximately 12% of children use some form of CAM, spending between $27 and $34 billion for these services out of their own pockets (Nahin et al, 2016).

Rather than emerging from the leadership of health care professionals, the growing popularity of CAM has been consumer driven. Several factors contribute to consumers' desire for CAM:

- *Dissatisfaction with the conventional health care system:* The impersonal nature of health care has grown with costs. Shorter hospital stays, several months' waiting periods to see a physician, hurried staff that barely have time to provide basic care, and horror stories of the adverse effects of medications are causing consumers to look for alternative approaches that are safer, less costly, and more responsive and personalized than conventional health care.
- *Increased empowerment of consumers in the health care system:* The Internet and growing assertiveness of consumers in all areas has affected health care. Consumers expect to have a voice in their care planning activities and to be able to utilize all available options for health promotion and disease management, including therapies outside mainstream medicine.
- *Unwillingness to "grin and bear" the effects of diseases:* Today's consumers are less willing than previous generations to live with symptoms that alter their lifestyles or to passively accept terminal diagnoses and wait to die. They want to have options and to be empowered to do everything conceivable to promote the best possible quality and quantity of their lives,

and they are willing to look to alternative healing measures to do so.
- *Shrinking world:* The rapid pace and ease of information sharing have enabled individuals to learn about diverse practices of cultures throughout the world.
- *Growing evidence of effectiveness:* The body of research supporting the effectiveness of alternative therapies increases almost daily. People hear testimonials from friends and family about the way they have been helped by acupuncture, herbs, and other forms of CAM. In addition, the media regularly report these findings, contributing to consumers' awareness of the body of evidence.

CAM practices and products are consistent with the values, beliefs, and philosophic orientations toward health held by many people (National Center for Complementary and Integrative Health [NCCIH], 2016a). With rare exceptions, consumers prefer natural approaches that afford them an active role in their care over high-tech interventions that relegate them to a passive, obedient role. They want to connect with their health care providers, have their individuality recognized, and gain education and skills to effectively make decisions and direct their care. Increasingly, consumers are seeking measures to enhance not just their bodies but also their minds and spirits. The quality of their lives is equally if not more important in comparison with the quantity of years they live. Consumers often discover that CAM promotes many principles of holistic care that they value, such as individual empowerment, self-care, attention to all facets of one's being, and a high quality of life.

PRINCIPLES UNDERLYING ALTERNATIVE HEALING

A wide range of healing therapies are encompassed in CAM, yet most are based on some common principles:
- *The body has the ability to heal itself.* Most conventional medicine works from the premise that the elimination of sickness requires an intervention "done to" the body (e.g., giving medications, surgery). In CAM, there is the assumption that the body has the potential to heal itself. Complementary and alternative healing therapies enhance the body's ability to self-heal.
- *Health and healing are related to a harmony of mind, body, and spirit.* The mind, body, and spirit are inseparable; what affects one affects all. Healing and the improvement of health demand that all facets of

a person be addressed, not merely a single symptom or system.

- *Basic, positive health practices build the foundation for healing.* Good nutrition, exercise, rest, stress management, and avoidance of harmful habits (e.g., smoking) are essential ingredients in health maintenance and the improvement of health conditions. Practitioners of healing therapies are more likely than conventional practitioners to look at total lifestyle practices rather than the diseased body part.

- *Approaches to healing are individualized.* The unique composition and dynamics of each person are recognized in CAM. Practitioners of healing therapies explore the underlying cause of a problem and customize approaches accordingly. It is rare in CAM to find a standing protocol that treats everyone with similar conditions alike.

- *Individuals are responsible for their own healing.* People can use a wide range of therapies, from conventional prescription drugs to herbal remedies, to treat illness. However, it is the responsibility of competent adults to seek health advice, make informed choices, gain necessary knowledge and skills for self-care, engage in practices that promote health and healing, and seek help when needed. Clients are responsible for getting their minds, bodies, and spirits in optimal condition to heal rather than look externally for a physician or nurse to heal them.

A holistic philosophy, promotion of positive health habits, and the client's responsibility for facilitating his or her own health and healing are common threads among healing therapies.

OVERVIEW OF POPULAR CAM HEALING THERAPIES

Hundreds of healing therapies are practiced throughout the world, with varying degrees of evidence to support their effectiveness. As the use of these therapies grew in the United States, the National Institutes of Health (NIH) established the Office of Alternative Medicine in 1992 to evaluate these complementary and alternative practices and products. In 1998, the Office of Alternative Medicine became a freestanding center within the NIH and was named the National Center for Complementary and Alternative Medicine. The name has now been changed to the National Center for Complementary and Integrative Health (NCCIH) to reflect the

---

> **BOX 11.1   Categories and Examples of Complementary Health Approaches**
>
> **Natural Products**
> Herbs (botanicals), vitamins, minerals, probiotics
>
> **Mind-Body Practices**
> Acupuncture, chiropractic and osteopathic manipulation, healing touch, hypnotherapy, massage therapy, meditation, movement therapies (Alexander technique, Feldenkrais method, Pilates, Rolfing Structural Integration, Trager psychophysical integration), relaxation techniques (breathing exercises, guided imagery, progressive relaxation), tai chi
>
> **Other Approaches**
> Ayurvedic medicine, homeopathy, naturopathy, traditional Chinese medicine

wider acceptance and use of CAM in mainstream health care. NCCIH has categorized CAM into several major fields of practice (Box 11.1); the center supports research and serves as a clearinghouse for information on alternative practices and products.

Consumers' growing use of CAM therapies as well as the increased integration of such therapies into conventional care places a demand on nurses to become familiar with these therapies. Some of the frequently used CAM therapies are discussed in the following sections.

Acupuncture

Practiced in China for more than 2000 years, acupuncture is a major therapy within traditional Chinese medicine. It is based on the belief that there are invisible channels throughout the body, called *meridians,* through which energy flows. This energy, called qi (pronounced "chee"), is considered the vital life force. It is believed that illness and symptoms develop when the flow of energy becomes blocked or imbalanced. Health is restored when the energy becomes unblocked; unblocking is achieved by stimulating acupuncture points on the meridian(s) affected (Figure 11.1).

The acupuncturist typically begins the treatment by taking a history, examining the tongue, and evaluating pulses. On the basis of where the acupuncturist assesses the energy imbalance to be, he or she places needles at specific points. The placement of the needles may have no obvious relationship to the area of the body that is symptomatic. Sometimes the acupuncturist applies heat

Fig. 11.1 Acupuncture meridians. (From Eliopoulos, C. [1999]. *Integrating alternative and conventional therapies.* St Louis: Mosby.)

TABLE 11.1	Ayurvedic Metabolic Body Types
Type	**Characteristics**
Vata	Unpredictable; moody; vivacious; hyperactive; imaginative; intuitive; impulsive; fluctuating energy levels; slender; prominent features and joints; eats and sleeps at varying times throughout day; prone to insomnia, premenstrual syndrome (PMS), muscular cramps, and constipation
Pitta	Predictable; orderly; efficient; perfectionist; intense; passionate; short-tempered; medium build; follows routine schedule; warm skin; prone to heavy perspiration, thirst, acne, ulcers, hemorrhoids, and stomach problems
Kapha	Relaxed; graceful; tendency toward procrastination; affectionate; forgiving; compassionate; sleeps long and deeply; cool, pale, and oily skin; eats slowly; prone to high cholesterol, obesity, allergies, and sinusitis

to the acupoints by burning a dried herb on the top of the needle or skin; this procedure is known as *moxibustion.* Electroacupuncture, a process in which a small current of electricity is applied to the tip of the needle, is another means of stimulating acupoints.

Pain relief is the most common reason people seek acupuncture treatment, and research supports its effectiveness for this problem (American Society of Anesthesiologists Task Force on Chronic Pain Management, 2010; Hillinger et al, 2017; Koog et al, 2014; Liang et al, 2017). The use of acupuncture for dental pain and chemotherapy-induced nausea and vomiting has also been supported by research. There is some evidence that acupuncture can be of help for nicotine withdrawal, asthma, stroke rehabilitation, carpal tunnel syndrome, and a growing list of other conditions.

Insurance companies vary in their coverage of acupuncture, so it is best for clients to call their individual insurer for determination of benefits. State health departments can be consulted for licensing requirements for acupuncturists in a given state.

Ayurveda

Although it has gained popularity because of the writings and lectures of Deepak Chopra, Ayurveda has existed in India for more than 5000 years. Ayurveda, which means "the science of life," is a system of care that promotes spiritual, mental, and physical balance. Noninvasive approaches are used to achieve balance; they include yoga, massage, diet, purification regimens, breathing exercises, meditation, and herbs.

Individuals are believed to have distinct metabolic body types called *doshas,* which are *vata, pitta,* and *kapha* (Table 11.1). Signs of illness occur when the delicate balance of the doshas is disturbed.

The treatment to restore balance is influenced by the body type a client possesses and could include the following:
- Cleansing and detoxification
- Palliation
- Rejuvenation through special herbs and minerals
- Mental hygiene and spiritual healing

Currently, there is no process for licensing or certifying Ayurvedic practitioners. Because some of the treatments have the potential to cause complications (e.g., dehydration from cleansing enemas, herb-drug interactions), finding a reputable trained practitioner is important. There is a need for continued research because scientific evidence for the effectiveness of Ayurvedic practices varies, and more rigorous research is needed to determine which practices are safe and effective.

Biofeedback

A popular mind-body intervention, biofeedback is a technique in which the client is taught to alter specific bodily functions (e.g., heart rate, blood pressure, muscle tension) by using various relaxation and imagery exercises. Machinery, such as electroencephalograms, electromyelograms, and thermistors, are used to measure and offer feedback about the function that the client is trying to alter. As the client becomes familiar with ways to successfully alter bodily responses, the equipment may no longer be necessary.

There are many conditions for which biofeedback can offer benefit, including urinary incontinence, anxiety, stress, irritable bowel syndrome, neck and back pain, and cardiac arrhythmias.

Chiropractic Medicine

Chiropractic medicine, a manipulative and body-based method, is a popular and widely accepted CAM therapy in the United States perhaps because it was developed here and has been practiced for more than a century. Chiropractors are licensed in every state, and most insurance companies pay for chiropractic treatments.

Chiropractic medicine is based on the belief that misalignments of the spine, called *subluxations*, put pressure on the nerves, leading to pain and disruptions in normal bodily function. The misalignment is treated by manipulation and adjustment of the spine. Typically, the chiropractor's hands do the alignment, although chiropractors increasingly are using heat, electrical stimulation, and other treatments.

Dietary Supplements

The past advice that vitamin and mineral supplements are unnecessary if one is eating well has been replaced with the recommendation that everyone should take a daily vitamin and mineral supplement. This shift in thinking has resulted from the realization that many people do not consume the proper nutrients through their diets. Pollutants, stress, and other factors that are more common today than in previous generations heighten the body's need for added protection. Also, unlike our ancestors, who consumed produce that was picked the same day, we tend to eat more processed foods and produce that may have been in transit for several days before reaching us; therefore, the foods we consume contain fewer vitamins and minerals. Given these factors, the National Research Council of the National Academy of Sciences is reevaluating the need to increase the recommended dietary allowances (RDAs).

Specific dietary supplements are thought to be beneficial for specific health conditions. However, too much of a good thing could prove harmful, and high doses of vitamins and minerals can lead to serious complications (Altizer et al, 2014; *Consumer Reports*, 2012; Guallar et al, 2013; Harvard School of Public Health, 2017). For example, high doses of folic acid can mask a vitamin B12 deficiency (a cause of dementia), and calcium in excess of 2500 mg/day can cause kidney stones and impair the body's ability to absorb other minerals. In addition, because new research may disprove earlier claims about supplements, nurses need to keep abreast of new findings so that they can use supplements wisely and educate consumers to do the same.

Herbs

Herbs are a major entity under the category of natural products. Plants have been used for medicinal purposes for nearly as long as humans have inhabited the earth. It is estimated that as many as 70,000 plant species have been used at one time or another by various cultures for medicinal purposes (Kennedy, 2017; PDR Staff, 2013; Pharmaceutical Press Editorial, 2013). Botanical medicine was a mainstream practice in the United States until the early nineteenth century, when medicine's shift toward a more scientific approach caused drugs to be viewed more favorably than herbs. But in the 1960s, when the movement toward natural health began to grow, interest in herbal products increased. The use and sales of herbal remedies have grown significantly since.

In reality, herbs are not that foreign to conventional medicine. Many modern drugs are derived from plants, including the following:

- Atropine from *Atropa belladonna*
- Digoxin from *Digitalis purpurea*
- Ipecac from *Cephaelis ipecacuanha*
- Reserpine from *Rauwolfia serpentina*

With more than 20,000 herbs and related products on the market, staying current of uses, dosage, interactions, and adverse effects is a near impossibility. However, nurses would be wise to become familiar with some of the most commonly used herbs (Box 11.2) and to know where to obtain information on other herbs when needed. Because of consumers' widespread use of herbs, questions regarding use of all supplements and education to ensure their safe use are significant nursing responsibilities.

BOX 11.2 Facts about Commonly Used Herbs

Cannabis (Marijuana)

Uses: Appetite stimulant, anorexic, antiemetic, and treatment of chronic pain, Crohn's disease, severe muscle spasms, and seizures.

Cautions: Can cause dizziness, fatigue, tachycardia, slower reaction times, impaired short-term memory, impaired judgment, anxiety, hallucinations, acute psychosis (in large doses). Further study is needed to determine short- and long-term risks. States vary in their laws concerning medicinal marijuana use; individuals should check with their own state laws regarding legality and conditions of use.

Chamomile

Uses: Sedative effect, calming an upset digestive tract, healing mouth ulcers caused by chemotherapy or radiation.

Cautions: Because it contains coumarin, it could affect coagulation, although clinical studies have not demonstrated this effect to date; if the client is using an anticoagulant and chamomile, monitoring is necessary. People are more likely to experience allergic reactions to chamomile if they are allergic to related plants in the daisy family, which includes ragweed, chrysanthemums, marigolds, and daisies.

Echinacea

Uses: Stimulates the immune system to treat or prevent colds, flu, and other infections.

Cautions: Although immunosuppressive effects with long-term use are inconclusive at present, it's best to limit to short-term use. It should not be used in people with autoimmune diseases. People are more likely to experience allergic reactions to echinacea if they have asthma or are allergic to related plants in the daisy family, which includes ragweed, chrysanthemums, marigolds, and daisies. Gastrointestinal side effects are common.

Feverfew

Use: Relief of migraines (although more evidence is needed).

Cautions: Contraindicated for clients with allergies to ragweed and other members of the Compositae family. People who have used feverfew for an extended period may have headaches, difficulty sleeping, nervousness, and joint and muscle stiffness when they stop taking it. Women who are pregnant should not use feverfew because it may cause the uterus to contract, increasing the risk of miscarriage or premature delivery.

Garlic

Uses: Lowers blood pressure; reduces "bad" cholesterol; stimulates immune system; heart tonic; antioxidant.

Cautions: Close monitoring necessary if taken by person using an anticoagulant because it can prolong bleeding time. Should not be used by women who are breastfeeding.

Ginger

Uses: Antiemetic. Studies are mixed on whether ginger is effective for nausea caused by motion, chemotherapy, or surgery. Research is being conducted on ginger's benefit for rheumatoid arthritis, osteoarthritis, or joint and muscle pain.

Caution: Few side effects are linked to ginger when it is taken in small doses. Powdered form can cause gas, bloating, heartburn, and nausea.

Ginkgo Biloba

Use: Believed to increase circulation to the brain and improve cognitive performance in persons with dementia; however, research has not shown ginkgo to be effective in improving memory or cognitive function.

Cautions: Close monitoring necessary if taken by person using an anticoagulant because ginkgo can prolong bleeding time; can reduce effectiveness of anticonvulsants. Should not be used by people who have fragile blood vessels and a tendency to easily bleed. Side effects of ginkgo may include headache, nausea, gastrointestinal upset, diarrhea, dizziness, and allergic skin reactions. More severe allergic reactions have occasionally been reported. Fresh (raw) and roasted ginkgo seeds should be avoided; they can cause serious adverse effects because they contain high amounts of ginkgotoxin (which is present only in small amounts in standardized ginkgo leaf extracts, which do not pose the same risk).

Ginseng

Uses: Improves resistance to stress; immune stimulant; general stimulant. Some studies have shown that Asian ginseng may lower blood glucose and may have beneficial effects on immune function.

Cautions: Can cause breast tenderness in some menstruating women. Asian ginseng may lower blood glucose levels; this effect may be seen more in people with diabetes. Therefore, people with diabetes should use extra caution with Asian ginseng, especially if they are using medicines to lower blood glucose or taking other herbs thought to have the same effect, such as bitter melon and fenugreek. Most common side effects are headaches and sleep and gastrointestinal problems.

Green Tea

Uses: Laboratory studies suggest that green tea may help protect against or may slow the growth of certain

BOX 11.2   Facts about Commonly Used Herbs—cont'd

cancers, but studies in people have shown mixed results. Some evidence suggests that the use of green tea preparations improves mental alertness, most likely because of its caffeine content. There are not enough reliable data to determine whether green tea can aid in weight loss, lower blood cholesterol levels, or protect the skin from sun damage.

Caution: There have been some case reports of liver problems in people taking concentrated green tea extracts, but this problem does not seem to be connected with green tea infusions or beverages. Although these cases are very rare and the evidence is not definitive, experts suggest that concentrated green tea extracts be taken with food and that people should discontinue use and consult a heath care practitioner if they have a liver disorder or experience symptoms of liver trouble, such as abdominal pain, dark urine, and jaundice. Green tea and green tea extracts contain caffeine, which can cause insomnia, anxiety, irritability, upset stomach, nausea, diarrhea, or frequent urination in some people. Green tea also contains small amounts of vitamin K, which can make anticoagulant drugs, such as warfarin, less effective.

Lavender
Uses: Treatment of anxiety, restlessness, and insomnia. Studies have shown mixed results. Most commonly used in aromatherapy. Some early results from research shows that lavender oil when combined with other herbal oils can aid in preventing hair loss in persons with alopecia areata.

Caution: Can cause drowsiness. Topical use of diluted lavender oil or use of lavender as aromatherapy is generally considered safe for most adults. However, lavender oil can be poisonous if taken orally, and applying lavender oil to the skin can cause irritation. There have been reports that topical use can cause breast growth in young boys.

Saw Palmetto
Uses: Thought to improve symptoms of benign prostatic hypertrophy; however, research concluded that it was no more effective than placebo.

Caution: Saw palmetto appears to be well tolerated by most users. It may have mild side effects, including stomach discomfort. Bleeding risk can be increased when it is taken by persons who are also using anticoagulants.

Soy
Uses: May slightly lower levels of low-density lipoprotein (LDL; "bad") cholesterol when taken daily. Some studies suggest that soy isoflavone supplements may reduce hot flashes in women after menopause; however, the results have been inconsistent.

Caution: Minor stomach and bowel problems such as nausea, bloating, and constipation are possible. The safety of the long-term use of soy isoflavones has not been established. Soy's possible role in breast cancer risk is uncertain. Until more is known about soy's effect on estrogen levels, women who have or who are at increased risk for development of breast cancer or other hormone-sensitive conditions (such as ovarian or uterine cancer) should be particularly careful about using soy and should discuss it with their health care providers.

St.-John's-Wort
Uses: Short-term treatment of mild to moderate depression. Although some studies have reported benefits for more severe depression, others have not; for example, a large study sponsored by NCCIH found that the herb was no more effective than placebo in treating minor, moderate, or major depression.

Cautions: Can cause photosensitivity, particularly in fair-skinned individuals; contraindicated when other antidepressants are used. Other side effects include anxiety, dry mouth, dizziness, gastrointestinal symptoms, fatigue, headache, and sexual dysfunction. Can interact with antidepressants, birth control pills, cyclosporine, digoxin, indinavir (and possibly other drugs used to control human immunodeficiency virus [HIV] infection), irinotecan (and possibly other drugs used to treat cancer), seizure-control drugs (e.g., dilantin and phenobarbital), and warfarin and related anticoagulants.

Valerian
Use: Sedative, but there is not enough evidence from well-designed studies to confirm this effect. Safe to use for short periods (4 to 6 weeks).

Caution: Can have mild side effects, such as headaches, dizziness, upset stomach, and tiredness the morning after its use. Should not be used with barbiturates.

Homeopathy

Homeopathy is a branch of medicine developed in the late eighteenth century by Samuel Hahnemann. It was widely practiced in the United States until the early 1900s, when modern (i.e., conventional) medicine discredited it as being unscientific and ineffective. Homeopathy remained popular in other parts of the world, however, and has regained popularity in our country.

The origin of the word *homeopathy* helps in understanding this therapy. In Greek, the word *homos* means

---

BOX 11.3 Principles Underlying Homeopathy

Law of Similars

This law builds on the idea of prescribing remedies that produce symptoms similar to those of the illness being treated, the same principle on which vaccines are based. In homeopathy, a dilute preparation is made from a plant or other biologic material; the more dilute the preparation, the higher its potency. The solution is typically added to a sugar tablet or powder for oral use or to a lotion or ointment for external use.

Law of Minimum Dose

This law, also known as the *principle of dilutions,* states that the lower the dosage of the substance, the greater its effectiveness. In the preparation of homeopathic remedies, substances are diluted and shaken vigorously; a portion of that substance is then diluted and shaken. This procedure is repeated to the point that the final substance is so dilute that no molecules of the original plant or substance remain. This process, known as *potentiation,* is believed to transmit some form of information or energy from the original substance to the final diluted remedy. It is believed that the substance has left its imprint or "essence," which stimulates the body to heal itself (this theory is called the "memory of water").

Law of Cure

This is the principle used to evaluate the effectiveness of a remedy. If the treatment is successful, symptoms should travel from vital to less vital organs of the body, move from within the body outward, and disappear in reverse order of appearance. If symptoms do not follow this sequence, a new or additional treatment is used. In homeopathic medicine, a worsening of symptoms after a remedy is given is considered a positive sign that healing is taking place.

"similar," and *pathos* means "suffering." At the foundation of homeopathy are the laws of *similars,* the *minimum dose,* and *cure* (Box 11.3).

Although the reason for their effectiveness is not fully understood, homeopathic remedies have been shown to be effective for a variety of conditions. People use homeopathy for a range of health concerns, from wellness promotion and disease prevention to the treatment of diseases and conditions such as allergies, asthma, chronic fatigue syndrome, depression, digestive disorders, ear infections, headaches, and rashes (NCCIH, 2016b).

The ideal way to use homeopathic remedies is to have a homeopath prescribe a customized remedy based on individual characteristics and symptoms. However, homeopathic practitioners are not plentiful, so the next best thing is to buy over-the-counter preparations that are labeled for their intended purpose (e.g., arthritis, headache, hay fever, cold).

Hypnotherapy

Although the use of trance states for healing purposes dates back to primitive cultures, hypnotherapy was not approved as a valid medical treatment until the 1950s. This mind-body therapy is now widely and successfully used for a wide range of conditions, including chronic pain, migraines, asthma, smoking cessation, and irritable bowel syndrome.

In the process of hypnosis the therapist first guides the client into a relaxed state and then creates an image that focuses attention to the specific symptom or problem that needs to be improved. The client must be in a state of deep relaxation to be receptive to a posthypnotic suggestion. Most people are capable of being hypnotized if they are willing.

Imagery

Imagery, another mind-body intervention, is the process of creating a "picture" (image) in the mind that can cause a specific bodily response. Hypnosis also uses imagery, but in hypnosis an image and suggestion are presented to the person, whereas in imagery the person creates an image on his or her own. The process of imagery begins with the client establishing a desired outcome (e.g., to relieve stress, enhance circulation, reduce blood pressure). The nurse or other practitioner assists the client in creating an image that helps achieve the outcome (e.g., the nurse may describe how the blood circulates through the body, help the client develop an image of how cancer cells can be eliminated, or suggest that the client think of a peaceful place where cares can "melt away") and guides the client in reaching a relaxed state. As an alternative to having someone guide him or her through an imagery exercise, a client can learn the process from books or use commercially prepared audiotapes.

Imagery is not a difficult mind-body healing therapy to master and can be easily implemented in virtually every practice setting.

Magnet Therapy

Although a mainstream therapy in Germany and Japan, the use of magnets has only lately become popular in the United States. The most common uses of magnet therapy are for pain and wound healing.

The mechanism by which magnets work is not completely understood and is being investigated. It is believed that magnets relieve pain by creating a slight electrical current that stimulates the nervous system and consequently blocks nerve sensations. Magnets are hypothesized to speed wound healing by dilating vessels and increasing circulation to an area. Distributors of magnet products make additional claims about the health benefits of magnets, ranging from improving attention deficit disorder to boosting the immune system, although these benefits are yet to be proven.

Magnets come in a variety of forms, strengths, and prices: magnet disks that can be strapped to limbs, magnet mattresses that one can sleep on, and magnet jewelry. To be effective for therapeutic purposes, the magnet should have a strength of at least 500 gauss (which is about eight times stronger than the magnets used for attaching things to a refrigerator door).

Preliminary scientific studies of magnets for pain have produced mixed results (NCCIH, 2016c). Overall, there is no convincing scientific evidence to support claims that magnets can relieve pain of any type. Some studies, including an NIH clinical trial for back pain, suggest the possibility of a small benefit from using magnets for pain. However, the majority of rigorous studies have found no effect on pain. More research on magnets for pain is needed before any firm conclusion can be reached.

Persons with pacemakers should not use magnets, and because the effects of magnets on fetal growth are not fully understood, they should not be applied to the abdomen of a pregnant woman.

Massage, Bodywork, and Energy Therapies

Massage for healing purposes has been used for thousands of years to maintain health. Many people today receive regular massages as an important component of their self-care to aid in stress management. In addition to promoting relaxation, massage can be beneficial for reducing edema, promoting circulation and respirations, and relieving pain, anxiety, and depression.

A form of manipulative and body-based method, massage is the manipulation of soft tissue through rubbing, kneading, rolling, pressing, slapping, and tapping movements. The term *bodywork* is applied to the combination of massage with deep-tissue manipulation, movement awareness, and energy balancing. Touch therapies include techniques in which the hands of the nurse or therapist are near the body, in the client's energy field. Examples of various types of massage, bodywork, and touch therapies are described in Box 11.4.

BOX 11.4   Types of Massage, Bodywork, and Touch Therapies

Alexander Technique
Teaches improved balance, posture, and coordination by using gentle hands-on guidance and verbal instruction

Feldenkrais Method
Teaches movement re-education by using gentle manipulations to heighten awareness of the body; based on belief that each person has an individualized optimal style of movement

Healing Touch
A multilevel energy healing program that incorporates aspects of therapeutic touch with other healing measures

Reflexology
Application of pressure to pressure points on the hands and feet that correspond to various parts of the body

Reiki
A therapy that uses techniques to direct universal life energy to specific sites

Rolfing (Structural Integration)
Use of manual manipulation and stretching of body's fascial tissues to establish balance and symmetry

Swedish Massage
Most prevalent form of massage; uses long strokes, friction, and kneading of muscles

Trager Approach
Use of gentle, rhythmic rocking and touch to promote relaxation and energy flow

Because therapeutic touch (TT) is a popular alternative healing therapy among nurses, it deserves some discussion. TT, a form of energy therapy, became popular in nursing in the 1970s with the work and research of Delores Krieger (Krieger, 1979; Nurse Healers Professional Associates, 2017). Krieger advanced the theory that people are energy fields and that obstructed energy could be responsible for unhealthy states. She proposed that the nurse could draw on the universal field of energy and transfer this energy to the client. This incoming energy could help the client mobilize his or her own inner resources for healing and help unblock the client's obstructed energy.

In TT, there is little direct physical contact between the practitioner and the individual being treated. Rather, TT is an energy-based therapy; the nurse enters the client's energy field to assess and treat energy imbalances.

In the first step of TT, the nurse centers herself or himself and focuses on the intent to heal (this is sometimes referred to as *healing meditation*). During this phase, the nurse quiets his or her mind and prepares physically and psychologically to connect with the client. This is considered a crucial step in the process to enable the nurse to be fully present in the moment with the client. Then the nurse passes his or her hands over the client's body to assess the energy field and mobilize areas in which energy is blocked or sluggish by directing energies to that area. TT is used to reduce anxiety, relieve pain, and enhance immune function.

Healing touch (HT) is an energy therapy that is an offshoot of TT. It combines additional healing approaches to the basic ones of TT to open energy blockages, seal energy leaks, and rebalance the energy field. There is a six-level educational program for HT. The Healing Beyond Borders (formally Healing Touch International) website offers a full description of their program in addition to a bibliography of recent research related to this therapy (http://www.healingbeyondborders.org/).

Reiki is a practice in which the Reiki practitioner (of which there are several levels) channels energy to others using a series of hand positions. It is believed that healing energy flows through the hands without the need for any special skills. Like other forms of energy work, Reiki is believed to be useful for pain management, wound healing, stroke rehabilitation, and general relaxation; however, research is insufficient to suggest that Reiki is an effective treatment for any condition. Despite the limited research supporting its effectiveness (Lee et al, 2008), the low risk of side effects, affordability, and desire

of a person to utilize this therapy make an ethical case for its use (Ferraresi et al, 2013; NCCIH, 2017d).

With the use of healing energy therapies, nurses need to be aware that some individuals may feel spiritual distress if they receive healing energy because they may be concerned about what and who the source of the energy is. For example, a Christian who believes that healing comes directly from Jesus Christ may react negatively to receiving healing energy that is drawn from a vague universal force. Assessing the client's spiritual beliefs, explaining the therapy clearly, and obtaining consent before offering the treatment are useful.

Meditation and Progressive Relaxation

Meditation, a mind-body intervention that involves the act of focusing on the present moment, has been used for centuries throughout the world. This practice gained considerable attention in the United States in the 1970s when Harvard Medical School cardiologist Herbert Benson published research on the relaxation response (Benson et al, 1974). Benson and his associates reported that after 20 minutes of meditation, participants' heart rates, respirations, blood pressure, oxygen consumption, carbon dioxide production, and serum lactic acid levels decreased. This discovery led to the use of meditation for a variety of conditions, including stress, anxiety, pain, and high blood pressure.

Progressive relaxation is another exercise that shares some of the benefits of meditation. Typically a person learns to guide himself or herself through a series of exercises that relax the body, such as tightening and relaxing various muscle groups. Many CDs are available in bookstores and health food stores that offer scripts to guide meditation and progressive relaxation exercises.

Naturopathy

An intense interest in natural cures in Europe during the nineteenth century led to the development of spas that offered natural treatments to promote health and healing. Soon the movement spread to the United States, and in 1896 the American School of Naturopathy was founded. Naturopathic physicians and treatment facilities using natural cures became popular in the early part of the twentieth century. For example, John Kellogg ran such a facility in Battle Creek in which he subsequently became famous for the natural breakfast cereals that he used. As time progressed, medications and high-tech interventions caused naturopathy to pale by comparison; however, as consumers seek more natural approaches, this form of alternative medicine is making a comeback.

Naturopathy is based on the principle that the body has inherent healing abilities that can be stimulated to treat disease. Naturopathic physicians assess and treat the cause of the disease rather than merely alleviate symptoms. They help clients identify unhealthy practices, encourage healthy lifestyle habits, and guide them in managing health problems using natural approaches, such as herbs, homeopathic remedies, diet modifications, dietary supplements, and exercise.

There are a limited number of accredited schools of naturopathic medicine (e.g., Bastyr University, Southwest College of Naturopathic Medicine and Health Sciences, National University of Natural Medicine, and National University of Health Sciences). A handful of states license naturopaths and require that they graduate from an accredited program. However, there are many individuals practicing as naturopaths who have obtained their education and experience through other means or who practice in states that do not require licensure; thus learning about the credentials of a naturopath before receiving services is beneficial for clients.

Prayer and Faith

Many people consider their faith to be an integral part of their total being rather than a therapy, but now there is scientific evidence supporting the therapeutic benefits of faith and prayer in health and healing. Hundreds of well-conducted studies have revealed that people who profess a faith, pray, and attend religious services are generally healthier, live longer, have lower rates of disability, recover faster, have lower rates of emotional disorders, and otherwise enjoy better health states than those who do not (Barnum, 2010; O'Brien, 2017; Tuck and Anderson 2014; University of Maryland Medical Center, 2015). Not only do the faith and religious practices of individuals themselves affect health and healing, but research also supports the benefit of intercessory prayer.

Nurses need to appreciate that many people believe in the healing power of prayer and may expect their health care providers to join them in prayer if requested. This fact does not suggest that nurses or other health professionals should be forced into prayer if it is contrary to their beliefs; rather, if there is no objection from either party, prayer by the client and health care provider can be used as a valuable healing measure.

Tai Chi

Tai chi is another practice from traditional Chinese medicine used to stimulate the flow of *qi,* the life energy. It is a combination of exercise and energy work that looks like a slow, graceful dance using continuous, controlled movements of the arms and legs. There is a specific sequence of steps to follow in doing tai chi, but fortunately there are many inexpensive videos that can be used in addition to classes that are offered to aid people in learning this practice.

Tai chi has some demonstrated benefits, including reduced falls, improved coordination in older adults, and better function in persons with arthritis (Jahnke et al, 2010; NCCIH, 2017e; Yang et al, 2014). Many people find that tai chi helps reduce stress and promotes a general sense of well-being.

Yoga

Yoga has changed from a mystical form of Hindu worship practiced more than 5000 years ago to what is now known as a system of exercises involving various postures, meditation, and deep breathing. The word *yoga* means "union"; the union of body, mind, and spirit is achieved through yoga. Research suggests that yoga has many beneficial effects, such as reducing stress, improving mood and sense of well-being, decreasing heart rate and blood pressure, increasing lung capacity, improving flexibility, and promoting relaxation (NCCIH, 2017f). Yoga can be adapted to any level and capability so that it can be easily used.

Conclusion

There are many other alternative healing modalities, and new ones are appearing regularly. Some may be safe and effective but lack sufficient experience or clinical research to support their claims; others may be worthless and merely an attempt to sell a product or service. Discretion is crucial. Assistance in gaining objective information regarding CAM therapies can be obtained from the NCCIHAM website (http://www.nccih.nih.gov) or by calling 1-888-644-6226.

NURSING AND COMPLEMENTARY AND ALTERNATIVE MEDICINE THERAPIES

A Holistic Approach. The use of natural or "alternative" healing measures is hardly new to nursing. From Florence Nightingale (1860), who wrote about the importance of creating an environment in which natural healing could occur, through contemporary nurse theorists who discuss human and environmental energy fields (Hover-Kramer, 2012; Meleis, 2017; Rogers, 1975), nurses have long realized that healing quite effectively occurs in ways not encompassed within the conventional biomedical system. Nursing also has promoted many of the same principles evident in CAM, particularly care of the body, mind, and spirit. In fact, this is the essence of holistic nursing (Box 11.5). Nurses must ensure that the integration of CAM into their practice is done within a holistic paradigm to truly make them healing therapies and not merely disconnected procedures within an already fragmented health care system.

Facilitating Use of Complementary and Alternative Medicine

Nurses need to integrate CAM into their nursing practice. This integration begins during the assessment process

---

BOX 11.5 Beliefs Guiding Holistic Nursing Practice

- The uniqueness of each individual is honored.
- Health is a harmonious balance of body, mind, and spirit.
- The needs of individuals' bodies, minds, and spirits are assessed and addressed in the caregiving process.
- Health and disease are natural parts of the human experience.
- Disease is an opportunity for increased awareness of the interconnectedness of body, mind, and spirit.
- Individuals have the capacity for self-healing; the nurse facilitates this process.
- Nurses empower individuals for self-care.
- Individuals' cultural values, beliefs, and practices are honored and incorporated into the caregiving process.
- Individuals have a dynamic relationship with their environment; the environment is part of the healing process.
- Nurses, through their presence and being, are tools of the healing process.
- Nurses engage in self-care and an ongoing process of unfolding inner wisdom.

Nurses can learn about holistic nursing and network with holistic nurses through the American Holistic Nurses Association (AHNA) website (http://www.ahna.org).

---

when the nurse explores clients' use of CAM practices and products. Because it is not unusual for clients to use them without the knowledge of their physicians, nurses may be the first health professional with whom clients have discussed this issue. Factors to assess include the following:

- CAM practices and products being used and their sources
- Appropriateness of use of CAM practices and products
- Side effects and risks associated with use of CAM
- Conditions for which CAM currently is not used that could benefit by its use

Through the assessment process, nurses may identify the need to educate clients about the appropriateness of the CAM products and practices they are using. For example, a client with a pacemaker who uses magnets needs to be advised against continuing this practice; likewise, a client who drinks ginseng tea at bedtime requires an explanation that his insomnia may be the result of the stimulant effects of the herb. There may be situations in which nurses identify that specific conditions could benefit from the use of CAM therapies. As client advocates, nurses could bring this possibility to the attention of the physician and other members of the health care team and make recommendations accordingly.

Nurses traditionally have been responsible for the coordination of client care. As CAM therapies are integrated into conventional care, nurses are the logical professionals to oversee the various parts and ensure that they are working in harmony for the client's benefit.

Nurses can learn to use many alternative healing measures to enhance nursing care. Among these are acupressure, aromatherapy, biofeedback, imagery, massage, and therapeutic touch. Nurses should seek whatever additional education and training are required to gain competency in these therapies and ensure compliance with state licensing laws.

Integrating Complementary and Alternative Medicine into Conventional Settings

Nurses can demonstrate leadership in helping conventional clinical settings integrate CAM therapies. In fact, nursing's holistic orientation and traditional coordination responsibilities make nurses logical for this role. Case Study 11.1 describes how one nurse accomplished this task.

CASE STUDY 11.1

Becky Blake, RN, recently joined the nursing staff in a combined coronary care and step-down unit. It did not take her long to note the expert technical skill of her colleagues, who could read monitors in a flash and respond to emergencies without missing a beat. The skill, efficiency, and organization of the nursing staff were evidenced by the lack of medication errors, infections, and pressure ulcers, coupled with the shortest length of stays of comparable hospital units in the area.

Yet there seemed to be something missing. Clients and their families often showed signs of anxiety and fear that were not addressed. Familiar faces reappeared as some clients were re-admitted because they failed to alter lifestyle habits that contributed to their conditions. The same nursing staff who cared for people with hearts damaged by the effects of smoking, poor diet, and stress were guilty of the same unhealthy practices themselves.

It came to a head for Ms. Blake one morning when she was at a bedside changing an intravenous bag and checking equipment. The client, a man in his fifties, pulled at her arm, looked Ms. Blake in the eyes, and tearfully said, "How do you think I'm going to do? I've been awake all night wondering if I'll be able to do my job, take care of my wife, see my grandkids grow up, do the things I like to do." For the first time, Ms. Blake saw beyond the body in the bed to a human being experiencing considerable emotional distress—distress that was hardly beneficial to his condition. "We have managed to get this man's heart repaired," she thought, "but we have not begun to help him heal the emotional and spiritual pain that this illness created." This began a journey for Ms. Blake of discovering measures to help clients that went beyond the conventional treatments that were regularly prescribed.

Ms. Blake found a local network of holistic nurses and began attending their meetings. Through this group, she learned of the difference between healing and curing and the importance of addressing the needs of body, mind, and spirit. She also heard nurses discussing their own need to be nurtured and committed to positive self-care practices. She met nurses who shared how they were using alternative healing practices and who led her to resources from which she could learn more.

In the months that followed, Ms. Blake attended several workshops and learned how progressive relaxation, meditation, therapeutic touch, and aromatherapy could be used to benefit the clients on her unit. As her understanding of holism grew, she recognized that stress reduction and improved health habits for her coworkers were sorely needed.

After planting seeds through informal discussions and sharing of articles, Ms. Blake requested a formal meeting with the interdisciplinary team on the unit. In this meeting, she described her areas of concern, which included the need to:

- Address clients' emotional and spiritual needs more effectively.
- Promote improved health habits of the staff.
- Develop practices that would reduce stress for clients, their families, and staff.

The staff concurred with these needs and expressed a desire to take actions to address them. Ms. Blake offered some suggestions:

- Coordinate with the staff development instructor to have classes offered on progressive relaxation, imagery, meditation, therapeutic touch, and stress reduction.
- Form an ad hoc committee to develop guidelines, policies, and procedures on how these healing therapies could be safely and legally implemented.
- Begin to include healing therapies into care plans.
- Arrange for the nutritionist to offer classes to staff on healthy eating.
- Add healthy snacks to the break room.
- Coordinate with the housekeeping and maintenance departments to introduce aromatherapy diffusers, plants, and piped-in music in the unit.
- Develop a system to remind staff to use stress reduction measures throughout their shift.
- Collaborate with the nutritionist, social worker, spiritual care counselor, and nursing clinical resources to provide group sessions for clients and their families on topics such as coping with illness, stress management, and promoting healthy lifestyle habits.
- Request that the quality improvement coordinator monitor and evaluate the effect of these interventions.

It did not take long for the effects of these new approaches to be realized. Clients requested fewer sedatives and analgesics. Surveys of clients and families revealed higher levels of satisfaction. Staff sick days were reduced, and there seemed to be a greater sense of team spirit and cooperation. Soon staff in other parts of the hospital began requesting that similar interventions be implemented in their units.

Using Complementary and Alternative Medicine Competently

As increasing numbers of consumers and clinical settings are interested in or actually using CAM therapies, nurses are challenged to become knowledgeable about the uses, limitations, and precautions associated with these new practices and products. Maintaining a resource library and becoming familiar with websites to stay current are beneficial measures.

Nurses must become familiar with cultural factors that can influence acceptance and use of alternative healing practices. For instance, some individuals may object to energy therapies (e.g., TT, HT) on the grounds that they associate them with occult practices, or they may have anxiety about meditation because they believe evil spirits could invade their minds. As comforting as a massage can be, some people who come from cultures that believe it is inappropriate to touch a person of the opposite sex could become distressed by this measure. Knowledge and sensitivity to personal and cultural preferences are essential.

Legal Considerations

The use of CAM could present some legal issues for which nurses need to be concerned. As growing numbers of practitioners of healing therapies advocate for recognition and separate licensure, some of the healing therapies once considered part of nursing care may require such separate licensure. Such is the case with massage. In some states, nurses may not provide a massage unless they are licensed as massage therapists. Acupressure and biofeedback are among the other areas in which the nurse could be challenged if using them without a license. Nurses need to clarify the therapies that fall within the realm of nursing practice and take a proactive role in ensuring that other disciplines do not attempt to limit them.

Another legal concern for nurses in the growing arena of CAM is the question of to whom the nurse is responsible when practicing CAM therapies. New, nonconventional practice settings are developing. For example, a nurse may be employed in a setting in which there is an acupuncturist, hypnotherapist, and homeopath. Some questions that could arise include: Who supervises the nurse? Can these therapists delegate responsibilities to the nurse? How does the nurse ensure that in such a practice setting diagnoses are not being made or treatments being prescribed that are beyond the scope of the CAM practitioners? Nurses need to begin to consider the implications of new practice models and to develop clear practice guidelines that ensure a legally sound practice.

SUMMARY

An opportunity exists for nursing to demonstrate leadership in the integration of CAM with conventional care. Representing the largest number of health care professionals, nurses can have a significant effect on implementing CAM throughout the health care system. Nurses' historical holistic orientation to care enables them to ensure that the integration of CAM and conventional services is done in a manner that addresses the client's body, mind, and spirit. Without such coordinated efforts, there is the risk that these new therapies will merely be additional ingredients in an already fragmented system of care. Nurses have shown that they can coordinate and promote comprehensive care like practitioners of no other discipline. Therefore, nursing is the logical discipline to be the hub of the wheel of integrative services.

REFERENCES

Altizer, K. P., Nguyen, H. T., Neiberg, R. H., Quandt, S. A., Grzywacz, J. G., Lang, W., et al. (2014). Relationship between nonprescribed therapy use for illness prevention and health promotion and health-related quality of life. *Journal of Applied Gerontology, 33*(4), 456–473.

American Society of Anesthesiologists Task Force on Chronic Pain Management. (2010). Practice guidelines for chronic pain management: an updated report by the American Society of Anesthesiologists Task Force on Chronic Pain Management and the American Society of Regional Anesthesia and Pain Medicine. *Anesthesiology, 112*(4), 810–833.

Barnum, B. (2010). *Spirituality in nursing* (3rd ed.). New York: Springer.

Benson, H., Beary, J. F., & Carol, M. P. (1974). The relaxation response. *Psychiatry, 37*(1), 37–46.

Consumer Reports. (2012). Vitamins and supplements: 10 dangers that may surprise you. *Consumer Reports, 77*(9), 18–23.

Ferraresi, M., Clari, R., Banino, E., Boero, E., Crosio, A., Dayne, R., et al. (2013). Reiki and related therapies in the dialysis ward: an evidence-based and ethical discussion to debate if these complementary and alternative medicines are welcomed or banned. *BMC Nephrology, 14*, 129. Retrieved from http://www.biomedcentral.com/1471-2369/14/129.

Guallar, E., Stranges, S., Mulrow, C., Appel, L. J., & Miller, E. R. (2013). Enough is enough: Stop wasting money on vitamin and mineral supplements. *Annals of Internal Medicine, 159*(12), 850–851.

Harvard School of Public Health. (2017). *Antioxidants: Beyond the hype*. Retrieved from http://www.hsph.harvard.edu/nutritionsource/antioxidants/.

Hillinger, M. G., Wolever, R. Q., McKernan, L. C., & Elam, R. (2017). Integrative medicine for the treatment of persistent pain. *Primary Care, 44*(2), 247–264.

Hover-Kramer D. (2012). *Healing touch: Essential energy medicine for yourself and others*. Boulder CO: Sounds True.

Jahnke, R., Larkey, L., Rogers, C., Etnier, J., & Lin, F. (2010). A comprehensive review of health benefits of qigong and tai chi. *American Journal of Health Promotion, 24*(6), e1–e25.

Kennedy, A. (2017). *Herbal Medicine: Natural Remedies*. Berkeley CA: Althea Press.

Koog, Y. H., Lee, J. S., Wi, H. (2014, April 25). Clinically meaningful nocebo effect occurs in acupuncture treatment: A systematic review. *Journal of Clinical Epidemiology (Online), 67*(8), 858–869. http://www.jclinepi.com/article/S0895-4356(14)00089-4/abstract.

Krieger, D. (1979). *The therapeutic touch*. Englewood Cliffs, NJ: Prentice Hall.

Lee, M. S., Pittler, M. H., & Ernst, E. (2008). Effects of reiki in clinical practice: a systematic review of randomized clinical trials. *International Journal of Clinical Practice, 62*(6), 947–954.

Liang, Y. D., Li, Y., Zhao, J., Wang, X. Y., Zhu, H. Z., & Chen, X. H. (2017). Study of acupuncture for low back pain in recent 20 years: A bibliometric analysis via CiteSpace. *Journal of Pain Research, 10*(4), 951–964.

Meleis, A. I. (2017). *Theoretical nursing: Development and progress* (6th ed.). Philadelphia: Lippincott.

Nahin, R. L., Barnes, P. M., & Stussman, B. J. (2016). Expenditures on Complementary Health Approaches: United Status. *National Health Statistics Reports, No. 95*. Hyattsville, MD: National Center for Health Statistics.

National Center for Complementary and Integrative Health. (2016a). *The use of complementary and alternative medicine in the United States*. Retrieved from https://nccih.nih.gov/research/statistics/2007/camsurvey_fs1.htm.

National Center for Complementary and Integrative Health. (2016b). *Homeopathy: An introduction*. Retrieved from https://nccih.nih.gov/health/homeopathy.

National Center for Complementary and Integrative Health. (2016c). *Magnets for pain*. http://nccih.nih.gov/health/magnet/magnetsforpain.htm.

National Center for Complementary and Integrative Health. (2017d). *Reiki*. Retrieved from https://nccih.nih.gov/health/reiki/introduction.htm#hed3.

National Center for Complementary and Integrative Health. (2017e). *Tai chi*. Retrieved from https://nccih.nih.gov/health/taichi/introduction.htm.

National Center for Complementary and Integrative Health. (2017f). *Yoga for health*. Retrieved from https://nccih.nih.gov/health/yoga/introduction.htm.

Nightingale, F. (1860). *Notes on nursing*. London: Harrison.

Nurse Healers Professional Associates. (2017). *TT facts*. Retrieved from http://therapeutic-touch.org/int-contacts/tt-facts/.

O'Brien, M. E. (2017). *Spirituality in nursing: Standing on holy ground* (6th ed.). Sudbury, MA: Jones & Bartlett.

PDR Staff. (2013). *PDR for Nonprescription Drugs, Dietary Supplements, and Herbs* (34th ed.). Houston, TX: PDR Network.

Pharmaceutical Press Editorial. (2013). *Herbal Medicines* (4th ed.). Gurnee, IL: Pharmaceutical Press.

Rogers, M. (1975). *An introduction to the theoretical basis for nursing* (3rd ed.). Philadelphia: FA Davis.

Tuck, I., & Anderson, L. (2014). Forgiveness, flourishing, and resilience: the influence of expressions of spirituality on mental health recovery. *Issues in Mental Health Nursing, 35*(4), 277–282.

University of Maryland Medical Center. (2015). *Spirituality*. Retrieved from http://www.umm.edu/altmed/articles/spirituality-000360.htm.

Yang, G., Wang, L., Zhang, Y., Liu, J. (2014). Clinical research evidence of tai chi: a systematic literature review. *The Journal of Alternative and Complementary Medicine, 20*(5), A62–A70.

ADDITIONAL RESOURCES

Ali A, Scoulios N, Ten N, Kanodia A. (2014). A national assessment of the usage, cost, and reimbursement of unconventional medical laboratory tests, *Journal of Alternative and Complementary Medicine, 20*(5): A3–A4.

Bauml, J., Xie, S., Farrar, J., Bruner, D., Stricker, C., Bowman, M., et al. (2014). Expectancy in real and sham acupuncture: does believing make it so? *The Journal of Alternative and Complementary Medicine, 20*(5), A9.

Caspi, O., & Baranovitch, O. (2009). When science meets medical tradition: what is needed for a dialogue on integrate medicine? *Journal of Alternative and Complementary Medicine, 15*(5), 579–583.

Cayleff, S. E. (2016). *Nature's Path: A history of naturopathic healing in America.* Baltimore: Johns Hopkins University Press.

Chen, Y. W., Hunt, M. A., Campbell, K. L., Peill, K. & Reid, W. D. (2015). The effect of Tai Chi on four chronic conditions—cancer, osteoarthritis, heart failure and chronic obstructive pulmonary disease: a systematic review and meta-analysis. *British Journal of Sports Medicine, 50*(7), 397–407. Retrieved from http://bjsm.bmj.com/content/early/2015/09/04/bjsports-2014-094388.short?g=w_bjsm_ahead_tab.

Easley, T., & Home, S. H. (2016). *The modern herbal dispensatory: A medicine-making guide.* Berkeley, CA: North Atlantic Books.

Elder, C. R. (2013). Integrating naturopathy: can we move forward? *The Permanente Journal, 17*(4), 80–83.

Eliopoulos, C. (2018). *Invitation to holistic health: A guide to living a balanced life* (4th ed.). Boston: Jones & Bartlett.

Fontaine, K. L. (2014). *Complementary & alternative therapies for nursing practice* (4th ed.). Upper Saddle River, NJ: Prentice Hall.

Griffith, C. (2016). *The comprehensive repertory for the new homeopathic remedies: A guide to strategic prescribing.* New York: Penguin Random House.

Kabat-Zinn, J. (2006). *Coming to our senses: Healing ourselves and the world through mindfulness.* New York: Hyperion.

Kotsirilos, V., Vietta, L., & Sali, A. (2011). *A guide to evidence-based integrative and complementary medicine.* New York: Churchill Livingstone.

Lee Yue-Wei, D. (2016). *Methods and advances in traditional Chinese medicine.* Philadelphia: Elsevier.

Lim, C. Y., Takano, A., Yang, S., & Lee, P. (2014). Ayurvedic medicine and the lung. *Respiration, 87*(5), 428–431.

Micozzi, M. S. (2015). *Fundamentals of complementary and alternative medicine* (5th ed.). St Louis: Saunders.

National Center for Complementary and Integrative Health. *Herbs at a glance.* Retrieved from https://nccih.nih.gov/health/herbsataglance.htm.

National Academy of Science. (2016). *Dietary reference intakes (DRIs).* Retrieved from https://fnic.nal.usda.gov/dietary-guidance/dri-nutrient-reports/guiding-principles-nutrition-labeling-and-fortification.

Patz, S. (2014). Holistic assessment person centered care. *Beginnings, 34*(1), 10–11.

Perez, M. A., Pinzon-Perez, H. (2016). *Complementary, alternative, and integrative health: A multicultural perspective.* San Francisco: Jossey-Bass.

Pursell, J. J. (2015). *The herbal apothecary: 100 medicinal herbs and how to use them.* Portland, OR: Timber Press.

Rhyner, H. H. (2016). *Llewellyn's complete book of Ayurveda: A comprehensive resource for the understanding & practice of traditional Indian medicine.* Woodbury, MN: Llewellyn Worldwide.

Schiller, C., & Schiller, D. (2013). *The aromatherapy encyclopedia.* Laguna Beach, CA: Basic Health Publications.

Selin, H. (Ed.), (2010). *Medicine across cultures: History and practice of medicine in non-Western cultures (Science across cultures: The history of non-Western science),* Norwell, MA: Kluwer.

Smith, G. (2017). *Complementary and alternative medicine for nurses and allied health professionals: A guide to the evidence and clinical applications.* New York: Routledge.

Stengler, M., Balch, J., Balch, R. Y. (2016). *Prescription for natural cures: a self-care guide for treating health problems with natural remedies including diet, nutrition, supplements, and other holistic methods* (3rd ed.). Hoboken, NJ: Wiley.

Sublett, C. M. (2014). Adding to the evidence base: streamlining biofeedback for urge incontinence. *Urol Nursing, 34*(1), 27–28.

12

Palliative Care

Jeri Ashley, MSN, RN, AOCNS, CHPN,
Patricia R. Keene, DNP, ACNP-BC, ACHPN

Palliative care: A team concept.

ⓔ Additional resources are available online at: *http://evolve.elsevier.com/Cherry/*

LEARNING OUTCOMES

After studying this chapter, the reader will be able to:

1. Describe the palliative care model and its effectiveness today.
2. Summarize the key elements and issues of palliative care.
3. Integrate palliative care knowledge and skills into the professional nursing role.

KEY TERMS

Advance care plan This is a <u>process</u> of examining one's thoughts and feelings about what gives one's life value. By determining what gives value to one's life, one is then able to determine the goals for their health care. For example, watching and understanding a 6 year old grandchild's baseball game could be a strong value for an elderly grandfather. This requires that the man have ears that can hear and a brain that can understand. Should this same patient have a catastrophic stroke and in light of his cited value, he would choose to not have his life artificially prolonged but rather to die in the comfort of his home with hospice care. This is an example of the <u>process</u> that a patient might go through to determine health care goals. Further, the advance care plan consists of two parts: the advance directive documenting decisions made for the future and listing the decision-makers who will decide for the patient if the patient is unable to do so.

Advance directive A <u>document</u> in which a person with decision-making capacity gives permission about future medical care and/or designates the person to make decisions for him/her if decision-making capacity is impaired or lost.

Decision-making capacity The ability of one to make decisions about their health care. They must be able to understand the facts, to appreciate the alternatives that may exist, and to communicate these decisions to the health care team.

Disease trajectory The decline that is seen as a particular disease progresses.

Double effect In the care of seriously ill and dying patients, the intent of any treatment is to relieve pain and suffering—not to hasten the patient's death; however, the patient's death is a foreseeable potential effect of the treatment. An example would be escalating doses of morphine to relieve a patient's pain with the double effect of depressing respirations, resulting in death.

End-of-Life Nursing Education Consortium (ELNEC) A national project funded by the Robert Wood Johnson Foundation.

Hospice care This is not only a type of care but also a philosophy of care that focuses on comfort for the patient and family at the end of life.

Informed consent Permission given by a patient or caregiver to treat a medical condition with understanding of the risks/benefits of a medical procedure, costs that may accrue, and alternative therapies.

Interprofessional team A group of professionals who work together to provide comprehensive care to the patient/family.

Palliative care Care that seeks to improve the quality of life of patients who are facing serious illness.

Patient Self-Determination Act (PSDA) A federal law that requires health care institutions to give patients a copy of their decision-making rights, determine whether patients have advance directives, and assist them in completing them. The PSDA promotes patients making their own decisions about the health care they want to receive or refuse.

Prognostication A physician's prediction about the course and outcome of a disease, often made with consideration of survival, symptoms, function, and quality of life with or without treatment.

PROFESSIONAL/ETHICAL ISSUE

Mrs. P. is an 85-year-old widowed female admitted to the hospital with end-stage Parkinson's disease, which was diagnosed 5 years ago. Her family reports that she has had three falls in the past 2 weeks and during the past 6 months has lost 20 pounds. The weight loss is more than 10% of her body weight. She scores 40% on the Palliative Performance Scale and was recently diagnosed with right lower lobe pneumonia. The family states that she is having difficulty communicating her needs and is having dysphagia. It was thought that her recent pneumonia was secondary to aspiration. Two of her daughters want to start enteral feedings via a percutaneous endoscopic gastrostomy tube. When asked about **advance directives**, the family reports that she does not have any. A third daughter indicates that she would not want artificial nutrition and that they had talked about it. The first two daughters are concerned that she would starve to death.

As the RN on the **palliative care** team, what steps will you take to help the family come to consensus about whether to provide artificial nutrition?

Schwarz and Tarzian (2009) demonstrate a method of analyzing situations that are ethically challenging (Table 12.1).

VIGNETTE

Christine Glover is a 32-year-old divorced female who has been undergoing aggressive cancer chemotherapy for 4 years. Her physician has just informed her that her disease continues to spread in spite of these therapies. He tells her that there are two primary options: a Phase I clinical trial and hospice care. She longs to see her young children settled in with her parents before she dies, but she suffers with constant pain and intermittent nausea, and gravitates between anxiety and deep periods of depression, which she hides as best as she can from her family. She struggles between the two options of care, but doesn't know what questions to ask related to treatment. How does she tell her children? How does she prepare her parents for the role of parenting their grandchildren? How can she prepare herself for what lies ahead? She feels the depression enveloping her again.

Questions to Consider While Reading this Chapter:

1. What patient experiences have you had related to serious illness?
2. What do you think is important to include in serious illness/end-of-life discussions?
3. Have you considered how you would like to live during serious illness?
4. Have you completed your advance directive?
5. How can nursing research affect end-of-life care?

CHAPTER OVERVIEW

Someone should tell us, right at the start of our lives that we are dying. Then we might live life to the limit, every minute of every day. Do it! I say. Whatever you want to do, do it now! There are only so many tomorrows.

Pope Paul VI, 1897-1978

Palliative care is one of the newest subspecialties. The focus of palliative care is to give comfort to patients with serious illness. It can begin with the diagnosis of a serious illness and continue to the death of the patient, followed by continued support of the family. The purpose of this chapter is to describe the benefits, barriers, and challenges of palliative care as well as to discuss the role of the palliative care nurse.

TABLE 12.1   Steps to Analyze Situations Seen as Ethically Challenging and to Explore the Context in Which These Situations Have Risen

Steps to Analyze Ethically Challenging Situations	Context of the Situation
1. Review the overall situation—identify what is going on in this case. 2. Identify the ethical dilemma(s).	1. Mrs. P. has a disease that is end stage (Parkinson's disease). 2. Mrs. P. no longer has capacity and is nonverbal. There are no advance directives. Daughters are in disagreement regarding mother's wishes for health care.
3. Gather all relevant facts: • Significant medical and social history • Involved family • Decision-making capacity • Existence of advance directives—written, appointed, or verbal—and any pertinent institutional policies • Surrogate or health care agent if **decision-making capacity** is absent	3. The patient has a history of decline starting 4 years earlier, culminating to her present state. She does not have decision-making capacity. She did tell one daughter that she did not want a feeding tube.
4. Identify the parties or stakeholders involved in the situation, including those who will be affected by the decision(s) made.	4. Stakeholders include the patient and three daughters.
5. Identify relevant legal data, including both state and federal laws.	5. There is no relevant legal data.
6. Identify religious or cultural issues.	6. No religious or cultural belief sidentified.
7. Identify specific conflicts of ethical principles or values. Identify and consider nursing guidelines and the profession's code and position statements.	7. Ethical principles involved are: autonomy, beneficence, maleficence, and double effect.
8. Identify possible options, their purpose, and their probable consequences to the welfare of the patient. Identify and make use of interdisciplinary and institutional resources, including ethics committee, social workers, chaplains, and other experienced colleagues.	8. Options include feeding tube placement, artificial hydration. Risks of providing artificial nutrition and hydration (ANH) include aspiration, third spacing of fluids, diarrhea/constipation.
9. Identify practical constraints, including institutional, legal, organizational, and economic.	9. The team recognized patient is unable to participate in the decision-making process. The daughters reported that they wanted what was best for their mother.
10. Review and evaluate the situation after action has been taken—debrief and support the staff.	10. The decision was made not to start fluids or place a feeding tube. The patient was offered food and fluids orally until she was unable to swallow. She was allowed to die a natural death.

From Schwarz, J. K., & Tarzian, A. J. (2010). Ethical aspects of palliative care. In Matzo, M., & Witt Sherman, D. W. (Eds.), *Palliative care nursing: Quality care to the end of life* (pp. 119-141). New York: Springer Publishing Company.

INTRODUCTION

The world of health care is constantly changing; yet for Western health care, the growth and advancement of new and innovative treatments are mind-boggling. And with these new therapies comes an increasing emphasis on care and rehabilitation of those with serious illness. Today, we live longer; by 2030 20% of the American population will be more than 65 years of age (Meier et al, 2010).

Palliative care was coined by Dr. Balfour Mount in 1974. It comes from the Latin root word *pallium,* which referred to an outer garment that cloaked a person. This derivation suggests that palliative care "covers" or "cloaks" the symptoms of serious illness, providing comfort and relief. Palliative care recognizes the same needs, stressors, symptoms, and suffering that a hospice patient might endure but supports and enhances the best quality of life during the time of diagnosis, treatment, and life with serious illness.

The World Health Organization defined palliative care in 1990:

Palliative care is an approach that improves the quality of life of patients and their families facing the problem associated with life-threatening illness, through the prevention and relief of suffering by means of early identification and impeccable assessment and treatment of pain and other problems, physical, psychosocial and spiritual (Sepúlveda et al, 2002).

The Hospice and Palliative Nurses Association (HPNA) has developed standards of practice for registered nurses. HPNA defines a palliative nurse as one who:

- Provides age-appropriate culturally, ethically, and spiritually sensitive care and support.
- Maintains a safe environment.
- Educates patients/families to identify appropriate settings and treatment options.
- Ensures continuity of care and safe transitions to the next appropriate setting.
- Coordinates care across settings and among caregivers.
- Manages information and protects confidentiality.
- Communicates promptly and effectively.

However, nurses must recognize the need for palliative care in all settings and in all specialties. Stjernswärd and colleagues (2007) recognize that palliative care should be seen as a public health issue and as such all health care clinicians would do well to become palliative care generalists. As stated in the American Nurses Association (ANA) *Code of Ethics for Nurses,* "Nursing care is directed toward meeting the comprehensive needs of patients and their families across the continuum of care. This is particularly vital in the care of patients and their families at the end of life to prevent and relieve the cascade of symptoms of suffering that are commonly associated with dying" (ANA, 2015).

THE NATURAL COURSE OF SERIOUS ILLNESS

As a patient's health declines, decisions about care must be made. With the initial diagnosis, palliative care can help guide therapy. With disease progression to an end-stage condition, hospice is an option of care. Prior to palliative care, the care model showed disease progression and then death. The palliative care continuum model of care (Figure 12.1) begins comfort care at the time of diagnosis: Early in the disease process therapies are aggressive, but as the disease progresses comfort care increases. Included in this model is the introduction of hospice care and bereavement services.

As patient decline occurs, palliative care or hospice care becomes the focus. Frequently the terms are used synonymously, which is incorrect because they differ. Both offer comfort care to the patient with serious illness, but in hospice care the disease is considered end stage with progression to death. Finestone and Inderwies (2008) discuss the benefits of hospice, one of which is to support both the patient and family. Support includes

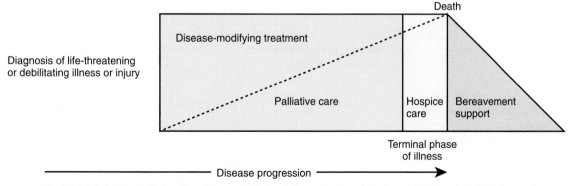

Fig. 12.1 Model for Palliative Care. (From *A National Framework and Preferred Practices for Palliative and Hospice Care Quality: A Consensus Report,* by the National Quality Forum, 2006, Washington, DC. Copyright [2006] © National Quality Forum.)

physical assistance but also emotional, psychologic, and spiritual support. Hospice is underutilized by much of the population, and this lack of use can be due to cultural beliefs, lack of understanding, fear, or decreased availability. Table 12.2 compares hospice and palliative care services.

Prognostication

Patients with serious illness question the time they have until death. Predicting a patient's death is not a simple task. Research shows that when physicians prognosticate, they are optimistic in predicting survival by up to as much as 300% (von Gunten, 2014). Physicians are faced with the task of telling a patient that their time to live is limited. This is difficult not only because of medical complexity but also because emotions come into play when there has been a patient-physician relationship. The disease process is distinguished by its severity and ability to be cured. Laboratory and diagnostic findings help to track the progress of the disease—is it improving or getting worse? Current functional status of the patient, including a history of falls, can be helpful for predicting as well. When functional status is examined, cognitive ability and the ability to perform activities of daily living are reviewed (Downing, 2011).

A number of tools are used to help with prognostication. The Palliative Performance Scale (PPS) (Table 12.3) and the Karnofsky Scale (Table 12.4) are two such tools.

TABLE 12.2   Comparison of Hospice and Palliative Care Services

Component	Palliative Care	Hospice
Focus of Care	To address the specific needs of patients and families experiencing serious illness	To address the specific needs of the dying patient and their family including bereavement services
Onset of Care	Begins at the time of diagnosis of a serious illness	Begins with a prognosis of 6 months or less
Medicare Benefit	Physicians (MDs) and nurse practitioners may bill	Yes
Beneficiary Entitled to Levels of Care	No specific levels of care	Yes Routine home care, respite care, general inpatient care, continuous care
Settings Where Care Delivered	All inpatient settings, outpatient, private practice, home care	Home, nursing home, residential, hospice, inpatient (on designated unit or designated beds)
Interprofessional Team Approach	Yes	Yes
Supplies and Symptom Management Medications Covered	No	Yes
Therapies Limited	No Palliative care is delivered with aggressive treatment and therapies.	Yes Therapies with significant burden but that may prolong life are restricted.
Quality Components Include Safety, Timeliness, Patient-Centered Care, Beneficial/Effective Care, Equity, and Efficiency	Yes	Yes
Expertise on Pain and Symptom Management	Yes	Yes
Appropriate at Any Age	Yes	Yes
Effective Initiation of Life Planning	Most effective	Effective if discussions occur prior to hospice or if earlier referrals to hospice

TABLE 12.3 Palliative Performance Scale

%	Ambulation	Evidence of Disease	Self-Care	Intake	Level of Consciousness
100	Full	Normal No disease	Full	Normal	Full
90	Full	Normal Some disease	Full	Normal	Full
80	Full	Normal with effort Some disease	Full	Normal or reduced	Full
70	Reduced	Can't do normal job or work Some disease	Full	As above	Full
60	Reduced	Can't do hobbies or housework Significant disease	Occasional assis- tance needed	As above	Full or confusion
50	Mainly sit/lie	Can't do any work Extensive disease	Considerable assis- tance needed	As above	Full or confusion
40	Mainly in bed	As above	Mainly assistance	As above	Full or drowsy or confusion
30	Bedbound	As above	Total care	Reduced	As above
20	Bedbound	As above	As above	Minimal	As above
10	Bedbound	As above	As above	Mouth care only	Drowsy or coma
0	Death	—	—	—	—

From Anderson, F., Downing, G. M., Hill, J., et al. (1996). Palliative performance scale (PPS): a new tool. *J Palliat Care, 12*(1):6. Copyright: Institut universitaire de gériatrie de Montréal.

TABLE 12.4 Karnofsky Performance Status Scale

Score	Criteria	Definitions
100	Normal, no complaints, no evidence of disease	Able to carry on normal activity and to work, no special care needed
90	Able to carry on normal activity, minor symptoms	
80	Normal activity with some symptoms	
70	Cares for self, unable to carry on normal activities	Unable to work; able to live at home and care for most personal needs; various degrees of assistance needed
60	Requires occasional assistance, cares for most needs	
50	Requires considerable assistance and frequent care	
40	Disabled, requires special care and assistance	Unable to care for self; requires equivalent of institutional or hospital care; disease may be progressing rapidly
30	Severely disabled; hospitalized but death not imminent	
20	Very sick; active supportive care needed	
10	Moribund; fatal processes are progressing rapidly	
0	Death	

From Callin, S. E., & Bennett, M. I. (2009). Assessment of mobility. In Walsh, T. D., Caraceni, A., Fainsinger, R., et al (Eds.), *Palliative medicine*. Philadelphia: Saunders.

The PPS is a more general tool that identifies functional decline and scores it. Scores are an indication about disease progression to death. The Karnofsky Scale is more appropriate for the patient with a cancer diagnosis.

It is helpful to compare the patient's status at 12 months, 6 months, and 1 month previously as well as the current status. The patient's ability to perform activities of daily living, a change in appetite, weight loss, anorexia/cachexia, and/or dysphagia all help paint the picture of serious illness with decline. Laboratory findings and diagnostic test results can also help validate the presence of serious illness. For example, by examination of laboratory data, one is able to assess the extent of organ decline.

After the nurse has gathered the objective and subjective data, a meeting with the patient and family is imperative. With *family* being defined by the patient, a family conference is invaluable. A group meeting allows everyone to hear the same thing at the same time from the health care provider. There is less room for misinterpretation as information is presented at a level understood by the patient and family. There must be time for questions. Information given must be realistic but should not take away hope.

There are different types of hope: hope for a cure; hope for more time; hope for no pain; hope for a good death. Physicians may shy away from specific time frames. What is helpful is if the patient/family can understand the "usual course of the illness." Some disease states follow a more predictable pattern—for example, metastatic cancer. Deaths due to heart failure, emphysema, or dementia, however, are not as easily predicted. With these disease states, it is helpful to review with the patient and family the decline that has already occurred. Plotting it on paper shows the decline and makes it more real. This discussion of prognostication does not end with one meeting but is ongoing as the disease progresses toward the end of life. Additionally, education is ongoing throughout the disease process for the patient and family.

Two Roads to Death. Ferris and colleagues (2003) describe two roads to death: the usual road and the difficult road. The usual road is what most would describe as a peaceful death, in which the patient begins sleeping more and being less and less responsive. He or she progresses to a comatose state and dies. Caregivers describe the death as peaceful and comfortable.

The difficult road, on the other hand, is one of restlessness with increased confusion and frequently with hallucinations. To avoid the difficult death, health care providers must view not only the physical aspects of patient care but also the emotional, spiritual, and psychosocial aspects. Physical pain can be medicated; however, emotional/spiritual pain is complicated and medications cannot always erase it. Health care providers must be open to listening and encouraging the patient to deal with difficult issues while able to do so.

When death occurs, it can be verified by the absence of heartbeat and respirations, fixed and dilated pupils, and absence of the corneal reflex. Other signs that are seen include a change in skin color and temperature. Frequently, eyes do not close completely and the jaw may remain open. Urine and stool may also be expelled. Depending on the setting, the patient is pronounced deceased by a nurse or physician.

Criteria for Palliative Care

For most institutions, a physician's order is required for hospice/palliative care services. Patients can be referred on admission as well as during their hospital stays. On admission, patients who have had multiple hospitalizations over a relatively short time for the same condition (e.g., heart failure, urinary tract infection, sepsis) should be considered. Things that may trigger a palliative care consult include (Weissman and Meier, 2011):

- Receiving a positive response when asking oneself the "surprise" question: "Would I be surprised if this patient died within 6 months to a year?"
- Patients who are receiving multifaceted care such as ventilator support, parenteral feedings, and assistance with functional needs
- A patient's place of residence in a long-term care facility (e.g., nursing home)
- The age of the patient
- Cognitive impairment
- Metastatic cancer
- Current or past enrollment in hospice care
- A patient who has not participated in advance care planning

Throughout a hospital stay, other triggers can indicate the need for a palliative care consult. These triggers may include the patient's desire to change health care providers, patient or family request for palliative care, and dissension about therapy/treatments being offered. Other triggers are a prolonged stay in the intensive care unit and symptoms that have not been controlled. Palliative care can assist with decisions about long-term use of feeding tubes, need for tracheostomy, dialysis, placement of a left ventricular assist device or automatic implanted cardioverter-defibrillator (AICD), and other life-prolonging therapies.

Palliative care can assist patients and their families with decision making regarding goals of care. For example, the initial intent of therapy may have been cure, but the disease was found to be widespread. The focus could then change to comfort. The patient may hear "There is nothing more we can do," but there is always care to be provided. It is the focus of the care that changes: the quality of time may now be the focus rather than the quantity.

Hospice Services

The term *hospice,* derived from the word "hospitality," can be traced back to medieval times, when it referred to a place of shelter and rest for weary or ill travelers on a long journey. The name was first applied to specialized care for dying patients by physician Dame Cicely Saunders, who began her work with the terminally ill in 1948 and eventually went on to create the first modern hospice—St. Christopher's Hospice—in London. She was also responsible for coining the term "total pain" to describe the full experience of physical, emotional, spiritual, and social distress and suffering of many hospice patients.

Saunders introduced the idea of specialized care for the dying to the United States in a lecture at Yale University. Her lecture on holistic hospice care launched a chain of events that resulted in the development of hospice care in the United States. This chain of events was spearheaded by Florence Wald, MS, RN, a former dean of Yale University School of Nursing.

Definition and Criteria for Hospice

Considered the model for quality, compassionate care at the end of life, hospice care involves a team-oriented approach of expert medical care focused on symptom management and is expressly tailored to the patient's wishes. Support is also extended to the family and loved ones. Generally, this care is provided in a number of settings. Medicare, private health insurance, and Medicaid in most states cover hospice care for patients. A patient is deemed an appropriate candidate for hospice care if he or she has a terminal diagnosis—that is, the patient has been assessed according to disease factors defined by

Medicare that determine a person's eligibility for hospice care. Example's of these factors include a patient's ability to breathe or patient's refusal of dialysis.

Hospice recognizes that the dying process is a part of the normal process of living and focuses on enhancing the quality of remaining life. Hospice affirms life and neither hastens nor works to postpone death. The hospice team is interdisciplinary and develops a care plan that meets each patient's individual needs for pain management and symptom control. Team members include the same disciplines as those for palliative care. Included in hospice responsibilities are managing the patient's pain and symptoms, assisting the patient with the emotional and psychosocial and spiritual aspects of dying, providing needed drugs, medical supplies, and equipment, coaching the family on caring for the patient as well as addressing family distress and suffering.

KEY ELEMENTS OF PALLIATIVE CARE

Eight Elements of End-of-Life Nursing Education Consortium

The End-of-Life Nursing Education Consortium (ELNEC) is a project started in February 2002 by Bettye Ferrell at City of Hope with a grant from the Robert Wood Johnson Foundation. The ELNEC core curriculum identifies eight modules: nursing care at the end of life, pain management, symptom management, ethical/legal issues, cultural considerations, communication, loss/grief/bereavement, and final hours. The goal of this project was to improve palliative care. Now there are ELNEC curricula for pediatrics, critical care, oncology, veterans, geriatrics, and advanced practice nursing. The newest model is integrating palliative oncology care into the Doctor of Nursing Practice. The ELNEC program went international in May 2008, again with the goal of educating nurses (http://www.aacn.nche.edu/ELNEC).

The Eight Domains of the National Consensus Project

The National Consensus Project (NCP) for Quality Palliative Care, which began in 2001, is a task force of organizations that strives to improve palliative care. The organizations involved are: American Academy of Hospice and Palliative Medicine (AAHPM), Center to Advance Palliative Care (CAPC), Hospice and Palliative Care Nurses Association, and National Hospice and Palliative Care Organization (NHPCO). NCP identifies eight practice domains for palliative care to follow:

- *Domain 1: Structure and Processes of Care.* This domain describes the use of the interprofessional team to work together assessing and planning care with patients and families.
- *Domain 2: Physical Aspects of Care.* This domain emphasizes the use of validated tools for assessment and the treatment of physical symptoms.
- *Domain 3: Psychological and Psychiatric Aspects of Care.* This domain stresses the need to address assessment and treatment of psychiatric concerns and diagnoses. Included also in this domain are the requirements of a bereavement program.
- *Domain 4: Social Aspects of Care.* This domain's focus emphasizes engaging patients and families in the patient's care and taking advantage of their strengths. The team social worker begins this process.
- *Domain 5: Spiritual, Religious, and Existential Aspects of Care.* This domain focuses on involving the chaplain in the plan of care throughout the disease trajectory. Spiritual and religious practices are encouraged as a means to obtain comfort.
- *Domain 6: Cultural Aspects of Care.* This domain focuses on the inclusion of cultural aspects when providing care and holds that the interprofessional team should be culturally competent.
- *Domain 7: Care of the Patient at the End of Life.* This domain emphasizes communication and physical signs and symptoms of the dying process. Again the patient/families/interprofessional team should be involved with scrupulous assessment and management of pain and other symptoms. Ongoing education for families about the dying process is of utmost importance.
- *Domain 8: Ethical and Legal Aspects of Care.* This domain addresses advance care planning and ethical/legal aspects. Advance care planning is seen as something that is ongoing and may change throughout the disease course. This domain reaffirms that ethical issues are common and must be addressed. The identification of complex legal and regulatory issues of palliative care is also addressed in this domain. (For more information, see https:// www.nationalcoalitionhpc.org/ncp-guidelines-2013/.)

BENEFITS OF PALLIATIVE CARE

Palliative care can be viewed as both a model of care and a philosophy of serving our patients. It is built of multiple components as expressed in the ELNEC's curriculum (ELNEC, 2013).

- The family is the unit of care and the patient defines family.
- The role of the nurse as an advocate is vital to the care of patients and their families.
- Culture is honored as an important aspect of the patient/family.
- Palliative care further carries an important focus to special populations such as the vulnerable, the prisoner, and the substance abuser.
- Serious illness affects all systems of care. Put another way: Where there are patients, there are patients who are suffering needlessly.
- Sensitivity to the reality of financial issues that affect quality of life is critical.
- Palliative care is not confined to just those with cancer and acquired immunodeficiency syndrome (AIDS), but to those with all life-threatening illnesses.
- The interprofessional care of the patient/family is integral to high quality palliative care.

To understand the benefits of palliative care, one must grasp the depth and breadth of symptoms, stress, and suffering of serious illness. This section examines a broad overview of these concepts; however, the reader is encouraged to continue to pursue more in-depth knowledge.

The numbers speak for themselves. We now live in a time of unprecedented numbers of older Americans who are living with chronic illnesses. In 2010, there were 403 million people 65 years or older, 12 times the number in 1900 (U.S. Census Bureau, 2014). Additionally, a baby born in the United States today can expect to live to 78 years old (U.S. Census Bureau, 2014). And with this longer lifespan comes an expectation that all illnesses can be treated, as many successes in public health and medical care have shown (Meier et al, 2010). However, "the sheer numbers of the elderly with chronic disability means an unprecedented number will experience prolonged functional dependency and frailty" (Meier et al, 2010). Approximately 57% of Americans 80 years and older report a severe disability (Meier et al, 2010). Individuals with five or more chronic illnesses account for 66% of

Medicare spending and are the largest consumers of health care (Meier et al, 2010).

Technology offers the ability to prolong life but does not consistently restore life to its former level of quality. Many Americans live with one or more chronic illnesses. And although these persons are living longer, many suffer from these illnesses that limit their lives (Meier et al, 2010). Furthermore, degenerative diseases have replaced communicable disease as the leading causes of death in the United States. Today, 54% of Americans die in acute care facilities surrounded by strangers and suffer from prolonged chronic illnesses and, in many cases, receiving futile treatment that may result in financial burden for the family (Grant and Dy, 2012).

The stress, symptoms, and suffering experienced in chronic illness by both the patient and the family also exact a tremendous burden. In 1995, the SUPPORT (Study to Understand Prognoses and Preferences for Outcomes and Risks of Treatment) study "demonstrated a lack of communication between patients, families, and health care providers about goals of care, a significant pain burden in seriously ill patients, and discrepancies between patient preferences for care and the aggressive care received" (SUPPORT Principal Investigators, 1995). This study became the impetus for increasing research and education in palliative care at the end of life.

Pain and Symptom Management

Pain and symptom management and communication are commonly recognized aspects of quality care for persons with serious illness. Dr. Nathan Cherny (2010) best delineates the impact of unrelieved pain in his description related to cancer:

> Unrelieved pain is incapacitating and precludes a satisfying quality of life; it interferes with functioning and social interaction, and is strongly associated with heightened psychological distress. It can provoke or exacerbate existential distress, disturb normal processes of coping and adjustment, and augment a sense of vulnerability contributing to a preoccupation with the potential for catastrophic outcomes. Persistent pain interferes with the ability to eat, sleep, think, interact with others, and is correlated with fatigue in cancer patients.

In palliative care, the prevalence of pain varies by diagnoses and demographics (Smith et al, 2010). And the fear of unrelieved pain expressed by patients and families is often reflective of what they have experienced (American Geriatrics Society, 2009). The experience of pain for the individual patient has multiple dimensions and includes such factors as the meaning of pain, knowledge of pain and pain management, expectation and goals of pain management, cultural beliefs, and the support received from family and others.

Pain is further complicated by the presence of other symptoms that can occur during serious illness: dyspnea, insomnia, constipation, nausea and vomiting, anxiety, depression, delirium, and fatigue. These symptoms seriously affect quality of life and may limit functional activity to the detriment of the patient's overall well-being. Through comprehensive assessment and manageent of patient and family, palliative care is able to improve quality of life as evidenced by these benefits:

- Relief of suffering
- Optimization of function
- Promotion of healing and comfort
- Fostering of appropriate hope
- Genuine coordination of care at times of transitions between health care providers
- Providing opportunity and assistance in exploring and preparing for hospice care as appropriate.

Suffering

In 1982, Dr. Eric Cassel published one of the earliest articles on suffering to enter the medical literature, and it opened discussions about suffering for professionals. In this article, he defines suffering as "a state of severe distress associated with events that threaten the intactness of a person" (Cassel, 1982). Suffering is the experience of a person, whereas pain and other symptoms are the result of physical body or organ changes. Suffering and pain can coexist together, although one can be present without the other. However, "the transition from pain to suffering can occur when pain is unrelieved and out of control or when the source of pain is unknown. The persistence of pain and uncertainty therefore can increase suffering" (Matzo and Sherman, 2015).

Relieving a patient's and family's suffering is central to the work of palliative care. Spiritual and existential distress is prevalent but also goes under-recognized in the hospice and palliative care populations (Pulchalski et al, 2009). Excellent pain and symptom management becomes the foundation for relief of suffering because active symptomatology can dominate a patient's life. However, once physical symptoms are resolved or controlled, spiritual assessment can reveal areas of loss, such as loss of hope, loss of meaning, loss of value, or loss of relationships (Quill et al, 2010). Once this suffering is discovered, practical strategies including counseling are methods to relieve it.

Family Caregiving

Family caregivers also benefit from palliative care services. The National Alliance for Caregiving defines a family caregiver as "someone who is responsible for attending to the daily needs of another person. He or she is responsible for the physical, emotional, and often financial support of another person who is unable to care for himself or herself due to illness, injury or disability" (National Alliance for Caregiving, 2013). The average period of caregiving is 4.6 years, with 31% of caregivers involved in caregiving for longer than 5 years. Weekly, the average time of caregiving is 20.4 hours, with females providing more caregiving time than males (National Alliance for Caregiving in Collaboration with AARP, 2009). The stresses of caregiving are multifactorial, including compassion fatigue with neglect of their own needs and health (Family Caregiver Alliance, 2006), role changes with stress (Dumont et al, 2008; Herbert et al, 2009), and the development of depression and other emotional complications (Family Caregiver Alliance, 2006). Matzo and Sherman (2015) define four general areas where strategies can successfully affect caregiving:

1. Setting realistic goals
2. Having difficult discussions
3. Finding help
4. Negotiating expectations

These strategies begin with a comprehensive family assessment, including an assessment of family strengths and weaknesses.

BARRIERS TO PALLIATIVE CARE

Four significant barriers form the basis for the growth and progress of palliative care for the future. First is the lack of a general understanding on the part health care professionals as well as the consumers of the role and nature of palliative care. With that strong linkage, patients and families and often health care providers believe "it's just not time yet," that is, "I'm not dying yet." The lack of recognition of the true nature of palliative care

prevents patients and families from obtaining the care they need to address needs of the whole person. Further, the lack of recognition of the negative impact of a disease condition on the whole person results in distress—physical, social, psychologic, and spiritual. The denial of death in our American culture also affects the lack of acceptance of palliative care. Woody Allen has been quoted as saying, "I don't want to achieve immortality through my work. I want to achieve it by not dying." The combination of this "stigma of death with widely held beliefs that modern medicine and hospitals can perform miracles in the battle against death" has meant that "hospitals and nursing homes have become the dominant site for gravely ill, dying people" (Meier, et al, 2010) with more than 70% of deaths in the United States occurring in an institution (Meier et al, 2010).

The second barrier to the growth and progress of palliative care is the limited numbers of palliative care–trained professionals. Although there has been remarkable growth of palliative care programs which has continued to the present, "these numbers have not matched the number of trained clinicians to lead and staff these programs" (Meier et al, 2010). As Meier and colleagues (2010) further report, "A number of strategies have been employed to improve medical and nursing education in palliative care, including the pursuit of subspecialty status for palliative medicine and nursing advocacy for changes in undergraduate and graduate accreditation standards; and numerous philanthropically funded efforts to train mid-career physicians and nurses."

The third barrier to palliative care growth and progress is the question, "How is palliative care paid for?" Although palliative care providers do bill Medicare and other payers for the care they deliver, the reimbursement is for time-intensive care and not procedural services. This reimbursement fails to cover the salaries of the professionals, much less the overhead expenses for running a business. As a result, the growth in hospital palliative care services has been financed "not by fee-for-service reimbursement to hospitals and providers but rather by hospitals operating budgets" (Meier et al, 2010). But first, these hospitals and their administrators must be persuaded of the value during economic times of decreased reimbursement. R. Sean Morrison and colleagues analyzed administrative data from eight hospitals with established palliative care teams from 2002 to 2004 and matched their patients with patients receiving usual care. "The palliative care patients who were discharged alive had an adjusted net savings of $1696 in direct costs per admission and $279 in indirect costs per day including significant reductions in laboratory and intensive care unit costs compared with usual care patients" (Morrison et al, 2008).

Communication is the fourth barrier, and it is a vital part of patient care; however, at the end of life it can be detrimental if poorly done. Patients and their families deserve appropriate information to help them make difficult decisions. As patients and families face serious illness, conversations must be kept simple. Trying to tell everything is overwhelming. Unfortunately, health care providers have not been educated in the delivery of difficult news.

COMMON CHALLENGES

Providing quality palliative care is not perfect and there are struggles. Giving up their independence can be devastating for patients as they decline. In a qualitative study, Smucker and colleagues (2014) described safety concerns from 17 hospices in 13 states. Hospice workers described harm from falls and uncontrolled symptoms, especially pain. Some of the factors identified as contributing to the safety issues included patients who were living alone and/or cognitively impaired, caregivers who were cognitively impaired, and caregivers with their own physical limitations. These barriers related to patient safety and independence need to be addressed.

Another common challenge is treating the patient for the family's sake. Families may want intravenous fluids, antibiotics, and other therapies. It is not easy helping them understand that these can be more of a burden than help and may hasten death. Frequently, the family/caregiver is not considering the best interest of the patient during decision making.

Withholding or withdrawing food and fluids or treatments is a challenge for palliative care providers. Withholding and withdrawing have both ethical and legal components. The principle of autonomy comes into play, and the individual ultimately has the right to refuse or accept a therapy. Ideally, the patients should speak for themselves, but unfortunately they may not be able to. Advance directives, if present, can speak for patients and their wishes. When therapies are considered, a time frame should also be discussed and the question asked, "Will the therapy be time sustaining or life prolonging?"

Families view food and fluids as an essential. They fear the patient will starve to death when food or fluids are withheld or not started. In truth, patients frequently stop eating gradually as they age or their disease progresses. Patients say "I'm not hungry" or "Food just doesn't taste good anymore." Families fear that their loved one is being starved by the health care provider. It is the progression of the disease that has caused decreased intake of food and fluids. Health care providers do not withhold nutrition from those patients who still want to eat. The introduction of artificial nutrition is just that: artificial! It is helpful to discuss the benefits and burdens of intravenous fluids and feeding tubes and the purpose of these therapies. Although both serve a useful purpose in the acute care setting for individuals whose prognosis is good, they are a burden for an individual who has a terminal illness. Historically, prior to the advent of intravenous therapy or tube feedings, patients ate and drank as long as they were able. When feeding became a burden, families continued to care for them, offering food and fluids, but not forcing them. The patient was allowed to die naturally. Further, it has not been found that artificial feedings prevent aspiration or improve wound healing (McDonald and Lesage, 2006).

PROFESSIONAL ISSUES IN PALLIATIVE CARE

The HPNA's *Scope and Standards of Practice* identifies the following specific areas of expertise for hospice and palliative care nurses (Dahlin and Glass, 2007):

1. Clinical judgment
2. Advocacy and ethics
3. Professionalism
4. Collaboration
5. Systems thinking
6. Cultural competence
7. Facilitator of learning
8. Communication

Certification

Currently, there are three levels of certification for the palliative care nurse. At the generalist level is the CHPN designation—certified hospice palliative nurse; for the palliative nurse administrator is the CHPA—certified hospice palliative administrator. The hospice palliative advanced practice nurse usually has specialty training or certification in palliative care. The advanced level certification is the ACHPN—advanced certified hospice palliative nurse.

At the institutional level, palliative care programs can now achieve recognition for high-quality palliative care through The Joint Commission. This voluntary certification is based on the National Consensus Project for Quality Care and the National Quality Forum's National Framework and Preferred Practices for Hospice and Palliative Care.

Quality Assessment and Improvement

The National Hospice and Palliative Care Organization is a hospice and palliative care national organization committed to social change for the care of patients at the end of life. As part of their mission, they are committed to the improvement of multiple areas of quality, including patient-centered measures related to management of pain within 48 hours of admission, avoiding unwanted hospitalizations, avoiding unwanted cardio-pulmonary resuscitation (CPR), and patient safety. In the area of bereavement, a survey has been designed to evaluate bereavement service and is completed by family members or primary caregivers. A post-death survey is completed by family members of hospice patients regarding their perceptions about the quality of the care given to their loved ones at end of life. Lastly, a staff job satisfaction survey has been designed specifically for hospice field staff.

The Center to Advance Palliative care is the nation's leading resource for palliative care program development. It provides multiple learning opportunities to assist health care institutions in building hospital programs from strategic planning, to funding, to operations, and sustainability. CAPC is a national organization dedicated to increasing the availability of quality palliative care service for people facing serious, complex illness. They have multiple references and resources available, including information on quality assessment and improvement.

Research

Research in palliative care is lacking, in part because it is a relatively new subspecialty but also because palliative researchers are faced with numerous ethical quandaries (Chen et al, 2014). Palliative care research must meet the same rigor as other disciplines, and barriers can include lack of funding, lack of staff, and lack of trained researchers. Obtaining subjects can also be a barrier, especially when patients/families as well as health care providers have poor understanding of palliative care. Because patients have life-limiting diseases, they may die before a study can be completed.

Ethical Concerns

Ethical challenges arise when the ethically appropriate course of action or range of choices is unclear, or when there are competing ethical claims that may not be reconcilable (Berlinger et al, 2013). For purposes of this chapter, the following four areas will be briefly examined: advance care planning, double effect, palliative sedation, and medically futile care.

Advance Care Planning. In December 1991, all hospitals, nursing facilities, hospice programs, and health maintenance organizations that serve Medicare or Medicaid patients were mandated to provide new patients with written information describing their rights under state law to make decisions about medical care, including their right of execute a living will or durable power of attorney for health care (Berlinger et al, 2013). This was the Patient Self-Determination Act (PSDA) of 1991. The living will or advance directive outlines one's decisions for health care for when one is unable to speak or decide. These documents were intended to foster communication between the doctor and the patient and at the same time, respect the patient's right to autonomy. Ethical dilemmas can arise because an advance directive "requires a person to predict accurately the final illness and what medical interventions might be available to postpone death and living wills require physicians to make decisions on the basis of their interpretation of the document, rather than a discussion of treatment options with a person acting on behalf of the patient" (Meier et al, 2010). The suggested solution now in practice is for the patient to appoint a health care agent or decision maker who can speak on the patient's behalf with detailed knowledge of his or her health care wishes.

Double Effect. Day to day, nurses face issues related to beneficence and nonmaleficence, or doing no harm. This principle becomes particularly important with seriously ill or dying patients who are often in a weakened condition, frail, frightened, and vulnerable. Nurses often become distressed when being requested to give opioid therapy to an actively dying patient.

Although these medications are intended to relieve pain and symptoms such as dyspnea, they also have a foreseeable risk of hastening death by respiratory depression.

Nash and Nelson (2012) have explained that according to the rule of double effect, an action with two possible effects—one good and one bad—is ethically acceptable if these four conditions are satisfied:

- The good effect has to be intended and therefore is not morally wrong.
- The bad effect is not intended but can be foreseen; that is, causing respiratory depression can result in death.
- The bad effect cannot be the means to the good effect. In this example, pain relief is not achieved by ending a patient's life.
- The symptom must be severe enough to warrant taking risks; that is, administering this dose at this time is needed to relieve the pain.

Palliative Sedation. At times in palliative care and particularly in patients receiving hospice care, patients present with intolerable symptoms that cannot be controlled by standard methods of pain management. Examples of symptoms that become intolerable are dyspnea, pain, and delirium with agitation. To appropriately manage these symptoms, palliative sedation can be considered. *Palliative sedation* is the use of sedating medications to relieve refractory or intolerable symptoms when other pharmacologic measures have failed. The education and informed consent discussion with the patient and/or the patient's decision maker includes the purpose of therapy, the expected outcomes, and how the patient and symptoms will be monitored. In consideration of the stress that family members are under during episodes of palliative sedation, continuing education and explanation of the patient's condition and status are important. Further, nursing and the interdisciplinary team require around-the-clock monitoring to ensure that symptoms are controlled, that limited numbers of breakthrough episodes are occurring, and that the need for increased medications are identified promptly.

Medically Futile Care. A medically futile treatment is a treatment option that offers no possibility of physiologic benefit related to diagnosis, prognosis, or the current medical condition. Ethically, a physician is not obligated to provide such a treatment; however, the physician should be aware of any state laws relevant to these decisions.

When decisions of medical futility are being made, a patient/family meeting is a critical strategy to ensure that all pertinent parties are involved in the decision-making process. These relevant parties include the physician, the patient and/or decision maker, the family, and members of the interdisciplinary team. Often, members of the hospital-based ethics committee are also involved.

The first step is to establish common ground of mutual understanding of the patient's condition. In this process the members of the interdisciplinary team ask open-ended questions of the patient/family to clarify that information is indeed understood. Once common ground is established, the next step is to determine and verbalize the patient's/family's goals and expectations of treatment. Then the physician explains the treatment options and, in the case of futile treatments, explains why a treatment cannot provide benefit. Lastly, the team clarifies the questions and misconceptions; and once these are clarified to the satisfaction of the patient/family, an explicit statement of the medical plan of action is made for everyone present to hear.

LEGAL CONCERN: RIGHT TO REFUSE TREATMENT

"The right to refuse is the belief that medical care is optional for adults with appropriate capacity" (Berlinger et al, 2013). The landmark cases of Quinlan and Cruzan and others have established that patients have a legal right to refuse life-sustaining medical treatment.

In April 1975, 21-year-old Karen Ann Quinlan suffered an anoxic brain injury. Her medical care included a tracheostomy, artificial ventilation, and a feeding tube with artificial nutrition and hydration. Her condition was later diagnosed as persistent vegetative state, at which time her father sought to be appointed by the courts as her legal guardian so that he could discontinue the respirator that assisted her breathing. Karen's physician refused to do so because this choice was not in accordance with medical standards of the day. After years and multiple court battles, the ventilator was removed, and she died several years later of an infection. The outcome of this woman's experience was the endorsement by the legal system of the use of hospital ethics committees to review decisions to withdraw life-sustaining treatments.

The second young woman to affect decisions to refuse medical treatment was Nancy Cruzan. She was 25 years old in January of 1983 when she was seriously injured in a motor vehicle accident. She was treated to restore her breathing and heartbeat both at the accident site and en route to the hospital, and she was admitted in a coma. A gastrostomy tube was inserted with her husband's permission. She was diagnosed as being in a persistent vegetative state.

Over time, her parents requested that the artificial nutrition and hydration be discontinued, but the hospital refused to do so without a court order. Once more, a series of court interventions were sought, including involvement of the U.S. Supreme Court. The legal outcome of this series of legal events was that the court stated that "incompetent patients need certain protections given when they cannot exercise their right of refusal"; therefore, it was appropriate at the state level "to impose additional safeguards in the form of the clear and convincing evidence standard in light of its interest in preserving life" (Nash and Nelson, 2012).

After this decision, the Cruzan family petitioned the state court in Missouri to grant the request to discontinue the artificial nutrition and hydration. The discontinuation was approved, and Nancy Cruzan died shortly thereafter. This case affects us today through the increased interest in advance care planning and health care decision makers and also "generated support for the Patient Self-Determination Act" of 1991 (Nash and Nelson, 2012).

SUMMARY

You matter because you are you, and you matter to the end of your life. We will do all we can not only to help you die peacefully, but also to live until you die.

Dame Cicely Saunders, 1918-2005; nurse, social worker, physician, founder of modern-day hospice

With the advancement of medical therapies comes the task of deciding when enough is enough. New therapies and devices are seen as a means of extending life by both the medical profession and patients. Unfortunately, this extension of life does not always carry with it quality of life. Difficult decisions arise when the disease has taken over. Health care providers must help patients and their families with these decisions as they face them or as they progress toward death, and comfort and quality of life must be the priority.

REFERENCES

American Geriatrics Society. (2009). American geriatric society clinical practice guidelines: pharmacological management of persistent pain in older persons. *Journal of the American Geriatric Society, 57*(8), 1331–1346.

American Nurses Association. (2015). *Code of ethics for nurses with interpretive statements.* Retrieved from http://www.nursingworld.org/MainMenuCategories/EthicsStandards/CodeofEthicsforNurses/Code-of-Ethics-For-Nurses.html.

Berlinger, N., Jennings, B., & Wolf, S. M. (2013). *The hasting center guidelines for decisions on life-sustaining treatment and care near end of life* (2nd ed.). New York: Oxford University Press.

Callin, S. E., & Bennett, M. I. (2009). Assessment of mobility. In T. D. Walsh, A. Caraceni, & R. Fainsinger (Eds.), *Palliative medicine.* Philadelphia: Saunders.

Cassel, E. J. (1982). The nature of suffering and the goals of medicine. *New England Journal of Medicine, 306*(11), 639–645.

Chen, E. K., Riffin, C., Reid, M. C., Adelman, R., Warmington, M., Mehta, S. S., et al. (2014). Why is high-quality research on palliative care so hard to do? Barrier to improved research from a survey of palliative care researchers. *Journal of Palliative Medicine, 17*(7), 782–787.

Cherny, N. I. (2010). Pain Assessment and cancer pain syndromes. In G. Hanks, N. I. Cherny, & N. A. Christakis (Eds.), *Oxford textbook of palliative medicine.* New York: Oxford University Press.

Dahlin, C., & Glass, E. (2007). *Hospice and palliative nursing: scope and standards of practice.* Silver Spring, Maryland: Hospice and Palliative Nurses Association and American Nurses Association.

Downing, C. M. (2011). "Who knows" 10 steps to better prognostication. In L. Emanuel, & S. L. Librach (Eds.), *Palliative care: Core skills and clinical competencies.* St. Louis: Saunders.

Dumont, I., Dumont, S., & Mongeau, S. (2008). End of life care and the grieving process: family caregivers who have experienced the loss of a terminal phase cancer patient. *Qualitative Health Research*, *18*(8), 1049–1061.

End-of-Life Nursing Education Consortium. (2013). *Core curriculum*. Retrieved from http://www.aacn.nche.edu/ELNEC.

Family Caregiver Alliance. (2006). *Caregiver assessment: principles, guidelines, and strategies for change, Report from a Consensus Development Conference* (Vol. I). Family Caregiver Alliance. Retrieved from http://www.caregiver.org/caregiver/jsp/content/pdfs/vl_consensus.pdf.

Ferris, F. D., von Gunten, C. F., & Emanuel, L. L. (2003). Competency in end-of-life care: last hours of life. *Journal of Palliative Medicine*, *6*(4), 605–613.

Finestone, A. J., & Inderwies, G. (2008). Death and dying in the US: the barrier to the benefits of palliative and hospice care. *Clinical Interventions in Aging*, *3*(3), 595–599.

Grant, M., & Dy, S. L. (2012). *UNIPAC #1: The hospice and palliative care approach to serious illness* (4th ed.). Glenview, Illinois: American Academy of Hospice Palliative Medicine.

Herbert, R. S., Schulz, R., Copeland, V. C., & Arnold, R. M. (2009). Preparing family caregivers for death and bereavement: insights from caregivers of terminally ill patients. *Journal of Pain and Symptom Management*, *37*(1), 3–12.

Matzo, M., & Sherman, D. W. (Eds.) (2015). *Palliative care nursing: Quality care at the end of life* (3rd ed.). New York: Springer Publishing Company.

McDonald, A., & Lesage, P. (2006). Palliative management of pressure ulcers and malignant wounds in patients with advanced illness. *Journal of Palliative Medicine*, *9*(2), 285–296.

Meier, D. E., Isaacs, S. L., & Hughes, R. G. (2010). *Palliative care: Transforming the care of serious illness* (3rd ed.). San Francisco: Jossey-Bass.

Morrison, R. S., Penrod, J. D., & Cassel, J. B., Caust-Ellenbogen, M., Litke, A., Spragens, L., et al. (2008). Cost savings associated with US hospital palliative care consultation programs. *Archives of Internal Medicine*, *168*(16), 1783–1790.

Nash, R. R., & Nelson, L. J. (2012). *Ethical and legal issues*. Glenview, Illinois: American Academy of Hospice and Palliative Medicine.

National Alliance for Caregiving in Collaboration with AARP. (2009). *Caregiving in the US*. Retrieved from http://www.caregiving.org/pdf/research/caregiving USAllAgesExecSum.pdf.

National Alliance for Caregiving. (2013). Care for the family caregiver: A place to start. Retrieved from http://www.caregiving.org/data/emblem_cfC10_Final12.pdf.

National Consensus Project for Quality Palliative Care. (2009). *Clinical practice guidelines for quality palliative care*. Retrieved from http://NationalConsensusProject.org.

National Consensus Project for Palliative Care. Retrieved from http://www.nationalconsensusproject.orgon. July 15, 2014.

National Quality Forum. (2006). *A national framework and preferred practices for palliative and hospice care quality: a consensus report*. Retrieved from http://www.qualityforum.org/Publications/2006/12/A_National_Framework_and_Preferred_Practices_for_Palliative_and_Hospice_Care_Quality.aspx.

Puchalski, C., Ferrell, B., Virani, R., Otis-Green, S., Baird, P., & Bull, J., et al. (2009). Improving the quality of spiritual care as a dimension of palliative care: the report of a consensus conference. *Journal of Palliative Medicine*, *12*, 885–904.

Quill, T. E., Holloway, R. G., Shah, M. S., et al. (2010). *Primer of palliative medicine* (5th ed.). Glenview, Illinois: American Academy of Hospice and Palliative Medicine.

Schwarz, J. K., & Tarzian, A. J. (2010). Ethical aspects of palliative care. In M. Matzo, & D. W. Sherman (Eds.), *Palliative care nursing: Quality care to the end of life*. New York: Springer Publishing Company.

Sepúlveda, C., Marlin, A., Yoshida, T., & Ullrich, A. (2002). Palliative care: the world health organization's global perspective. *Journal of Pain and Symptom Management*, *24*(2), 91–96.

Stjernswärd, J., Foley, K. M., & Ferris, F. D. (2007). The public health strategy for palliative care. *Journal of Pain and Symptom Management*, *33*(5), 486–493.

Smith, A. K., Cenzer, I. S., Knight, S. J., Puntillo, K. A., Widera, E., Williams, B. A., et al. (2010). The epidemiology of pain during the last 2 years of life. *Annals of Internal Medicine*, *153*(9), 563–569.

Smucker, D. R., Regan, S., Elder, N. C., & Gerrety, E. (2014). Patient safety incidents in home hospice care: the experiences of hospice interdisciplinary team members. *Journal of Palliative Medicine*, *17*(5), 540–544.

SUPPORT Principal Investigators. (1995). A controlled trial to improve care for the seriously ill hospitalized patients: the study to understand prognoses and preferences for outcomes and risks of treatment. *Journal of the American Medical Association*, *274*(20), 1591–1598.

U.S. Census Bureau. (2014). *65+ in the United States: 2010*. Washington, DC: US Government Printing Office.

von Gunten, C. F. (2014). Prognosis: how long do we wait for the doctor? *Journal of Palliative Medicine*, *7*(6), 634–635.

Weissman, D. E., & Meier, D. E. (2011). Identifying patients in need of a palliative care assessment in the hospital setting: a consensus report from the center to advance palliative care. *Journal of Palliative Medicine*, *14*(1), 17–23.

Wilner, L. S., & Arnold, R. (2014, November 12). *The palliative performance scale. Fast facts and concepts*. Retrieved from http://www.eperc.mcw.edu/EPERC/FastFactsIndex/ff_125.htm. http://www.mypcnow.org/#!fast-facts/c6xb

13

Workforce Advocacy for a Professional Nursing Practice Environment

Mary Jo Assi, DNP, RN, NEA-BC, FNP-BC, FAAN,
Cheryl Peterson, MSN, RN, Debra D. Hatmaker, PhD, RN, FAAN

A changing workplace requires nurses to embrace workforce advocacy to ensure quality care delivery and a healthy work environment.

ⓔ Additional resources are available online at: *http://evolve.elsevier.com/Cherry/*

LEARNING OUTCOMES

After studying this chapter, the reader will be able to:

1. Identify issues that affect the practice of professional nursing in the health care workplace.
2. Identify available resources to assist in improving the workplace environment.
3. Define the role of nurses in advocating for safe and effective workplace environments.
4. Describe workforce strategies that support efficient and effective quality patient care, and promote improved work environments for nurses.

KEY TERMS

Patient advocacy The nurse and the nursing profession's powerful voice at the local, state, and national levels in supporting policies that protect consumers and enhance accountability for quality by promoting safer health care systems. Patient advocacy is a cornerstone of the nursing profession, and patients depend on the nurse to ensure that they receive quality care. Workforce advocacy is a component of patient advocacy.

Workforce advocacy An array of services and tools designed to help nurses promote an optimal professional work environment and support their professional and personal development. Elements of workforce advocacy include staffing, workflow design, personal and social factors, physical environment, and organizational factors.

Workplace issues An array of complex issues nurses face in the workplace on a daily basis. These issues affect the nurse, the patient, the organization, and the profession. Examples include the nursing shortage, adequate staffing levels, errors in health care delivery, and violence in the workplace.

PROFESSIONAL/ETHICAL ISSUE

Victoria Larson graduated from nursing school last year and has worked in the postpartum unit of Southwest Regional Hospital since graduating and passing the National Council Licensure Examination (NCLEX). The postpartum unit uses couplet care in which the mother and baby are in the same room and cared for by one nurse. Over the last several months, Victoria has gained a great deal of confidence in caring for the mothers and babies together; however, she knows she still needs many more years of experience to become the expert nurse she aspires to be. Today, when Victoria arrives on the unit for her 7 AM to 7 PM shift, she becomes alarmed when she sees that the charge nurse has assigned her to six mother-baby sets. The typical assignment is three mother-baby sets but occasionally the nurse may be assigned four mother-baby sets when staffing is low. But six sets seems very unreasonable to Victoria, and she does not believe she can safely take care of this number of new mothers and babies. What options, if any, does Victoria have regarding this assignment that she believes to be unsafe? Discuss how she should approach the situation with her supervisor and what questions she should ask.

VIGNETTE

As a new graduate, 26-year-old Elena Gonzalez is searching for her first position as a registered nurse (RN) in a large metropolitan city. As part of her education, she learns about the importance of a nurse's role in advocating for a workplace conducive to delivering safe and effective quality health care. She also understands that the workplace is filled with complex issues—nursing shortages, staffing issues, potential exposure to bloodborne diseases—affecting the nurse, the patient, the organization, and the profession. Elena receives offers from various organizations. However, she wisely chooses not to accept a job on its "face value" and decides to investigate her opportunities more thoroughly. Using the Internet, she searches the websites of hospitals in her target area. She is looking for the answers to questions such as:

- Are any organizations within my area recognized as Magnet hospitals?
- Which organizations have shared governance models?
- What are the content and length of orientation for new nurses?
- What is the organization's philosophy regarding staff mix designations?
- Does the organization have a conflict resolution process?
- What is the organization's turnover rate, and what is the average time that nurses are employed in the organization?

Answers to these questions can be found on health care organizations' websites or from their nurse recruiters or nurse educators. Armed with answers to these and other questions, Elena decides to accept a position with a large tertiary care center that she believes has created an environment most supportive of ensuring the delivery of quality patient care. However, she knows that with the acceptance of this position, her role as a workforce and patient advocate has not ended; rather, it has only just begun.

Questions to Consider While Reading this Chapter:

1. What workforce advocacy strategies can Elena use to promote quality patient care and a safe work environment?
2. What is the value of shared governance to Elena's individual nursing practice?
3. If Elena becomes concerned about floating assignments, what questions can help guide her decision about accepting such assignments?
4. What online resources are available to help Elena learn more about important workplace issues and workforce advocacy?
5. How can Elena improve the marketability of her nursing expertise?

CHAPTER OVERVIEW

In today's modern health care system, nurses are faced with many workplace issues. These complex issues affect not only the nurse but also the patient, the organization, and the profession. This chapter attempts to identify a few select critical issues facing nurses and the nursing profession, including the nursing shortage, appropriate staffing, patient safety and advocacy, and workplace rights and safety. Workforce advocacy is defined, and its specific strategies are highlighted. To be successful and accountable professionals, nurses must recognize current issues and know where to seek support for workforce advocacy.

PROMOTING WORKFORCE ADVOCACY AND A PROFESSIONAL PRACTICE ENVIRONMENT

Professional nurses are experiencing involvement and control in the work environment that was unheard of 20 years ago. Important research is validating the contribution and value of registered nurses in the following areas:

- Preventing hospital readmissions (McHugh and Ma, 2013; Tubbs-Cooley et al, 2013)
- Decreasing adverse events and shorter length of stay (Frith et al, 2012; Kalisch et al, 2012; Martsolf et al, 2014)
- Decreasing patient mortality (Aiken et al, 2014; Duffin, 2014; Spetz et al, 2013)

Within this context of the important contributions that nurses make to patients, hospitals, and health care in general, we find nurses challenged to deliver care against all kinds of barriers and with dwindling resources. Nurses' strong commitment to patient care and their role as patient advocates often place them in direct conflict with those who have more control, such as physicians and administrators. How a nurse reacts to such conflicts within the workplace and continues to advocate to improve patient care is a necessary focus for the profession—a focus called **workforce advocacy**.

As we visit Elena Gonzalez 6 months after she assumed her new position, we find that she has become involved in advocating for a safe work environment. Elena and the other nurses working on the medical unit are concerned because there is a limited amount of safe patient handling equipment available. Their patients often have mobility issues, and the nurses are worried about suffering musculoskeletal injuries when transferring and repositioning patients. Where will they find information about ergonomic safety and other workplace safety issues? Are there regulations that require hospitals to implement safety measures to protect their staff against debilitating musculoskeletal injuries? What legal rights do nurses have to demand safe patient handling equipment? Is there an avenue to work with hospital administrators to decrease the costs associated with unsafe practices and to move toward a user-friendly work environment? All of these questions are related to workforce advocacy.

For more than a century, the American Nurses Association (ANA) and its state affiliates have advocated for the professional nurse and quality patient care. Through research, continuing education, and knowledge sharing among today's nursing community, ANA offers powerful resources to nurses seeking to overcome workforce challenges and realize opportunities. In 2003, ANA's commitment to workforce advocacy was advanced with the creation of services and tools designated to help individual nurses self-advocate in their professional and personal development (Box 13.1). Five opportunities and challenges for workforce advocacy programs are

---

BOX 13.1   Workforce Advocacy Ecosystem Model

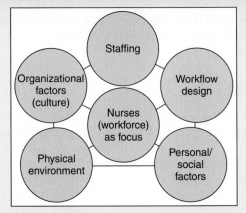

- *Staffing:* Refers to job assignments, including the volume of work assigned to individuals, the professional skills required for particular job assignments, the duration of experience in a particular job category, and work schedules
- *Workflow design:* Pertains to on-the-job activities of health care workers, including interactions among workers and the nature and scope of the work
- *Personal and social factors:* Refer to individual and group factors, such as stress, job satisfaction, and professionalism, in addition to skills that may be underdeveloped in the nursing population, such as financial literacy
- *Physical environment:* Includes aspects of the workplace, such as light, aesthetics, and sound; these elements will be crucial to address the needs of a maturing workforce and offer solutions to health care employers
- *Organizational factors:* Structural and process aspects of the organization as a whole, such as the use of teams, divisions of labor, shared beliefs, and an increasing leadership capacity among nurses

Adapted from Hickam D. H., Severance S., Feldstein A., et al. (2003). *The effect of health care working conditions on patient safety. Evidence Reports/Technology Assessments No. 74.* (AHRQ Publication No 03-E031, Rockville, MD: Agency for Healthcare Research and Quality; http://www.ahrq.gov.) Retrieved from http://www.ncbi.nlm.nih.gov/books/NBK36875/; and from http://www.nursingworld.org/MainMenuCategories/ThePracticeofProfessionalNursing/workforce/Workforce-Advocacy/Workforce-Ecosystem-2.html.

BOX 13.2   Five Opportunities and Challenges for Workforce Advocacy Programs

1. Identify mechanisms within health care systems that provide opportunities for RNs to affect institutional policies.
   - Shared governance
   - Participatory management models
   - Magnet hospital recognition
   - Statewide staffing regulations
2. Develop conflict resolution models for use within organizations that address RNs' concerns about patient care and delivery issues.
   - Identification of the reporting loop
   - Appointment of a final arbiter in disputes
3. Seek legislative solutions for workplace problems by reviewing issues of concern to nurses in employment settings and introducing appropriate legislation, such as the following:
   - Whistle-blower protection
   - "Safe harbor" peer review

- Support for rules outlining strong nursing practice standards
4. Develop legal centers for nurses that could provide legal support and decision-making advice as a last recourse to resolve workplace issues.
   - Provide fast and efficient legal assistance to nurses
   - Earmark precedent-setting cases that could affect case law and health care policy
5. Provide RNs with self-advocacy and patient advocacy information, such as the following:
   - Laws and regulations governing practice
   - Use of applicable nursing practice standards
   - Conflict resolution and negotiation techniques
   - State and national reporting mechanisms that allow RNs to report concerns about health care organizations and/or professionals

From American Nurses Association. (n.d.). Five opportunities/challenges for workforce advocacy programs. Retrieved from http://www.nursingworld.org/MainMenuCategories/ThePracticeofProfessionalNursing/workforce/Workforce-Advocacy/Opportunities-for-Advocacy-Programs.html; adapted from the Texas Nurses Association: Workplace advocacy program, and originally posted at http://www.CenterforAmericanNurses.

---

highlighted in Box 13.2. Other examples of workforce advocacy and specific workplace issues are discussed in the following sections.

NURSING SHORTAGES AND WORKFORCE CHALLENGES

The nursing profession has a long history of cyclic shortages, which have been documented since World War II. The most recent shortage, in the early 2000s, was eased by the downturn in the U.S. economy that occurred in the middle to late 2000s (Thrall, 2009). This easing in the shortage was largely due to the reentry of many retired nurses into the workforce because of economic pressures, nurses who had planned to retire who were holding on to their positions, some nurses working part-time who had taken full-time positions, and the fact that hospitals were treating fewer patients because many people were delaying procedures or not seeking care owing to loss of insurance (American Hospital Association, 2008; Buerhaus, 2008).

The focus on the nursing shortage that began in the early 2000s generated many positive results: an unexpected number of young people entered the nursing workforce from 2002 to 2009, causing faster growth in the supply than anticipated. There are several reasons for this increased supply, including higher levels of career and job satisfaction. Although the current numbers suggest that the United States is graduating sufficient nurses to meet demands, the landscape is more complicated. Data reveal that certain geographic areas may experience nursing shortages and that the loss of experienced nurses to retirement should compel employers to plan to retain experienced nurses while mentoring new nurses in their roles (AMN Healthcare, 2017; Health Resources and Services Administration [HRSA], 2017).

Future RN Employment Opportunities

Professional nursing is the largest U.S. health care occupation according to the Bureau of Labor Statistics (U.S. Department of Labor, 2016a). Employment of registered nurses is expected to grow by 16% from 2014 to 2024, much faster than the average for all occupations. RN employment will be affected by:

- The need to replace experienced nurses who leave the occupation. Almost 40% of registered nurses are older than 50 and the number of nurses leaving the workforce is growing steadily each year, from around

40,000 in 2010 to an expected nearly 80,000 by 2020 (Auerbach et al, 2015).

- Technologic advances in patient care that result in more patients' accessing the health care system and needing more specialized care.
- Increasing emphasis on preventive care.
- The rapid growth in the older population, who are much more likely than younger people to need nursing care.
- An increased emphasis on employment opportunities for nurses in case management and care coordination, such as Advanced Practice Registered Nurses (APRNs), which include Family Nurse Practitioners, Pediatric Nurse Practitioners, and Adult-Gerontology Acute Care Nurse Practitioners.

Employment will not grow at the same rate in every setting—hospital employment will grow more slowly because many procedures and types of care are shifting to outpatient and home health settings, more sophisticated procedures can safely be done outside the hospital, and home health and long-term care facilities will see employment growth because of the aging population.

Although current projections suggest that the United States will have a small surplus of RNs nationally, these estimates mask large geographic disparities. State-by-state analysis show both projected deficits of RNs in some states and large variations in supply in other states (HRSA, 2017). There have been layoffs by some hospitals at the same time that "registered nurse" ranks as the most advertised position nationwide. Health care employers must confront the reality of an aging population and increased access to care due to health care reforms while there is a "graying" of the nursing workforce. Planning for an adequate workforce will remain one of the most critical challenges of the new century. The following sections take a closer look at the challenges to ensuring an appropriate supply of nurses to meet the nation's health care needs.

Health Care as a Challenging Work Environment

In an examination of nursing workforce numbers, it is important to consider the nurses' work environment. In a 2017 job satisfaction and career plans survey of RNs, results showed that 83% of nurses stated they are satisfied with their career choice (AMN Healthcare, 2017). Despite the high level of career choice satisfaction,

respondents were less optimistic about their current jobs: Only 60% said they are satisfied, 55% said they worry that their jobs are affecting their health, and 38% said they often feel like resigning. Nursing has always been a stressful job; however, the dramatic changes in health care today create an added layer of uncertainty. Workplace challenges as indicated by this survey charge health system leaders to redesign work environments so that they are able to attract, retain, and develop the best RN workforce.

Nursing School Enrollments and Recruitment

Numerous efforts were undertaken over the past decade to recruit more students into nursing—efforts that have been largely successful. Professional nursing associations and health care companies educated the public regarding the shortage and the benefits of a nursing career. The Johnson & Johnson Campaign for Nursing's Future, a multiyear $30 million national initiative, was designed to enhance the image of the nursing profession, recruit new nurses and nurse faculty, and help retain nurses currently in the profession (Johnson & Johnson, 2017). Unfortunately, even when attempts to recruit more people into nursing have been successful, most schools and universities find themselves unable to expand their nursing programs to accept the qualified applicants because they are faced with a serious shortage of nursing faculty. National and statewide efforts have resulted in increases in nursing school enrollments for 16 consecutive years, yet these increases will not balance out the growing demand for nursing services and the need to replace retiring RNs (American Association of Colleges of Nursing [AACN], 2017a).

Along with the need to recruit into the profession, nursing must continue to examine the ways in which new nurses are introduced into the nursing work culture. Adequate orientation, mentoring, and preceptor programs are essential to introduce and retain new nurses.

Educational Preparation

During past shortages, employers have hired RNs regardless of their degree preparation. The current and projected demands for RNs require not simply more RNs, but more RNs of the right type and right educational and skill mix to handle increasingly complex care demands. Demand has intensified for more baccalaureate-prepared nurses with critical thinking, leadership, quality improvement, case management, and health promotion skills, who are capable of delivering care across a variety of health care settings. Demand has also increased for experienced RNs; for nurses in key clinical specialties, such as critical care, emergency department (ED), operating room, and neonatal intensive care; and for master's and doctorally prepared RNs in advanced clinical specialties, teaching, and research.

In October 2010, the Institute of Medicine (IOM, 2011) released its landmark report, *The Future of Nursing: Leading Change, Advancing Health,* initiated by the Robert Wood Johnson Foundation, which called for increasing the number of baccalaureate-prepared nurses in the workforce to 80% by 2020 (as of 2016, only 54% of RNs in the nursing workforce were prepared at the baccalaureate or graduate degree level [Campaign for Action, 2017]). This and other evidence-based recommendations contained in the report state that to respond "to the demands of an evolving health care system and meet the changing needs of patients, nurses must achieve higher levels of education" (IOM, 2011).

Faculty Shortages

One of the most critical problems facing nursing and nursing workforce planning is the aging of nursing faculty (AACN, 2017b). AACN's 2016 survey of baccalaureate nursing programs showed a 7.9% national faculty vacancy rate. The shortage of faculty is contributing to the current nursing shortage by limiting the number of students admitted to nursing programs. AACN reported that 64,067 qualified applicants were turned away from baccalaureate and graduate nursing programs in 2016, and an insufficient number of faculty was a major reason cited by schools for not accepting all qualified applicants (AACN, 2017b). Faculty salaries continue to be a major contributor to the faculty shortage. Academic institutions, especially those faced with budget cuts, generally cannot compete with nonacademic employers when it comes to salary benefits for faculty.

Nurse Retention

Past nursing shortages have demonstrated that the retention of professional nurses is a key to any organization's success. The ability of an organization to retain nurses depends primarily on the creation of an environment conducive to professional autonomy. Nurses want to work in an environment that supports decision making and effective nurse-physician relationships, which are critically important to patient safety. Although some progress has been achieved, RNs' perceptions of the hospital workplace environment demonstrate a need for improvement (Nei et al, 2015). A meta-analysis of 106 primary studies found the strongest predictors of nurse turnover intentions to be job strain, role tension, work-family conflict, job control, job complexity, rewards and recognition, and team cohesion.

Aging Workforce and Retention

As the nation works to enlarge the supply of professional nurses through education, strategies must be developed to retain the older, expert professional nurse. The following statistics detail the extent of the aging workforce issue:

- 50% of RNs are age 50 or over (National Council of State Boards of Nursing, 2015).
- In terms of nursing faculty, average age of doctorally-prepared nurse faculty is 57 and that for master's-prepared is 55 years (AACN, 2017B).

There has been little research to test the effectiveness of recruitment and retention strategies with older nurses. In a qualitative study of influences on the older nurse to continue bedside practice, the investigators found that the most pervasive and most difficult experiences for older nurses involved dealing with stress, frustration, constant change, physical and mental declines, and intergenerational conflict (Stichler, 2013). Although nursing literature is replete with the many positive aspects of continuing in nursing, suggestions on ways to keep older nurses practicing include better ergonomics and health care facility design to decrease the time nurses spend walking and reduce the physical demands of their work with aids such as mechanical lifts, decentralized supply storage, and better lighting at the bedside (Stichler, 2013).

Although many organizations have added on-site daycare and sick care for children of younger nurses, organizations may need to consider adding adult daycare to assist older nurses who are caring for aging parents. Creative staffing plans with shorter shifts and identified respite periods may help extend the work life of aging nurses. Technology has provided many workplace accessories that reduce the physical demands on nurses that can result in injury or stress, especially to aging nurses.

The American Organization of Nurse Executives (AONE, 2010) has developed *AONE Guiding Principles for the Aging Workforce*, which encourages health care facilities to develop benefits that will entice older nurses to stay in the organization, such as flexible work schedules, programs involving both experienced and newer nurses to promote knowledge transfer, environmental modifications with an emphasis on injury prevention, and phased retirement or rehiring post-retirement. Organizations that strategically plan for an aging workforce will be best positioned to deliver quality health care to their customers.

Emerging Workforce Recruitment and Retention

In addition to planning for retention of an aging workforce, health care is challenged to become the employer of choice for the younger emerging workforce. A number of studies have focused on the work and management expectations of today's young worker, who expects balance and perspective in the workplace. In a study focused on Generation Y nurses (those born after 1980), recognition was reported as a key motivator. The younger nurses identified their needs as stability, flexible work schedules, recognition, opportunities for professional development, and adequate supervision (Lavoie-Tremblay et al, 2010). Elena, the young nurse described at the beginning of the chapter, will be searching for opportunities to gain advanced training, education, and certification as she seeks to make herself more marketable in her professional nursing role. She expects feedback on her performance to help refine her skills and build her confidence. She also expects her manager to take a personal interest in her, to know her name, and to help her build a competitive portfolio. Many managers are unaware of these expectations in emerging workforce employees and contribute to the hastened exit of such employees from the workplace by not attending to their personal and career needs.

Nursing Salaries

RN salaries show a consistent pattern in alignment with nursing shortages. The hospital RN shortages of the 1960s, 1970s, 1980s, and early 1990s were transitory until wage increases brought the demand and supply of RNs into equilibrium. Unfortunately, during the 1990s nursing salaries remained flat—low salaries

definitely contributed to the nursing shortage. Another concern with nursing salaries is the small opportunity for significant salary increases as nurses gain more experience.

Fortunately, a sharp increase in RN wages occurred in 2002 and 2003. This increase reflects the acceleration in demand for RNs that occurred from 2001 to 2004. Since 2014, the average staff nurse wages have beat inflation. The Bureau of Labor Statistics (U.S. Department of Labor, 2016a) reported that the median salary for a registered nurse in May 2016 was $68,450. The best paid 10% of RNs made more than $102,990, whereas the bottom 10% earned less than $47,120. In 2016, the highest median salaries were earned by nurses working in government, hospitals, and home health care.

Work Environment

In the late 1990s, studies focused on the work environment as a significant contributor to the difficulty in recruiting and retaining RNs (Nolan et al, 1999). Primary factors for nurse turnover were workload and staffing patterns. Other issues identified were insufficient supply of qualified managers and experienced staff, increased market demand, and inappropriate staffing. In a later survey, the need for more qualified nurses in leadership positions was identified as supporting healthy work environments (AMN Healthcare, 2017). The importance of addressing the work environment is clear—efforts at increasing the overall supply of nurses are unlikely to be successful if retention strategies are not developed.

Most health care employers now understand the importance of directing their attention to improving the workplace. Nursing school enrollments are at capacity, and it is vital to retain nurses in an effort to boost overall supply. Research has shown the positive impact of a healthy work environment on staff satisfaction, retention, improved patient outcomes, and organizational performance (Aiken et al, 2009; Sherman and Pross, 2010). In a study exploring the mechanism by which reducing patient-to-nurse ratios improves outcomes, Aiken and colleagues (2011) found that decreasing the number of patients per nurse improved mortality and failure to rescue, predominantly in hospitals rated as having a good work environment. Hospitals with a poor work environment derived no benefit from reducing patient-to-nurse ratios.

Several national initiatives have been undertaken to promote positive and safe work environments for nurses. In one of the first efforts, the Nursing Organizations Alliance, a coalition of more than 65 national nursing organizations, developed its *Principles and Elements of a Healthful Practice/Work Environment* (Nursing Organizations Alliance, 2004), which provides a framework for organizations to improve nurses' work environments. The American Association of Critical Care Nurses promotes a "healthy work environment" as one of their three major advocacy issues and has developed standards along with measurement tools (AACN, 2014). The Joint Commission (TJC) also noted more than a decade ago, "if the staffing levels and work environments are not safe for the nurses, they will not be safe for the patients" (TJC, 2002).

SAFE STAFFING

Many nurses across the country are concerned about the inadequacies of staffing to meet patient care needs. In a survey of almost 220,000 RNs from 13,000 nursing units in more than 550 hospitals that had a response rate of 70%, nurses reported that 54% of nurses in adult medical units and EDs did not have sufficient time with patients; that overtime had increased during the past year, with 43% of all RNs working extra hours because the unit was short-staffed or busy; and that inadequate staffing had affected unit admissions, transfers, and discharges more than 20% of the time (ANA, 2014a).

A landmark study by Aiken and colleagues (2002) found that in hospitals with fewer nurses per patient, surgical patients were more likely to experience higher death rates from failure to rescue (insufficient nursing care) and death from complications. The same study also found that nurses working in institutions plagued by insufficient staffing and workforce shortages were more likely to experience emotional exhaustion and greater job dissatisfaction. Subsequent research has reinforced the importance of appropriate nurse staffing and positive patient outcomes (ANA, 2017; Avalere Health, 2015).

Given concerns about resources and shifting health care landscape, challenges continue with regard to determining optimal staffing and how to appropriately use unlicensed personnel to assist in the delivery of care to patient populations who are more acutely ill, who require high-tech care, and whose lengths of stay are being reduced to keep costs in check. Federal regulations require hospitals to "have adequate numbers of licensed registered nurses, licensed practical [vocational] nurses, and other personnel to provide nursing care to all patients as needed" (U.S. Department of Health and Human Services, 2011). With such nebulous language, it has been left to the states to ensure that staffing is appropriate to meet patients' needs safely. Three general approaches to ensure sufficient nurse staffing have been utilized at the state level (ANA, 2013a):

- Require hospitals to have a nurse-driven staffing committee to create staffing plans that reflect the needs of the patient population and match the skills and experience of the staff. ANA endorses this approach through its *Principles for Nurse Staffing, Second Edition,* which provides recommendations on optimal staffing and requires nurses to be an integral part of the nurse staffing plan development and decision-making process (ANA, 2012). Such an approach provides for flexible staffing levels that can account for the intensity of patient needs, number of admissions, discharges, and transfers during a shift, level of experience of nursing staff, layout of the unit, and availability of resources (e.g., ancillary staff, technology) (ANA, 2013a). As of 2017, seven states require hospitals to have staffing committees responsible for plans and staffing policy—Connecticut, Illinois, Nevada, Ohio, Oregon, Texas, and Washington.

- Require facilities to disclose staffing levels to the public and/or a regulatory body. As of 2017, five states require some form of disclosure/public reporting—Illinois, New Jersey, New York, Rhode Island, and Vermont.

- Enact legislation to mandate specific nurse-to-patient ratios. As of 2017, California is the only state with specified nurse-to-patient ratios.

Under the California rules, one nurse will care for not more than five patients in medical-surgical units, four patients in specialty care and telemetry units, and three patients in step-down units. Research studying the effectiveness of California's staffing law showed that California hospitals increased nurse staffing levels over time significantly more than comparison state hospitals did; however, findings related to patient safety measures were mixed, with significantly decreased rates associated with failure to rescue and significantly increased rates of infections due to medical care in some California hospitals than in comparison state hospitals; and there were no statistically significant changes in rates of either respiratory failure or postoperative sepsis (Mark et al, 2013).

As nurses consider staffing, they will be faced with many decisions, including how to determine appropriate staffing when considering RN positions, how to promote safe staffing in their own settings, and even being faced with patient care assignments that they feel to be potentially unsafe. When considering a position, nurses should ask the questions regarding safe staffing that are listed in Box 13.3. Resources to help nurses' decision making relative to adequate staffing and mandatory overtime are p shown in Box 13.4. Box 13.5 identifies questions to help

---

BOX 13.3   Questions to Ask About Safe Staffing Before Accepting Employment

1. Who is the chief nursing officer, to whom does she or he report, and does she or he have authority over staffing?
2. Who controls the staffing budget?
3. Is the level of staffing an active and ongoing discussion in the organization, and do staff nurses have input?
4. Does the organization have a shared governance model?
5. When, where, and how is staffing input obtained from staff nurses?
6. How do ratios in the organization compare with recommendations of national and regional organizations, such as the American Organization of Nurse Executives and the American Association of Critical-Care Nurses?
7. What are the content and length of orientation for new nurses?
8. What is the philosophy regarding staff mix designations?
9. What is the frequency of floating to other nursing units?
10. What are the criteria used by the organization in determining competency of cross-trained staff?
11. What resources does the organization use to supplement staff during peak census?
12. If concerns arise about the adequacy of staffing, where and to whom is it appropriate to voice those concerns?
13. How are overtime, on-call time, and cancellation of regularly scheduled shifts handled?
14. Does the organization mandate overtime? If so, can the staff nurse refuse to participate without repercussions?
15. What is the turnover rate, and what is the average longevity of staff nurses?
16. What opportunities for advancement exist in the organization, such as clinical ladders or other systems of recognition?
17. Where does the organization expect discussions about staffing or practice issues to take place?
18. Is there a conflict resolution process in place?

From American Nurses Association. (n.d.). Questions to ask about safe staffing before accepting employment. Retrieved from https://www.nursingworld.org/practice-policy/workforce/questions-to-ask-about-safe-staffing-before-accepting-employment/.

BOX 13.4   Resources for Decision Making Related to Adequacy of Staffing and Mandatory Overtime

Guidebooks

ANA Principles for Nurse Staffing, 2nd Edition: Directs RNs on how to determine the level of nurse staffing for any setting. It focuses on patient acuity systems, the basics of workload measurement, patient classification, unlicensed assistive personnel, the role of professional judgment, and the development of principles.

ANA's Principles for Delegation: Provides the principles and guidelines for delegation of tasks to others. Its purpose is to define relevant principles and provide RNs with practice strategies when delegating patient care to nursing assistive personnel. It also covers needed definitions and the essentials of care provision and related nurse education.

Principles for Nursing Documentation: Focuses on managing the increasingly complex requirements of documenting patient care activities in both paper and electronic formats.

These three documents are available as a *Principles for Practice* set at http://www.nursesbooks.org.

Other Resources

ANA's Nurse Staffing website:
https://www.nursingworld.org/practice-policy/advocacy/state/nurse-staffing
ANA's Position Statements Regarding Workplace Advocacy:
https://www.nursingworld.org/practice-policy/advocacy/state/nurse-staffing

BOX 13.5 Questions to Ask in Making the Decision to Accept a Staffing Assignment

1. *What is the assignment?*

   Clarify the assignment. Do not assume. Be certain that what you believe is the assignment is indeed correct.

2. *What are the characteristics of the patients being assigned?*

   Do not just respond to the number of patients; make a critical assessment of the needs of each patient, his or her age, condition, other factors that contribute to special needs, and the resources available to meet those needs. Who else is on the unit or within the facility that might be a resource for the assignment? Do nurses on the unit have access to those resources? How stable are the patients, and how long have they been stable? Do any patients have communication and/or physical limitations that will require accommodation and extra supervision during the shift? Will there be discharges to offset the load? If there are discharges, will there be admissions, which require extra time and energy?

3. *Do I have the expertise to care for the patients?*

   Am I familiar with caring for the types of patients assigned? If this is a float assignment, am I cross-trained to care for these patients? Is there a buddy system in place with staff who are familiar with the unit? If there is no cross-training or buddy system, has the patient load been modified accordingly?

4. *Do I have the experience and knowledge to manage the patients for whom I am being assigned care?*

   If the answer to this question is no, you have an obligation to articulate limitations. Limitations in experience and knowledge may not require refusal of the assignment but rather an agreement regarding supervision or a modification of the assignment to ensure patient safety. If no accommodation for limitations is considered, the nurse has an obligation to refuse an assignment for which she or he lacks education or experience.

5. *What is the geography of the assignment?*

   Am I being asked to care for patients who are in proximity for efficient management, or are the patients at opposite ends of the hall or on different units? If there are geographic difficulties, what resources are available to manage the situation? If my patients are on more than one unit and I must go to another unit to provide care, who will monitor patients out of my immediate attention?

6. *Is this a temporary assignment?*

   When other staff are located to assist, will I be relieved? If the assignment is temporary, it may be possible to accept a difficult assignment, knowing that there will soon be reinforcements. Is there a pattern of short staffing, or is this truly an emergency?

7. *Is this a crisis or an ongoing staffing pattern?*

   If the assignment is being made because of an immediate need on the unit, a crisis, the decision to accept the assignment may be based on that immediate need. However, if the staffing pattern is an ongoing problem, the nurse has the obligation to identify unmet standards of care that are occurring as a result of ongoing staffing inadequacies. This may result in a request for "safe harbor" and/or peer review.

8. *Can I take the assignment in good faith? (If not, you will need to get the assignment modified or refuse the assignment.)*

   Consult your individual state's nurse practice act regarding clarification of accepting an assignment in good faith. In understanding good faith, it is sometimes easier to identify what would constitute bad faith. For example, if you had not taken care of pediatric patients since nursing school and you were asked to take charge of a pediatric unit, unless this were an extreme emergency, such as a disaster (in which case you would need to let people know your limitations, but you might still be the best person, given all factors for the assignment), it would be bad faith to take the assignment. It is always your responsibility to articulate your limitations and to get an adjustment to the assignment that acknowledges the limitations you have articulated. Good faith acceptance of the assignment means that you are concerned about the situation and believe that a different pattern of care or policy should be considered. However, you acknowledge the difference of opinion on the subject between you and your supervisor and are willing to take the assignment and await the judgment of other peers and supervisors.

From American Nurses Association. (n.d.). *Questions to ask in making the decision to accept a staffing assignment.* Retrieved from https://www.nursingworld.org/practice-policy/workforce/questions-to-ask-in-making-the-decision-to-accept-a-staffing-assignment-for-nurses.

the staff nurse decide whether to accept an assignment. These questions are designed to help the staff nurse think critically about the assignment, so if there is a problem, the nurse can be clear in telling the manager what makes her or him uncomfortable with the assignment.

Floating and Mandatory Overtime

As concerns about nursing shortages ebb and flow so too does the use of floating and mandatory overtime as strategies for addressing immediate nurse staffing issues. When the availability of nursing staff tightens, employers may (1) require that professional nurses "float" to other patient care units for which they have little or no orientation, experience, or support and (2) implement mandatory overtime and/or mandatory on-call requirements. Particularly with regard to mandatory overtime, such strategies can be challenging, given research findings that nurses' work schedules are associated with patient mortality. For example, one study found that pneumonia deaths were significantly more likely in hospitals where nurses reported schedules with long work hours and lack of time away from work (Trinkoff et al, 2011). In addition, findings related to nursing fatigue and sleep deprivation showed that nurses are more likely to report clinical decision regret, which occurs when their behaviors do not align with professional nursing practices standard or expectations (Scott et al, 2014).

Nurses believe that an employers' ability to mandate last-minute overtime or to use peer pressure as a negative motivator relieves the employers' sense of urgency to find safer and more appropriate staffing. Although nurses are fully cognizant and concerned about inadequate staffing, they may also be resentful that they bear the personal, professional, and legal burden for this problem by having to work overtime. Although the growing research on overtime and medical errors has caused many facilities to drop their use of mandatory overtime and even to limit hours of voluntary overtime, it continues to be a concern. Excessive and recurrent use of overtime, at times used as a staffing strategy, has made it necessary for states to pursue legislation limiting its use. See the ANA website at for more information and resources on mandatory overtime (http://www.nursingworld.org).

PATIENT ADVOCACY

Patient advocacy is a cornerstone of the nursing profession, and patients depend on nurses to ensure that they receive proper care. Although nurses have always advocated for their patients, it has only been during the past 30 years that the recognized role of the nurse as patient advocate has begun to clearly emerge. Today's health care systems have created an environment in which errors and adverse events are attributed to complex systems and complicated uses of technology. This complex environment demands that the nursing profession assert

Professional nurses are struggling to deliver patient care against all kinds of barriers and with dwindling resources.

its powerful voice in the role of patient advocate by supporting public policies that protect consumers and enhance accountability for quality by promoting safer health care systems.

Patient Safety

Institute of Medicine. A major IOM report on patient safety, *To Err Is Human*, focused a great deal of attention on patient safety when it reported that between 44,000 and 98,000 patients die in U.S. hospitals each year from preventable medical errors (Kohn et al, 2000). Subsequently, the IOM released its report, *Keeping Patients Safe: Transforming the Work Environment of Nurses*, which examined patient safety from the perspective of the work environment in which nurses provide patient care (Page, 2004). The second report provided evidence of the critical role nurses have in the health care system and found that the typical work environment of nurses is characterized by many serious threats to patient safety. These two reports have spurred the development of nursing-focused quality and safety programs.

The National Database for Nursing Quality Indicators. The National Database for Nursing Quality Indicators (NDNQI) is a national nursing quality measurement program that enables hospitals to compare measures of nursing quality against national, regional, and state norms for similar units and hospitals. NDNQI was instituted by the ANA as a tool for nursing quality measurement, novel research, and collaborative learning through data collection at the nursing unit level that allows for empirical linkages between nursing care and patient outcomes. Indicators such as patient falls, physical restraints, nosocomial infections, nursing care hours provided per patient day, and RN satisfaction surveys are used for quality improvement, reporting requirements (e.g., TJC, Magnet Recognition Program), staff retention efforts, budget allocation, and research.

Quality Safety and Education for Nurses. Recognizing the need to strengthen nurses' competencies in the science of patient safety and quality, the Quality Safety and Education for Nurses (QSEN) project was developed to prepare nurses with the knowledge, skills, and attitudes necessary to continuously improve the quality and safety of the health care systems

in which they work (QSEN Institute, 2012). The QSEN competencies are presented in more detail in Chapter 22.

High Reliability Organizations. An increased focus on patient safety that has led to interest from health care leaders in adapting the principles of high reliability to hospital and health care organizations. High reliability organizations (HROs) are organizations in which harmful events rarely occur despite the potential for errors resulting in catastrophic outcomes (Ulrich and Kear, 2014). Many organizations are adopting methods used in high reliability science to create safer work and practice environments and reducing the likelihood that patients will come to harm through error or defects in the provision of care (Chassin and Loeb, 2013).

Whistle-Blower Protection

Nurses want the assurance that if they are acting within the scope of their practice, they will be able to speak up for their patients through appropriate channels without fear of retaliation. State and federal whistle-blower protection legislation seeks to prohibit health care organizations from retaliating against the professional nurse who in good faith discloses information or participates in agency investigations. Specifically, whistle-blower protection protects nurses who speak out about unsafe situations from being fired or subjected to other disciplinary actions by their employers.

In Texas two nurses filed a complaint against a physician citing unsafe medical practice. The case made national headlines in 2009 when both nurses were charged by the sheriff's department with harassment and ultimately fired from their hospital jobs. Charges against one of the nurses were dropped. The second nurse endured a 4-day trial and was found not guilty. The nurses filed a federal civil suit against their accusers, alleging violation of civil rights, among other violations, and won a $750,000 settlement. ANA and the Texas Nurses Association strongly supported the nurses, advocating for the importance of protecting whistle-blowers from prosecution. Ultimately, the county sheriff, county attorney, and hospital administrator were charged and received jail sentences for their roles in trying to silence the two nurses. In addition to a $5000 fine, the physician received 60 days in

BOX 13.6   Things to Know about Whistle-Blowing

- If you identify an illegal or unethical practice, reserve judgment until you have adequate documentation to establish wrongdoing.
- Do not expect those that are engaged in unethical or illegal conduct to welcome your questions or concerns about this practice.
- Seek the counsel of someone you trust outside of the situation to provide you with an objective perspective.
- Consult with your state nurses association or legal counsel if possible before taking action to determine how best to document your concerns.
- Remember that you are not protected in a whistle-blower situation from retaliation by your employer until you blow the whistle.
- Blowing the whistle means that you report your concern to the national and/or state agency responsible for regulation of the organization for which you work or, in

- the case of criminal activity, to law enforcement agencies as well.
- Private groups, such as The Joint Commission or the National Committee for Quality Assurance, do not confer protection. You must report to a state or national regulator.
- Although it is not required by every regulatory agency, it is a good rule of thumb to put your complaint in writing.
- Document all interactions related to the whistle-blowing situation, and keep copies for your personal file.
- Keep documentation and interactions objective.
- Remain calm, and do not lose your temper, even if those who learn of your actions attempt to provoke you.
- Remember that blowing the whistle is a very serious matter. Do not blow the whistle frivolously. Make sure you have the facts straight before taking action.

American Nurses Association. (2011). *Things to know about whistle-blowing.* Retrieved from https://www.nursingworld.org/practice-policy/workforce/things-to-know-about-whistle-blowing/.

jail and 5 years of probation and surrendered his medical license. These actions sent a powerful message in support of whistle-blower protection. Box 13.6 provides an overview of things to know about whistle-blowing. Nurses should check with their state nurses association to assess the status of whistle-blower protection in their state.

NURSE AND WORKPLACE SAFETY

Nurses are battling to provide safe, quality care for patients in an environment that is inherently dangerous. The occupational safety and health of nurses is an ongoing concern for individual nurses as well as professional nursing associations because of numerous hazards that exist in the health care workplace. See the Centers for Disease Control and Prevention (CDC), National Institute for Occupational Safety and Health (NIOSH) web page for detailed information about current health hazards that exist in the health care workplace (http://www.cdc.gov/niosh/topics/healthcare). The following sections focus on four key hazards of concern to nurses: bloodborne pathogens, ergonomic injuries, workplace violence, and fatigue.

Exposure to Bloodborne Pathogens

Nurses and other health care professionals are at major risk for exposure to bloodborne diseases, including hepatitis B, hepatitis C, and human immunodeficiency virus–acquired immunodeficiency syndrome (HIV-AIDS). In 1991, the Occupational Safety and Health Administration (OSHA) issued the bloodborne pathogens standard to protect health care workers from this risk (NIOSH, 2017). The standard was revised by the Needlestick Safety and Prevention Act of 2000 (CDC, 2016). The law requires the use of safer needle devices to protect from sharps injuries. Additionally, the law requires employers to solicit the input of nonmanagerial employees responsible for direct patient care who are potentially exposed to sharps injuries in the identification, evaluation, and selection of effective engineering and work-practice controls. This law also requires employers to maintain a sharps injury log to contain, at a minimum, the brand of device involved in the incident, the department or work area where the exposure incident occurred, and an explanation of how the incident occurred.

Despite this legislation, safer practices related to handling of sharps have not been universally adopted. A decade after the law was enacted, one study demonstrated a

6.5% increase in sharps injuries in operation room settings (Jagger et al, 2010). And although the federal legislation requires that nurses and other direct care workers help evaluate and select safe needle devices, a 2011 survey reported that 43% of nurses who had access to safe needle devices did not know whether nurses were involved in the selection process, and 19% reported that nurses were not involved (ANA, 2014a). See the ANA website at for more information and resources about needlestick safety (http://www.nursingworld.org).

Ergonomic Injuries

The latest data from the U.S. Department of Labor, from 2016, indicate that individuals working in health care experienced the highest rate of musculoskeletal nonfatal injuries and illnesses (musculoskeletal disorder [MSD]), followed by the manufacturing and retail industries (U.S. Department of Labor, 2016b). Nurse aides, orderlies, and attendants reported the highest incidence of MSDs and were ranked second in overall MSDs requiring days away from work, with RNs ranked ninth (U.S. Department of Labor, 2016b).

The extent of MSDs among the U.S. nursing workforce is distressing because it is estimated that 12% of nurses leave the profession annually as a result of back injuries, and more than 52% complain of chronic back pain (Gallagher, 2013). Two decades of research have demonstrated that use of a single approach (e.g., engineering controls, administrative changes, or worker training) to reduce the incidence of MSDs has been ineffective. There has been a shift toward evidence-based practices, such as a comprehensive program that creates no-lift policies, secures appropriate safe patient handling and mobility technology, and trains staff on usage, with a comprehensive tracking system of MSD injuries that includes ongoing evaluation of the program.

Over the past decade, ANA has led major initiatives aimed at reducing workplace injuries, including the *Safe Patient Handling and Mobility Interprofessional National Standards* (ANA, 2013b). These standards, developed by an interprofessional work group of subject matter experts, outline the role of employers and health care workers in safe patient handling and mobility. For more information about these standards, see the Handle with Care resources on the ANA website at www.nursingworld.org. As of 2014, 11 states had

adopted legislation to implement safe patient handling programs in health care facilities (ANA, 2013b). Federal legislation has been introduced to Congress intended to create a national occupational safety and health standard to reduce injuries to both patients and health care workers (Government Printing Office, 2013).

Experts strongly suspect that workplace injuries are highly underreported. Nurses have cited various reasons for not reporting workplace injuries. According to ANA's *2011 Health and Safety Survey* (ANA, 2014a), 68% of nurses who did not report their injuries chose not to do so because they did not think the injury was significant. Other common reasons were being too busy (14%) and not having anyone to cover them (26%).

Every organization should have specific policies concerning reporting of workplace injuries and illness. ANA provides a number of resources and information concerning nurses' health and safety rights. OSHA's record-keeping standard requires employers to keep a log of workplace injuries and to keep the OSHA 300 Log available to employees and their representatives (OSHA, 2013). The OSHA standard also prevents discrimination against employees who report a work-related injury, illness, or fatality.

Incivility, Bullying, and Violence in the Workplace

OSHA has reported that between 2002 and 2013 health care workers had four times the risk of experiencing a violence-related workplace injury requiring time off from work than individuals in the overall workforce (OSHA, 2015). This statistic does not include trauma experienced from verbal and less severe physical abuse. It is important to recognize that the spectrum of workplace violence also includes peer-to-peer "lateral violence," defined as acts of incivility or bullying behavior between colleagues. These behaviors, which include covert or overt acts of verbal and nonverbal aggression, have been reported to result in psychologic distress severe enough to cause some nurses to leave the profession (ANA, 2015; Dillon, 2012).

Reports in the literature underscore the fact that underreporting of workplace violence is very common and may stem from the perception by health care workers that physical and verbal abuse is just "part of the job." Data obtained from nurses (RNs and licensed practical nurses [LPNs]) in a state-wide population-based study showed that almost half (49.8%) of nurse respondents experienced physical violence over the course of their careers, with 81.8% reporting verbal abuse as the most common type of violence experienced (Texas Department of State Health Services, 2016). In the first national study of ED nurses and perceptions of workplace violence, investigators determined that violence against ED nurses is prevalent (Gacki-Smith et al, 2009). More than 25% of nurses who participated in this study reported experiencing physical violence more than 20 times in the past 3 years, and almost 20% reported experiencing verbal abuse more than 200 times during the same period. Another study found that more than 50% of nurses who responded to the survey were fearful of being physically injured at the workplace but were unprepared to handle violent behavior should it be directed toward them by a patient, family member, visitor, or coworker (Speroni et al, 2014). Greater than 25% of nurse respondents in this study said they had never received any training about workplace violence prevention.

The ANA convened a panel of nurses from all areas of practice to develop a white paper, *Workplace Violence, Incivility and Bullying*, which outlines the responsibilities and actions that both individuals and organizations must undertake to create and maintain a violence-free workplace (ANA, 2015). Nurses in all settings must proactively advocate for interventions that ensure personal safety and a safe work environment. Workplace violence prevention programs must include a zero tolerance policy for workplace violence, verbal and nonverbal threats, and actions; must ensure that no employee who reports or experiences workplace violence faces reprisals; must have detailed record keeping to assess risk and measure progress; must develop a comprehensive plan for maintaining security in the workplace; must demonstrate management commitment from leadership; and must provide periodic employee education about violence prevention in the workplace (ANA, 2017).

Nurse Fatigue

Because the nature of health care can be physically and emotionally taxing and can require 24/7 scheduling in some settings, nursing can be a challenging profession. Nurses may work long and variable hours, forgoing adequate rest and sleep, which may result in fatigue. Restorative sleep is critical to the health of the nurse and to ensure that the nurse can provide the highest quality patient care possible (Trinkoff et al, 2011). In an integrative review of the literature that involved 22 studies, Smith-Miller and colleagues (2014) found that more than 70% of nurse participants reported feeling fatigued often or very often.

Inadequate sleep is known to negatively affect performance and mood and may result in an increase in risk-taking behavior, impairment of communication skills, and deficits in short-term and working memory (Killgore et al, 2012). In addition to the increased risk for work-related errors, the effects of fatigue on the health and well-being of the nurse are well documented. Shift work and long hours have been linked to a multitude of health-related disorders, including diabetes, cardiovascular disease, depression, sleep disturbances, and physical injuries (Bae and Fabry, 2014; Bannai and Tamakoshi, 2014).

In 2013, ANA convened a professional issues panel that included nurses from all areas of the professional nursing community to address the safety and health issues related to nurse fatigue (ANA, 2014b). The resulting position statement outlined responsibilities of both nurses and employers and included a substantive list of recommendations ranging from limitation of hours worked (to no more than 40 hours in one week and 12 hours in one shift), to elimination of mandatory overtime, to redesign of work schedules to minimize the occurrence of fatigue in the workplace (ANA, 2014b). Both the nurse and the employer have ethical responsibilities to ensure the safety and well-being of those who work in health care settings and the patients they care for. The nurse must take the steps necessary to ensure that he or she has adequate rest prior to the start of a work shift, and the employer must develop and maintain policies and procedures that support a healthy work environment and adequate rest.

Advocating for a Safer Workplace

ANA has emerged as a leader in health care worker health and safety, working in collaboration with other nursing organizations, including the American Association of Occupational Health Nurses, the Association of periOperative Registered Nurses, the Emergency Nurses Association, and labor unions representing health care workers. These organizations advocate for administrative controls, such as adequate staffing and health and safety committees; engineering controls, such as ventilation and safer needlestick devices; and personal protective equipment, such as respirators and synthetic gloves that prevent exposure to hazardous substances and/or prevent illness or injury from unavoidable exposure. Although the health care industry can be a dangerous place to work, many of the risks are avoidable and dangerous exposures preventable.

MAGNET RECOGNITION PROGRAM AND PATHWAYS TO EXCELLENCE

The American Academy of Nurses, an ANA affiliate, undertook a national study of 163 acute care hospitals in the early 1980s to identify the factors associated with retaining qualified nurses during a nursing shortage (McClure et al, 1983). The ANA's credentialing arm, the American Nurses Credentialing Center (ANCC), used the study findings to create the Magnet Recognition Program, which includes best practice standards to improve nurse satisfaction and the work environment of nurses as well as to reduce turnover rates.

Magnet program standards were originally called the 14 forces of magnetism; as the model evolved with the 2008, 2014, and 2019 manuals, these standards were collapsed into five domains with a greater emphasis on outcomes: Transformational Leadership, Structural Empowerment, Exemplary Professional Practice, New Knowledge and Innovation, and Empirical Outcomes (ANCC, 2017a). Research has consistently shown that Magnet hospital nurses have higher levels of autonomy, more control over the practice setting, and better relationships with physicians (Aiken et al, 2008, 2009; Armstrong et al, 2009; Kramer et al, 2011) as well as lower mortality rates (McHugh et al, 2013). Nurses advocating for a strong workplace should advocate for their hospital to achieve Magnet status. For more information about the *Magnet Recognition Program,* go to https://www.nursingworld.org/organizational-programs/magnet/.

Some organizations may choose to pursue Pathways to Excellence designation. Based on the Texas Nurse-Friendly Program originally developed for small/rural hospitals, the standards were revised by the ANCC to meet national criteria and were renamed the Pathway to Excellence program. Pathway practice standards were developed according to evidence-based practices and expert nurse input that promote and support a positive practice environment (ANCC, 2017b). For more information

about the Pathway to Excellence Program, go to http://www.nursecredentialing.org/pathway.

SHARED GOVERNANCE

Introduced in the 1970s, *shared governance* has been identified by RNs as a cornerstone of excellence in nursing practice (Brody et al, 2012). Shared governance provides an organizational framework for nurses in direct care to engage in creating and sustaining an optimal nursing practice and work environment, ensuring that nurses are active participants in decision making and have shared accountability for the outcomes of those decisions. Magnet Recognition Program standards support the formation of formal shared governance or decision-making models as foundational to professional practice. In organizations that do not have shared governance, it is important that nurses have access to and input into decisions that affect nursing practice and patient outcomes. Box 13.7 identifies questions that should be asked about shared governance or participatory management models when nurses are trying to identify the organization that would be most conducive to the delivery of quality nursing care.

BOX 13.7 Questions to Ask about Shared Governance Models

- Are nurses encouraged to participate in shared governance?
- How do nurses become involved in the shared governance process?
- What is the ratio of staff nurses to managers involved in shared governance within the organization?
- Is adequate work time allowed to participate in governance councils?
- How does the organization communicate shared governance decisions with staff nurses?
- How did shared governance improve nursing care delivery in the organization?
- Do nurses feel shared governance within their organization is beneficial to their practice?
- Does the organization have outcomes data related to shared governance?
- If so how have those data affected changes in nursing practice?

From American Nurses Association. (n.d.). Questions to ask about shared governance models. Retrieved from https://www.nursingworld.org/practice-policy/workforce/questions-to-ask-about-shared-governance-models-in-nursing/.

CONFLICT RESOLUTION

All organizations should provide nurses with access to conflict resolution procedures that define the processes they should follow if they are in disagreement with the organization's policies and/or leadership. Examples include open-door policies, ombudsman programs, and dispute-resolution processes. When seeking dispute resolution, the nurse may use a third party or resources internal to the organization to assist in the resolution. Some states have processes that can help resolve patient care or professional issues. These processes include peer review, safe harbor, and mandatory reporting.

■ SUMMARY

This chapter has covered a variety of significant workplace issues and has identified workforce advocacy strategies for a nurse to use to improve the workplace environment and quality of patient care. A rapidly changing health care environment, significantly affected by an aging workforce and a nursing shortage, creates a challenge for all nurses.

Nurses must be aware of the issues facing the profession and know where to seek assistance, information, and resources to address workplace issues. Working together with the resources of organizations such as the American Nurses Association, nurses can create a workplace that promotes career satisfaction and quality patient care.

REFERENCES

Aiken, L. H., Clarke, S. P., Sloane, D. M., Sochalski, J., & Silber, J. H. (2002). Hospital nurse staffing and patient mortality, nurse burnout, and job dissatisfaction. *JAMA, 288*(16), 1987–1993.

Aiken, L. H., Clarke, S. P., Sloane, D. M., Lake, E. T., & Cheney, T. (2009). Effects of hospital care environment on patient mortality and nurse outcomes. *The Journal of Nursing Administration, 39*(Suppl 7–8), S45–S51.

Aiken, L. H., Cimiotti, J. P., Sloane, D. M., Smith, H. L., Flynn, L., & Neff, D. F. (2011). Effects of nurse staffing and education on patient deaths in hospitals with different nurse work environments. *Medical Care, 49*(12), 1047–1053.

Aiken, L. H., Buchan, J., Ball, J., & Rafferty, A. M. (2008). Transformative impact of Magnet designation: England case study. *Journal of Clinical Nursing, 17*(24), 3330–3337.

Aiken, L. H., Sloane, D. M., Bruyneel, L, Van den Heede, K., Griffiths, P., Busse, R., et al. (2014). Nurse staffing and education and hospital mortality in nine European countries: A retrospective observational study. *Lancet, 383*(9931), 1824–1830.

American Association of Colleges of Nursing. (2017a). *Nursing Shortage Fact Sheet*. Washington DC: American Association of Colleges of Nursing. Retrieved from http://www.aacnnursing.org/Portals/42/News/Factsheets/Nursing-Shortage-Factsheet-2017.pdf.

American Association of Colleges of Nursing. (2017b). *Nursing Faculty Shortage Fact Sheet*. Washington DC. Retrieved from http://www.aacnnursing.org/Portals/42/News/Factsheets/Faculty-Shortage-Factsheet-2017.pdf.

American Association of Critical Care Nurses. (2014). *AACN's Healthy Work Environments Initiative*. Retrieved from https://www.aacn.org/nursing-excellence/healthy-work-environments.

American Hospital Association. (2008). *New report details impact of economic downturn on patients and hospitals*. Retrieved from http://www.aha.org/presscenter/pressrel/2008/081119-pr-econimpact.shtml.

American Nurses Association. (2012). *Principles of Nurse Staffing* (2nd ed.). Retrieved from http://www.nursesbooks.org/ebooks/download/ANA_Principles_Staffing.pdf.

American Nurses Association. (2013a). *Nurse Staffing Plans & Ratios*. Retrieved from http://www.nursingworld.org/MainMenuCategories/Policy-Advocacy/State/Legislative-Agenda-Reports/State-StaffingPlansRatios.

American Nurses Association. (2013b). *Safe Patient Handling and Mobility*. Retrieved from http://nursingworld.org/Safe-Patient-Handling-and-Mobility.

American Nurses Association. (2014a). *2011 ANA health and safety survey*. Retrieved from http://www.nursingworld.org/2011HealthSurveyResults.aspx.

American Nurses Association. (2014b). *Nurse Fatigue*. Retrieved from http://www.nursingworld.org/MainMenu-Categories/WorkplaceSafety/Healthy-Work-Environment/Work-Environment/NurseFatigue.

American Nurses Association. (2015). *Incivility, bullying and workplace violence*. Retrieved from http://www.nursing-world.org/Bullying-Workplace-Violence.

American Nurses Association. (2017). *Nurse staffing*. Retrieved from http://www.nursingworld.org/MainMenuCategories/Policy-Advocacy/State/Legislative-Agenda-Reports/State-StaffingPlansRatios.

American Nurses Credentialing Center. (2017a). *ANCC Magnet Recognition Program®*. Retrieved from http://www.nursecredentialing.org/Magnet.

American Nurses Credentialing Center. (2017b). *ANCC American Nurses Credentialing Pathway to Excellence®*. Retrieved from http://www.nursecredentialing.org/pathway.

American Organization of Nurse Executives. (2010). *AONE Guiding Principles for the Aging Workforce*. Retrieved from http://www.brewer.org/resources/aging-workforce.

AMN Healthcare. (2017). *Survey of registered nurses: Viewpoints on retirement, education and emerging roles.* Retrieved from https://www.amnhealthcare.com/2017-rnsurvey/.

Armstrong, K., Laschinger, H., & Wong, C. (2009). Workplace empowerment and Magnet hospital characteristics as predictors of patient safety climate. *Journal of Nursing Care Quality, 24*(1), 55–62.

Auerbach, D. I., Buerhaus, P., & Staiger, D. (2015). Will the RN workforce weather the retirement of the Baby Boomers? *Medical Care, 53*(10), 850.

Avalere Health LLC. (2015). *Optimal nurse staffing to improve quality of care and patient outcomes.* Retrieved from http://www.nursingworld.org/Avalere-White-Paper-on-Nurse-Staffing.

Bae, S. H., & Fabry, D. (2014). Assessing the relationships between nurse work hours/overtime and nurse and patient outcomes: systematic literature review. *Nursing Outlook, 62*(2), 138–156.

Bannai, A., & Tamakoshi, A. (2014). The association between long working hours and health: A systematic review of epidemiological evidence. *Scandinavian Journal of Work, Environment & Health, 40*(1), 5–18.

Brody, A. A., Barnes, K., Ruble, C., & Sakowski, J. (2012). Evidenced-based practice councils: potential path to staff nurse empowerment and leadership growth. *The Journal of Nursing Administration, 42*(1), 28–33.

Buerhaus, P. I. (2008). Current and future state of the U.S. nursing workforce. *JAMA, 300*(20), 2422–2424.

Campaign for Action (2017). *Transforming nursing education.* Retrieved from https://campaignforaction.org/issue/transforming-nursing-education.

Centers for Disease Control. (2016). *Needlestick Safety and Prevention Act 2000.* Retrieved from http://www.cdc.gov/sharpssafety/pdf/Neelstick%20Saftety%20and%20Prevention%20Act.pdf.

Chassin, M. R., & Loeb, J. M. (2013). High reliability health care: getting there from here. *The Milbank Quarterly, 91*(3), 459–490.

Dillon, B. L. (2012). Workplace violence: Impact, causes, and prevention. *Work, 42*, 15–20.

Duffin, C. (2014). Increase in nurse numbers linked to better patient survival rates in ICU. *Nursing Standard, 28*(33), 10.

Frith, K. H., Anderson, E. F., & Tseng, F., & Fong, E. A. (2012). Nurse staffing is an important strategy to prevent medication error in community hospitals. *Nursing Economic$, 30*(5), 288–294.

Gacki-Smith, J., Juarez, A. M., Boyett, L., Homeyer, C., Robinson, L., & MacLean, S. L. (2009). Violence against nurses working in US emergency departments. *The Journal of Nursing Administration, 39*(7–8), 340–349.

Gallagher, S. (2013). *Implementation guide to the safe patient handling and mobility interprofessional national standards.* Silver Spring, MD: American Nurses Association.

Government Printing Office. (2013). *113th Congress 1st session H.R. 2480, nurse and healthcare worker protection act of 2013.* Retrieved from http://www.gpo.gov/fdsys/pkg/BILLS-113hr2480ih/pdf/BILLS-113hr2480ih.pdf.

Institute of Medicine. (2011). *The Future of nursing: leading change, advancing health.* Washington, DC: National Academies Press.

Jagger, J., Berguer, R., Phillips, E. K., Parker, G., & Gomaa, A. E. (2010). Increase in sharps injuries in surgical settings versus nonsurgical settings after passage of national needlestick legislation. *Journal of the American College of Surgeons, 210*(4), 496–502.

Johnson & Johnson. (2017). *Campaign for nursing's future.* Retrieved from https://www.discovernursing.com/.

Kalisch, B. J., Tschannen, D., & Lee, K. H. (2012). Missed nursing care, staffing and patient falls. *Journal of Nursing Care Quality, 27*(1), 6–12.

Killgore, W. D., Grugle, N. L., & Balkin, T. J. (2012). Gambling when sleep deprived: don't bet on stimulants. *Chronobiology International, 29*(1), 43–54.

Kohn, L., Corrigan, J., & Donaldson, M. (2000). *To err is human: Building a safer health system.* Washington, DC: National Academies Press.

Kramer, M., Maguire, P. A. T., Brewer, B. B. (2011). Clinical nurses in Magnet hospitals confirm productive, healthy unit work environments. *Journal of Nursing Management, 19*(1), 5–17.

Lavoie-Tremblay, M., Leclerc, E., Marchionni, C., & Drevniok, U. (2010). The needs and expectations of Generation Y nurses in the workplace. *Journal for Nurses in Staff Development, 26*(1), 2–8.

Mark, B. A., Harless, D. W., Spetz, J., Reiter, K., & Pink, G. (2013). California's minimum nurse staffing legislation: results from a natural experiment. *Health Services Research, 48*(2), 435–454.

Martsolf, G. R., Auerbach, D., Benevent, R., Stocks, C., Jiang, H. J., Pearson, M. L., et al. (2014). Examining the value of inpatient nurse staffing: an assessment of quality and patient care costs. *Medical Care, 52*(11), 982–988.

McClure, M., Poulin, M., Sovie, M. D., et al. (1983). Magnet® hospitals: attraction and retention of professional nurses: Task

Force on Nursing Practice in Hospitals, American Academy of Nursing. *American Nurses Association Publications,* (G–160), i–xiv, 1–135.

McHugh, M. D., Kelly, L. A., Smith, H. L., Wu, E. S., Vanak, J. M., & Aiken, L. H. (2013). Lower mortality in magnet hospitals. *Medical Care, 51*(5), 382.

McHugh, M. D., & Ma, C. (2013). Hospital nursing and 30 day readmissions among Medicare patients with heart failure, acute myocardial infarction and pneumonia. *Medical Care, 51*(1), 52–59.

National Institute for Occupational Safety and Health, Centers for Disease Control and Prevention. (2017). *NIOSH Workplace safety and health topics: health care workers.* Retrieved from https://www.cdc.gov/niosh/topics/healthcare/default.html.

Nei, D., Snyder, L. A., & Litwiller, B. J. (2015). Promoting retention of nurses: a meta-analytic examination of causes of nurse turnover. *Health Care Management Review, 40*(3), 237–253.

Nolan, M., Lundh, U., & Brown, J. (1999). Changing aspects of nurses' work environment: a comparison of perceptions in two hospitals in Sweden and the UK and implications for recruitment and retention of staff. *The Journal of Nursing Research, 4*(3), 221–233.

Nursing Organizations Alliance. (2004). *Principles and elements of a healthful practice/work environment.* Retrieved from http://www.aone.org/resources/healthful-practice-work.pdf.

Occupational and Safety and Health Administration. (2013). *OSHA injury and illness recordkeeping and reporting requirements.* Retrieved from https://www.osha.gov/recordkeeping.

Occupational and Safety and Health Administration. (2015). *Workplace violence in healthcare.* Retrieved from https://www.osha.gov/Publications/OSHA3826.pdf.

Page, A. (Ed.). (2004). *Keeping patients safe: Transforming the work environment of nurses, Institute of Medicine.* Washington, DC: National Academies Press.

Quality and Safety Education for Nurses Institute. (2012). *Project Overview.* Retrieved from http://qsen.org/about-qsen/project-overview/.

Scott, L. D., Arslanian-Engoren, C., & Engoren, M. C. (2014). Association of sleep and fatigue with decision regret among critical care nurses. *American Journal of Critical Care, 23,* 13–23.

Sherman, R., & Pross, E. (2010). Growing future nurse leaders to build and sustain healthy work environments at the unit level. *Online Journal of Issues in Nursing, 15*(1), Manuscript 1. Retrieved from http://nursingworld.org/MainMenuCategories/ANAMarketplace/ANAPeriodicals/OJIN/TableofContents/Vol152010/No1Jan2010/Growing-Nurse-Leaders.aspx/.

Smith-Miller, C. A., Shaw-Kokot, J., Curro, B., & Jones, C. B. (2014). An integrative review: fatigue among nurses in acute care settings. *Journal of Nursing Administration, 44*(9), 487–494.

Speroni, K., Fitch, T., Dawson, E., et al. (2014). Incidence and cost of nurse workplace violence perpetrated by hospital patients or patient visitors. *Journal of Emergency Nursing, 40*(3), 218–228.

Spetz, J., Harless, D. W., Herrera, C. N., & Mark, B. A. (2013). Using minimum nurse staffing regulations to measure the relationship between nursing and hospital quality of care. *Medical Care Research and Review, 70*(4), 380–399.

Stichler, J. F. (2013). Healthy work environments for the ageing nursing workforce. *Journal of Nursing Management, 21,* 956–963.

Texas Department of State Health Services. (2016). *Workplace violence against nurses in Texas.* file:///C:/Users/SON/Downloads/DSHS-Report-HB2696%20(3).pdf.

The Joint Commission. (2002). *Health care at the crossroads: Strategies for addressing the evolving nursing crisis.* Oakbrook Terrace, IL: The Joint Commission on Accreditation of Healthcare Organizations.

Thrall, T. H. (2009). The return of the RNs. *Hospitals & Health Networks, 83*(4), 22–24.

Trinkoff, A. M., Johantgen, M., Storr, C. L., Gurses, A. P., Liang, Y., & Han, K. (2011). Nurses' work schedule characteristics, nurse staffing, and patient mortality. *Nursing Research, 60*(1), 1–8.

Tubbs-Cooley, H. L., Cimiotti, J. P., Silber, J. H., Sloane, D. M., & Aiken, L. H. (2013). An observational study of nurse staffing ratios and hospital readmission among children admitted for common conditions. *BMJ Quality & Safety, 22*(9), 735–742.

Ulrich, B., & Kear, T. (2014). Patient safety and patient safety culture: Foundations of excellent health care delivery. *Nephrology Nursing Journal, 41*(5), 447–456, 505.

U.S. Department of Health and Human Services, Health Resources and Services Administration. (2017). *Supply and demand projections of the nursing workforce: 2014-2030.* Retrieved from https://bhw.hrsa.gov/sites/default/files/bhw/nchwa/projections/NCHWA_HRSA_Nursing_Report.pdf

U.S. Department of Health and Human Services, Centers for Medicare and Medicaid Services. (2011). *§482.23 Condition of participation: Nursing services.* Retrieved from http://www.gpo.gov/fdsys/granule/CFR-2011-title42-vol5/CFR-2011-title42-vol5-sec482-23/content-detail.html.

U.S. Department of Labor, Bureau of Labor Statistics. (2016a). *Occupational outlook handbook (2016-2026).* Retrieved from http://www.bls.gov/ooh/healthcare/registered-nurses.htm.

U.S. Department of Labor, Bureau of Labor Statistics. (2016b). *Survey of occupational injuries and illnesses.* Retrieved from https://www.bls.gov/iif/osch0060.pdf.

14

Collective Bargaining and Unions in Today's Workplace

Barbara Cherry, DNSc, MBA, RN, NEA-BC

Collective bargaining is a method to achieve power sharing in the workplace.

(e) Additional resources are available online at: *http://evolve.elsevier.com/Cherry/*

LEARNING OUTCOMES

After studying this chapter, the reader will be able to:

1. Use terms associated with collective bargaining correctly in written and oral communications.
2. List key events in the historical development of collective bargaining and unions.
3. Recognize questionable labor or management practices in the workplace.
4. Analyze collective bargaining as a method to achieve power sharing in the workplace.
5. Evaluate current conflicts and controversies associated with collective bargaining by professional nurses.

KEY TERMS

Arbitration The process of negotiation sanctioned in the United States by the National Labor Relations Board. It is the method used for formal talks between management and labor within modern business, industry, and service organizations. "Binding arbitration" means that all parties must obey the arbitrator's recommendations.

Collective bargaining The process whereby workers organize under the representation of a union in order to share a degree of power with management to determine selected aspects of the conditions of employment.

Grievance A term associated with a negative workplace event that results in an allegation by an employee that he or she has not been treated fairly and equitably. Grievances can occur in union and non-union settings. In a union setting, a grievance generally arises when two parties, such as an employee and a manager, interpret contract provisions differently.

Grievances often involve job security or safety, which is a union priority, or job performance or discipline, which is a management priority.

Industrial unionism A type of union in which there is a single union for all workers in a corporation. For example, all people who work in an automobile manufacturing company may be grouped together under the United Auto Workers (UAW). It is possible that the industrial union, with its massive numbers of union members, is the strongest possible collective group.

Labor A group composed of those who work for others to receive a salary.

Management The group of people within a business or company who plan, organize, lead, or control the activities of employees who have agreed to work to receive a salary.

Occupational unionism A type of union in which each occupation within a given company has separate unions; these occupational groups might join others of like work across boundaries and across the country. White collar workers coming from a background of higher education and some measure of job security tend to prefer occupational unionism and organizing with like-minded professionals. In general, nurses prefer occupational unionism.

Picketing A form of protest in which people (called picketers) congregate outside a place of work or location where an event is taking place. Often this is done in an attempt to dissuade others from going in ("crossing the picket line"), but it can also be done to draw public attention to a cause.

Right-to-work laws Statutes enforced in 22 U.S. states, mostly in the southern and western United States, allowed under provisions of the Taft-Hartley Act, which prohibit agreements between unions and employers that make membership or payment of union dues or "fees" a condition of employment, either before or after hiring.

Secret ballot elections To establish a union in a workplace, a majority of employees must express support for the union. The employees prove majority through a secret ballot election conducted by the National Labor Relations Board.

Strike A work stoppage caused by the refusal of a large portion of employees to perform work; usually takes place to enforce demands relating to employment conditions or to protest unfair labor practices. A sympathy strike occurs when one union stops work to support the strike of another union.

Unfair labor practices Actions that interfere with the rights of employees or employers as identified under the National Labor Relations Act. An unfair labor practice can be something as simple as suspicion by an employee that he or she was assigned to an unpopular task unfairly, or it can be as complex as the identification of a pattern of many employees receiving discriminatory treatment in the workplace because of being union supporters. Unfair labor practices are a frequent source of either strikes or the initiation of union activity within a setting.

Union A group of workers who band together to accomplish goals related to conditions of employment.

PROFESSIONAL/ETHICAL ISSUE

Samuel Lennon is a registered nurse in the cardiovascular lab at University Hospital. He is currently experiencing extreme stress and internal conflict because the nurses are going through a union organizing effort. What he thought would be a fairly easy process to vote in a union to represent the nurses with a strong voice to improve their nurse-to-patient ratios has turned into a tension-filled, adversarial situation. Before the union efforts started, Samuel had a good relationship with his nurse manager; now they are pitted against each other because they have very different perspectives about unions. He is also feeling tension and distrust with the same nurses he had supportive working relationships with only a few weeks ago; but they are now against one another because of opposing views about unions. His once collegial relationships with the pharmacists and physical therapists on his unit have also become strained. Samuel is now having a great deal of self-doubt about the unionizing efforts and especially what some of his colleagues perceive to be the potential for patient abandonment in the event of a strike. Samuel's greatest concern is how this very difficult situation is affecting patient care.

How can Samuel resolve his feelings and ethical concerns about the unionizing effort yet remain true to the original goals of unionization?

VIGNETTE

Addison Mitchell graduated in June from nursing school. She passed the National Council Licensure Examination (NCLEX) and can now call herself a registered nurse (RN). As she drives to the hospital on the first day of her new job, she is feeling a sense of pride and joy, mixed with sheer fright, as she realizes that this is the world-class place she has chosen for her first job. She had always dreamed of working at this hospital, and she will now have a chance to become a seasoned nurse at one of the finest hospitals in the country.

Addison is realistic enough to know that her feelings of joy may not last because her new job is likely to be very stressful, but she is unaware that she is on the verge of walking into a challenging situation. As she enters the drive leading to the hospital parking area, picketers are there with signs about unfair working conditions and she quickly learns that nurses are involved in organizing to be represented by a union.

As Addison walks to the building with her new name tag that reads "Registered Nurse," she is approached by a person asking her to sign a card.

Addison replies, "I'm sorry. I'm new here. I need to get my feet on the ground, and then I will be happy to talk to you about the card." Addison begins to feel very anxious because she does not have a good understanding of union organizing efforts or the issues the nurses are facing.

Addison does not yet know that she will be approached many times in the coming days by coworkers who will tell her how she should feel and what she should do. She has much to consider before making a decision between two alternatives that she does not fully understand.

Questions to Consider While Reading this Chapter:

1. What questions should the nurse ask about collective bargaining and labor relations?
2. What does signing a card mean, and what questions should Addison ask before signing?
3. How can Addison establish good relationships with both nurse managers and staff nurses in an atmosphere in which collective bargaining has put these two groups in adversarial positions?
4. What skills and information will Addison need to navigate and make effective decisions in this hospital?
5. What provisions in a union contract are in a patient's best interest as well as a nurse's?
6. What resources are available to Addison to help her learn more about labor and management issues occurring in the hospital?

CHAPTER OVERVIEW

Collective bargaining is a very complex and often an emotionally charged issue. Because the future of nursing may be influenced by our collective and individual efforts to be fairly represented and to have a voice in the conditions of our work, it is important to understand the costs and benefits of collective action as well as the motives of those who would represent nursing. This chapter attempts to present a balanced view of collective bargaining and unionization in the hope that students, staff nurses, and nurses in managerial positions will use the information to make effective decisions when confronted with collective bargaining issues.

DEVELOPMENT OF COLLECTIVE BARGAINING IN AMERICA

Early Activities

During the late nineteenth century, when the Industrial Revolution was a force throughout North America, a cadre of thinkers arose who believed that workers needed to join together to protect themselves from circumstances such as long work hours, child labor, and unhealthy factory conditions. These early groups sought such basic conditions as safety in work situations, adequate pay for hours worked, and the right not to be arbitrarily dismissed. This banding together of workers to accomplish goals was termed *trade unionism*. The technique was successful in many instances and remains with us today.

Federal Legislation

As a result of these early efforts at unionization, Congress passed the National Labor Relations Act (NLRA) in 1935. Under the terms of the NLRA, employees were given the right to self-organize, to form labor unions, and to bargain collectively. As part of the 1935 NLRA, the National Labor Relations Board (NLRB) was established to implement provisions of the NLRA. The NLRB is an independent federal agency that continues to play a vital role in labor-management relations and, working through 26 regional offices in major U.S. cities, the agency conducts union elections and prosecutes unfair labor practices.

With employees' rights protected by federal legislation, collective bargaining now occurs in companies across the country. Employees can legally organize themselves into units recognized under terms of the NLRA without fear of being fired for belonging to a union or for participating in union activities, such as collective bargaining. Typical goals in collective bargaining activities are to establish reasonable working conditions and to make formal agreements between employees and management for wages and health and retirement benefits. Unions can vary by the group or groups of employees represented. Industrial unionism is a single union representing all workers in a company whereas occupational unionism is a separate union representing a distinct occupation within a given company.

However, exemptions to the 1935 NLRA were established for nonprofit companies. This provision meant that employees of nonprofit hospitals, such as nurses, were not protected under the NLRA and therefore were not legally protected for participation in collective bargaining activities. Hospitals' employees may have been excluded from protection by the NLRA because it was believed that services provided were so essential that organizing activities would be contrary to the public's interest. Eventually, in 1974, legislation allowed for the inclusion of nonprofit hospitals in coverage under provisions of the NLRA. Nurses could form collective bargaining units. The 1974 amendments also included the requirement for a 10-day written notice of the intent to picket or to strike. This notice would give the health care facility time to prepare and would protect the relative health and safety of the public.

Development of Collective Bargaining in Nursing

Formal unionization in nursing began in 1946 when the American Nurses Association (ANA) endorsed collective bargaining as a way to gain economic security and influence employment issues for nurses. While the ANA worked to pave the way for collective bargaining, it also struggled with its role in representing nurses who were part of unions as well as nurses who did not support unionization. To help resolve ANA's role in representing different interests of nurses, a national nurses union—United American Nurses (UAN)—was established as an ANA affiliate to create an independent voice for union nurses. In 2009, the UAN dropped its affiliation with the ANA and merged with the California Nurses Association/National Nurses Organizing Committee and the Massachusetts Nurses Association to form National Nurses United (NNU).

According to the most current estimates available, approximately 17% of the nation's RNs are members of unions (Department of Professional Employees, 2015). NNU is the largest nursing union in the United States,

representing over 150,000 registered nurses (NNU, 2018). Other unions that represent nurses include some ANA state affiliates, Service Employees International Union, and the American Federation of State, County and Municipal Employees.

THE COLLECTIVE BARGAINING PROCESS

Collective bargaining is a method of equalizing power. As such, it involves negotiation and administrative agreements between employees and employers. Because the individual employee, or even a small group of employees, has limited power to bargain with the employer, banding together in a union gives the employees a stronger voice to negotiate with management. The goals of collective bargaining are achieved by imposing rules regarding how employers must treat employees represented by a union. The union movement in the United States is involved with strengthening a worker's position in the relationship between management and labor.

Nurses and nurse managers need to understand the steps involved in the union organizing and election process as well as what are considered appropriate or inappropriate management responses and labor responses. Because union organizing involves power sharing and sometimes a temporary sense of distrust between direct-care nurses and management, it can become an anxious and emotional process. Knowing the allowable patterns for the process of union organizing can help alleviate some stress.

The following discussion is an overview of the general steps in the union organizing process based on information taken from the *Basic Guide to the National Labor Relations Act* (NLRB, 1997). The reader will see that careful attention is given to ensuring fairness for employer, employees, and the unions that may be involved in an election to determine whether employees agree to unionize.

Although this discussion provides a general overview of the union election process, readers are encouraged to visit the NLRB website (http://www.nlrb.gov) for more detailed information about the union election process.

The Preformal Period in Union Organizing

The goal of collective bargaining is the equalization of power between labor (e.g., direct-care nurses) and management. To initiate collective bargaining activities, an organizing drive is instituted by union forces, who attempt to create an official NLRB-sanctioned bargaining unit in a particular institution. The bargaining unit is either accepted or rejected through an election process in which non-management employees (direct-care nurses) vote. If accepted, the bargaining unit will be made up of union members who are workers at the unionized facility and will be designed to protect the workers against arbitrary treatment and unfair labor practices.

A union organizing drive may be initiated when nurses in a particular health care facility contact a union because they feel a need for help in negotiating with their employer. The stimulus for this initial contact is usually not frivolous. There is typically a pervasive feeling among the nurses on a particular unit or in the health care facility as a whole that working conditions are unsatisfactory and that there is no possibility of making improvements under the existing management circumstances.

It is helpful at this point to examine what is to be gained by those petitioning the NLRB for an election for union representation. For a group of nurses, a newly formed union will:

- Have the power to make certain demands of the employer, especially regarding salary, benefits, and nurse-to-patient ratios.
- Provide some degree of political power on a local level.
- Require nurses to pay dues to the union.

For the union organization, a newly formed union will:

- Give the organization additional power by adding more members and more bargaining units, especially if the union is part of a larger national union.
- Increase monetary support for the union organization through dues paid by nurses. The additional money can be used to pay union officials' salaries, organize other bargaining units, or contribute to political causes or candidates.

Once a union has been contacted by nurses and told that there is some interest in establishing a collective bargaining unit, union forces try to determine whether efforts to organize the majority of nurses in the facility will be successful. This determination is made through a process of "signing cards." Union authorization cards help the union organizer, a person who works for the union, to decide whether there is enough interest

in unionization on the part of nurses employed in the facility. Once signed by the nurse, the union authorization card designates the union as his or her bargaining agent. The signed authorization card is legally binding on the employee, despite any claims the union may make to the contrary. *It is very important for the nurse to understand that his or her signature on a union authorization card is automatically authorizing the union to serve as his or her legal representative.*

If 30% of employed nurses sign cards, signaling an interest in representation by the union, the employer and the NLRB are officially notified, and the employer must refrain from anti-labor action, such as firing those who favor the union (NLRB, 1997). If 50% plus 1 of the nurses who are eligible to vote (non-management nurses) responds in the affirmative to accept union representation, then nurses in the facility become represented by the union and are unionized.

Right-to-Work Laws. An important exception to note here is that there are 24 states with right-to-work laws that allow employees to work without being compelled to join a union. A nurse in a right-to-work state can choose not to become a union member yet receives the benefits resulting from the union contract. Thus, in right-to-work states, union member nurses may work alongside non–union member nurses, possibly creating tension between the two groups. The 28 right-to-work states are Alabama, Arizona, Arkansas, Florida, Georgia, Idaho, Indiana, Iowa, Kansas, Kentucky, Louisiana, Michigan, Mississippi, Missouri, Nebraska, Nevada, North Carolina, North Dakota, Oklahoma, South Carolina, South Dakota, Tennessee, Texas, Utah, Virginia, West Virginia, Wisconsin, and Wyoming.

Allowable Actions during the Union Organizing Effort. To follow the process effectively, a nurse should be aware of details of what is and is not allowed and what is and is not likely to occur during union organizing efforts. When a specific union, such as National Nurses United, initiates organizing activities in a particular facility, an organizer goes to the facility. The organizer, who may be called a *business agent* or *field representative,* is responsible for developing and implementing plans to ensure success of the unionizing effort.

To form a core support group in the facility, the organizer locates respected leaders in the workplace. Meetings are then held in nonwork settings such as homes or restaurants to gain initial information about grievances and workplace inequities. This information is used as a basis for campaign literature. To gain additional supporters, discussion and card signing take place in areas in the actual facility: locker rooms, bathrooms, lunch areas, lounges, and less visible work areas. Now, e-mail and social media—Twitter and Facebook—are being used effectively as means for union organizers to communicate with employees (Carlson, 2014).

As the union drive surfaces to gain management's attention, organizers begin to distribute cards more openly. At this point, the union organizer sends a registered letter to the employer with the names of employees on the organizing committee. Management will probably have already become aware of organizing activities through clues such as employee behavior changes during this period. There will be times when individuals seem distracted or when there is an increase in the number or aggressive quality of complaints about workplace conditions. Conversely, there may be a feeling of distancing between labor and management and an air of unnatural silence among employees.

Although peaceful strikes and picketing may occur for the purpose of publicity or seeking recognition, the NLRB prohibits certain behaviors during the pre-election period. The union may not:

- Inflame racial prejudices.
- Lie about loss of jobs if the union loses the election.
- Forge documents or signatures.
- Meet or distribute literature in work areas during work times.
- Hold meetings within 24 hours of an election.
  During the pre-election period, management may not:
- Solicit spying.
- Photograph employees engaged in union activities.
- Visit employees in their homes.
- Lie about what will happen if the union is the victor in an election.
- Question employees about their preferences regarding union activity.

The Election Process

There are several steps in the election process. Either the union or the employer must petition the NLRB for an election. Once this petition is made, the request is passed along to the regional NLRB director. Within 48 hours, the union must submit proof of its claim that 30% of eligible nurses are interested in forming a collective bargaining

unit. Eligible nurses are generally considered to be nurses who are engaged in patient care and are not in management positions. Normally, for a 10-day period, literature will be distributed to eligible employees. The union and the employer may circulate literature; however, both sides must cease such activities 24 hours before the election.

On the day designated for the election, the three parties (the NLRB, union representatives, and employer representatives) meet to review the list of those eligible to vote. A secret ballot election is then conducted by the National Labor Relations Board. The three parties then count ballots, and in case of a true tie, a victory for the employer is declared. However, any votes in dispute will be set aside for a later recount. Objections must be made within 5 working days after the election and may be made on the grounds of problems with the conduct of the election or unfair labor practices.

Post Election

After the election, in the case of a union victory, federal law guarantees workers the right to collectively bargain and strike. Nurses may subsequently change a bargaining agent or remove the union representation by having 30% of nurses sign cards. An election would follow, requiring a vote of 50% plus 1 in favor of the change (NLRB, 1997).

The NLRA mandates that under the rules of collective bargaining, meetings between management and labor be held at reasonable times for the purpose of conferring in good faith. Mandatory topics for arbitration include wages; the establishment of rules about the use of labor, such as hours of work and nurse-to-patient ratios; individual workers' rights; resolution of grievances; and methods of enforcement, interpretation, and administration of the union agreement. Negotiations between union and management occur in cycles following the initial year of collective bargaining. Negotiations are held before a contract is ratified (approved) by both union and management and again just before the contract expires.

Principles to Guide Fairness during Union Organizing

In an unprecedented collaboration between a major U.S. health care employer and unions, a set of guiding principles was established to ensure a fair process for union organizing efforts. The principles, which can serve as a guide for employers and unions across the country, help ensure that health care employees are able to make informed decisions regarding unionization without undue influence or pressure from either side. On the basis of these seven principles, employers as well as unions should agree in writing how they will (Catholic Healthcare Association of America, 2009):

- Demonstrate respect for each other's organization and mission.
- Provide workers with equal access to information from both sides.
- Adhere to standards for truthfulness and balance in their communications.
- Create a pressure-free environment.
- Allow workers to vote through a fair and expeditious process.
- Honor employees' decision regardless of the outcome.
- Create a system for enforcing these principles during the course of an organizing drive.

UNIONS AND PROFESSIONAL NURSING

Professionalism versus Unionization

Nurses in the workplace are buffeted by cost cutting, nursing shortages, shuffled duties, concerns about patient safety and quality care, and hospital reorganizations that bring job insecurity and uncertainty. Despite these troublesome working conditions, it is often problematic for nurses to come to grips with their feelings related to the emotionally charged issues associated with unionization. Many nurses may be reluctant to become involved with what they view as trouble-making groups who exaggerate the issues just to win the contest against the adversary, which is management. It is difficult to reconcile feelings of professionalism and service with the perceived connotations of strife and discord associated with unions.

In addition, nurses who try to update their thoughts about unionization through reading finds that it becomes difficult to find objective reading material. Few experienced authorities on collective bargaining can remain neutral or objective. It is challenging to read about unionization without encountering biased language and the attempt to paint one side or the other in extremely unflattering terms. This situation does not help clear away the fog of conflict surrounding unionization decisions for nurses.

Questions to Answer

Four major questions need to be answered as nurses consider unionization.

1. Are there relevant gains to be made for the nursing profession and for improved patient care through collective bargaining—or is this a myth?
2. Should nurses, who frequently are called on to supervise the work of others, be classified for collective bargaining purposes as management or labor?
3. Will nurses be too reluctant to strike? This is one of the most powerful tools that a union has at its disposal. There is concern that strikes by nurses could negatively affect patient care and destroy the public's image of nursing. More importantly, the strike is contrary to nursing ethics and licensure to do no harm and avoid patient abandonment.
4. How will nursing unions affect other members of the interprofessional team (e.g., physical therapy, dietary, pharmacy), which is essential for quality patient care? Will the nurses' collective bargaining contract create inequities for other professionals?

These questions are addressed in more detail in the following sections.

Gains for the Nursing Profession and Patient Care?

When considering unionization, nurses need to seriously reflect on issues that affect the practice of professional nursing and on the patient care environment beyond the aspects that unions typically address during negotiations (wages and benefits, work hours, worker safety, and resolution of grievances). The primary triggers that spark interest in being represented by a union often are forgotten in the challenges confronted by nurses during the union organization process. Consider the following issues that may prompt a group of nurses to seek union representation:

- Physicians not seeing critical patients in a timely manner, putting patients at risk
- Lack of administrative support for collegial, professional relationships among nurses, physicians, and other interprofessional team members
- Deficient patient handoff procedures that cause errors, frustration, interdepartmental conflicts, and delay in care
- Inadequate addressing of nursing staff continuing education and unit-specific competencies
- Self-scheduling being designed around staff needs, not patient and unit needs

Nurses are cautioned that gains in wages and benefits may be achieved through unionization but the nursing practice environment may suffer. In one large study using the National Sample Surveys of Registered Nurses for 2004 and 2008, union representation was negatively associated with job satisfaction (Seago et al, 2011). The researchers in this study point out that a cause for this finding may be that union nurses could be more vocal about expressing their concerns, or the dissatisfaction may have led to the unionization. Another study comparing 84 union and 84 non-union hospitals in the United States found that hospitals with unions have significantly lower patient satisfaction (Koys et al, 2015).

Another professional practice issue to consider is that open dialog between nurses and their managers regarding patient care issues and concerns is limited in a unionized facility. For example, the manager cannot discuss performance issues or concerns with a nurse directly; the union representative must serve as the intermediary between the nurse and the manager. This added layer to address the nurse's performance increases costs to the facility for both management time and legal expense.

When faced with union organizing efforts, nurses need to carefully consider all factors, including the professional practice environment. Box 14.1 presents a list of questions the nurse should ask when confronted by a union organizing effort.

Promoting a Positive Work Environment. Regardless of whether the nurse works in a union environment, there are several strategies he or she can use to develop and encourage sound relationships between management and labor to promote a positive work environment:

- Assess your knowledge of the labor laws and practices in your area; seek to understand the unique culture of the facility; and seek help before union activity begins or grievances are filed.
- Understand what protections are already in place through laws and regulations to protect your rights as a nurse (e.g., whistle-blower protection, staffing regulations, safe patient handling laws).
- Identify and be proactive in situations in which nurses or managers disrespect others, ignore serious staff and patient care concerns, or neglect appropriate communication and follow-up.
- Participate in education and training that will improve your labor relations skills in union and non-union environments.
- Be proactive in solving issues that compromise patient care; embrace your role in achieving timely outcomes that truly improve care.
- Develop an understanding of and respect for the health care facility's financial challenges and become part of the solution for more cost-effective care.

Management or Staff?

One of the difficult issues for nursing in relation to collective bargaining is that in the eyes of the NLRB certain nurses are singled out as management or supervisory personnel and are not allowed NLRA protection, which applies only to nonmanagement employees. Charge nurses and shift supervisors have traditionally been considered part of management rather than labor. But what about nurses who routinely supervise others who act merely as extenders of care? Are these nurses acting exclusively on behalf of the company that employs them, or are they routinely carrying out their responsibilities as professional nurses?

The definition of *manager* or *supervisor* is problematic even in non–health care settings. In nursing, things become even more complicated. Most experienced RNs are involved in some type of supervisory or management work. For example, most staff nurses who ordinarily

---

BOX 14.1   Questions to Ask when Confronted by a Union Organizer

- What measures has the union successfully used to improve quality of care and promote national patient safety goals?
- Will the union guarantee in writing that it will be getting employees a specified wage increase and better benefits or be liable to employees if it doesn't?
- How much are union dues? What portion of union dues goes to paying union salaries?
- Are there special union assessments? If so, how much are they and how often are they imposed?
- What are the consequences if employees violate the union constitution and/or bylaws?
- Will the union guarantee in writing that employees will not be permanently replaced during an economic strike?
- Will the union pay wages to employees if they are called on to strike?
- Will union members be expected to picket at other unionized facilities in the event of a strike or an informational picket?

provide bedside care have been called on to be in charge of a particular unit for a particular working shift. Does this mean that the nurse should no longer be considered nonmanagement?

Another trend that affects decisions about supervisory status is the increasing use of unlicensed personnel in health care workplaces. More nurses could now be classified as supervisory because they direct the activities of unlicensed workers. In 1994, in *NLRB v. the Health Care and Retirement Corporation,* the U.S. Supreme Court ruled that nurses do indeed direct the work of others and therefore are not eligible for protection under the NLRA. This case was important to the nursing profession because had the ruling been upheld, it would have dramatically lowered the numbers of nurses who could act as "laborers" and engage in collective bargaining. However, in 1997 the decision of the U.S. Court of Appeals for the Ninth Circuit helped clarify this point. The court ruled that RNs who performed charge nurse duties were not management and therefore were eligible for collective bargaining protection. In another case, *Providence Alaska Medical Center v. NLRB,* the ruling recognized that the judgment used by RNs in assigning patients and coordinating patient care was part of their professional role rather than part of any statutory supervision as defined by the NLRA.

Beyond the issue of recognizing who is management and who is staff, there is the uncomfortable prospect of pitting nurse managers against their colleagues in the workplace. A definite schism occurs when managers and staff are placed on opposite sides of the table. Bad feelings arise. For example, a nurse manager represents management but is not insulated in an executive office. In addition, the nurse manager must often assume duties routinely performed by staff nurses in the event of a strike. This situation can lead to lingering negative feelings even after the strike is resolved.

Techniques frequently used by nurse managers to maintain smooth and efficient job performance in their work settings may be relatively ineffective when unionization or collective bargaining initiatives occur. For example, the nurse manager who believes that open communication in both upward and downward directions is useful for problem solving may become frustrated during unionization initiatives. Union tactics may involve coaching nurses at staff levels to use the "silent treatment" and not cooperate with nurse managers' attempts to communicate.

To Strike or Not?

Strikes can have very powerful effects. One can best understand the economic effect of a strike by noting that hospitals become concerned over lost revenues when the average daily census drops only a few percentage points. A hospital could possibly have to turn away patients because of a strike and could lose that market share permanently, resulting in long-term losses to the hospital. Thus a strike or the threat of a strike can be effective in gaining concessions (e.g., salary increases, better benefits) from management in an effort to avoid the strike completely or to end it as soon as possible. However, it is important to note that in some states, collective bargaining contracts may contain "no strike" clauses, prohibiting the collective bargaining unit from having the power of the strike.

Nursing is a trusted profession, and for many nurses, the strike is a symbol of negative behavior. To safeguard nursing's image and allow hospitals to react effectively in safeguarding patient care, a 10-day notice of intent to strike is required. On receipt of such notice, the NLRB attempts to mediate, and the hospital in question is encouraged to decrease census and halt elective admissions. Schedules are developed for covering the emergency department, operating room, and intensive care areas.

As nurses are confronted with making decisions about unionization, it is important to consider the many issues that would affect their personal economic welfare, their practice environment, and the quality of patient care they are able to provide. There are no easy answers because the issues and challenges vary depending on each organization's unique set of circumstances. To successfully negotiate unionization initiatives and make good decisions, nurses are encouraged to learn more about collective bargaining and unions.

Nursing Unions and Interprofessional Teamwork?

Nursing may be the only professional occupation in a health care setting to be represented by a union (i.e., occupational unionism). Unfortunately, having unionized nurses working alongside employees, such as pharmacists and therapists, who are not represented by unions, may create ill will between the two groups. The benefit package for nurses represented by a union can be different from—and likely better than—the benefit package for other employees. As employment and practice issues arise, nurses have union representation as their go-between to work with management, whereas other disciplines work directly with management to resolve issues. The union contract for nurses' benefits will increase the overall costs to the organization, forcing the organization to cut in other areas not controlled by the union, such as benefits for non-unionized health professionals. Imagine how the relationship between two professionals might be strained if the nurse represented by the union has more paid time off and more frequent salary increases than a colleague he or she works with on a daily basis; plus the non-nursing professional knows that the cost of the union contract may be the reason he or she is not able to get a salary increase. Relationships between interprofessional team members is a very important issue as nurses consider unionization!

SUMMARY

This chapter has provided a history and overview of the collective bargaining process and addressed some important issues for nurses to consider as they face questions regarding unionization. These important issues include the role of unionization in addressing the professional practice environment and quality care, the questions surrounding management versus labor in collective bargaining, and the controversy of the strike as a strategy to gain concessions from the employer. The role of unions in the future of health care may hinge on cooperation versus conflict, on relative productivity gains in union versus non-union facilities, and on the success of human relations practices in union as well as non-union workplaces. Nurses live in a new era in health care and will need to continue to grow in their knowledge of unions and collective bargaining.

REFERENCES

Carlson, J. (2014). 2014 likely to be busy year for unions. *Modern Healthcare, 44*(3), 8.

Catholic Healthcare Association of America. (2009). *Respecting the just rights of workers: guidance and options for Catholic health care and unions.* Retrieved December 27, 2017 from http://www.usccb.org/issues-and-action/human-life-and-dignity/labor-employment/upload/respecting_the_just_rights_of_workers.pdf.

Department of Professional Employees, AFL-CIO. (2015). *Nursing: A profile of the profession.* Retrieved December 27, 2017 from http://dpeaflcio.org/programs-publications/issue-fact-sheets/nursing-a-profile-of-the-profession/#_edn35.

Koys, D. J., Martin, W. M., Lavan, H., & Katz, M. (2015). Union density and hospital outcomes. *Hospital Topics, 93*(3), 69–76.

National Labor Relations Board. (1997). *Basic Guide to the National Labor Relations Act.* Washington, DC: U.S. Government Printing Office.

National Nurses United. (2018). *About us.* Retrieved December 27, 2017 from https://www.nationalnursesunited.org/about.

Seago, J. A., Spetz, J., Ash, M., Herrera, C. N., & Keane, D. (2011). Hospital RN job satisfaction and nurse unions. *The Journal of Nursing Administration, 41*(3), 109–114.

15

Information Technology in the Clinical Setting

Teresa M. Stephens, PhD, RN, CNE,
Tami H. Wyatt, PhD, RN, CNE, ANEF, FAAN

Electronic health records offer nurses and other team members information when, where, and how they need it.

ⓔ Additional resources are available online at: *http://evolve.elsevier.com/Cherry/*

LEARNING OUTCOMES

After studying this chapter, the reader will be able to:

1. Describe key attributes of electronic health record systems and their influence on patient safety and quality care.
2. Explain "meaningful use" criteria as applicable to electronic health records.
3. Critique various types of point-of-care technology and their use in the clinical setting.
4. Assess how future trends in technology will affect health care delivery.
5. Use established criteria to evaluate the content of health-related sites found on the Internet.

KEY TERMS

Decision support tools Software programs that process data to produce or recommend decisions by linking with an electronic knowledge base controlled by established rules for combining data elements; the knowledge base and rules mimic the knowledge and reasoning an expert health professional would apply to data and information to solve a problem.

Electronic health record (EHR) The longitudinal electronic record of patient health information generated by one or more encounters in any care delivery setting; has the ability to support other care-related activity such as evidence-based decision support, quality management, and outcomes reporting (American Health Information Management Association [AHIMA], 2012).

EHR (electronic health record) interoperability EHR systems that have the ability to share and transfer patient data seamlessly across health care systems and settings in a standardized manner that protects the reliability, confidentiality, privacy, and security of the information.

EHR "meaningful use" A defined set of EHR capabilities and standards that EHR systems must meet to ensure that their full capacity is realized and for the users (hospitals and physician/provider practices) to qualify for financial incentives from Medicare.

Health information technology The use of various forms of technology to improve the

Thanks to Leslie H. Nicoll, PhD, MBA, RN, and Cynthia K. Russell, PhD, APN, for their contributions to this chapter in previous editions.

quality of health services to individuals and communities.

Information technology The hardware and software that enable information to be stored, retrieved, communicated, and managed.

Point-of-care technology Technologies that allow real-time data retrieval, documentation, and decision support at the bedside or wherever direct care is provided.

PROFESSIONAL/ETHICAL ISSUE

Katherine is a recent registered nurse–bachelor of science in nursing (RN-BSN) graduate working in the post-anesthesia care unit of a small, community-based hospital. She receives a new patient and begins reviewing the patient's history and medication orders. This patient, a 68-year-old male with multiple comorbidities, has just returned from a hernia repair procedure. Katherine notes he has multiple drug allergies, and she is unfamiliar with one of his prescribed pain medications. She uses her mobile device to access a drug database to check for any interactions and/or contraindications. As she is reviewing this information, her shift supervisor enters the room and demands that she put her phone away. Katherine explains what she is doing and expresses her concern over the prescribed medications. The supervising nurse tells Katherine that it is not her responsibility to question a doctor's orders. She continues to inform Katherine that it is against hospital policy for nurses to use a cell phone during work hours.

Discuss how Katherine might address this situation in a professional manner to advocate for the use of mobile devices as knowledge support in the quest to enhance the quality and safety of patient care.

VIGNETTE

Victoria Ellis is finally living her dream. After four hard years in school, Victoria is working at a university medical center. Although she graduated from a well-respected nursing program, she is apprehensive about her new role, especially documenting care and accessing pertinent information. In nursing school, all of her clinical experiences were in facilities that used electronic health records (EHRs), but as a student, Victoria's access to the EHRs was limited. She could not log onto the system herself, she could not chart, and she could access only limited screens such as lab values, assessment information, and vital signs.

Victoria learned in school that EHRs are a vital information technology tool in health care today, but according to her limited experience, an EHR seems like it is nothing more than a paper chart on a computer. So, what is all the hype about EHRs, information technology, and health care?

Questions to Consider While Reading this Chapter:

1. What are the potential benefits of electronic health records to nurses, other health care providers, and patients?
2. What are the barriers to a universal U.S. health information technology infrastructure?
3. What is meant by "meaningful use" of EHRs?
4. How might advanced point-of-care technology influence health care at the bedside?
5. How does health information technology affect consumer health?

CHAPTER OVERVIEW

Today's clinical setting is filled with a multitude of technologic tools and equipment that are used by all health care providers. Nurses are likely to encounter voice communication systems, handheld mobile devices, robotic pharmacy dispensaries, wearable technologies, and complex computers and EHRs. These records present data in graphs, tables, and charts that may reveal a different story from that told by words and numbers alone. Transforming patient data into meaningful bits of information is merely one advantage of health information technology (HIT). These data can also be shared with other facilities, creating a comprehensive patient record, thereby reducing duplicate services and tests and creating continuity in care. In this chapter, we explore the important role of HIT in today's clinical environment, barriers to and opportunities with advanced HIT, and ways to educate consumers about health information on the Internet.

HEALTH INFORMATION TECHNOLOGY ACROSS THE GLOBE

Health information technology, or technology used to promote the health and well-being of patients and the community, is ever-increasing as technology rapidly advances. Consumer-driven demands for greater knowledge and access about care options have driven many of the technology integrations within health care settings, including nursing academia and practice. Additionally, regulatory and accrediting bodies are requiring or strongly recommending the integration of technology into all aspects of nursing academia and practice. Expansion of the Internet is also responsible for promoting access to health resources and information. Global integration of technology has advanced the possibilities for networking, education, provider consultation, and disaster response without regard to geographic limitations.

Health Information Technology in the United States

Health information technology has been a hot topic for more than two decades, specifically in relation to the need for improved quality and safety of patient care. The United States is currently challenged to implement EHRs universally across all settings, from hospitals to ambulatory care settings to home health agencies and nursing homes. For EHR systems to have the greatest impact on cost and quality, they must be interoperable with the ability to exchange information across systems and settings in a standardized manner that protects the reliability, confidentiality, privacy, and security of the information.

Within the United States, there are two major influences on the adoption of EHRs: the federal government and America's health insurance plans. Both of these entities can set certain requirements regarding EHRs as a condition of payment for services. In the past, measuring adoption rates of EHRs in the United States was a challenge because it depended on self-reporting. However, the Centers for Medicare & Medicaid Services (CMS) now offers incentive programs for providers—hospitals and physician/provider practices—that qualify and adopt certified EHRs that meet meaningful use criteria (CMS, 2017).

ELECTRONIC HEALTH RECORDS

An EHR is a system that captures, processes, communicates, secures, and presents data about the patient. In addition to capturing patient data, other components of an EHR include clinical rules, patient education materials, evidence-based practice guidelines, and payer rules related to reimbursement. When these elements work together in an integrated fashion, the EHR becomes much more than a patient record—it becomes a knowledge tool. The system is able to integrate information from multiple sources and provide decision support; thus the EHR serves as the primary source of information for patient care and quality improvements in the health care system.

Key Functions of the EHR

The Institute of Medicine (IOM) (2003) recommends that EHR systems offer the following eight functionalities: (1) health information and data capture; (2) results/data management; (3) provider order entry management; (4) clinical decision support; (5) electronic communication and connectivity among providers, the health care team, and patients; (6) patient support; (7) administrative process support; and (8) reporting and population health management. Table 15.1 provides more detailed information about these core functionalities.

Clinical decision support is of particular relevance to nursing practice because it contributes to safety and quality by providing automatic reminders about preventive practices, such as immunizations, drug alerts for dosing and interactions, and electronic resources for data interpretation and clinical decision making. Current efforts focus on the creation of nursing process–based clinical decision support tools to better promote effective communication in and among health care teams to facilitate continuity and individuality of care (Müller-Staub et al, 2016).

Another component of the EHR relevant to safety and quality is computerized provider order entry (CPOE), defined as the "process by which a health care provider (i.e., physician, nurse practitioner, physician's assistant, or physical or occupational therapist) directly enters orders for client care into a hospital information system" (Hebda et al, 2017). CPOE contributes to safety and quality by eliminating lost orders and illegible handwriting; generating related orders automatically (e.g., a laboratory test needed to monitor a specific medication); monitoring for duplicate or contradictory orders; and reducing time to fill orders (Hebda et al, 2017; IOM, 2003). The success of CPOE depends on the user's

TABLE 15.1   Core Functionalities for Electronic Health Record Systems As Recommended by the Institute of Medicine

Health information and data	Information to make sound clinical decisions, such as past medical history, laboratory tests, allergies, current medications, and consent forms
Results management	Electronic reports of laboratory results and radiology procedures with automated display of previous results; electronic consultation reports
Order entry and order management	Computerized provider order entry with or without decision support to eliminate lost orders and illegible handwriting, generate related orders automatically, monitor for duplicate or contradictory orders, and reduce time to fill orders
Decision support	Enhance clinical performance by providing reminders about preventive practices, such as immunizations, drug alerts for dosing and interactions, and clinical decision making
Electronic communication and connectivity	Electronic communication between health care team members and other care partners, such as radiology and laboratory personnel, and connectivity to the patient record across multiple care settings
Patient support	Computer-based patient education and home monitoring where applicable
Administrative processes	Scheduling systems, billing and claims management, insurance eligibility, and inventory management
Reporting and population health management	Meeting of public and private sector reporting requirements at the federal, state, and local levels; addressing of internal quality improvement initiatives

Data from Institute of Medicine. (2003). Key capabilities of an electronic health record system: Letter report. Washington, DC: National Academies Press. Retrieved from http://www.nap.edu/openbook.php?record_id=10781.

understanding of specific functionality issues, such as current paper workflows, backlogs, and workarounds.

In addition to providing the core functions as noted earlier, the EHR must be efficient and must offer additional support, the nature of which depends on each institution or facility and the type of services provided (e.g., ambulatory or inpatient services). For example, an inpatient facility EHR needs to integrate with nursing services, pharmacy, operating room management systems, and laboratory information systems, to name a few. To view sample screens from an EHR, see Figures 15.1 and 15.2.

Fig. 15.1 Selected Screen from a Patient's EHR. (Courtesy of Epic.)

	1/20/15
	1348
🖵 Shift Event	
Discharge Planning	
Additional information relevant for discharge planning	
Advance Directives (For Healthcare)	
🖵 Advance Directive	
Information Provided on Healthcare Directives	
Healthcare Agent Appointed	
Healthcare Agent's Name	
Healthcare Agent's Phone Number	
Pre-existing DNR/DNI Order	
Patient Requests Assistance	
Care considerations	
Name patient prefers to be called	
Time of arrival to unit	
Do you have a caregiver preference	
Describe any social factors influencing your treatment	
Describe any ethnic/cultural factors influencing your	
Describe any educational factors influencing your	
Other respectful considerations	

Fig. 15.2 Selected Screen from a Patient's EHR. (Courtesy of Epic.)

EHR Data Management

A fully functional EHR is a complex system. Consider a single data element (datum), such as a person's weight. The system must be able to capture, or record, the weight, then store it, process it, communicate it to others, and present it in a usable format, such as a bar graph or chart. All of this must be done in a secure environment that protects the patient's confidentiality and privacy. The complexity of these issues and the development of the necessary systems help explain why adoption of fully functional EHR systems has been slow.

Data Capture. *Data capture* refers to the collection and entry of data into an EHR. The origin of the data may be local or remote from patient-monitoring devices, direct from the individual recipient of health care, or even from others who have information about the recipient's health or environment, such as relatives, friends, and public health agencies. Data may be captured by multiple means, including key entry, pattern recognition (e.g., voice, handwriting, or biologic characteristics), and medical device transmission.

Storage. *Storage* refers to the physical location of data. In EHR systems, data need to be distributed across multiple systems at different sites. For this reason, common access protocols, retention schedules, and universal identification are necessary.

Access protocols permit only authorized users to obtain data for legitimate uses. The systems must have backup and recovery mechanisms in the event of failure. Retention schedules address the maintenance of data in active and inactive forms as well as the permanence of the storage medium. A person's identity can be determined by many types of data in addition to common identifiers, such as name and number. Universal identifiers or other methods are required for integrating health data of an individual distributed across multiple systems at different sites.

Information Processing. EHR functions provide for effective retrieval and processing of data into useful information. These include decision support tools, such as alerts and alarms for drug interactions, allergies, and abnormal laboratory results. Reminders can be provided for appointments, critical path actions, medication administration, and other activities. The systems also may provide access to consensus- and evidence-driven diagnostic and treatment guidelines and protocols. The nurse could integrate a standard guideline, protocol, or critical path into a specific individual's EHR, modify it to meet unique circumstances, and use it as a basis for managing and documenting care. Outcome data communicated from various caregivers and health care recipients themselves also may be analyzed and used for continual improvement of the guidelines and protocols. Data may also be downloaded into statistical software programs for more sophisticated analysis for research purposes. Organizations are increasingly using EHRs for electronic surveillance to monitor trends and indications of potential critical incidents to prompt preventive and/or responsive actions in advance of an actual disease outbreak.

Information Communication. *Information communication* refers to the interoperability of systems and linkages for exchange of data across disparate systems. To integrate health data across multiple systems at different sites, identifier systems (unique numbers or other methodology) for health care recipients, caregivers, providers, payers, and sites are essential. Local, regional, and national health information infrastructures that tie all participants together using standard data communication protocols are key. There are hundreds of types of transactions or messages that must be defined and agreed to by participating stakeholders. Vocabulary and code systems must permit the exchange and processing of data into meaningful information. EHR systems must provide access to point-of-care information databases and knowledge sources, such as pharmaceutical formularies, referral databases, and reference literature.

Security. Computer-based patient record systems provide better protection of confidential health information than paper-based systems because such systems incorporate controls designed to ensure that only authorized users with legitimate uses have access to health information. Security functions address the confidentiality of private health information and the integrity of the data. Security functions must be designed to ensure compliance with applicable laws, regulations, and standards. Security systems must ensure that access to data is provided only to those who are authorized and have a legitimate purpose for its use. Security functions also must provide a means of auditing for inappropriate access. Three important terms must be clearly understood:

- *Privacy* refers to the right of an individual to keep information about himself or herself from being disclosed to anyone else. If a patient has had an abortion and chooses not to tell a health care provider this fact, the patient would be keeping that information private.
- *Confidentiality* refers to the act of limiting disclosure of private matters. Once a patient has disclosed private information to a health care provider, that provider has a responsibility to maintain the confidentiality of that information and not to reveal the information to others who do not have a legitimate need to know.
- *Security* refers to the means to control access and protect information from accidental or intentional disclosure to unauthorized persons and from alteration, destruction, and loss. When private information is placed in a confidential EHR, the system must have controls in place to maintain the security of the system and not to allow unauthorized persons access to the data (Computer-Based Patient Record Institute [CPRI], 1995).

Information Presentation. The wealth of information available through EHR systems must be managed to ensure that authorized caregivers (including nurses) and others with legitimate uses have the information they need in their preferred presentation form. For example, a nurse may want to see data organized by source, caregiver, encounter, problem, or date. Data can be presented in detail or summary form. Tables, graphs, narrative, and other forms of information presentation must be accommodated. Some users may need to know only of the presence or absence of certain data, not the nature of the data itself. For example, blood donation centers draw blood for testing for human immunodeficiency virus, hepatitis, and other conditions. If a donor has a positive test result, the center may be given not the specific information regarding the test but only general information that a test result was abnormal and that the donor should be referred to a health care provider.

EHRs and "Meaningful Use"

The American Recovery and Reinvestment Act of 2009 directed the "meaningful use" of EHR systems for hospital and physician practice settings and provided for financial incentives from the CMS to providers who adopt and use EHRs that meet the meaningful use standards. "Meaningful use" refers to a complex set of capabilities and standards to be met by EHR use in a series of three stages over several years (HealthIT.gov, 2015).

Stage 1 meaningful use (2011-2012) criteria primarily addressed the capture of health information, access to comprehensive patient health data, exchange of clinical information among the health care team, and reports for quality improvement and public reporting requirements. Stage 2 criteria, effective in 2014, focused on continuous quality improvement at the point of care and structured information exchange (for example, the electronic exchange of diagnostic test results) (U.S. Federal Register, 2012). Stage 3, implemented in 2017, focuses on using certified EHR technology (CEHRT) to improve health outcomes and also serves to introduce the final rule, which modified Stage 2 to ease reporting requirements and align with other quality reporting programs

In order for a provider (hospital or physician/provider practice) to qualify for the EHR incentive program through CMS, its EHR must be certified, confirming that it meets the required meaningful use standards and structure of patient data to be easily retrieved and transferred for the promotion of patient care. A certified health product list (CHPL), providing information on products and modules certified for the Medicare and

Medicaid EHR incentive programs, is available on the HealthIT.gov website.

Meaningful use, as described by the Medicare and Medicaid EHR incentive programs, utilizes technology to meet the quality and safety goals of patient care. These goals are grouped into five primary patient care domains (HealthIT.gov, 2015):

1. Improve quality, safety, and efficiency
2. Engage patients and families in their health care
3. Improve care coordination
4. Improve public and population health
5. Ensure privacy and security for personal health information

Although great progress in EHR adoption and usage has been made, the full capacity has not yet been realized. This situation may be due in part to barriers that impede the universal adoption of EHRs in the United States, which is discussed in the following section.

Opportunities for and Barriers to Adoption of EHRs in the United States

Clearly, the movement toward meaningful use EHRs along with financial incentives is designed to promote universal adoption of EHRs in the United States. This movement creates not only opportunities but also some barriers for independent health care providers. Meeting the guidelines for meaningful use EHRs is strenuous and often costly for community-based ambulatory services and small rural inpatient centers. Nonetheless, federal dollars have been allocated for this endeavor, and incentive money is available for facilities and providers meeting the criteria for meaningful use. As previously noted, revisions to Stage 2 have helped alleviate some of the issues affecting reporting ability.

The power of sharing data across health care settings surpasses the benefits to an individual patient. Obviously, patients benefit when their different providers have access to the same comprehensive patient record. Shared records promote continuity of care across systems and potentially reduce costs by eliminating duplicate diagnostic testing and services. Moreover, much can be learned when data are shared across systems. Aggregate data from such systems can be evaluated and predict outcomes in a particular population, disease, complication, or extended hospital stay. The ability to predict outcomes from data entered across systems, termed *mining data* or *examining trends,* can be highly beneficial for examining population health outcomes.

Great strides have been made in the use of EHRs to increase patient and provider communication, decrease errors, and streamline the workflow process. However, despite the evidence for these positive results, there is continued resistance from providers, including nurses (Gomes et al, 2016). The integration of technology, including the use of EHRs, will continue to change the practice of nursing, prompting the need for more research to explore patient-centered care practices within this new paradigm.

EHRs and the Health Insurance Portability and Accountability Act

Because of the increase in the number of EHRs in the 1990s and the anticipated penetration of EHRs in health care, experts advocated for standardized protocols and clinical practice guidelines to ensure privacy and security. The Health Information Portability and Accountability Act (HIPAA) was signed into law in 1996. HIPAA regulations focus on the privacy and security of patient data, including standard formats for transmitting electronic patient information. By April 2005, health care institutions had to comply with federal HIPAA regulations.

The HIPAA requires that every organization or facility that gathers or collects personal health information (PHI) to name an individual as a privacy officer and to develop policies and procedures to ensure the privacy and security of PHI. The protection of PHI extends to every employee, new hire, and patient. Those found in violation of HIPAA regulations may be subject to criminal penalties and civil monetary penalties.

POINT-OF-CARE TECHNOLOGY

With advancing technologies and the movement toward universal use of EHRs, there is a greater demand for HIT at the point of care. This means HIT directly at the bedside or within close proximity to the area where services are delivered. Point-of-care technology is no longer nonessential but is paramount to delivery of safe, efficient, high-quality patient care with access to patient data and evidence-based guidelines. The technology must provide access to past and current patient data, references, policies, procedures, and evidence-based literature to guide clinical decisions at the point of care. A variety of technology tools support point-of-care decision making and documentation, such as handheld computers, tablets, and smartphones.

It is nearly impossible to visit a health care facility or office and not see providers using mobile technology. These small devices are as robust as laptops or desktop computers but are more convenient for on-the-go health care providers. These systems have wireless Internet capability so that patient information and other resources can be accessed anywhere, anytime, within the confines of the firewall-protected health care environment to maintain privacy, security, and confidentiality of the data. Small laptops also allow providers to access pertinent information at the point of care. These laptops are usually secured to a mobile cart, so they have names like *computer on wheels (COWs)*, *mobile point-of-care (MPOC)*, and *computer at bedside (CAB)*.

Smartphones and tablets promote evidence-based clinical decision making at the point of care. These palm-sized computers can store medical applications and access health care journals, calculators, databases, and more through their wireless capabilities. One of the greatest advantages of smartphones is the convenient and quick access to references and tools for patient education and care. For example, nurses can teach patients about tracking their health by using tools on smartphones or display pictures that show proper procedures. A variety of applications are available for managing chronic disease, diet, exercise, and lifestyle choices (Wyatt and Krauskopf, 2012).

Point-of-care technology is an essential component of nursing as it shifts from a practice that relies on memory to one that emphasizes continuous use of as-needed resources. This means that nurses must transform from being technical experts to knowledge workers and must rely on the ever-increasing and reliable computer memory versus the overburdened and fallible human memory. Computer-based alerts and reminders provided by point-of-care technology are helpful in detecting and preventing potential adverse drug events related to drug-drug interactions and abnormal laboratory values.

Mobile devices, such as tablets, are being used in many organizations as standards of care to promote safety and quality via enhanced communications among team members. One example is the use of tablets for virtual handoffs. The virtual handoffs use video technology to include the patient and his/her family in the introductions and initial conversations about the transfer, reducing anxiety and promoting rapport. Nurses have found these virtual first encounters helpful in confirming patient information and promotion of accountability (Santa and Roach, 2017).

Mobile health applications (apps) are increasingly being used in the clinical environment by providers and patients. One example is the use of mobile apps for home monitoring of infants recently discharged from the neonatal intensive care unit. Home monitoring has traditionally depended on the parents' ability to assess, record, and report significant data, which often results in delay and/or noncompliance in reporting of critical information that leads to complications, even deaths. With the use of mobile technology, data are collected via the app and securely transferred to the EHR, where nurses and caregivers can immediately review and revise the plans of care. Mobile apps have been found to greatly enhance the home monitoring of such infants to minimize delays in care and reduce at-home mortality (Erickson et al, 2017).

As today's health care environment focuses on safe, efficient, effective, and high-quality care, access to patient data, standardized protocols, and clinical practice guidelines through point-of-care technology has become the standard for patient care. Nurse scientists are increasingly focusing their research efforts on the benefits of using secured mobile devices that are compliant with the HIPAA. These research efforts are widely being translated into clinical environments to improve the quality and safety of patient care and contribute to the efficiency and satisfaction of our nursing staff.

Telehealth

A discussion about technology at the point of care would be incomplete without mentioning *telehealth*—the use of telecommunications technology to assess, diagnose, and, in some cases, treat persons who are at a distance from the health care provider. Nurses, physicians, radiologists, psychiatrists, and others use this technology via telephone, computers, interactive videos, and teleconferencing. In many instances, telehealth makes possible the delivery of health care services to underserved populations, such as rural communities, older adults, and prisoners, who may have difficulty accessing necessary services. Demonstrated benefits of telehealth include improved quality of care, enhanced continuity of care, increased availability of experts, improved access to care, improved decision making and time savings, and higher-quality records related to the incorporation of digital information (Hebda et al, 2017).

The home care arena is seeing significant changes as a result of telehealth. Telehome care devices used to be as simple as blood pressure cuffs. Today, devices such as automated blood pressure monitors, glucose testing meters, electrocardiograms, peak flow meters, pulse oximeters, weight scales, and two-way digital transport systems are used. The devices offer data recording, audible alarms or reminders, and data uploading in addition to reports on disease progression and trends. They are used for diverse patient populations, including persons with heart failure, hypertension, diabetes, asthma, chronic obstructive pulmonary disease, cystic fibrosis, depression, and bipolar disorder.

These advances in technology that enhance and improve health care delivery systems are only as effective as the persons who consume the technology, namely, health care personnel and patients. Without the skill set to use point-of-care technologies, EHRs, and telehealth, patients will not benefit from the advanced technology. Further, patients must possess skills to evaluate and critique technologies and information that influence their health.

INFORMATION LITERACY FOR NURSES

The Association of College and Research Libraries (ACRL) defines *information literacy* (IL) as the "ability to identify an information need; find and evaluate information; assess information; use information ethically; and document (ACRL, 2013). It is dangerous to assume that nurses can rely on memory alone when practicing in a complex and dynamic health care environment; therefore, IL skills are necessary for the provision of safe and quality care as well as evidence-based practice. The IL skills that equip the nurse for the timely retrieval of information necessary to plan, deliver, and evaluate evidence-based care also support independent lifelong learning. Additionally, many leading organizations, including the Institute of Medicine and accrediting bodies, promote the use of technology by nurses at all levels of practice to prevent errors, to enhance care coordination and communication, and to support clinical decision making.

Unfortunately, there is great discrepancy in the levels of IL skills possessed by both new and experienced nurses. As a result, many nurses turn to less reliable sources (e.g., coworkers) for critical information. Like critical thinking, IL is a concept that must be emphasized within both academic and practice settings. The emphasis includes removing barriers to accessing online information at the point of care and providing ongoing training to nursing

staff to improve these competencies (Carter-Templeton et al, 2014).

The ACRL published the Information Literacy Competency Standards for Nursing in 2013. These standards are based on the nursing profession's fundamental values of evidence-based practice and translational research. According to these standards, the information-literate nurse is one who: (1) defines and articulates the need for information, (2) accesses needed information effectively and efficiently, (3) critically evaluates the procured information and its sources, and as a result, decides whether or not to modify the initial query and/or seek additional sources and whether to develop a new research process, (4) individually or as a member of a group, uses information effectively to accomplish a specific purpose, and (5) understands many of the economic, legal, and social issues surrounding the use of information and accesses and uses information ethically and legally (ACRL, 2013).

CONSUMER HEALTH INFORMATION TECHNOLOGY

Web 2.0 tools, such as social media, collaboration sites, interactive websites, and Internet bulletin boards or blogs, encourage individuals to be more involved and more knowledgeable about their own health. The information that patients and families glean from such sites can be a challenge for providers because as patients are better informed, health care providers are required to answer more directed questions. Further, the health care provider must inform patients how to be good consumers of health information. Because providers are seen as the experts, it is the providers' responsibility to ensure that patients are well informed about how to evaluate content and protect the privacy of others while engaged in discussion via either the Internet or other forms of wireless connection.

Health consumers of all ages are increasingly turning to social media for information about health promotion such as healthy eating, exercise, and ways to reduce stress (Thielst, 2011). Consumers often access YouTube, Facebook, Twitter, and LinkedIn to learn more about health, health prevention, and health promotion. Web 2.0 tools are designed to allow any Internet user to become an author of content. With the growing number of Internet users, content is also expanding exponentially so that one can find information about virtually anything, including the most obscure illnesses, home remedies, procedures, and medications. For this reason, information accessible on the Internet may not necessarily be accurate or created by experts. Consumers of information on the Internet, especially health information, must be knowledgeable consumers and must evaluate the credibility and accuracy of the source. The following section provides valuable information about how to find and evaluate web-based information.

Finding Information on the Internet

Effective and efficient Internet searching is a must in today's information-overloaded society. Purposeful use of a variety of strategies can improve search results; Table 15.2 provides an example of these search strategies:

- Quick and dirty searching can be useful if you are looking for information in an unfamiliar area. Type your search term into a search engine such as Google (http://www.google.com). Review your results to see which ones sound most promising.
- Advanced searching allows you to set specific limits on your searches. For instance, at Google's advanced search (http://www.google.com/advanced_search), you can limit your searching to educational (.edu), organizational (.org), or governmental (.gov) domains, as well as by language, file type, and date. Another advanced search option is http://www.googlescholar.com, where you are more likely to find information related to

research and evidence-based practice. Limiting your searches in this way can help ensure that your results are more credible, authoritative, useful, and current.

- Brute force is a method of searching in which you type in what you think might logically be a web address and see what happens. Sometimes you will receive an error message, but sometimes you find precisely what you are looking for.
- Link searching can be helpful once you find a relevant website. Explore links from the site you find that connect to other relevant sites.
- Professional associations and societies are a good starting point for professionally oriented information. Scientific and research information usually requires literature resources that can be found in scholarly databases, such as MEDLINE and the Cumulative Index to Nursing and Allied Health Literature (CINAHL).

It is important to be persistent and purposeful in searching. No one search strategy or search engine works for all purposes every time. Although search engines have improved over time, it can still be a challenge to find what you need on the Internet.

Evaluating Information Found on the Internet

As you access information on the Internet, it is imperative that you perform a critical evaluation of what you have obtained. The Internet is open to anyone with

TABLE 15.2 Illustration of Search Strategy Effectiveness for "Never Events"*

Type of Search	Site	Results
Quick and dirty	http://www.google.com	54,200—majority of results were newspaper articles and general websites and articles that list never events but do not provide useful information
Advanced	http://www.google.com/advanced_ search	For *.gov* = 1830 For *.org* = 6520 For *.edu* = 406
Brute force	Searched http://www.neverevents.com	Page returned that said "Page coming soon"
Link searching	Using the *.gov* advanced search: • First result is Centers for Medicare & Medicaid Services (CMS) • Second result is the Agency for Healthcare Research and Quality (AHRQ)	From first result—no links From second result—many helpful links, including: • What's New in Never Events • Editor's Picks for Never Events including those from the AHRQ, journal articles, books/reports, newspaper/magazine articles, tools/toolkits, and web resources

*The term being explored is *never events,* which Medicare defines as preventable errors for which Medicare will no longer reimburse organizations if they occur.

access to a computer, and material that looks official may actually be posted by persons without formal education in an area. Some of the information you access may also contain inaccuracies. The affiliation of a website is important to note immediately: *.edu* is an educational institution; *.org* is a nonprofit organization; *.com* is a commercial enterprise; *.net* is an Internet service provider; *.gov* is a governmental body; and *.mil* is military. There are several forms that can assist you in your evaluation. Table 15.3 shows a website evaluation form

---

TABLE 15.3 Website Evaluation Form

Website title:
Web URL:
Date visited:
Brief description of the contents of the site:

CRITERIA AND TYPES OF EVIDENCE	HOW CRITERION IS MET	RATING				
		1 Low	2	3	4	5 High
1. Authority with regard to topic—Who is responsible for the site? Author of site (individual or institutional affiliation, organization) Credentials, expertise, experience Contact information (name, e-mail, postal address) URL type suggests reputable affiliation						
2. Objectivity—Is the purpose of the site clear, including any particular viewpoint? Statement of purpose and scope Intended audience Information presented as factual or opinion, primary or secondary in origin Criteria for inclusion of information Disclosure of sponsorship or underwriting						
3. Accuracy—Is the information accurate?						
4. Currency—Is the information current? Facts compare with related print or other online sources Links provided to quality web resources						
5. Usability—Is the site well designed and stable? Site organization logical and easy to maneuver Content readable by intended audience Information presented is error free (spelling, punctuation) Readily identifiable link back to the institutional or organizational home page Site reliably accessible Pages loaded quickly						
Subtotal for each of the five criteria						
ASSESSMENT OF WEBSITE						
Rating based on the total number of points: 5-9 points: poor 10-14 points: fair 15-19 points: good 20-25 points: excellent	Your personal assessment—Would you recommend this site? Why or why not?					

Courtesy Kent State University Libraries and Media Services, Kent, OH. Available online at http://www.library.kent.edu/files/webevalform.pdf.

from Kent State University that offers five criteria and examples of the types of evidence that should factor into your rating of a website.

FUTURE HEALTH INFORMATION TECHNOLOGY TRENDS

With technology advancing at warp speed, it is difficult to imagine the future, but some of our current technologies offer some insight about the possibilities. To better understand how technology will shape health care, let us review some of the ways technology is currently shaping our lives.

- Social media will no longer be a source of informal content. Social media will develop into social platforms with more legitimate data sources than websites (Accenture, 2014).
- Cloud computing (e.g., applications and data stored and accessed through the Internet) will dominate the computing world (Accenture, 2014).
- Patient-centered care driven by rapid change and unlimited opportunity will include advancements in gene therapy, immuno-oncology, personalized medicine, artificial intelligence, and wearable digital devices (World Economic Forum, 2018).

- Gaming will continue to expand health technologies by promoting health maintenance, physical activity, and cognitive skills that may lead to improved health behavior (Safavi, 2014).
- Smart watches will continue to expand their features and become as ubiquitous as smartphones (Forbes. com, 2014).
- Mobile technologies that promote health (mHealth) will continue to advance, allowing patients and providers to communicate routinely (Jayanthi, 2014).
- The availability of sensors and wearable health monitoring technologies will continue to increase, offering more options to continuously assess individuals (Jaynathi, 2014).

Security is paramount for health care data. Future health information technologies will integrate more biometric technology for authentication and security. Biometric technologies use human characteristics, such as fingerprints, retinas, irises, voices, and facial patterns, to authenticate or grant access to data or information. More and more health care information systems are including biometric options to provide an additional layer of security. It is almost incomprehensible to imagine health care in 2025 when one considers the evolution in technology and how technology has shaped health care since the invention of the stethoscope.

▊ SUMMARY

As a profession, nurses must understand and manage information technology, promote the meaningful use of EHRs, and teach patients how to use health information wisely. As the largest group of organized health care professionals in the United States, nurses have a responsibility to patients and society to continually improve and refine their competencies and knowledge base related to HIT. Findings of multiple studies confirm that nurses in every role and at each level of education and practice exhibit large gaps in knowledge of and competencies in information technology.

Technology is an essential resource for nurses in their important role of tracking, interpreting, and improving quality of care, in addition to translating research into practice. Technology continues to change and evolve at an ever-increasing pace. Be a lifelong learner. Take in-person or online classes. Arrange groups in your place of employment to learn more about health information technology in the clinical setting. Review the resources that are available to you, and evaluate them to ensure they are valid, current, and based on evidence. If the resources are not valid, take action within your facility to replace outdated or inaccurate resources. If the sources are valid, integrate them into your everyday practice.

REFERENCES

Accenture. (2014). *Accenture Technology Vision*. Retrieved from https://www.accenture.com/t20160316T224443__ w__/fr-fr/_acnmedia/PDF-10/Accenture-Technology-Vision_2014.pdf.

American Health Information Management Association. (2012). *Resources: Glossary of terms*. Retrieved from http://www.myphr.com/healthliteracy/glossary.aspx.

Association of College and Research Libraries. (2013). *Information literacy competency standards for nursing*. Retrieved from http://www.ala.org/acrl/standards/nursing.

Carter-Templeton, H., Patterson, R., & Mackey, S. (2014). Nursing faculty and student experiences with information literacy: A pilot study. *Journal of Nursing Education and Practice, 4*(1), 208–217.

Centers for Medicare & Medicaid Services. (2017). *Medicare and Medicaid electronic health record incentive program*. Retrieved from https://www.cms.gov/Regulations-and-Guidance/Legislation/EHRIncentivePrograms/index.html?redirect=/EHRIncentivePrograms/.

Computer-Based Patient Record Institute. (1995). *Guidelines for establishing information security policies at organizations using computer-based patient records: Work group on confidentiality, privacy and security*. Schaumburg, IL: Computer-Based Patient Record Institute.

Erickson, L., Hunt, C., & Blizzard, P. (2017). Leveraging technology to improve care and patient outcomes. *American Nurse Today, 12*(9), 303-311.

Forbes.com. (2014). *Smartwatches, Google glass, and the wearable technology chocolate box*. Retrieved from http://www.forbes.com/sites/rajsabhlok/2013/12/05/smartwatches-google-glass-and-the-wearable-technology-chocolate-box/.

Gomes, M., Hash, P., Orsolini, L., Watkins, A., & Mazzoccoli, A. (2016). Nurses' beliefs about using an electronic health record and their ability to incorporate professional and patient-centered nursing activities in patient care. *Computers, Informatics, Nursing, 34*(12), 578–586.

HealthIT.gov. (2015). *Meaningful use definition & objectives*. Retrieved from http://www.healthit.gov/providers-professionals/meaningful-use-definition-objectives.

Hebda, T., Hunter, K., & Czar, P. (2017). *Handbook of informatics for nurses & healthcare professionals* (6th ed.). Upper Saddle River, NJ: Pearson-Prentice Hall.

InformationWeek. (2014). *3 trends are reshaping healthcare IT*. Retrieved from http://www.informationweek.com/healthcare/leadership/3-trends-are-reshaping-healthcare-it/d/d-id/1113460.

Institute of Medicine of the National Academies. (2003). *Key capabilities of an electronic health record system: Letter report*. Washington, DC: National Academies Press. Retrieved from http://www.nap.edu/openbook.php?record_id=10781.

Jayanthi, A. (2014). 10 biggest technological advancements for healthcare in the last decade. *Becker's Hospital Review*. Retrieved from https://www.beckershospitalreview.com/healthcare-information-technology/10-biggest-technological-advancements-for-healthcare-in-the-last-decade.html.

Müller-Staub, M., de Graaf-Waar, H., & Paans, W. (2016). An internationally consented standard for nursing process-clinical decision support systems in electronic health records. *Computers, Informatics, Nursing, 34*(11), 493–502.

Safavi, K. (2014). 3 trends are reshaping healthcare IT. Information Week IT Network, 01.16.2014. Retrieved from http://www.informationweek.com/healthcare/leadership/3-trends-are-reshaping-healthcareit/d/d-id/1113460.

Thielst, C. B. (2011). Social media: Ubiquitous community and patient engagement. *Frontiers of health services management, 28*(2), 3–14.

U.S. Federal Register. (2012). *Medicare and Medicaid Programs; Electronic Health Record Incentive Program-Stage 2*. Retrieved from https://www.federalregister.gov/articles/2012/03/07/2012-4443/medicare-and-medicaid-programs-electronic-health-record-incentive-program-stage-2.

World Economic Forum. (2018). 5 key trends for the future of healthcare. (website). https://www.weforum.org/agenda/2018/01/this-is-what-the-future-of-healthcare-looks-like.

Wyatt, T. H., & Krauskopf, P. B. (2012). E-health and nursing: Using smartphones to enhance nursing practice. *Online Journal of Nursing Informatics, 16*(2). Retrieved from http://ojni.org/issues/?p=1706.

16

Emergency Preparedness and Response for Today's World

Rebecca R. Keck, DNP, RN, NEA-BC,
Elizabeth E. Weiner, PhD, RN-BC, FACMI, FAAN

Partnering to respond to disaster.

(e) Additional resources are available online at: *http://evolve.elsevier.com/Cherry/*

LEARNING OUTCOMES

After studying this chapter, the reader will be able to:

1. Describe the interaction between local, state, and federal emergency response systems.
2. Summarize the roles of public and private agencies in preparing for and responding to a mass casualty event.
3. Compare and contrast chemical, biologic, radiologic, nuclear, and explosive agents and treatment protocols.
4. Access resources related to disaster preparedness on the Internet.
5. Communicate effectively (using correct emergency preparedness terminology) in regard to a mass casualty incident.
6. Describe the need for personal preparedness for individuals and households.

KEY TERMS

Active shooter An individual actively engaged in killing or attempting to kill people in a confined and populated area; in most cases, active shooters use firearms and there is no pattern or method to their selection of victims.

All-hazards approach A process approach for all sectors to prepare for any emergency or disaster that may occur.

Biologic agents Microorganisms or toxins from living organisms with infectious or noninfectious properties that produce lethal or serious effects in plants and animals.

Chemical agents Solids, liquids, or gases with chemical properties that produce lethal or serious effects in plants and animals.

Crisiz standard of care A substantial change in usual health care operations and the level of care it is possible to deliver, which is made necessary by a pervasive (e.g., pandemic influenza) or catastrophic (e.g., earthquake, hurricane) disaster.

This change in the level of care delivered is justified by specific circumstances and is formally declared by a state government, in recognition that crisis operations will be in effect for a sustained period.

Disaster condition A significant natural disaster or human-caused event that overwhelms the affected state, necessitating both federal public health and medical care assistance.

Emergency As defined in the Stafford Act, any occasion or instance for which, in the determination of the president, federal assistance is needed to supplement state and local efforts and capabilities to save lives and protect property, public health, and safety; includes emergencies other than natural disasters.

Emergency Management Assistance Compact (EMAC) An organization authorized by the U.S Congress through which a state impacted by a disaster can request and receive assistance from other member states quickly and efficiently (EMAC, 2017).

Incident command system (ICS) A multiagency operational structure that uses a model adopted by the fire and rescue community. The ICS can be used in any size or type of disaster to control response personnel, facilities, and equipment.

Lead agency As defined by the FBI, the federal department or organization assigned primary responsibility to manage and coordinate a specific function—either crisis management or consequence management. Lead agencies are designated on the basis of their having the most authority, resources, capabilities, or expertise relative to accomplishment of the specific function.

Major disaster As defined under the Stafford Act, any natural catastrophe (including any hurricane, tornado, storm, high water, wind-driven water, tidal wave, tsunami, earthquake, volcanic eruption, landslide, mudslide, snowstorm, or drought) or, regardless of cause, any fire, flood, or explosion in any part of the United States that in the determination of the president causes damage of sufficient severity and magnitude to warrant major disaster assistance under the Stafford Act to supplement the efforts and available resources of states, local governments, and disaster relief organizations in alleviating the damage, loss, hardship, or suffering caused thereby.

Mass casualty incident (MCI) A disaster situation that results in a large number of victims who need the response of multiple organizations.

Mitigation Those activities designed to alleviate the effects of a major disaster or emergency or long-term activities to minimize the potentially adverse effects of future disasters in affected areas.

Pandemic Outbreak of disease that affects populations worldwide; for example, pandemic influenza causes serious illness worldwide.

Preparedness Activities that build capability and capacity to address potential needs identified by the threat and vulnerability study.

Recovery Activities designed to return responders and the facility to full normal operational status and to restore fully the capability to respond to future emergencies and disasters; activities traditionally associated with providing federal supplemental disaster relief assistance under a presidential major disaster declaration.

Response Activities to address the immediate and short-term effects of an emergency or disaster. Response includes immediate actions to save lives, protect property, and meet basic human needs.

Scene assessment The act of reviewing the location of an event to look for information that might help to determine treatment options.

Terrorist attack As defined by the FBI, a violent act or an act that is dangerous to human life, in violation of the criminal laws of the United States or of any state, and intended to intimidate or coerce a government, the civilian population, or any segment thereof in furtherance of political or social objectives.

Triage Process of prioritizing which patients are to be treated first; first action in any disaster response.

PROFESSIONAL/ETHICAL ISSUE

Jeannette Fraser, RN, worked in the emergency department (ED) of a major hospital system when, during her shift in the ED, an explosion occurred at a large factory near the city. As soon as the hospital determined that a disaster occurred with multiple injuries, the hospital's emergency operations plan (EOP) was activated. Fortunately, less than 1 month before the explosion, Jeannette had participated in a large-scale disaster drill conducted by the hospital in partnership with agencies from across the city, including the fire department, the police department, and the city's emergency operations center. Although extremely anxious, Jeannette knew exactly what to do and went to work in her assigned role to triage victims who were coming into the ED. Jeannette knew that the entire hospital staff was more successful in managing the disaster and helping victims because of the well-coordinated EOP that was in place.

Now Jeannette has moved to another state and accepted a nursing position in the outpatient clinic of a large academic medical center. As part of her orientation, Jeannette asks her supervisor about the facility's EOP and the supervisor replies, "I am sure we have a written plan in the policy manual, but I really don't know much about it. This is a very safe community, so we don't need to worry about anything happening here. And besides, if something did happen, the victims would go to the hospital, and it would not affect us." This response from her supervisor leaves Jeannette feeling very concerned and wondering whether she should get involved in helping the clinic understand the importance of having a good EOP that is coordinated with the hospital and other community agencies.

Think about Jeannette's situation as you consider the following questions:

- In the event of a major disaster, is it conceivable that victims might go to an outpatient or community-based clinic for treatment?
- What are some strategies Jeannette can use to persuade the clinic managers of the importance of having an up-to-date EOP in place?
- When might nurses in an ambulatory clinic be considered "first responders"?
- What local, state, and/or federal resources are available to help communities develop EOPs?

VIGNETTE

Jane Wolverton works as a staff nurse on a medical-surgical unit at the Culverton General Hospital. She is in a patient's room giving an intravenous (IV) medication when the news program announces that there has been a major explosion at a chemical plant. The plant has 400 workers, including her husband.

Questions to Consider While Reading this Chapter:

1. How do we prepare for mass casualty events that will overwhelm the resources of our health facility?
2. How do we plan for a catastrophic event to ensure that the response offers the best care possible given the resources at hand? How are response efforts coordinated so that the needs of the local area are met?
3. How do hospitals organize themselves to manage disaster situations while continuing to communicate with other external agencies?
4. How does the response differ when the hospital suffers damage and cannot function normally?
5. Where can I find current information about this ever-changing area?

CHAPTER OVERVIEW

The purpose of this chapter is to describe the various components of our nation's local, state, and federal National Response Framework and how these components interrelate in the event of a mass casualty incident (MCI). The problems associated with natural or terrorist disasters when the health care system is damaged or rendered ineffective because of the event are reviewed. The kinds of agents that may be used in a terrorist attack are described along with the activities and response systems related to the preimpact and impact phases of a disaster. Readers will be particularly interested to note how standard triage and patient care priorities change when care is provided during an MCI. Additionally, readers are encouraged to closely review the list of key terms to understand and be able to use emergency preparedness terminology and explore the online resources about emergency preparedness and disaster management found throughout the chapter.

THE NATIONAL IMPERATIVE FOR EMERGENCY PREPAREDNESS

During the past two decades, we have seen many mass casualty events on U.S. soil, some from natural disasters and some as a result of terrorist attacks. Examples of terrorist attacks include the bombing of the Alfred P. Murrah Federal Building in Oklahoma City in 1995; the attacks on the U.S. embassies in Kenya and Tanzania in 1998; the attack in 2000 on the U.S.S. *Cole,* an American warship refueling in Yemen; and the anthrax scare in 2002. None of these events, however, had the same effect as the events of September 11, 2001, when the United States experienced devastating, well-coordinated attacks in New York City and Washington, D.C., that led to the deaths of more than 3000 people.

Later events have kept the threat of terrorism alive. The Boston Marathon bombings in 2013 killed three people and injured an estimated 264 others, who were treated in 27 local hospitals (Kotz, 2013). This event vividly demonstrated the need to have coordinated efforts among first responders: law enforcement/fire, medical and mental health services, emergency management, and related local and federal agencies. The brutal beheadings of journalists by Islamic extremists remind all of us that the ever-changing world is difficult to protect.

The disasters unfolding in this century are frequently associated with global instability, economic decay, political upheaval and collapse of government structure, violence and civil conflicts, famine, and mass population displacements (Veenema, 2003a). The growing complexity and nature of disasters create considerable challenges for individuals responsible for disaster planning and related responses. The need for formalized plans for preparedness, mitigation, response, recovery, and evaluation is essential to minimizing the impact to individuals and society at large. Nurses serve in vital roles in planning development and overall response.

Although a great deal of attention has been focused on preparing for an MCI related to a terrorist attack, the United States has suffered major damage from natural disasters. Hurricane Katrina has become the classic example of massive system failure in emergency response. Most of the destruction was due to storm surge, and further flooding took place in New Orleans as the levee system catastrophically failed. Although the death toll from this event did not reach the level seen at the World Trade Center in New York City, the damage to the health care systems in the affected areas was substantial. It became evident very quickly that the response systems in place could not be effective in dealing with the destruction of the health care infrastructure, and in fact, the health care agencies themselves were sites of mass casualties. The extensive need for immediate and long-term shelters for large numbers of victims also highlighted the need for nurses to have knowledge and skills in how to meet the needs of victims with psychologic and chronic diseases in a sheltered environment. The year 2017 proved to be a devastating one for catastrophic hurricanes impacting numerous southern states (Florida, Texas, Louisiana), Puerto Rico, the Caribbean, Cuba, and Mexico. In particular, Hurricane Irma forced large-scale evacuations as it developed from a tropical storm to a category 5 hurricane. These natural disaster events caused infrastructure damage to power, water supply, gas, homes, industry, and health care facilities. Once again coordinated local, state, and federal responses were key in preparation for and response to these events. Postevent evaluations still indicate a need for further refinement in emergency operations planning and response.

Emergency management plans must address adequate response systems that can be used regardless of the cause of the MCI. A more reasonable approach has been the movement to plan and improve responses to a variety of hazards, called an all-hazards approach. Nurses have traditionally received disaster education as a part of community health content within nursing education programs as it related to natural disasters; however, the education has been focused on responding to a disaster site of victims when the health care system is still intact.

The same is true for other health care professional education programs. In addition, they have not routinely received education related to dangerous biologic agents or chemical agents or to nuclear, explosive, or radiologic hazards. It is imperative that all health care providers become knowledgeable about how to provide care for victims of all types of hazards and in situations in which the health care system itself either has been damaged or destroyed or has no contact with the other parts of the community.

It is recognized by all federal agencies that the most serious knowledge deficit for health care providers is in the area of bioterrorism attacks and pandemic flu events. Unlike the other hazards, these situations place the health care providers in a position of being first responders. Traditionally, first responders to emergencies have been the law enforcement, firefighters, and emergency medical technicians who respond with ambulances. In a biologic event (covert or natural transmission), however, victims first appear in emergency departments, physicians' offices, nurse-managed clinics, or even in school health settings. Health care professionals need to be able to identify symptoms, patterns of similar events, and other irregularities. If they fail to recognize or report significant events, a biologic event could go unrecognized until it is of epidemic proportions.

The same principles of responding to a bioterrorist event are pertinent for coping with a natural biologic outbreak, such as a pandemic flu event or severe acute respiratory syndrome (SARS). It is these types of diseases and exposures that are becoming the target of education not only for the health care community but also for the general community at large so as to foster cooperation to prevent spread of a disease that would eventually become pandemic and a mass casualty event.

THE BASICS OF EMERGENCY PREPAREDNESS AND RESPONSE

Nurses have significant experience in dealing with natural disasters and are familiar with the work of the Red Cross in bringing disaster relief to affected areas. A disaster condition is defined as a significant natural disaster or human-caused event that overwhelms the affected state and necessitates both federal public health and medical care assistance (Federal Emergency Management Agency [FEMA], 2014a). The disaster condition must be of significant impact to warrant federal resources. Understanding the responsibilities of the multiple agencies that respond to a disaster is imperative to be able to communicate with patients, families, and other health care providers.

In some situations, the number of victims is so large that multiple organizations are called to respond. When casualties occur at this level, the event is termed a mass casualty incident (MCI) or mass casualty event (MCE). Although the situation may be unfamiliar for some nurses, it is important to remember that the nursing fundamentals practiced in other settings and during smaller crises are generally still applicable. Traditionally, triage that is practiced in most health care agencies categorizes patients into low risk, intermediate care, and critically ill (those who need immediate care to save their lives). With such large numbers, however, there is a paradigm shift to crisis standards of care in which priorities change into doing the greatest good for the greatest number of people. Care is given to those patients who have the greatest chance of survival. This type of triage typically places nurses in ethical situations in which they experience discomfort, particularly if patients are triaged and tagged to receive only pain management rather than the typical extensive treatment that might be provided during normal health care conditions. Furthermore, the public responds to the visible tags placed on patients and can provide added stress when calling out to health care providers to provide further care.

Community disaster plans need to clearly define the care processes to be used when the needs shift from those of one patient to the needs of the populations (Hanfling et al, 2012). Nurses may also find themselves in positions in which there is a lack of necessary resources, and they will then have to come up with creative solutions. Powers (2010) describes examples of such adaptability by the Australian team in the Maldives after the tsunami in 2004, with such actions as using rigid plastic drink bottles as sharps containers at each patient's bed area and using the large, rigid containers that transport medical supplies as privacy screens and walls between treatment areas. Busby and Witucki-Brown (2011) described such actions and decisions by nurses and other responders as developing situational awareness about MCIs.

Terrorism has created the need for us to prepare against a variety of different agents. A standardized nomenclature has been developed for five categories using the acronym CBRNE, which stands for chemical, biologic, radiologic, nuclear, and explosive. Table 16.1 describes the similarities and differences related to the CBRNE agents and provides information about treatment protocols for each agent.

PHASES OF DISASTER

Powers (2010) describes three phases of the disaster continuum: preparedness, relief response, and recovery. In the preparedness phase, activities are focused on planning, preparedness, prevention, and warning. After the impact, all efforts are directed to responding to the disaster, initiating the emergency management system, and mitigating the effects of the hazard. During the recovery phase, which usually begins 72 hours after the disaster and may continue for 2 to 3 years, a network of activities is designed to enhance rehabilitation and reconstruction. Evaluation of the disaster preparedness and response plan is a major activity that needs to be included in the recovery phase.

Nursing as a profession has a long history of being creative and visionary in its continuous efforts to meet the needs of patients and their families. Nursing leadership, in tumultuous times such as during a disaster continuum or at a mass casualty incident, will require significant amounts of the same creativity and vision (Veenema, 2003b). Thus, it is important for nurses to understand the phases of a disaster, described in the following sections, to know what actions are necessary in each phase.

Preparedness Phase

In January 2001, The Joint Commission's disaster preparedness standards were modified to introduce the concepts of emergency management and community involvement in the management process. These modifications call for accredited organizations to take an "all-hazards" approach to disaster planning—reviewing, analyzing, and addressing all hazards that are determined to be credible and serious threats to the community. Following the terrorist attacks on September 11, 2001, The Joint Commission (TJC) made an additional modification to the standard requiring organizations to communicate and coordinate with one another (TJC, 2013).

Every disaster, regardless of the cause, begins as a local event. Each locale has the responsibility for responding to the emergencies within its community first. Thus, the heaviest burden falls on the local community when a mass casualty occurs. Assistance from state and federal levels is appropriated when the local system is unable to provide the necessary level of care. It is imperative, then, that communities plan for the services that will be needed in a time of disaster and train providers within each agency about responding to all hazard types of MCEs.

TABLE 16.1 CBRNE Agents

Agents	Action	Advantages	Disadvantages	Treatment
Chemical	Agents injure or kill through variety of means: vesicant, nerve, blood, respiratory	Spread easily through air; cause immediate effects; require decontamination	Less toxic than biologic agents; need to be used in large quantities; subject to dispersion by wind; terrorists need to protect themselves; require trained HAZMAT teams	Dependent on agent used; in some cases there are agent-specific medications; require decontamination; require use of personal protective equipment by personnel
Biologic	Disease-causing organisms (bacteria, viruses, toxins)	Available; small quantities can have large effect; spread through large areas; can remain in air or on surfaces; difficult to prepare against	Delayed effects; production hazardous to terrorists; difficult to develop	Dependent on agent used; most cause flu-like symptoms; plague and smallpox most contagious; timing of specific treatment critical; in some cases there are vaccines
Radiologic	Ionizing radiation is able to strip electrons from atoms, causing chemical changes in molecules; expression may be delayed; radiation depends on time, distance, shielding, and quantity of radioactive material	Available; psychologic effect likely to be substantial; often used in conjunction with explosive devices ("dirty bombs")	Delayed effects of radiation materials; difficult to shield against	Dirty bomb causes immediate effects (radiation burns, acute poisoning) and long-term effects (cancer, contamination of drinking water); decontamination must occur before patient care can be safely provided by the health care worker
Nuclear	Depends on yield of nuclear weapon, but consists of blast range effects, thermal radiation, nuclear radiation, and radioactive fallout	Requires decontamination; contamination can remain for many years; psychologic effect likely to be substantial	Large, heavy, and dangerous weapons; hazardous to terrorists; make weapons of this type expensive and difficult to make	Symptomatic treatment of thermal burns, shrapnel injuries, and radioactive fallout; depends on distance from source and time of exposure
Explosive	Most common method for terrorists; capable of violent decomposition; pressure, temperature changes, and propellants cause injury and/or death	Available materials to construct explosive device; large devices can be placed in abandoned vehicles; smaller device can be placed on the body of a person willing to commit suicide by igniting the device	Volatile ingredients could cause premature explosion of device, thus creating danger for terrorists; government agencies have improved training and processes for identifying incendiary devices	Symptomatic; often requires treatment for burns

Efforts must be directed toward the interrelationship of roles and responsibilities of agencies and services that will be needed at the time of a disaster. Key elements of a community preparedness program include the following:

- Assessing the community for risks and determining the types of events that may occur
- Planning the emergency activities to ensure a coordinated response effort
- Building the capabilities that are necessary to respond to the consequences of the events

There must be agreements between agencies within the community and between neighboring communities for such entities as emergency response units, hospitals, long-term care facilities, clinics, and health departments to be able to provide mutual aid and transfer of people and materials during a time of disaster. The IOM report *Crisis Standards of Care* emphasizes that integrated planning for coordinated response by state and local governments, emergency medical services, health care organizations, and health care providers in the community is critical to successfully responding to disasters (Hanfling et al, 2012).

Agreements should be in place that address issues related to credentialing health care providers who may be shared among institutions. The Medical Reserve Corps (MRC) was initiated in 2002 to improve the health and safety of communities across the country by organizing and utilizing public health, nursing, medical, and other volunteers to serve their communities. There are currently 993 MRC units and 207,783 volunteers throughout the United States and its territories (Division of the Civilian Volunteer Medical Reserve Corps, 2017). Part of the requirements for membership in the MRC is to complete an emergency response curriculum. Several of the MRC units are associated with universities (Culley, 2010).

The MRC is the responsibility of the local area, with many states receiving funding to establish the network of volunteers. They function as a way to locally organize and utilize volunteers who want to donate their time and expertise to prepare for and respond to emergencies and promote healthy living throughout the year. MRC volunteers supplement existing emergency and public health resources. There are situations (such as Hurricane Katrina) for which local units deployed outside of their region to respond to the additional needs that were not being met. (Visit https://mrc.hhs.gov for more information about how to volunteer to participate in the MRC system.)

Plans and contracts also need to be developed with school systems, YMCAs buildings, and other large facilities to provide shelter for large numbers of victims. The interface with volunteer agencies, such as the Red Cross, also needs to be arranged. Each agency should have a well-developed emergency operating plan (EOP) that includes its responsibilities and capabilities for responding to an MCI, an identified chain of command, and a plan for interaction with other community agencies. Agency personnel should be knowledgeable about their role in the EOP and should receive education concerning the ways to respond to all types of hazards.

Several federal-level programs are designed to assist communities in planning their emergency response to an MCI and to provide assistance during a time of disaster. Agency and community EOPs should outline their relationship with the federal system. The National Response Framework is a guide to how the nation conducts an all-hazard response—from the smallest incident to the largest catastrophe—using a comprehensive, national, all-hazards approach to domestic incident response (FEMA, 2014b). Figure 16.1 illustrates the relationship among local, state, and federal response systems. The following is a description of the key components of the federal response system.

Metropolitan Medical Response System. The Metropolitan Medical Response System (MMRS) program builds a cadre of specialty trained responders and equipment in local or sub-state jurisdictions. The system is coordinated with area and statewide planning systems and integrates the efforts of all of the emergency response teams. The MMRS includes plans for expanding hospital-based care, enhancing emergency medical transport and emergency department capabilities, locating specialized pharmaceuticals to respond to an MCI, managing mass fatalities, and providing mental health care for the community, victims, and health care providers. Scenarios designed to test the effectiveness of the MMRS in the community in providing an integrated response to an MCI are conducted on a regular basis.

National Disaster Medical System. The National Disaster Medical System (NDMS) is a federally coordinated system that augments the nation's medical response capability during times of major peacetime disasters and provides support to the military and the Department of Veterans Affairs medical systems in caring for casualties evacuated back to the United States from armed conventional conflicts overseas (U.S. Department of Health and

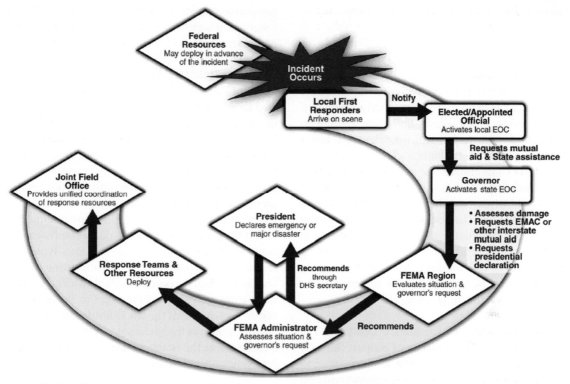

Fig. 16.1 Emergency response flows from the community to the state to the federal level. *DHS,* Department of Homeland Security; *EMAC,* Emergency Management Assistance Compact; *EOC,* emergency operations center; *FEMA,* Federal Emergency Management Agency. (Department of Homeland Security. (2008). National response framework. Retrieved from www.fema.gov/pdf/emergency/nrf/nrf-overview.pdf.)

Human Services [USDHHS], 2017). The National Response Framework utilizes the NDMS under Emergency Support Function #8, Health and Medical Services, to support the federal medical response to major emergencies and federally declared disasters, including national disasters, major transportation accidents, technologic disasters, and acts of terrorism. For more information about becoming involved in NDMS visit the website (http://www.phe.gov/Preparedness/responders/ndms.)

Disaster Medical Assistance Teams. Disaster Medical Assistance Teams (DMATs) are regionally organized teams of health care professionals and administrative staff designed to be the rapid-response component to support local medical care needs until federal resources can be deployed; DMATs can be sent into areas outside their own regions to assist in providing care for ill or injured victims at the location of a disaster or emergency. DMATs provide triage, medical or surgical stabilization,

and continued monitoring and care of patients until they can be evacuated to locations to receive definitive medical care. Specialty DMATs can also be deployed to address, for example, mass burn injuries, pediatric care requirements, and chemical injury or contamination. For more information about DMATs, visit the website (https://www.phe.gov/Preparedness/responders/ndms/ndms-teams/Pages/dmat.aspx.)

Commissioned Corps. The Commissioned Corps emergency response teams are managed by the Office of the Surgeon General and are part of the U.S. Public Health Service. These teams are an additional asset capable of responding in times of extraordinary need when the public health needs exceed the capability of the local or state agencies. The Commissioned Corps comprises more than 6500 health care professionals who can be deployed to respond to a disaster, either as a large group or in small numbers, to support the DMAT's effort.

For more information, visit the website (https://www.surgeongeneral.gov/corps/index.html).

Strategic National Stockpile. The Centers for Disease Control and Prevention (CDC) host a Strategic National Stockpile (SNS) that has large quantities of medicine and medical supplies to protect the American public if there is a public health emergency severe enough to cause local supplies to be depleted. The SNS has a national repository of antibiotics, chemical antidotes, antitoxins, IV administrations, airway supplies, and other medical-surgical items. A 12-hour "push-pack" of supplies can be deployed within 12 hours of the decision to activate the SNS. The community emergency plan should include procedures to receive the push-pack. Follow-up pharmaceutical or medical supplies can be shipped within 24 to 36 hours if required. This supply can be tailored to the specific needs of the event if the needs are known at that time (CDC, 2017a).

Emergency Management Assistance Compact. The Emergency Management Assistance Compact (EMAC) was authorized by the U.S Congress to allow states to request and receive assistant from other states impacted by a governor-declared disaster. This program allows states to quickly and efficiently request and receive assistance from other member states in the form of personnel, equipment and other supplies for emergency response and recovery efforts (EMAC, 2017).

Using Response Resources. Community emergency operating plans must include strategies for the community's interaction with these various state and federal response teams and systems to efficiently use the services and materials provided for mass casualty response. Hospital EOPs should include descriptions of the federal responses and how they will be incorporated into the emergency operations. Developing community "crisis standards" was the focus of the IOM reports of 2009 and 2011, which outline the critical components that need to be in place at each level (Hanfling et al, 2012).

Individual Citizen Preparedness. Although not formally part of emergency operations, individuals and households play an important role in the overall emergency management strategy. Individuals can contribute by reducing hazards in and around their homes, preparing emergency supply kits and household emergency plans, and

monitoring emergency communications carefully. The government website Ready provides additional disaster response information (http://www.ready.gov).

Relief Response Phase

Response Activities. Response activities are first initiated during the impact phase of disasters. These activities begin at the time of the event and are focused on providing the first emergency response to victims of the disaster, stabilizing the situation, and giving adequate treatment to victims. This phase requires the interaction of emergency responders from fire and police departments, emergency medical services, hazardous materials teams, health care agencies, health departments, and to enable the group to triage, provide assistance, conduct a scene assessment and stabilize the scene. Typically, the first unit responding establishes an incident command post from which to coordinate the activities. However, as other units arrive and as the cause of the incident becomes known, one of the law enforcement agencies may assume control as the lead agency if there is suspicion of a crime before the establishment of a community-based emergency operations center (EOC).

National Incident Management System. Emergencies breed chaos, and it is essential that order be brought to the situation for an effective response. The National Incident Management System (NIMS) provides a systematic proactive approach to guide departments and agencies at all levels of government, nongovernmental organizations, and the private sector to work seamlessly during disaster situations (FEMA, 2017). The system is designed to expand from one person or agency performing all roles to having hundreds of people involved in the process. An efficient NIMS requires a hierarchic chain of command led by the incident manager or commander. Assigned personnel who refer to specific job action sheets consistently follow job assignments. An NIMS is established at the scene of the disaster and includes representatives of all agencies needed to provide the emergency services.

At the time of a mass casualty, each hospital system initiates its emergency response plans. Structures may vary from hospital to hospital, but most are using the system called the hospital incident command system (HICS). The assumption is that in a time of crisis, communication will be improved if all disaster responders begin from a common structure. The HICS defines responsibilities, reporting channels, and common terminology for hospitals, fire departments, local governments, and other agencies (California Emergency Medical Services Authority, 2017). The HICS can be customized for organizations of varying sizes. (The 2014 [5th edition] of the *HICS Guidebook* can be downloaded online at no charge, at https://emsa.ca.gov/disaster-medical-services-division-hospital-incident-command-system/.)

Regardless of the structure of the NIMS, the ultimate aim is to coordinate the safe and effective response of emergency resources to an incident. In the HICS, there is only one incident commander, supported by clearly identified levels in the command structure. The hierarchy of command is important so that there is no confusion as to who reports to whom or about who is managing the incident. The chain of command is established to allow for communication to flow from the top down or the bottom up. (FEMA provides online training modules about the incident command system for hospitals and health care providers, at https://training.fema.gov/is/courseoverview.aspx?code=IS-100.HCb.)

Personal Protection and Safety. Personal protection and safety are important regardless of the situational factors causing an MCI. What is important to note, however, is that situational factors dictate how to be personally protected and safe. Protecting the lives of emergency responders takes precedence over other incident issues, because if emergency responders are exposed or injured, they will not be able to provide care to others.

Because of the varied routes of exposure from CBRNE agents, personal protective equipment (PPE) must be designed to impede the most vulnerable route(s), thereby blocking the agent from entering the body. Specially designed PPE is available in a variety of levels, each level designed to meet specific protection needs:

- *Level A* equipment consists of a totally encapsulated chemical resistant suit, including supplied air. As a result, maximum respiratory and skin protection is provided. This level of equipment is used to protect against liquid splashes or in situations in which agents are still unidentified.
- *Level B* equipment is a chemical splash–resistant suit with hood and self-contained breathing apparatus (SCBA). It provides maximum respiratory protection but less skin protection than level A equipment.
- *Level C* equipment is chemical-resistant clothing with a hood and an air-purifying respirator. The respirator can remove all anticipated contaminants and concentrations of chemical materials, thus providing adequate protection against airborne biologic agents and radiologic materials.
- *Level D* protection may consist of a uniform or scrubs and is appropriate when it has been determined that no respiratory or skin hazard is present.

Although each level provides some protection, it is important to understand the limitations of all PPE. Typically, first responders to community emergencies are firefighters, police, and emergency medical technicians. These professionals have traditionally been trained in the effective use of PPE and can be a good community resource. In addition, hospital infection control personnel can be an excellent resource for the use of PPE. As health care providers assume the care of patients who may have been contaminated, it is important to note whether they have been decontaminated and require no further protective equipment or what additional level of protection is required.

Communication within the Health Care Facility. At the initial time of the event, when news stories are first breaking, staff, patients, and families may hear of the incident before the EOP and HICS have been initiated. In this case, it is crucial for the facility information officer to take charge of communicating with the news media and for administrators to initiate a plan to communicate within the health care facility. Crisis intervention strategies to prevent group panic must be instituted immediately. Communication officers need to:

- Determine the effects the crisis will have on the audience.
- Speak clearly and simply about the facts.
- Be direct, honest, and to the point.
- Reassure and calm the audience.

Regular updates of information (every 30 minutes) need to be planned and distributed to all hospital units as quickly as possible. Patients and families need to be informed of measures that will be taken with the initiation of the EOP, such as early discharge or relocation of less ill patients to other areas of the hospital or to other facilities. Family members may not be able to leave the hospital to return home; if so, arrangements must be made to care for them, including providing medications that they take regularly.

LESSONS LEARNED FROM MASS CASUALTY INCIDENTS

Although preparation for all types of causes of MCIs (natural or human-caused) is necessary, nurses must understand the actions needed when the health care agency is damaged and how health care providers must function during these times. Issues related to use of personnel, rotation and resting of personnel, use of family or volunteers, methods of evacuation, and care of hospital staff and families must be included in emergency preparedness preparations and education. Alterations in the standard of care during an MCI need to be understood. Hospitals are viewed by the community and employees as places of safe haven when a disaster strikes. Incoming staff will be limited, and decisions about how care will be provided must be made. Places to provide rest and measures to encourage staff to rest should be determined early in the MCI. Mechanisms for staff to contact their families or significant others should be initiated as soon as possible. Arrangements need to be made for the care of children, other dependents, and pets for those staff members who will be staying at the hospital for extended periods.

In addition, measures must be included to provide information to the staff for those who are not able to locate their family because of the disaster. The role of the information liaison office of the HICS is most important for this function. In addition to these considerations, mass causality incidents have the potential to create widespread civil unrest and violence, which may follow immediately following the event. Safety/security resources, if available, should be put in place as quickly as possible. Personal safety and the safety of others must remain at the forefront in response efforts. This principle is particularly true for vulnerable populations such as women, children, elderly, and those with disabilities.

Staff need to be prepared to cope with power outages and damage to the institution. All hospitals are equipped with emergency generators, and most hospital staff members assume that these will be operational. Emergency plans and drills must include scenarios of how to adapt care if the generators are not functioning. It is important that the staff delivering care have the skill set to know how they will function in these situations. Lessons learned from previous disasters emphasize the necessity to include the care delivery staff in this level of detail. Some examples of decisions that have had to be made were how to:

- Deliver medications when the usual pumps were not functioning.

- Decide what medications would be given when the medication supply was depleted.
- Provide ventilation and suctioning without electricity.

Nurses and staff on the nursing units need to be prepared for these situations. Composing unit-based scenarios for discussion can be helpful in preparing for an MCI.

Japan is perhaps the most well-prepared country in the world for any disaster, yet the experience of the Great East Japan earthquake in March 2011 caused Japanese authorities to understand that past assumptions and lessons learned were not particularly valid (Yamamoto, 2011). This was a compound disaster beginning with an earthquake at a magnitude of 9.0 that resulted in a devastating tsunami with a consequent nuclear crisis involving the release of radioactive materials into the environment. Earlier, it had been recommended to prepare a 3-day supply of food and other necessities to survive a disaster. However, during this event, responders learned that this supply was not enough; it was 1 to 2 weeks before there was enough food and water to go around, and even shelters ran short of food and supplies. Shelters also had to take care of community patients, yet they did not have adequate medical supplies.

BIOLOGIC CAUSES OF MASS CASUALTY

Pandemic Influenza

Nurses also need to be prepared to respond to MCIs that result from biologic agents. Although terrorist dissemination of biologic agents was initially the focus of emergency preparedness efforts following the World Trade Center attack, the natural dissemination of biologic agents such as influenza has been the priority for disaster preparedness efforts for communities. A *pandemic influenza* is a global outbreak that occurs when a new influenza virus emerges in the human population, causing serious illness and death as it spreads worldwide. The United States has had three previous pandemic flu experiences: In 1918, 50 million died worldwide and 675,000 died in the United States; in 1957, 1 to 2 million died worldwide and 70,000 died in the United States; and in 1968, 700,000 died worldwide and 34,000 died in the United States (CDC, 2018).

Tracking and predicting pandemic flu is an important component of the response to this potential serious threat to the nation's health. The most up-to-date information for flu tracking and reporting is now found on the CDC and World Health Organization (WHO) websites. Health care providers are directed to these websites to determine the flu outbreaks in their own areas and those within the region, country, and the world. Although most people believe that flu transmission is a local problem, it has become a global issue with the amounts of international travel and transmission that now occur.

It is important to note that in 2009, when the H1N1 flu virus reached global proportions and was declared an international flu pandemic, academic and pharmaceutical communities united to develop and produce a vaccine within months of its initial detection. The H1N1 vaccine was demonstrated to be effective in diminishing the transmission of the flu. Interestingly, although the H1N1 flu vaccine was readily available, many people, including health workers, did not avail themselves of it. Research indicated that there were cultural differences in the value placed on receiving the flu vaccine and that many people believed their chances of contracting the disease was small or the side effects of the vaccine outweighed its benefits (Seale et al, 2011).

It needs to be emphasized that although antivirals might be helpful in the event that vaccines are not available in the early stages of a pandemic, the current supply of antiviral medication would be grossly inadequate to meet our projected needs if all of the population were to choose to utilize these medications. Depending on the type of virus or bacteria, it is estimated that as a result of production limitations, new vaccines may not be available until 4 to 6 months after the pandemic actually starts. Unfortunately, regular flu shots are designed for a specific strain of flu and thus do not provide immunity to the various types of flu such as H5N1 and H1N1.

The CDC and the WHO have developed surveillance mechanisms to determine phases of pandemic alert, which include decisions on when to move from one phase to another. The CDC has also developed competencies for response to a pandemic flu epidemic. For more information visit the WHO influenza website (http://www.who.int/influenza/en/) or the CDC website (http://www.cdc.gov/flu/professionals).

As with other MCIs, planning is aimed at saving the largest number of people. It is likely that flu varieties would strike nearly simultaneously in many different geographic regions and cause multiple waves of disease lasting 4 to 6 weeks in communities. Thus, local communities need to make their plans self-sufficient because other areas would be dealing with the same problem. Control methods include isolation, quarantine, and restrictions. Limitations include suspension of large public gatherings, school closures, and social distancing.

The term *social distancing* refers to keeping people as far apart as possible to limit the possibilities of spreading germs. The most commonly recommended type of social distancing that has proved to be effective for H1N1 virus has been keeping anyone suspected of the illness at home until 24 hours after the fever has subsided. Health care providers are advised to treat patients symptomatically without encouraging them to come to offices or emergency departments. Many health care facilities set up separate screening facilities for those who have flu-like symptoms.

As a health care provider, you need to take the time to become familiar with your institution's preparedness plan. Most have a plan specific to the threat of pandemic flu. Know what your role is, how you would be notified, and where and how you would report if an emergency is declared.

Being prepared means that you and your family need to be prepared as well. Practice good health hygiene, and follow the general principles of sound public health. Teach family members how to cover their mouths when coughing, how to appropriately dispose of used tissues, and how and when to wash their hands. Develop contingency plans to address school and business closures, unavailability of public transportation, and disruption in social activities. Grocery stores and gas stations may not be open during their typical hours. That means that personal stockpiling of food and medications would help you and your family get through this event with minimal contact with others. Ideally, the goal is to keep the number of people infected within range of existing medical capabilities.

For current information regarding the status of any pandemic flu in the United States, visit the CDC's Influenza web page (http://www.flu.gov); planning guides for federal, state, business, and local authorities as well as individuals are available at this website. Global updates can be found at the WHO website (http://www.who.int/influenza).

Ebola

A later world threat is the 2014 Ebola epidemic, which affected multiple countries in West Africa. Symptoms of Ebola include: fever, severe headache, muscle pain, weakness, diarrhea, vomiting, abdominal pain, and unexplained hemorrhage (CDC, 2017b). The infection can be spread through direct contact with blood or body fluids of a person ill with Ebola, objects contaminated with the virus, or infected animals. Although the risk of an Ebola outbreak in the United States is very low, the CDC and its partners are taking precautions to prevent it. The Emergency Operations Center has been activated, and teams of public health experts have been sent to West Africa in an effort to control the transmission of the disease before it hits pandemic proportions. For the most current information about Ebola, visit the WHO website (http://www.who.int/csr/disease/ebola/en/).

HUMAN CAUSES OF MASS CASUALTY: ACTIVE SHOOTER EVENTS

The federal government defines an active shooter as "an individual actively engaged in killing or attempting to kill people in a confined and populated area, typically through the use of firearms" (Federal Bureau of Investigations [FBI], 2015). The FBI (2014) analyzed 160 active shooter incidents from 2000 through 2013 to look for common elements that might guide law enforcement officials in more effective prevention and response efforts. In the 160 events, 486 individuals were killed and 557 were wounded. This represents an average of 11.4 incidents annually from 2000 to 2013, with an average of 6.4 incidents annually from 2000 to 2006 and an average of 16.4 events annually from 2007 to 2013 (FBI, 2014).

Active shooter events can take place in a wide variety of locations, including schools, health care facilities, and office settings. The U.S. Department of Homeland Security (2008) offers recommendations for response to an active shooter, which are shown in Table 16.2.

With the recognition of the increased active shooter threat and the swiftness with which active shooter incidents unfold, there is greater emphasis on the importance of training and exercises. It is important, too, that training and exercises include not only an understanding of the threats faced but also the risks and options available in active shooter incidents.

TABLE 16.2 Recommended Response to an Active Shooter

1. Evacuate (RUN)	2. Hide Out (HIDE)	3. Take Action Against the Active Shooter (FIGHT)
If there is an accessible escape path, attempt to evacuate the premises. Be sure to: • Have an escape route and plan in mind • Evacuate regardless of whether others agree to follow • Leave your belongings behind • Help others escape, if possible • Prevent individuals from entering an area where the active shooter may be • Keep your hands visible • Follow the instructions of any police officers • Do not attempt to move wounded people • Call 911 when you are safe	If evacuation is not possible, find a place to hide where the active shooter is less likely to find you. Your hiding place should: • Be out of the active shooter's view • Provide protection if shots are fired in your direction (e.g., an office with a closed and locked door) Try not to trap yourself or restrict your options for movement To prevent an active shooter from entering your hiding place: • Lock the door • Blockade the door with heavy furniture If the active shooter is nearby: • Lock the door • Silence your cell phone and/or pager • Turn off any source of noise (e.g., radios, televisions) • Hide behind large items (e.g., cabinets, desks) • Remain quiet If evacuation and hiding out are not possible: • Remain calm • Dial 911, if possible, to alert police to the active shooter's location • If you cannot speak, leave the line open and allow the dispatcher to listen	As a last resort, and only when your life is in imminent danger, attempt to disrupt and/or incapacitate the active shooter by: • Acting as aggressively as possible against him/her • Throwing items and improvising weapons • Yelling • Committing to your actions

From U.S. Department of Homeland Security. (2008). *Active shooter: how to respond.* Retrieved from http://www.dhs.gov/xlibrary/assets/active_shooter_booklet.pdf.

SUMMARY

Preparing for an MCI requires a complex set of activities. All nurses need to be aware of the emergency response system at the local, state, and federal levels and to know how to interface with the systems. They should be involved in developing and evaluating the emergency response plans for their health care agencies and communities. Consider Jane in the opening vignette. Her understanding of the resources available in the community's emergency response system will help her better cope with the disaster facing her family and the hospital where she works. Just as in Jane's situation, disaster can strike anytime, and preparation for an effective emergency response is absolutely critical to ensure the very best outcome for everyone involved. Nurses are well positioned to serve in leadership roles within health care agencies during the time of a disaster because of their excellent communication and collaboration skills.

REFERENCES

Busby, S., & Witucki-Brown, J. (2011). Theory development for situational awareness in multi-casualty incidents. *Journal of emergency nursing, 37*(5), 444–452.

California Emergency Medical Services Authority. (2017). *Disaster medical services: Hospital incident command system (HICS)*. Retrieved from https://emsa.ca.gov/disaster-medical-services-division-hospital-incident-command-system-resources/.

Centers for Disease Control and Prevention. (2018). Influenza (Flu). Retrieved from https://www.cdc.gov/flu/.

Centers for Disease Control and Prevention. (2017a). *Strategic national stockpile*. Retrieved from http://www.cdc.gov/phpr/stockpile/stockpile.htm.

Centers for Disease Control and Prevention. (2017b). *2014-2016 Ebola outbreak in West Africa*. Retrieved from http://www.cdc.gov/vhf/ebola/outbreaks/2014-west-africa/index.html.

Culley, J. M. (2010). The role of the Medical Reserve Corps in nursing education. *Journal of nursing education, 49*(12), 708–711.

Division of the Civilian Volunteer Medical Reserve Corps. (2017). *About the medical reserve corps*. Retrieved from https://mrc.hhs.gov/pageviewfldr/About.

Emergency Management Assistance Compact. (2017). *EMAC*. Retrieved from https://www.emacweb.org.

Federal Bureau of Investigation. (2015). Critical incident response group, "Active shooter event: Quick reference guide". Retrieved from https://www.fbi.gov/file-repository/active-shooter-event-quick-reference-guide_2015.pdf.

Federal Bureau of Investigation. (2014). *A study of active shooter incidents in the United States between 2000-2013*. Retrieved from http://www.fbi.gov/news/stories/2014/september/fbi-releases-study-on-active-shooter-incidents.

Federal Emergency Management Agency. (2014a). *A guide to the disaster declaration process and federal disaster assistance*. Retrieved from https://www.fema.gov/pdf/rrr/dec_proc.pdf.

Federal Emergency Management Agency. (2014b). *NRF resource center*. Retrieved from https://training.fema.gov/nrfres.aspx.

Federal Emergency Management Agency. (2017). *National incident management system*. Retrieved from http://www.fema.gov/national-incident-management-system.

Hanfling, D., Altevogt, B. M., Viswanathan, K., & Gostin, L. O. (2012). *Crisis standards of care: A systems framework for catastrophic disaster response*. Retrieved from https://www.nap.edu/catalog/13351/crisis-standards-of-care-a-systems-framework-for-catastrophic-disaster.

Kotz, D. (2013, April 24). Injury toll from Marathon bombs reduced to 264. *The Boston Globe*. Retrieved from http://www.bostonglobe.com/lifestyle/health-wellness/2013/04/23/number-injured-marathon-bombing-revised-downward/NRpaz5mmvGquP7KMA6XsIK/story.html.

Powers, R. (2010). Introduction to disasters and disaster nursing. In R. Powers, & E. Daily (Eds.), *Disaster Nursing International* (pp. 1–11). Cambridge, NY: Cambridge University Press.

Seale, H., Kaur, R., Wang, Q., Yang, P., Zhang, Y., Wang, X., et al. (2011). Acceptance of a vaccine against pandemic influenza A (H1N1) virus amongst healthcare workers in Beijing, China. *Vaccine, 29*(8), 1605–1610.

The Joint Commission. (2013). *New and revised requirements address emergency management oversight*. Retrieved from http://www.jointcommission.org/assets/1/18/JCP0713_Emergency_Mgmt_Oversight.pdf.

U.S. Department of Health and Human Services. (2017). *National disaster medical system*. Retrieved from https://www.phe.gov/Preparedness/responders/ndms/Pages/default.aspx.

U.S. Department of Homeland Security. (2008). *Active shooter: How to respond*. Retrieved from http://www.dhs.gov/xlibrary/assets/active_shooter_booklet.pdf.

Veenema, T. G. (2003a). Essentials of disaster planning. In T. G. Veenema (Ed.), *Disaster nursing and emergency preparedness for chemical, biological, and radiological terrorism and other hazards* (pp. 3–30). New York: Springer Publishing Company.

Veenema, T. G. (2003b). Leadership and coordination in disaster healthcare systems: The federal disaster response network. In T. G. Veenema (Ed.), *Disaster nursing and emergency preparedness for chemical, biological, & radiological terrorism and other hazards* (pp. 31–61). New York: Springer Publishing Company.

Yamamoto, A. (2011). Experiences of the great East Japan earthquake March 2011. *International nursing review, 58*(3), 332–334.

17

Nursing Leadership and Management

Barbara Cherry, DNSc, MBA, RN, NEA-BC

All *nurses—regardless of their role or setting—must step up as leaders to promote healthier patients and happier staff.*

ⓔ Additional resources are available online at: *http://evolve.elsevier.com/Cherry/*

LEARNING OUTCOMES

After studying this chapter, the reader will be able to:

1. Discuss the responsibility of being a leader in any role or setting where professional nursing is practiced.
2. Relate leadership and management theory to nursing leadership and management activities.
3. Differentiate among the five functions of management and essential activities related to each function.
4. Integrate principles of patient-centered care in professional nursing practice.
5. Implement effective team-building skills as an essential component of nursing practice.
6. Implement the nursing process as a method of problem solving and planning.
7. Apply principles and strategies of change theory in the management role.

KEY TERMS

Authority The legitimate right to direct others, given to a person by the employer through an official position, such as manager or administrator.

Health care organization Any business, company, institution, or facility (e.g., hospital, home health agency, ambulatory care clinic, health insurance company, nursing home) engaged in providing health care services or products.

Leadership The act of guiding or influencing people to achieve desired outcomes; occurs any time a person attempts to influence the beliefs, opinions, or behaviors of an individual or group (Hersey and Blanchard, 1988).

Management Coordination of resources, such as time, people, and supplies, to achieve outcomes; involves problem-solving and decision-making processes.

Organizational chart A visual picture of the organization that identifies lines of communication and authority.

Productivity The amount of output or work produced (e.g., home visits made) by a specific amount of input or resources (e.g., nursing hours worked).

Resources Personnel, time, and supplies needed to accomplish the goals of the organization.

PROFESSIONAL/ETHICAL ISSUE

Marybeth Rodgers graduated from nursing school 5 years ago and worked at a renowned academic medical center in a busy medical-surgical unit since graduation. She recently took a job as a staff RN in a small community hospital closer to her home to reduce her commute time and give her more time with her family. Marybeth was very confident in her skills and knowledge to care for adult medical-surgical patients because of her experience over the past 5 years, but she knew she would have a lot to learn in this new setting. After a few weeks working on her new unit in the community hospital, she began to sense that one of her nurse colleagues was resentful toward her. Initially the nurse was refusing to help her when she had questions, but she has now begun to openly criticize Marybeth with statements such as "I guess you think you are smarter than everyone else because you worked at that academic medical center downtown" and "I think you are just lazy and don't want to think for yourself; after all, you had all those medical students to think for you." Marybeth senses that she is being talked about by the other nurses and is being excluded from some conversations. She is coming to deeply regret her decision to move to the community hospital; she is having trouble sleeping and now dreads coming to work every day. Marybeth is deeply concerned about reporting the situation to the nurse manager because she knows that the nurse who is causing the problems has worked on the unit for many years and seems well-liked by the supervisor and other nurses. What are Marybeth's options for addressing this situation? What does the American Nurses Association (ANA) Code of Conduct tell us about a nurse's ethical obligation to support colleagues? What resources can Marybeth access to learn more about disruptive behaviors and how to handle them?

VIGNETTE

Nancy Brown, a new registered nurse (RN), has accepted a position in a busy outpatient dialysis unit. During nursing school, Nancy worked in the facility as a patient care technician, and she is confident in her clinical skills because of this experience. Mary, the nurse manager of the dialysis unit, has scheduled Nancy to attend the new-nurse orientation. Although Nancy thinks to herself, "I know what the RNs do around here;

I'd like to jump right in without attending orientation," she readily accepts the assignment.

The nurse manager begins the orientation program with a discussion about the mission of the organization and the RN's responsibility to ensure that quality patient care is provided in a safe and cost-effective manner. As Nancy progresses through the orientation program, her confidence quickly fades. She becomes overwhelmed as she listens to a description of her new responsibilities as an RN. The RN's duties involve much more than the expected physical assessment and developing and implementing care plans. Some of Nancy's many new responsibilities as a staff RN are to:

- Supervise patient care technicians and manage assignments and supply use for a group of patients.
- Meet with the interprofessional team, including the social worker, dietitian, nephrologist, nurse manager, and the patient and family, to develop the patient's care plan and then follow up to coordinate and implement the plan.
- Serve on a task force charged with developing and implementing a zero-tolerance policy for bullying and incivility in the workplace.
- Perform chart audits to review nursing documentation, identify problems, develop recommendations, and report to the quality improvement committee.

As Nancy is trying to assimilate the information being presented, she almost fails to hear Mary say that within 6 months of employment, all staff RNs are expected to begin orientation for the charge nurse position to provide backup coverage. At the end of the orientation, Nancy has a new perspective about professional nursing practice—it seems to be as much about managing the delivery of patient care as actually giving the care!

Questions to Consider While Reading this Chapter:

1. What skills will assist Nancy as she begins her new role as a staff RN with many leadership and management responsibilities?
2. Why is it important for the nursing staff to understand the mission and values of the organization to provide direct patient care?
3. What type of team-building skills will help Nancy as she learns to work with the interprofessional team and coordinate the patient's plan of care with a diverse group of health professionals?

4. What resources are available to help Nancy learn and enhance her management and leadership skills?

CHAPTER OVERVIEW

During nursing school, students are often more concerned with developing clinical knowledge and skills and are less concerned with management and leadership skills. However, immediately after graduation the new nurse is placed in many situations that require leadership and management skills—managing a group of assigned patients, serving on a task force or committee, supervising unlicensed assistive personnel and licensed vocational nurses (LVNs) or licensed practical nurses (LPNs), or addressing difficult situations such as incivility and bullying. In addition to providing safe, evidence-based, high-quality clinical care, the challenges for RNs today are to manage nursing units that are constantly admitting and discharging higher-acuity patients, to motivate and coordinate a variety of diverse health professionals and paraprofessionals, and to look for ways to improve the work environment to support healthier patients and happier staff.

Regardless of the position or area the nurse is employed in, the health care organization will expect the professional nurse to have leadership skills to:

- Make good clinical decisions based on safety, quality, cost, legal, and ethical aspects of care.
- Promote evidence-based practice. (See Chapter 6.)
- Lead quality improvement initiatives in the work environment. (See Chapter 22.)
- Coordinate patient care activities for the interprofessional team.
- Promote team morale, patient satisfaction, and overall productivity.
- Support compliance with governmental regulations and accreditation standards.

As the reader can easily visualize, leadership and management activities are a primary responsibility for the RN. In fact, professional nursing within a health care organization has as much to do with managing the delivery of care as it does with actually providing that care. This chapter presents key leadership and management concepts that will guide the nurse to grow and develop in this important aspect of the professional practice role.

Throughout this chapter, the term *organization* is used to refer to the hospital, home health agency, post–acute care facility, long-term care facility, ambulatory clinic, managed care company, or any other area in which a nurse might be employed to practice professional nursing. Legal and ethical issues are a critical component of leadership, although it is not within the scope of this chapter to discuss these issues. The reader is encouraged to review Chapter 8 regarding legal issues and Chapter 9 regarding ethical issues.

LEADERSHIP AND MANAGEMENT DEFINED AND DISTINGUISHED

Leadership Defined

Leadership occurs any time a person attempts to influence the beliefs, opinions, or behaviors of a person or group (Hersey and Blanchard, 1988). Leadership is a combination of intrinsic personality traits, learned leadership skills, and characteristics of the situation. The function of a leader is to guide people and groups to accomplish common goals. For example, an effective nurse leader is able to inspire others on the health care team to make patient-centered care an important aspect of all care activities.

It is important to note that even though leaders may not have formal authority granted by the organization, they are still able to influence others. The job title "nurse manager" does not make a nurse a leader. Today's complex health care environment requires that *every* nurse—regardless of his or her role or setting—provide leadership to advance excellence in nursing practice and patient care.

Management Defined

Management refers to the activities involved in coordinating people, time, and supplies to achieve desired outcomes and involves problem-solving and decision-making processes. Managers maintain control of the day-to-day operations of a defined area of responsibility to achieve established goals and objectives. Managers plan and organize what is to be done, who is to do it, and how it is to be done. A manager has:

- An appointed management position within the organization with responsibilities to perform administrative tasks, such as planning staffing, performing employee performance reviews, controlling use of supplies and time, and meeting budget and productivity goals

- A formal line of authority and accountability to ensure that safe and effective patient care is delivered in a manner that meets the organization's goals and standards

Leadership versus Management

Although leadership and management are intertwined and it is difficult to discuss one without the other, these concepts are different. Leadership is the ability to guide or influence others, whereas management is the coordination of resources (time, people, supplies) to achieve outcomes. People are led, whereas activities and things are managed. Leaders are able to motivate and inspire others, whereas managers have assigned responsibility for accomplishing the goals of an organization. A good manager should also be a good leader, but this may not always be the case. A person with good management skills may not have leadership ability. Similarly, a person with leadership abilities may not have good management skills. Leadership and management skills are complementary; both can be learned and developed through experience, and improving skills in one area will enhance abilities in the other.

Power and Authority

Leadership and management require power and authority to motivate people to act in a certain way. Authority is the legitimate right to direct others and is given to a person by the organization through an official position, such as nurse manager. For example, a nurse manager has the authority to direct staff nurses to work a specific schedule. *Power* is the ability to motivate people to get things done with or without the legitimate right granted by the organization. The primary sources of power are as follows (Hersey et al, 1979):

- *Reward power* comes from the ability to reward others for complying and may include such rewards as salary, desired assignments, and acknowledgment of accomplishments.
- *Coercive power,* the opposite of reward power, is based on fear of punishment for failure to comply. Sources of coercive power include withholding of pay increases, undesired assignments, verbal and written warnings, and termination.
- *Legitimate power* is based on an official position in the organization. Through legitimate power, the manager has the right to influence staff members, and staff members have an obligation to accept that influence.

- *Referent power* comes from the followers' identification with the leader. The admired and respected nurse is able to influence other nurses because of their desire to emulate him or her.
- *Expert power* is based on knowledge, skills, and information. For example, nurses who have expertise in areas such as physical assessment or technical skills or who keep up with current information on important topics will gain respect from others.
- *Information power* is based on a person's possession of information that is needed by others.
- *Connection power* is based on a person's relationship or affiliation with other people who are perceived as being powerful.

An individual may also have informal power resulting from personal relationships, being in the right place at the right time, or unique personal characteristics, such as attractiveness, education, experience, drive, or decisiveness. By understanding the authority of an assigned position and the sources of formal and informal power, the nurse will be better able to influence others to accomplish goals.

Formal and Informal Leadership

Both formal and informal forms of leadership can exist in every organization. Formal leadership is practiced by the nurse who is appointed to an approved position (e.g., nurse manager, supervisor, director) and given the authority to act by the organization. Informal leadership is exercised by the person who has no official or appointed authority to act but is able to persuade and influence others. The informal leader, who may or may not be a professional nurse, may have considerable power in the work group and can influence the group's attitude and significantly affect the efficiency and effectiveness of workflow, goal setting, and problem solving.

The nurse manager must learn to recognize and effectively work with informal leaders. Informal leadership may be positive if the informal leader's purpose is congruent with that of the nursing unit and organizational goals. For example, the informal leader of a patient care group may be highly supportive of a new nursing care delivery model being implemented on the unit, and as a result, the other team members will be more willing to accept the change. However, an informal leader who is not supportive of the nursing unit's goals can create an uncomfortable work environment for the nurse manager and the entire team. Following are some strategies the nurse manager can use to work with informal leaders:

- Identify the informal leaders in the work team and develop an understanding of their source of power. (See sources of power in the previous section.)
- Involve the informal leaders and other staff members in decision-making and change-implementation processes.
- Clearly communicate the goals and work expectations to all staff members.
- Do not ignore an informal leader's attempt to undermine teamwork and change processes. Coaching and counseling the person and setting clear expectations may be required.

LEADERSHIP THEORY

Understanding the development and progression of leadership theory is a necessary building block for developing leadership and management skills. Researchers began to study leadership in the early 1900s in an attempt to describe and understand the nature of leadership. The following sections review a few key leadership theories. Readers are encouraged to learn more about leadership and management theories, especially as they advance in their nursing career.

Leadership Trait Theory

Early leadership theory centered on describing the qualities or traits of leaders and has been commonly referred to as *trait theory* (Stogdill, 1974). Leadership trait theory was based on the assumption that leaders were born with certain leadership characteristics. Traits found to be associated with leadership include intelligence, alertness, dependability, energy, drive, enthusiasm, ambition, decisiveness, self-confidence, cooperativeness, and technical mastery (Stogdill, 1974). Although trait theories have been important in identifying qualities that distinguish today's leaders, these theories have neglected the interaction between other elements of the leadership situation. Trait theories also have failed to recognize that leadership traits can be learned and developed through experience. However, by keeping in mind these traits associated with effective leadership, the new nurse can identify areas in which he or she should improve and develop.

Transformational Leadership

In a contemporary concept of leadership, Burns (1978) identified and defined transformational leadership. Burns contends that there are two types of leaders: (1) the transactional leader, who is concerned with day-to-day operations, and (2) the transformational leader, who is committed to organizational goals, has a vision, and is able to empower others with that vision. The transformational leader is able to guide employees to feel pride in the work of the organization and to inspire them to be actively engaged to achieve the mission and goals of the organization. Transformational leaders spend time teaching and coaching, seek differing perspectives when faced with problems to solve, have a passion for excellence, and seek new ways to improve the work environment. Box 17.1 compares characteristics of Burns's (1978) transformational and transactional leadership styles.

Studies have reported that nurse managers who demonstrate more transformational leadership characteristics achieve higher levels of staff satisfaction and work group effectiveness (Bormann and Abrahamson, 2014; Burke et al, 2017). The implication for nurse managers is that transformational leadership is very effective in increasing staff satisfaction and work effectiveness. Readers are encouraged to read more about

---

BOX 17.1   Comparison of Transformational and Transactional Leaders

Transformational Leaders	Transactional Leaders
• Identify and clearly communicate vision and direction	• Focus on day-to-day operations and are comfortable with the status quo
• Empower the work group to accomplish goals and achieve the vision	• Reward staff for desired work ("I'll do X in exchange for you doing Y.")
• Impart meaning and challenge to work	• Monitor work performance and correct as needed or
• Are admired and emulated	• Wait until problems occur, and then deal with them
• Provide mentoring to individual staff members based on need	

transformational leadership and to seek out transformational leaders as mentors. However, it is important to note that even the most effective transformational leaders fail unless they possess the day-to-day management skills of transactional leaders (Bass et al, 1987).

LEADERSHIP SKILLS AND PRACTICES

Three major types of skills and practices are required for effective leadership (Hersey and Blanchard, 1988):

- *Technical skills*—for nurses, this type includes clinical expertise and nursing knowledge.
- *Human skills*—the ability and judgment to work with and lead people in a compassionate, caring way.
- *Conceptual skills*—the ability to understand the complexities of the overall organization and to recognize how and where one's own area of management fits into the overall organization.

At the staff nurse level of management, a considerable amount of technical skill and clinical expertise is needed because the nurse generally is involved in direct supervision of patient care and may be required to help train and mentor nurses. As one advances from lower levels to higher levels in the organization, more conceptual skills and practices are needed. Box 17.2 provides examples of technical, human, and conceptual practices required for nurse leaders.

MANAGEMENT THEORY

Behavioral theories emerged to explain aspects of management based on behaviors of managers, leaders, and followers. Three prevalent management behavior styles were identified by Lewin (1951) and White and Lippit (1960): authoritarian, democratic, and laissez-faire. Box 17.3 presents characteristics of these management styles, which vary in the amount of control exhibited by the manager and the amount of involvement that the staff has in decision making. At one extreme, the autocratic manager makes all decisions with no staff input and uses the authority of the position to accomplish goals. At the opposite extreme is the laissez-faire manager, who provides little direction or guidance and will forgo decision making. Democratic management is also often referred to as *participative* management because of its basic premise of encouraging staff members to participate in decision making.

Depending on the situation, the nurse manager may need to use different types of management styles. For example, autocratic management might be appropriate in an emergency situation, such as treating a patient in cardiac arrest. However, in structuring the weekend call schedule for a home health agency, a participative style of management would be more effective.

BOX 17.2 Effective Leading and Managing: Technical, Human, and Conceptual Practices

Technical Practices
- Keep your own clinical skills and knowledge current.
- Act as a willing expert resource and teacher for clinical problems.
- Use sound clinical judgment and critical thinking.

Human Practices
- Maintain honesty and integrity in work and relationships—trust is essential for effective leadership.
- Create a teaching and learning environment—earn a reputation for exceptional teaching and mentoring.
- Develop and role model a commitment to excellence.
- Create an open, nonthreatening environment—share information, keep staff informed, and encourage them to discuss issues.
- Become a proactive problem solver—knowing how to solve problems is more important than knowing all the answers.

- Maintain a confident, positive outlook—identify areas in which you are weak, and seek help to learn and grow.

Conceptual Practices
- Make a commitment to support the mission, vision, and goals of the organization.
- Accept the realities of complex health care systems, which are under pressure to improve patient safety and quality while reducing costs.
- Understand the needs of external customers (patients, families, physicians, referring facilities) and internal customers (staff, administrators, and other departments).

BOX 17.3   Management Styles

Autocratic/Authoritative	Democratic/Participative	Laissez-Faire
• Determines policy and makes all decisions • Ignores subordinates' ideas and suggestions • Dictates the work with much control • Gives little feedback or recognition for work • Makes fast decisions • Successful with employees with little education or training	• Encourages staff participation in decision making • Involves staff in planning and developing new ideas and programs • Believes in the best in people • Communicates effectively, and provides regular feedback • Builds responsibility in people • Works well with competent, highly motivated people	• Does not provide guidance or direction • Unable or unwilling to make decisions • Does not provide feedback • Initiates little change • Communicates by memos or e-mail • May work well with professional people

Today's health care system requires the use of a democratic or participative management style that involves the staff in patient safety, quality improvement, patient-centered care, and cost reductions. Health care settings are driven to become increasingly cost-effective while continuing to improve quality, customer satisfaction, and positive patient outcomes. Staff directly involved in the challenges presented by patient care often can suggest the most workable, practical solutions.

Organizational Theory

Just as leadership and management theories evolved to provide a framework for understanding leadership and management, organizational theory evolved to provide a framework for understanding complex organizations. A brief review of systems theory and chaos theory can provide readers with insight into the value of using organizational theory to understand management processes within today's dynamic, complex health care organizations.

Systems Theory. The systems theory views the organization as a set of interdependent parts that together form a whole (Thompson, 1967). The interdependent nature of the parts of the organization suggests that anything that affects the functioning of one part of the organization will affect the other parts. Open systems theory suggests that the organization not only is affected by internal changes among any of its parts but also is directly influenced by external environmental forces, and vice versa—the internal forces will affect the external environment. In contrast to open systems theory, closed systems theory

Leadership, management, and organizational theories provide the building blocks for effective nursing management practices.

CASE STUDY 17.1

The hospital in which William Scoggins, RN, works has reduced the number of RNs employed by the hospital and now requires that the remaining RNs work overtime "at the request of administration." The quality of patient care, patient safety, and the individual nurses' professional practice and personal health have been negatively affected by this change. William and his fellow RNs seek advice from their state nurses association about their professional responsibility to work mandatory overtime. The state nurses association is responding to the situation, which is occurring more frequently across the state and nation, by proposing legislation to mandate hospitals to have effective staffing plans and to limit mandatory overtime. The state government may now require hospital administrators to respond to the need for increased staffing levels.

views the system as being totally independent of outside influences, which is an unrealistic view for health care organizations. To be successful, today's health care organizations must be able to continually adapt to internal and external changes.

Consider the example in Case Study 17.1 to help explain systems theory. As internal forces in one department (hospital administration) mandated changes that affected another area (RNs and patient care), internal forces (RNs) pushed for changes from the external environment (state nurses association and state government). The external environment may now force changes to the organization (hospital administration).

Systems theory has provided nurses with a framework to view nursing services as a subsystem of the larger organization and to realize the interrelatedness and interdependence of all the parts of the organization. The nurse will be wise to consider open systems theory and the effect a change in one area will have in another area, internal as well as external to the organization.

Chaos Theory. Chaos theory is a more recently developed organizational theory that attempts to account for the complexity and randomness in organizations. Despite the implications of the word *chaos,* the theory actually suggests that a degree of order can be attained by viewing complicated behaviors and situations as predictable. Nurse managers may wish for balanced and steady work environments, but in reality they are dealing with

what seems, at best, a chaotic system. Chaos theory says that variation is a normal part of managing health care systems. On the basis of chaos theory, a nurse manager knows that staff absences due to illness, sick children, and family emergencies are a fact of life, which require the nurse manager to have backup plans in place in the event that staff members "call in" and are unable to report for their assigned shifts. Other examples of variation in health care are cultural diversity, a constantly fluctuating patient census, and staffing shortages. Until nurses understand that these variations are a normal, predictable state in the organization that should be planned for, they may continue to experience excessive anxiety with the daily events that occur in health care organizations (McGuire, 1999).

MANAGEMENT FUNCTIONS

Classic theories of management suggest that the primary functions of managers are planning, organizing, and controlling (Stogdill, 1974). Leaders in nursing management have added two more functions to this list and now recognize five major management functions (Figure 17.1) as necessary for the management of nursing organizations: (1) planning, (2) organizing, (3) staffing, (4) directing, and (5) controlling (Marquis and Huston, 2017). These management functions are interrelated; different phases of the process occur simultaneously, and the processes should be circular, with the manager always working toward improving quality, patient safety, and staff and customer satisfaction. Because understanding these five management functions is essential for success as a nurse, they are discussed in further detail.

Planning

Planning, the first management function, involves several steps: (1) identify goals and objectives to be achieved; (2) identify resources needed (e.g., people, supplies, equipment); (3) determine action steps; and (4) establish a timeline for the action steps and goal achievement. All management functions are based on planning. *Without effective planning, the management process will fail.* Effective planning requires the nurse to understand the organization's mission, philosophy, strategic plan, goals, and objectives.

Mission and Philosophy. The *mission* statement, the foundation of planning for any organization, describes

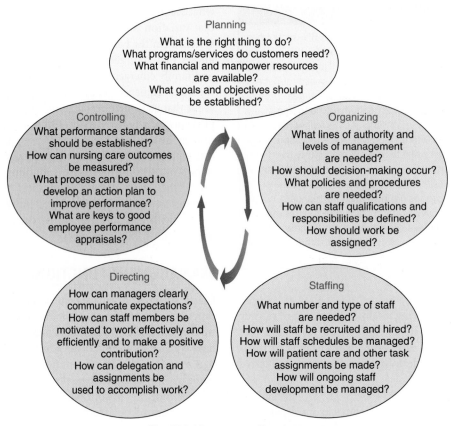

Planning
What is the right thing to do?
What programs/services do customers need?
What financial and manpower resources are available?
What goals and objectives should be established?

Controlling
What performance standards should be established?
How can nursing care outcomes be measured?
What process can be used to develop an action plan to improve performance?
What are keys to good employee performance appraisals?

Organizing
What lines of authority and levels of management are needed?
How should decision-making occur?
What policies and procedures are needed?
How can staff qualifications and responsibilities be defined?
How should work be assigned?

Directing
How can managers clearly communicate expectations?
How can staff members be motivated to work effectively and efficiently and to make a positive contribution?
How can delegation and assignments be used to accomplish work?

Staffing
What number and type of staff are needed?
How will staff be recruited and hired?
How will staff schedules be managed?
How will patient care and other task assignments be made?
How will ongoing staff development be managed?

Fig. 17.1 Management Functions.

the purpose of the organization and the reason it exists. Most health care organizations exist to provide high-quality patient care, but emphasis may be placed on different concepts, such as research, teaching, preventive care, spiritual care, and community service. The *philosophy* is the set of values and beliefs that guides the actions of the organization and thus serves as the basis of all planning. New nurses should be aware of the mission and philosophy of the employing organization and should understand the relationship between their own personal value system and that of the organization. Box 17.4 provides an example of an organization's mission and philosophy statements.

Strategic Planning. Strategic planning is long-range planning, extending 2 to 5 years into the future. It results from an in-depth analysis of (1) the business, community, regulatory, and political environment outside the organization; (2) customer and patient needs; (3) technology changes; and (4) strengths, problems, and weaknesses internal to the organization. The purposes of strategic planning are to:

- Identify strategies to respond to changes in customer needs, technology, health care legislation, the business environment, and the community.
- Dedicate resources to important services and new programs.
- Eliminate duplication, waste, and underused services.
- Establish a timeline for goal achievement.

The *strategic plan* is a written document that details organizational goals, allocates resources, assigns responsibilities, and determines time frames. Development of the strategic plan is generally coordinated by upper-level managers, who engage employees at all levels in the strategic planning process. Consider the example in Case Study 17.2.

BOX 17.4   Sample Mission, Values, and Philosophy Statement

The mission of Community Hospital is to provide high-quality, cost-effective health services that patients and families recommend, employees are proud of, and the community values.

The philosophy and values of Community Hospital are:

- We are committed to professional and individual excellence, with support for personal and professional growth.
- We believe in ethical and fair treatment for *all* through a commitment to relationships based on fairness and trust with our patients and our employees.
- Teamwork is consistently demonstrated as we work together to provide ever-improving quality care.
- Compassion is our highest priority; we will always provide care and comfort to people in need with respectful and dignified treatment at all times.
- Innovation in service delivery is accomplished by investing in the development of new and better ways to deliver health care.

CASE STUDY 17.2

Susan Huffington, RN, nurse manager for the Quality Care Home Health Agency, noticed that the office had been receiving several calls per week for skilled nursing care for pediatric oncology patients. The agency did not provide services for pediatric patients. Susan reported the situation to the administrator. Susan soon was involved in gathering information about the number of home health agencies that offered pediatric oncology care, the standards of nursing care recommended for pediatric oncology patients, how pediatric oncology patients were receiving home care, how many pediatric patients in the area might need such services, and what reimbursement was available for such services. Within the next few months, the management team for Quality Care Home Health Agency decided that as part of the agency's strategic plan, a program for pediatric oncology services would be developed.

Goals and Objectives. Goals and objectives state the actions necessary to achieve the strategic plan and are central to the entire management process. Goals should be measurable, observable, and realistic. Objectives are more specific and detail how a goal will be accomplished with an established target date.

CASE STUDY 17.3

Michele Walker, RN, has recently been appointed as nurse manager in a 150-bed long-term care facility. The mission and philosophy of the organization are to "respect the dignity and worth of the individual and to provide care that will help restore the individual to the best possible state of physical, mental, and emotional health while maintaining his or her sense of spiritual and social well-being." Kenneth Cole, Administrator, has asked Michele to develop a set of goals that she views as priorities to accomplish in the next year. After gathering data about resident needs, costs, and staffing levels and meeting with the medical director, direct-care staff, and staff members in rehabilitation therapy, social services, dietary, and maintenance, Michele develops the following goals:

1. Increase by 25% over 12 months the level of satisfaction related to emotional well-being and socialization expressed by residents and family members on the quarterly quality of life satisfaction survey. This will be accomplished by improving coordination of care activities among nursing, therapy, and social services.
2. Reduce resident falls by 50% over 6 months through the implementation of an evidence-based guideline for falls prevention.
3. Increase by 30% over 12 months the number of nursing staff who achieve national certification as gerontologic nurses through the American Nurses Credentialing Center. To accomplish this goal, the facility will offer certification review courses over the next 6 months.

Together Michele and Kenneth review the goals, agree that they fit with the overall organizational plan, and address the needs identified in Michele's facility assessment activities.

Goals and objectives serve as the manager's road map. Organization-wide goals are established in the strategic planning process, and then unit goals that support the organization-wide goals are developed. Nurse managers should be able to clearly articulate the goals of both the organization and the nursing unit. Additionally, goals and objectives must be communicated to everyone who is responsible for their attainment. Consider the example in Case Study 17.3.

Operational Planning. The nurse manager is most likely to be responsible for operational planning or the short-range planning that encompasses the day-to-day activities of the organization. For example, short-range planning for a medical-surgical unit in a hospital might include maintaining an overall patient-to-staff ratio of 5:1, with 70% of the staff being RNs. As part of accomplishing organizational goals and objectives, the nurse manager involved in operational planning must be concerned with the:

- Number, acuity, type, and location of patients to be cared for.
- Qualifications and competencies of nursing and other health care staff.
- Type and amount of supplies and other physical resources available.
- Allocation of resources (e.g., staff, supplies, time) to meet budgetary goals.

The nurse manager also must plan for a variety of other activities, such as staff development, regulatory compliance, and quality improvement and patient safety projects. (See Chapter 22.)

Organizing

Organizing is the second management function. At the organizational level, organizing is necessary to establish a formal structure that defines the lines of authority, communication, and decision making within an organization. The formal organizational structure helps establish the roles and responsibilities of each level of management. The **organizational chart** provides a visual picture of the organization and identifies lines of communication and authority. All nurses should be familiar with the organizational chart of their employing institution. Organizing also involves developing policies and procedures to help outline how work will be done and establishing position qualifications and job descriptions to define who will do the work.

At the unit level, nurses must determine how to best organize the work activities to meet goals. Organizing involves:

- Using resources (e.g., staff, supplies, time) wisely.
- Assigning duties and responsibilities appropriately.
- Coordinating activities with other departments.
- Effectively communicating with subordinates and superiors to ensure a smooth workflow.

Models for staffing and organizing the delivery of patient care are discussed in Chapter 21.

Staffing

Staffing is the third management function. The provision of health care is labor-intensive, with a workforce that is made up of people with a variety of education and skill levels (e.g., professional nurses, physicians, pharmacists, social workers, therapists, dietitians, licensed vocational or practical nurses, technicians, and unlicensed assistive personnel). Hiring and managing staff to accomplish the work of the institution are important functions for all levels of managers.

Marquis and Huston (2017) have described steps in the staffing function as follows:

1. Determine the number and type of staff needed on the basis of goals and budget requirements.
2. Recruit, interview, select, and assign personnel according to job description and performance standards.
3. Get new employees off to a good start by offering excellent orientation, training, and socialization programs.
4. Implement an ongoing staff-development program to ensure that employees at all levels have opportunities to develop personally and professionally and to enhance their knowledge and skill levels.
5. Implement creative and flexible scheduling based on patient care needs, employee needs, and **productivity** requirements.

The staffing process most likely will prove to be one of the most time-consuming and challenging functions for the nurse manager; however, it is probably the nurse manager's most important job. Little can be accomplished without the right people properly trained to do the work in an environment that promotes collegial, productive relationships among the health care team.

Nursing leaders are highly concerned with recruiting and retaining a talented RN workforce. Factors positively associated with RNs' work satisfaction are presented in Box 17.5. These factors are based on research studies and provide managers with information about how they can increase nurse satisfaction and thus reduce nursing turnover and improve recruitment and retention efforts. Staff schedules (days and shifts staff are assigned to work) and patient assignment schedules (patient care assignments for which each staff member is responsible during his or her workday) are key to nurse satisfaction, recruitment, and retention.

While meeting staff and patient scheduling needs, the nurse manager must also accomplish organizational staffing and productivity goals. *Productivity* is the amount of work produced through the use of a specific amount of resources; it is measured as output divided

---

BOX 17.5 Factors Influencing Nurses' Job Satisfaction and Dissatisfaction

Sources of Satisfaction	Sources of Dissatisfaction
• Leaders who inspire vision and have a passion for excellence in nursing practice • Empowerment and trust to make decisions and support for decisions that are made • Positive environment with opportunities to learn from mistakes • Transparent sharing of unit clinical and operational data • Fairness of the work schedule and salary • Meaningful connections with leaders and ongoing feedback about performance • Sincere thanks and positive recognition • Leaders who role-model professionalism through dress and communication • Guidance, mentorship, and opportunities for professional development and advancement • Opportunity to be involved in change processes and problem solving • Respectful relationships among staff and physicians, peers, administrators, and other departments	• Supervisors who are uninvolved and unsupportive • Tolerance for bullying and incivility • Poor communication and unclear expectations • Vague, inconsistent rules and regulations • No thanks or recognition • Not being informed about changes or involved in the change process • No commitment to professional development • No help from managers during crisis • Inadequate feedback about performance • Excessive workload negatively affecting quality and increasing stress for the nurse

Data from Burke, D., Flanagan, J., Ditomassi, M., & Hickey, P.A. (2017). Characteristics of nurse directors that contribute to registered nurse satisfaction. *J Nurs Adm, 47*(4), 219-225; Wieck, K. L., et al. (2009). What nurses want: the nurse incentives project. *Nurs Econ, 27*(3), 169-201; Hairr, D. C., Salisbury, H., Johannsson, M., & Redfern-Vance, N. (2014). Nurse staffing and the relationship to job satisfaction and retention. *Nurs Econ, 32*(3), 142-147; and Dotson, M. J., Dave, D. S., Cazier, J. A., & Spaulding, T. J. (2014). An empirical analysis of nurse retention: what keeps RNs in nursing? *J Nurs Adm, 44*(2), 111-116.

---

by input. For example, the number of nursing hours worked over a 24-hour period divided by the patient census is a standard productivity measurement used by many hospitals. From a practical perspective, the nurse caring for eight medical-surgical patients during one shift has a higher productivity ratio than the nurse caring for only five patients of similar acuity. Other examples of productivity measurements include number of home visits completed and number of procedures performed. Productivity is a method of measuring and tracking the amount of labor costs as compared with the amount of work produced and is a factor in staffing decisions.

Directing

Directing is the fourth management function. After managers have planned what to do, organized how to do it, and staffed positions to do the work, they must direct personnel and activities to accomplish goals. Directing involves issuing assignments and instructions that allow workers to clearly understand what is

expected, in addition to guiding and coaching workers to achieve planned goals. Directing requires the nurse to:
• Clearly communicate performance expectations.
• Create a motivating climate and team spirit.
• Model expected behaviors.
• Facilitate feedback.

Communicating Performance Expectations. It is the manager's responsibility to monitor how well staff are performing their jobs. The first step is to ensure that staff clearly understand job expectations. Consider the following:
• Does the staff member know what problems and issues should be reported to the supervisor and how and to whom to report?
• Does the staff member know how to perform clinical procedures correctly or how and where to seek help when necessary?
• Does the nurse clearly understand the expectations for documenting clinical care?

- Does the nurse know how and when to report to physicians and/or involve other members of the interprofessional team?
- Is the staff member able to meet patient care needs for the number of patients assigned during a typical shift?
- Does the nurse know how to communicate effectively with patients as well as family members?

These questions represent only a sample of issues that the nurse manager will consider when striving to communicate performance expectations.

Communicating performance expectations is an ongoing process that begins in new-employee orientation and continues throughout the term of employment. An important step in communicating expectations is to directly observe employees performing their jobs; through direct observation, the manager can identify strengths and weaknesses and determine areas where performance expectations need to be addressed. The next step is to communicate expectations in a respectful two-way process in which the manager seeks first to understand the staff member's perspective, feelings, and knowledge about the issue and then to clarify the expectations in a nonjudgmental, nonthreatening way. The final step is to determine issues that may be preventing the employee from meeting performance expectations and to work with that employee to develop a mutually agreed-upon plan so that he or she can achieve expectations.

Creating a Motivating Climate. Motivation is the inner drive that compels a person to act in a certain way. The amount and quality of work accomplished by a person are a direct reflection of his or her motivation. A great deal of research has been undertaken to better understand human motivation. Most researchers agree that motivation is complex and involves a combination of extrinsic, or external, rewards, such as money, benefits, and working conditions, in addition to intrinsic, or internal, needs for recognition, self-esteem, and self-actualization. Box 17.5 summarizes factors that influence nurses' job satisfaction and dissatisfaction.

Positive encouragement and support from the nurse manager are essential to create a motivating work climate. An effective method to demonstrate encouragement and support is a technique known as "management by walking around," in which the nurse manager literally walks around the unit with the primary purpose of interacting positively with the staff. Just as it implies, management by walking around allows the nurse manager to interact with many different staff on a day-to-day basis, promote quality patient care, and build positive relationships with not only staff but also patients, families, and the interprofessional team.

Positive reinforcement in the form of a sincere "Thank you, you did a good job" is one of the most powerful yet most often underused motivational resources available to the manager. To be effective, positive reinforcement should (1) be specific with praise given for a particular task done well or goal accomplished; (2) occur as close as possible to the time of the achievement; (3) be spontaneous and unpredictable (praise given routinely tends to lose its value); and (4) be given for a genuine accomplishment (Peters and Waterman, 1982). Management by walking around puts the manager in a position to observe the employee's work performance and offer immediate praise for a job well done.

Role Modeling. Positive role modeling is another effective tool the nurse can use to create a positive team spirit and promote high-quality patient care. Positive role modeling simply means that the nurse performs the job in such a way that he or she demonstrates ideal performance as a professional nurse, with the hope that others will follow the example. Obviously, nurses must be role models for excellence in patient care; similarly, nurses must also model caring and respectful relationships with the entire interprofessional health care team along with an enthusiastic attitude to promote camaraderie and team spirit.

Several other skills are essential as nurses function in the directing role, including effective communication and conflict management skills (see Chapter 19), delegation skills (see Chapter 20), and team-building skills (discussed in section "Team Builder").

Controlling

The purpose of controlling, the fifth management function, is to ensure that employees accomplish goals while maintaining a high quality of performance. Controlling requires the nurse to:

- Establish performance or outcome standards.
- Determine action plans to improve performance.
- Evaluate employee performance through performance appraisals and feedback.

Establishing Performance Standards. *Performance standards* describe a model of excellence for work activities and serve as the basis of comparison between actual and desired work performance. For example, performance standards in an ambulatory outpatient clinic might include that (1) every patient is informed about all laboratory results within 48 hours, whether normal or abnormal, and (2) all diabetic patients must remove their shoes and socks for a complete foot examination each time they come to the clinic. Nurses can draw on several resources for establishing performance standards, such as:

- Written organizational policies and procedures
- Standards for the practice of professional nursing developed by the ANA and published in *Nursing: Scope and Standards of Practice* (ANA, 2015a)
- Standards for professional nursing specialty practices, such as *Home Health Nursing: Scope and Standards of Practice* (ANA, 2014) and *Genetics/Genomics Nursing: Scope and Standards of Practice* (ANA, 2016).
- Evidence-based practice guidelines

Nurses should continually look for ways to improve individual, team, and organizational performance to achieve established standards of care. Chapter 22 provides more discussion about performance standards and presents an excellent process for measuring performance and planning for improvement.

Evaluating Employee Performance. Evaluating employee performance occurs through the formal annual evaluation process and through frequent feedback and coaching provided to employees. A manager should never wait until the annual performance review to discuss problems or deficiencies with a staff member. Consistent, ongoing feedback and coaching about job performance clarify expectations, improve the quality of work, and allow the manager to correct problems before they become serious. Feedback and coaching can occur in brief, spontaneous interactions or in planned sessions with the employee. Box 17.6 presents useful tips for effective coaching.

Ongoing documentation about an employee's job performance is an essential management responsibility. Each health care organization has specific policies related to documentation of employee performance and annual performance evaluations. The result of routine performance evaluations should be mutual goal setting designed to meet the employees' training, educational, and professional development needs.

Balancing the Five Management Functions

The management functions of planning, organizing, staffing, directing, and controlling provide the nurse with a practical set of skills to guide the implementation of management activities. The new nurse will be challenged to maintain the different stages of management that occur in the span of just one day. In addition to managing different phases of the process that are occurring simultaneously, the nurse also must function in many different management roles described in the following section.

BOX 17.6 Tips for Effective Coaching

- Discuss situations in a neutral way—avoid judgmental language that will put the other person on the defensive.
- Encourage the other person to provide his or her perspective about the situation (e.g., "What did you think about your exchange with Dr. Jones?").
- Encourage the person to reflect on his or her performance through open-ended questions, such as:
  - What are your main concerns?
  - What would you like to see happen next?
  - What can you learn from this situation?
  - What is confusing to you?
  - What are some things you could do differently next time?

- Be specific and provide clear examples when possible (e.g., "Next time you are dealing with a difficult family member, consider . . . ").
- Share your own experiences if they are relevant and might help.
- Be sincere. Provide coaching and feedback with the clear intent of helping the person improve.
- Be realistic. Focus on factors that the person can control.
- Thank the employee for listening.
- Ask for feedback from your coworkers, subordinates, and peers about your own performance, and listen when it is offered.

Data from Grensing-Pophal, L. (2000). Give-and-take feedback, *Nurs Manage, 31*(2), 27-28; and Harvard Business Essentials. (2000). *Manager's toolkit: the 13 skills managers need to succeed*, Boston: Harvard Business School Press.

ROLES OF THE NURSE LEADER AND MANAGER

Nurses assume various roles as they function in leadership and management positions. The first step to being an effective nurse leader is to clearly understand the job description, roles and responsibilities, and policies and procedures related to the position in which the nurse is employed or assigned. The following discussion presents information about roles that a nurse will assume in any position.

Patient Satisfaction and Customer Service Provider

Over the past few years, patient satisfaction has moved to the forefront of the nurse's agenda. Nursing shortages, reduced length of stay, more complex patient needs, and national concerns about the quality and safety of patient care have contributed to this growing concern about patient satisfaction. With the advent of health care reform, patient satisfaction is now tied directly to financial rewards for hospitals. Medicare reimbursement rewards inpatient hospitals for providing quality care to include patient satisfaction based on the hospital's scores on the Hospital Consumer Assessment of Healthcare Providers and Systems (HSAHPS), a standardized patient satisfaction survey that addresses these seven core dimensions:

- Communication with nurses
- Communication with doctors
- Responsiveness of hospital staff
- Pain management
- Communication about medicines
- Cleanliness and quietness of hospital environment
- Discharge information

From how quickly call lights are answered to the extent of family support provided, nurses are challenged to meet a wide spectrum of patient needs to include promoting good communication with the health care team and the patient and family. The complex health care environment has created a competitive marketplace in which home health agencies, hospitals, ambulatory clinics, and even hospice agencies compete for patients. To survive and thrive in this competitive environment, the nurse must keep patient satisfaction and customer service, which include safety and quality care, first and foremost as the motivator of all plans and activities.

Team Builder

A *team* is a group of people organized to accomplish the necessary work of an organization. Teams bring together a range of people with different knowledge, skills, and experiences to meet customer needs, accomplish tasks, and solve problems. Team members may be unit secretaries, nursing assistants, social workers, dietitians, therapists, physicians, licensed vocational or practical nurses, and RNs. A team should have clearly defined goals and should be empowered to make decisions within its realm of responsibility. Team building should create *synergy* (the ability of a group of people working together to accomplish significantly more than each person working individually).

Bringing people together to work as a group does not necessarily make them a team. To create synergy, teams must have defined goals and objectives, a commitment to work together, good communication, and a willingness to cooperate. Team members should be encouraged to communicate with one another to identify effective work division and solutions to problems so that synergy is accomplished. The nurse, as team builder, must serve as a role model to encourage and help develop team principles of respect, cooperation, commitment, and a willingness to accomplish shared goals. As a role model for team members, the nurse should:

- Show respect for all members of the team and value their input.
- Clearly define team goals ("What do we want to accomplish?").
- Clearly establish the decision-making authority within the realm of the team.
- Encourage team members to develop a sense of stewardship (or ownership) for the success of the team.
- Exhibit a personal commitment to team goals.
- Encourage team members to willingly help one another.
- Provide the resources necessary to accomplish goals (e.g., time for team meetings, information, supplies).
- Teach members to exchange constructive feedback for the purpose of meeting team goals.
- Provide relevant and timely feedback to the team.

The leader's behaviors have a significant effect on the behaviors of the team. The nurse as leader must have an astute self-awareness of his or her own emotional patterns and an understanding that negative moods can have a negative influence on relationships with staff members. Learning to recognize and manage one's emotional patterns and negative moods is an important step in team building. The nurse who is enthusiastic, caring, and supportive can generate those same feelings among all team members, which will carry over to patient care.

Resource Manager

Resources include the personnel, time, and supplies needed to provide patient care and operate the organization. Resources cost money and are always in limited supply. Unfortunately, no health care organization can afford the luxury of an unlimited number of staff or supplies to accomplish the required work. With health care facilities' focus on cost containment, it is essential that nurses develop an understanding of and expertise in resource management.

Each of the management activities—planning, organizing, staffing, directing, and controlling—comes into play in the role of resource manager. The nurse needs to learn and develop skills in the following areas:

- Planning for the necessary resources (primarily staff and supplies) to manage the unit
- Organizing the resources to meet identified goals
- Staffing appropriately as determined by patient needs and the budget plan
- Directing to maintain resource allocations within budgetary guidelines
- Controlling by analyzing financial reports and making adjustments where necessary

Budget and financial reports are the primary tools for resource management. Because budget and financial management is a very minimal part of the nursing school curriculum, nurses must take initiative for on-the-job training about the organization's budget and financial management processes. Nurses are encouraged not to be unsettled by financial and budget reports and conversations and, instead, to get involved. They should not be afraid to say "I don't understand. Please explain." Nurses should review budget and financial reports, ask questions, talk to seasoned nurse managers, talk to the organization's finance department staff, and even consider taking an accounting or finance course at the local college. Understanding financial and budget management is one of the most useful and powerful tools one can have as a nurse leader. Another resource is Chapter 18 of this text, which provides more detailed information about budgets.

Decision Maker and Problem Solver

Problem solving and decision making are essential skills for professional nursing practice. Not only are these skills required in clinical patient care, they also are vital components of effective leadership and management. The nurse leader is continually engaged in decision making and problem solving while managing the work unit.

Nursing Process as a Guide for Decision Making and Problem Solving.
The nursing process, familiar to nurses for addressing patient care needs, can be applied to all management activities requiring decision making and problem solving. The nursing process as a problem-solving process, using assessment, analysis and diagnosis, planning, implementation, and evaluation, has proved effective in managing the complex decisions required in nursing practice.

Assessment. During the assessment stage, it is important for the nurse to separate the problem from the symptom by gathering information about the problem or situation. It often is appropriate to involve others—especially those close to the situation—who may be able to provide a different viewpoint or information the manager lacks. For example, the nurse manager who is concerned about increasingly high absenteeism among the staff needs to investigate the situation carefully. What is causing the absenteeism? Are there problems on the unit creating an unhappy work environment? Are several staff members coincidentally having personal problems? Are absentee policies being unfairly administered? The nurse manager must correctly assess and diagnose the problem before developing solutions.

Analysis and diagnosis. During the analysis stage, the decision maker uses information gathered in the assessment phase to identify the specific problem to be solved. At this stage, the manager must also decide whether the situation is important enough to require intervention and whether it is within his or her authority to intervene.

Planning. During the planning stage, the goal is to identify as many options as possible and then objectively weigh the options as to possible risks and consequences and positive and negative outcomes, including patient outcomes and staff satisfaction as key considerations. The decision maker should be flexible, creative, and open to suggestions from other staff and peers when reviewing options. Preconceived ideas and rigid thinking, such as "there is only one way to do this job" or "that's the way we have always done it," should be avoided. It is also important to remember that decisions made with input from those who will be affected by the decision are more likely to result in positive outcomes. Cost, quality, and legal and ethical aspects of care should also be carefully considered.

Implementation. The implementation stage should include effective communication, delegation, and supervision. (See "Stages of Change" presented later in this chapter.) It is important for the nurse to show positive support for the decision outcome and to encourage cooperation and support among all staff. Persons higher in the organizational structure may mandate some decisions, and although not able to control that decision, the nurse can influence a positive outcome.

Evaluation. The evaluation stage is necessary to ensure that the implemented plan effectively resolved the problem or the decision situation. Considerable time and energy may be spent on identifying the problem, generating possible options, and selecting and implementing the best solution. However, time for follow-up evaluation must also be allocated. It is important to establish early (during the planning stage) how and what evaluation and monitoring will take place, who will be responsible, and when it will be accomplished.

Resources for Decision Making and Problem Solving. Staff input should be included in each stage of the decision-making problem-solving process. Additionally, the nurse might seek help from others who are more experienced and knowledgeable in specific areas. Even the most experienced nurses will not be able to effectively solve every problem, nor will any nurse have all the answers. The key is to understand and incorporate the decision-making problem-solving process into all activities; know when and how to access resources; and to learn and improve as successes and failures are experienced.

Change Agent

This text frequently has referred to the changing health care environment, and true to that concept, change is an inevitable occurrence in health care. Whether working with individuals, groups, or the entire organization, the professional nurse is certain to be involved in managing change. The nurse as the change agent is responsible for guiding people through the change process. To successfully engage in change, the nurse must first be willing to

confront the demand for change; staff cannot be expected to embrace change if their nurse leader has not done so.

People often feel threatened by change and may react, especially at first, with resistance and hostility. Change that is carefully planned and implemented slowly with all people continually informed and involved will be more successful in reaching the desired outcome (or change). Change often creates a wide range of feelings among staff and managers, including fear, achievement, loss, pride, stress, and dissatisfaction. The successful change agent understands the very real nature of these emotions and manages the change process such that all involved experience at least some degree of success and pride in the outcome.

In his classic work on change, Lewin (1951) identified the following rules that should be followed when change is necessary:

1. Change should be implemented only for good reason.
2. Change should always be planned and implemented gradually.
3. Change should never be unexpected or abrupt.
4. All people who may be affected by the change should be involved in planning for the change.

Change may be indicated for several reasons, such as solving an identified problem, implementing a new program, improving work efficiencies, and adjusting to new mandates from regulatory agencies. Even though a strong reason for change may exist, it almost always is met with some resistance. Resistance is demonstrated by refusal to cooperate with a course of action or by active opposition to the change. The effective change agent recognizes that resistance is a natural response to change and does not waste time or energy attempting to eliminate it. Instead, the effective change agent identifies and implements effective change strategies to overcome resistance.

Stages of Change. Effective change strategies can be developed through the three classic stages of change identified by Lewin (1951). These stages are:

1. *Unfreezing stage*—The change agent promotes problem identification and encourages the awareness of the need for change. People must believe that improvement is possible before they are willing to consider change. The change agent's responsibilities are to:
    - Gather information about the problem.
    - Accurately assess the problem.

- Decide whether change is necessary.
- Make others aware of the need for change.

2. *Moving stage*—The change agent clarifies the need to change, explores alternatives, defines goals and objectives, plans the change, and implements the change plan. The change agent's responsibilities are to:
   - Identify areas of support and resistance.
   - Set goals and objectives.
   - Include everyone affected in the planning.
   - Develop an appropriate change plan with target dates.
   - Implement the change plan.
   - Be available to help, support, and encourage others through the process.
   - Evaluate the change and make modifications if necessary.

3. *Refreezing stage*—The change agent integrates the change into the organization so that it becomes recognized as the status quo. If the refreezing stage is not completed, people may drift into old behaviors. The change agent's responsibilities are to:
   - Require compliance with the changed processes.
   - Find ways to engage the staff to support the change.
   - Adopt new policies that may be required to support the change.
   - Support and encourage others until the change is viewed no longer as new but as part of the status quo and is well integrated into daily work.

In alignment with Lewin's (1951) three stages of change (i.e., unfreezing, moving, and refreezing), involvement and education are key to successful change.

Involvement. The importance of involving all individuals, groups, or departments affected by the change cannot be overstated. Involvement consists of clear, two-way communication and a concerted effort to garner information and feedback from all affected parties about the need for change. The effective change agent understands that a change in one area almost always affects another group or department (remember systems theory?).

Education and Training. Education and training also are important components of effective change. People must have appropriate education and training to understand and comply with new policies, procedures, work processes, duties, or responsibilities. Early in the change process, the change agent must consider the training needs of all individuals, groups, and departments. Education and training can reduce fear of the unknown and allow the staff to feel prepared and comfortable with taking on new or different responsibilities.

Clinical Consultant

Staff members look to the nurse leader as a resource for clinical advice. For example, the nurse leader is frequently called on to assess difficult or unusual patient cases and guide the staff nurse to make appropriate nursing judgments. In this role, the nurse serves as a role model for excellence in nursing care and clinical judgment and provides ongoing training and education.

Staff Developer

The nurse should be ever mindful of the need for learning and training opportunities to enhance professional and personal growth for all employees he or she supervises as well as for himself or herself. Accessing resources and planning staff development activities that meet the needs of individual staff members, including RNs, LPNs or LVNs, nursing assistants, and clerical staff, is a very important role for the nurse.

Mentor

As the nurse develops into an effective leader, he or she should accept the responsibility to act as a mentor to new nurses, helping them develop effective leadership and management skills. Mentorship is key to developing our future nurse leaders and managers.

Corporate Supporter

The nurse, as a corporate supporter, has a responsibility to embrace the mission, goals, and objectives of the employing organization. In this role as corporate supporter, the nurse is a professional representative for the organization and is committed to supporting and accomplishing organizational goals.

CREATING A CARING AND RESPECTFUL ENVIRONMENT

Perhaps the most important responsibility for the nurse is to create an environment of caring—for patients, families, and other staff members. Staff members who work in an environment in which they feel respected and cared for are able to pass that feeling of caring on to their patients and colleagues. Caring for the staff members can be demonstrated by:

- Offering sincere positive recognition for both individuals and teams.
- Praising and giving thanks for a job well done.
- Spending time with staff members to reinforce positive work behaviors.
- Meeting the staff members' personal needs whenever possible, such as accommodating scheduling needs for family events.
- Providing guidance and support for professional and personal growth.
- Maintaining a positive, confident attitude and a pleasant work environment.

Staff members who feel that their work is valued and they are respected and cared about as individuals are able to further contribute to a positive, caring environment in which to provide excellent patient care. Creating a caring environment in the highly technical, fast-paced, and extremely stressful settings in which nurses work can be a significant challenge. However, it is a challenge that is at the heart of nursing if we are to promote the very best in patient care.

Addressing and Preventing Bullying and Incivility

Unfortunately in today's workplace, disruptive behaviors, also referred to as bullying, lateral violence, or incivility, are all too common among nurses, physicians, managers, and others. Bullying is defined as the "repeated, unreasonable actions of individuals directed toward an employee (or employees) which are intended to intimidate, degrade, humiliate or undermine; or which create a risk to the health or safety of the employees" (Washington State Department of Labor and Industries [WSDLI], 2011). Examples of bullying behaviors are unwarranted or invalid criticism, unjustified blame, profane or disrespectful language, being gossiped about or being the target of rumors, being yelled or shouted at in a hostile way, being sworn at or verbally abused, being assigned undesirable work differently from the rest of your colleagues, and being "put down" or humiliated in front of others (WSDLI, 2011). Incivility may be considered a milder form of bullying and, according to the ANA (2015b), "may take the form of rude and discourteous actions, of gossiping and spreading rumors, and of refusing to assist a coworker." Incivility is considered a precursor of bullying. These unacceptable behaviors may occur among coworkers or may come from the manager against the employee or from other members of the health care team.

The negative effects of bullying and incivility are significant. Nurses who are victims may have problems with their physical health (e.g., sleep disturbances, depression, musculoskeletal problems) and experience feelings of self-blame, reduced self-esteem, and work withdrawal (WSDLI, 2011). The extreme result of bullying for nurses is that they may leave the profession completely. Bullying causes distress and low morale among other staff, results in lower productivity and higher costs for the organization, and may also lead to concerns about patient safety and quality of care.

Nurses must provide the leadership to *STOP* bullying in the workplace. Nurses, especially new nurses, must understand that under no circumstances should bullying behaviors be tolerated. Managers have the ultimate responsibility to ensure that such behaviors will not be tolerated and will be immediately addressed and stopped. Following are some important steps to address bullying from an individual level (WSDLI, 2011):

- Recognize that bullying is occurring.
- Realize that the victim is *not* the source of the problem.
- Recognize that bullying is about control and has nothing to do with the victim's performance.
- Keep a record of the nature of the bullying (dates, times, places, what was said or done and who was present).
- Know and follow the organization's policy on bullying and incivility in the workplace.

Each nurse must strive to establish healthy interpersonal relationships with his or her colleagues and all members of the health care team and must demonstrate professional, caring communication to continually reinforce civility and a respectful work environment (ANA, 2015b).

Actions that employers can take to prevent bullying include (1) implement and enforce zero-tolerance anti-bullying policies; (2) have training in place to ensure everyone is aware of what bullying is and how it must be reported; and (3) create culture of respect and an expectation of professional demeanor for all. The reader is encouraged to learn more about bullying from articles in nursing journals and ANA's Position Statement, *Incivility, Bullying and Workplace Violence*, available on the ANA website (http://www.nursingworld.org).

SUMMARY

In every area of health care, the professional nurse is expected to provide leadership and management expertise to help manage complex and ever-changing health care organizations. The multifaceted set of theories, functions, roles, and skills presented in this chapter may at first seem overwhelming to the novice nurse. However, by learning and understanding the principles and concepts involved, the graduate nurse can become a successful nurse leader and manager.

Leadership, management, and organizational theories provide a framework on which to build effective nursing management practices. Although there is no one "best" leadership theory, professional nurses should maintain an awareness of their own behavior and how the key elements of the leadership situation influence outcomes.

The management functions planning, organizing, staffing, directing, and controlling provide the nurse with a defined, practical set of skills to guide management activities. Professional nurses can apply these management functions to perform effectively in various management roles, including customer service provider, team builder, resource manager, change agent, clinical consultant, staff developer, mentor, and corporate supporter.

Developing effective leadership and management skills is an ongoing process that continues throughout one's career as a professional nurse. Nurses in management positions should routinely analyze personal strengths and weaknesses in each of these management roles and identify areas in which learning and development are needed. Box 17.7 provides resources for individual assessments of leadership styles. Modeling effective nurse managers and reading relevant professional journal articles and books can increase leadership and management knowledge and skills. Management and leadership roles are challenging and exciting and present a wonderful opportunity to grow professionally and personally.

BOX 17.7 Resources for Individual Leadership Assessments

Consider the following excellent resources for conducting personal leadership assessments and identifying opportunities to build personal leadership skills:
- *The Leadership Challenge with LPI: Leadership Practice Inventory,* by James M. Kouzes and Barry Z. Posners (publisher Jossey-Bass)
- *Strength Finders 2.0,* by Tom Rath with access code for online assessment (publisher Gallup Press)
- *The New Leadership Challenge: Creating the Future of Nursing,* with online leadership assessments, by Sheila C. Grossman & Theresa M. Valiga. (publisher FA Davis)

REFERENCES

American Nurses Association. (2014). *Home health nursing: Scope and standards of practice* (2nd ed.). Washington, DC: American Nurses Association.

American Nurses Association. (2015a). *Nursing: Scope and standards of practice* (3rd ed.). Washington, DC: American Nurses Association.

American Nurses Association. (2015b). *Position Statement: Incivility, Bullying and Workplace Violence.* Retrieved from http://www.nursingworld.org/DocumentVault/Position-Statements/Practice/Position-Statement-on-Incivility-Bullying-and-Workplace-Violence.pdf.

American Nurses Association. (2016). *Genetics/genomics nursing: Scope and standards of practice* (2nd ed.). Washington, DC: American Nurses Association.

Bass, B. M., Avolio, B. J., & Goodheim, L. (1987). Biography and the assessment of transformational leadership at the world-class level. *Journal of Management, 13*(1), 7–19.

Bormann, L., & Abrahamson, K. (2014). Do staff nurse perceptions of nurse leadership behaviors influence staff nurse job satisfaction? The case of a hospital applying for Magnet® designation. *The Journal of Nursing Administration, 44*(4), 219–225.

Burke, D., Flanagan, J., Ditomassi, M., & Hickey, P. A. (2017). Characteristics of nurse directors that contribute to registered nurse satisfaction. *The Journal of Nursing Administration, 47*(4), 219–225.

Burns, J. (1978). *Leadership.* New York: Harper & Row.

Dotson, M. J., Dave, D. S., Cazier, J. A., & Spaulding, T. J. (2014). An empirical analysis of nurse retention: what keeps RNs in nursing? *The Journal of Nursing Administration, 44*(2), 111–116.

Grensing-Pophal, L. (2000). Give-and-take feedback. *Nursing Management, 31*(2), 27–28.

Harvard Business Essentials. (2004). *Manager's toolkit: The 13 skills managers need to succeed.* Boston: Harvard Business School Press.

Hairr, D. C., Salisbury, H., Johannsson, M., & Redfern-Vance, N. (2014). Nurse staffing and the relationship to job satisfaction and retention. *Nursing economic$, 32*(3), 142–147.

Hersey, P., & Blanchard, K. (1988). *Management of organizational behavior: Utilizing human resources* (4th ed.). Englewood Cliffs, NJ: Prentice-Hall.

Hersey, P., Blanchard, K. H., & Natemeyer, W. E. (1979). Situational leadership, perception and impact of power. *Group & Organization Management, 4*(4), 418–428.

Lewin, K. (1951). *Field theory in social sciences.* New York: Harper & Row.

Marquis, B. L., & Huston, C. J. (2017). *Leadership roles and management functions in nursing* (9th ed.). Philadelphia: Wolters Kluwer/Lippincott.

McGuire, E. (1999). Chaos theory: learning a new science. *The Journal of Nursing Administration, 29*(2), 8–9.

Peters, T., & Waterman, R. H. (1982). *In search of excellence.* New York: Harper & Row.

Stogdill, R. M. (1974). *Handbook of leadership: A survey of theory and research.* New York: The Free Press.

Thompson, J. D. (1967). *Organizations in action.* New York: McGraw-Hill.

Washington State Department of Labor and Industries. (2011). *Workplace bullying and disruptive behavior: What everyone needs to know.* Retrieved from http://www.lni.wa.gov/safety/research/files/bullying.pdf.

White, R. K., & Lippit, R. (1960). *Autocracy and democracy: An experimental inquiry.* New York: Harper & Row.

18

Budgeting Basics for Nurses

Barbara Cherry, DNSc, MBA, RN, NEA-BC

The budget serves as the financial guideline that enables the clinical team to provide quality patient care.

Ⓔ Additional resources are available online at: *http://evolve.elsevier.com/Cherry/*

LEARNING OUTCOMES

After studying this chapter, the reader will be able to:

1. Understand the basic terminology of budgeting in the health care industry.
2. Contribute to the budget development process for a nursing or clinical department.
3. Contribute to the capital budget development process for a nursing or clinical department.
4. Explain aspects of monitoring financial performance against an operational budget.
5. Understand the overall contributions nurses can make in a health care organization's budget process.

KEY TERMS

Budget Financial plan for the allocation of the organization's funds and a control for ensuring that results comply with the plan.

Budget assumptions Statements that reflect issues affecting the future performance of the organization; used as the framework for developing the budget; budget assumptions address questions such as the following: Are supply prices likely to increase or decrease? What salary range will ensure that the organization is able to recruit and retain quality employees? What are the competitors offering in terms of new services? Is the patient census likely to increase or decrease over the next year?

Capital expenditures Amount spent on items that will have long-term (greater than 1 year) value to an organization; typically includes buildings and equipment.

Expense An event or item that requires the outlay of money for purchase or the incurrence of an obligation for future payment; major expenses for health care organizations include employee salaries, medical supplies and equipment, and facility maintenance.

Fiscal year A 12-month period used for calculating annual (yearly) financial reports in business; the fiscal year does not have to constitute the calendar year (January to December) but may be any 12-month period (e.g., August through July) established and maintained consistently by the business.

Full-time equivalent (FTE) The number of hours worked or paid that is equal to that expected of a full-time employee working a 40-hour workweek; annual work hours for 1 FTE equal 2080 hours, and monthly work hours equal 173.33 hours. One FTE position may be occupied by one employee working full time or shared by two or more employees working part time.

Incremental budgeting An approach to budget development that extrapolates from the prior period's budget and adjusts for future growth or decline in revenues or expenses to determine the budget for the next period.

Revenue Money that a health care organization receives in exchange for providing health care or other related services through normal business activities; synonymous with income.

Salaries, wages, and benefits (SWB) Budget category that typically includes direct payment for hours worked, bonuses, accrued paid-time-off, health benefits, employer portion of payroll taxes, and workers' compensation.

Supplies Materials used in performing tasks within the organization; typically include clinical disposables, pharmaceuticals, and office supplies.

Variance The difference between the planned budget and the actual results.

Variance analysis The process of analyzing the differences in the planned budget results and the actual results; involves quantitative and qualitative analysis.

Zero-based budgeting An approach to budget development that begins as though the budget were being prepared for the first time.

PROFESSIONAL/ETHICAL ISSUE

Claire Ramsey, RN, works in the critical care unit of a large academic medical center. A new staffing policy for the hospital has been implemented and requires that either nurses are sent home or their shifts are cancelled in advance if the patient census is low. The nurse must either take paid time off to receive pay for the cancelled shift or can choose not to be paid for the cancelled shift. One of Claire's colleagues, Jonathan, is very vocal about his dislike of this policy and expresses to others that the hospital is "cheating" the nurses by cancelling shifts; he often remarks how unfair management is because, as he points out, the managers' shifts are never cancelled, and the hospital has "plenty of money" regardless of the number of patients on the unit. Claire is becoming uncomfortable with Jonathan's discussions because they seem to be leading to low morale and dissatisfaction among some of the nurses. She really likes her job and does not want to see the unit morale deteriorate over a policy that she herself does not understand and that she believes is not well understood by many other nurses, including Jonathan.

- Discuss the reasons from a budgeting perspective that the shift cancellation policy was implemented for this hospital.
- What steps can Claire take to help herself and her colleagues learn more about the staffing policy and why it was implemented?
- How should Claire respond to Jonathan when he begins to vocalize his objections about the policy to her?

VIGNETTE

Justine Scott, RN, sat in the staff meeting being led by the nurse manager for the cardiac telemetry unit where she has worked for the last 6 months since graduating from nursing school. As Justine listened to the nurse manager discuss the unit's budget, she felt as if she were hearing a foreign language. The nurse manager discussed "variances for labor and supply costs that were most likely due to increased patient acuity and patient census above budgeted levels." The nurse manager explained the importance of accurately identifying reasons for the budget variances to ensure appropriate resources are allocated to their unit to support quality patient care. The nurse manager then requested input from the staff nurses regarding their observations about supply usage and overtime costs and how they might be better controlled. In the final topic for the staff meeting, the nurse manager requested input from the staff on "equipment needs to be considered as the unit's capital budget request is developed." As a new nurse, Justine noticed that staff meetings seemed to center more on discussions regarding the "budget" than on clinical issues. She realized that the budget must be extremely important to support patient care and resolved to learn more about budgets, the financial terminology used by her nurse manager, and what she could do as a staff nurse to support the nurse manager in this seemingly important area of nursing practice.

Questions to Consider While Reading this Chapter:

1. Who should be concerned about unit or departmental budgets?

2. What is the primary purpose of developing a unit or departmental budget?
3. How can nurses and nurse managers improve clinical care with better budgeting skills?
4. What resources are available to help nurses learn more about budgets in the health care setting?

CHAPTER OVERVIEW

The budget serves as the financial guideline that enables a health care organization to achieve its goal of providing high-quality patient care services. Just as nurses learn about clinical guidelines for the care of patients with various diseases, it is also essential that nurses have a working knowledge of the guidelines that ensure that the organization is able to operate in a stable financial environment through effective budget management. As nurses advance into management positions, they may have financial responsibility for a business unit and must be competent to serve as the bridge between the clinical setting and financial managers who have no clinical background. Additionally, the focus on cost and quality initiatives in today's health care settings requires that even staff nurses have a basic understanding of the budget. "The education and evolution of nurses as business managers is critical to building a strong RN workforce" (Talley et al, 2013). This chapter introduces the basic concepts of budgeting in health care organizations; for a deeper understanding of budgeting, nurses are encouraged to continue to build their knowledge by using a health care finance text and/or other resources noted on the Evolve site.

WHAT IS BUDGETING?

As a nursing student, you are probably more aware of budget concepts than you realize. When you decided to become a registered nurse (RN), you had a goal to graduate from nursing school within a specified time period. You had to make a budget plan by predicting your expenses for that period, such as tuition, books, and living expenses. You also predicted your revenue from sources such as student loans, part-time jobs, savings, and parental and spousal support. After predicting your expenses and your revenues, you most likely planned your budget for how much you could spend on a weekly or monthly basis during this time and eventually achieve your goal of graduating from nursing school. Similarly, health care organizations develop budgets for a specified period by determining what goals they want to achieve, predicting expenses and revenues, then planning the annual budget and monitoring it on a monthly basis. For example, a hospital may plan its annual budget to maintain staffing and supplies to operate its current number of beds, provide a raise for all staff, and open a new outpatient surgical center.

Basically the health care organization's budget is a document that details how financial resources will be allocated to ensure that the organization is able to conduct its daily business and achieve strategic goals. The budget itemizes the organization's predicted expenses and expected revenues for a given period of time. More important, budgets require ongoing attention to ensure that the organization's financial needs are met. Just as nursing students most likely have to make decisions to adjust their budgets during nursing school to meet unexpected changes in revenues or expenses, the health care organization invariably experiences the same challenges during the year. Thus the budget becomes a dynamic action plan that guides the allocation of resources and expenditures and influences the nurse manager's decision making on a day-to-day, week-to-week, or month-to-month basis.

Budgets perform four basic functions to make certain the organization can achieve its strategic goals and permit continued operations from an economic point of view. The four budgeting functions are: (1) planning, (2) coordinating and communicating, (3) monitoring progress, and (4) evaluating performance. The following sections describe each of these budget functions.

Planning

Planning is the most important function of the budgeting process. During the planning phase, managers first decide on the goals to achieve for a specified period and identify resources (e.g., staff, supplies, equipment) needed to achieve those goals. Next, they predict revenues and expenses based on those goals and develop budget assumptions to use in planning the budget. Budget assumptions allow the managers to answer various questions that will have an effect on the budget, such as the following:

- What should nursing salaries be in the coming year to reward and retain nurses, and to remain competitive with other health care organizations in the area?
- How will new services being offered by other health care organizations in the area affect our organization?

Budgets are most often developed for a 1-year period on the basis of predicted amounts of services. For example, hospitals predict patient census for the coming year and then allocate funds for nursing salaries based on the predicted census.

Consider the following example: The hospital management team has decided to establish a chest pain center as part of the emergency department (ED). In planning the annual budget for the ED and its new chest pain center, the managers have developed the following assumptions:

- The chest pain center will see 12 patients every 24 hours. Of the 12 patients, 75% of the daily census (8 patients) are patients directed from the current ED census, and 25% (4 patients) are patients new to this hospital.
- Four beds will be dedicated to the chest pain center and will require remodeling of an underused section of the current ED.
- The chest pain center will be staffed with RNs dedicated to the center.

The management team has planned to include the following expenses in the annual budget for the new chest pain center: salaries for nurses and support staff, supplies, monitoring equipment, equipment maintenance, funds for marketing the new program, and funds to remodel an area in the current ED for the program. Managers also need to think about the other areas that will be affected by the new chest pain center, such as the cardiac catheterization suite, echocardiography resources, laboratory, electrocardiography resources, and materials management, which all deserve budgetary consideration as a result of the wide-reaching effect of this seemingly small service expansion.

Historically, nursing has had limited input into fiscal (or financial) planning and development of the organization's budget. Administrators with no clinical background and little understanding of nursing values, beliefs, and care requirements traditionally made decisions about resource allocations related to nursing. Today, participating in the budget process to determine resource allocation is a fundamental responsibility of nurse leaders. Involving staff nurses in the budget planning is also highly recommended. Managers and staff who participate in budget planning are more likely to be cost-conscious and to appreciate how their unit should function to meet the overall financial goals.

Coordinating and Communicating

Although not commonly associated with budgets, coordination and communication are very important functions of budgeting. The budget process, by necessity, requires that many different groups within an organization come together to discuss the resources necessary to accomplish the goals of a business unit. Therefore, one can think of the budget process as the best opportunity to discuss concerns about resource allocation with the organization's leaders, who are capable of resolving issues.

Consider the new chest pain center described earlier. To plan how the center will establish itself as a center of excellence for emergency care of patients with chest pain, many groups must coordinate and communicate to ensure success for the new business unit:

- Nurses and physicians with experience in caring for patients with chest pain offer input about equipment and supply needs, room layout and design, staffing models, electronic health record needs, and support staff;
- Financial managers offer input about reimbursement rates and other financial considerations related to caring for this population;
- Marketing professionals offer input about how the program can be advertised to inform the community about the new service.
- Hospital administrators and department managers offer input as to how this new center will affect other areas of business both inside and outside the hospital.

Monitoring Progress

Monitoring progress is one of the most vital functions of the budget—and the function that the nurse manager is most involved with on a daily basis. It is through the comparison of actual financial performance against expected, or budgeted, performance that an organization measures the effectiveness of its budget. Ongoing monitoring of the budget allows timely corrective action or, if the budget plan is right on target, the knowledge that no adjustments are required.

Consider the chest pain center again. The budget was developed on an anticipated volume of 12 patients every 24 hours, and staffing was implemented to serve this volume of patients. At the end of its first month of operation, the nurse manager reviews the budget information and sees that the actual patient volume is averaging only 8 patients per 24 hours, and the associated revenue for the center is approximately 70% of the planned revenue. The nurse manager has several issues to consider: Does staffing need to be reduced to better reflect the number of patients being treated by the center? Are the patients being seen of higher acuity (i.e., sicker) and thus require a higher intensity of nursing care? Is the low volume a reflection of the newness of the program, which is not yet widely appreciated in the community, and so as its reputation grows, will the volume also grow? If no immediate changes are made, how will the reduced revenue affect the financial status of the center? Fortunately, the nurse manager can consult others involved in developing the budget to address these important issues and make decisions to ensure the success of the center.

The difference between the planned budget and the actual results is called a *variance*. A **variance** is favorable when the results are better than expected, and unfavorable when the results are worse than expected. The lower than planned revenue in the chest pain center is an example of an unfavorable variance. *Variance analysis,* the process by which deviations from budgeted amounts are examined, is discussed in more detail later in the chapter.

Evaluating Performance

Budget results can also be used as part of the manager's performance evaluation, including the staff bonus structure for some health care organizations. Evaluating the manager's performance on the basis of budget results is becoming more widely used because of the

growing trend toward accountability and compliance in the business world. By looking at the budget results for a given period, an evaluator can determine the manager's overall success in achieving goals. Nurse managers are frequently evaluated according to their effectiveness in managing nursing overtime costs and supply use, both of which are reflected in the nursing unit's budget. Performance evaluations based on budget results can motivate managers to effectively control budgets and will serve as a basis for salary decisions and career advancement for these managers. Even though a manager is the captain of the unit and is ultimately accountable for the unit's budgetary performance, a lack of staff ownership of and involvement in the unit's operation usually leads to problems for the manager.

TYPES OF BUDGETS

The three types of budgets for which a nurse manager typically has responsibility are operational, labor, and capital budgets. The components of these budgets are presented in Box 18.1 and are discussed in more detail in the following sections.

Operational Budget

The operational, or operating, budget represents revenues and expenses for an operational unit, such as a product line, unit, department, or overall organization. The chest pain center previously discussed is considered a product line; an example of a nursing unit is the intensive care

BOX 18.1	Three Types of Budgets
Operating budget	Allocates funds for daily expenses, such as salaries, utilities, repairs, maintenance, and patient care supplies
Labor budget	A subset of the operating budget; allocates funds for salaries, overtime, benefits, and staff development and training
Capital budget	Allocates funds for construction projects and/or long-life medical equipment, such as cardiac monitors, defibrillators, and computer hardware

BOX 18.2   Examples of Typical Expenses and Revenues for a Health Care Organization

Expenses	Revenues (Payments From)
• Salaries	• Medicare
• Benefits (paid time off; health insurance)	• Medicaid
• Patient care supplies	• Private insurance
• Overhead expenses	• Individuals (self-pay)
• Utilities	• Grants
• Administrative costs	• Charitable or philanthropic donations
• Maintenance	
• Housekeeping	

unit or medical-surgical unit; an example of a department is dietary or human resources. The expenses in the operational budget are those necessary to operate on a daily basis (i.e., salaries and supplies), and the revenues are those paid to the organization from various payer sources (Box 18.2). (See Chapter 7 for more information about sources of payments for health care services.)

Labor Budget

The labor budget is a subset of the operational budget. Its purpose is to provide detailed documentation of salaries, wages, and benefits with respect to the operational unit. Factors that affect the personnel budget include salary rates, overtime, benefits (e.g., paid time off, health insurance), staff development and training, and employee turnover. The labor budget is virtually always the largest expense item in an operational budget for a health care organization because salaries for nurses, other professional staff (pharmacists, physical therapists, etc.) and support staff (e.g., nursing assistants, unit secretaries, transportation staff) compose the greatest percentage of expenses in the budget. The labor budget is also used to provide managers with a *productivity metric,* which is the amount of work produced (i.e., hours of nursing care per patient-day) by a specific amount of input or resources (i.e., nursing hours worked).

The productivity metric is necessary to give managers a measurement of the number of nursing hours worked in comparison with the amount of patient care provided. Low productivity (high nursing hours worked with low patient census) is not desirable

because it means higher staff salaries combined with lower revenues for patient care services. High productivity (high patient census with low nursing hours) means that there are fewer staff to take care of more patients, so the unit may not be able to provide safe, quality patient care. Most health care organizations have a recommended productivity measure that allows for a balance between financial efficiency and quality and safety of patient care. To achieve this balance, nurses must be at the table during budget planning to ensure that the patient quality and safety are discussed along with productivity and financial efficiency.

One of the primary difficulties encountered in managing the labor budget is accurately predicting future staffing needs. Because budgets are based on a predicted amount of services (i.e., patient census), variances between actual staffing levels and budget levels occur if the facility experiences an unanticipated increase or decrease in patient services. Another concern related to the budget and labor expense is balancing the patient acuity, or degree of patient illness, with the nurse-to-patient ratio.

An important aspect of labor budgeting is understanding the 12-month historical trend for labor hours and patient-days. As a general rule, organizations expect nurse managers to control the number of hours worked by staff and not the actual salary expense. Wage levels, benefit costs, and other related expenses are typically controlled at the leadership level. The operational aspect of scheduling staff (measured in worked hours) to meet the needs of patient volume (measured by patient census) is best controlled and budgeted at the unit or departmental level.

Capital Budget

The capital budget represents funds allocated for construction projects and major equipment purchases (e.g., cardiac monitor, defibrillator, computer hardware), typically referred to as capital expenditures. The capital budget is developed separately from the operating budget because payments for capital purchases are spread out over multiple years. The main requirements for a purchase or acquisition to be considered as part of the capital budget is that it has a useful life expectancy of more than 1 year and it costs more than a minimum dollar amount established by the organization, typically $500 to $2000.

The term *capital* simply refers to the funds used to purchase long-term investments, such as major medical equipment, computer systems, and newly constructed buildings. A capital budget item is an expensive purchase that will be used by the organization for many years. Capital budget items are often referred to as *capital assets, long-term investments, capital investments,* or *capital acquisitions.* These capital assets are treated differently from the operating budget expense because of their multiyear value. Because capital purchases are often considered investments, they are scrutinized more carefully during the budgeting process.

Planning capital budget requests tests the nurse manager's long-range planning skills. The nurse manager must be able to look 1 year to several years into the future to identify capital budgeting needs and to bring those needs to the attention of senior management. The unit or department need for a capital purchase must be weighed against the financial implications for the organization's entire capital budget. The nurse manager along with input from his or her staff has a critical role in helping to plan the capital budget, justify priorities, and ensure that the needs of the facility and patients are met. Staff nurses are vital to a successful capital planning process because their "frontline" equipment needs must be made known to management for purchase consideration.

Budget Methods

There are two basic methods for budgeting: the *incremental* approach and the *zero-based* approach. Both approaches have particular strengths and weaknesses and both are completely sound approaches in most situations.

Incremental Budgeting. Incremental budgeting is the more commonly used method, primarily because it is relatively simple to apply to most circumstances. The incremental approach is simply a forward trend of recent performance with adjustments for future growth or decline in revenues or expenses. For example, in this approach, the nursing unit's budget is based on the actual costs from the previous budget period with a small increase for planned salary raises and the higher cost of supplies. It is also possible that the incremental budget might include a decrease in all expenses.

Zero-Based Budgeting. Zero-based budgeting is used far less frequently than incremental budgeting. This method builds a budget from the assumption of no volume and no resources allocated; in other words, it is developed as though the budget were being prepared for the first time. Each budget cycle begins with a critical review of budget assumptions and proposed revenues and expenditures. Then core resources necessary for one unit of service are identified, and from there, resource allocation is determined on a variable basis tied to volume.

Again, consider the chest pain center. If the nurse manager were developing a zero-based budget, he or she would start each new budget planning cycle by:

- Determining the revenue and expenses for caring for one patient with chest pain.
- Predicting the average patient volume for the center.
- Calculating the total revenues and expenses for the budget period.

In developing the budget, the nurse manager understands that whereas one nurse is necessary to care for one patient, that nurse may also be able to care for two or three other patients at the same time. Thus, the cost of nursing salaries varies according to the volume of patients being treated in the center.

This process works somewhat differently in support departments that do not provide a revenue-generating service such as patient treatment. Examples of departments that are necessary to support treatment and care delivery processes but are not revenue generating include nursing administration and human resources. In such support departments, expenses do not vary with patient volume. Thus, these departments base their budgets not on a variable volume of patient visits but, rather, on a set core of expenses to run the department.

DEVELOPING A BUDGET

Developing a budget is actually a continual process. Organizations are constantly making projections for future budgets, implementing current budgets, and analyzing month-to-month variances in relation to the budget. The current budget usually covers a 12-month period, also known as the organization's *fiscal year.* The development of the budget for the new fiscal year occurs a few months ahead of the start of the new fiscal year so that the budget can be developed and approved at all levels before it becomes effective. For example, if the organization's fiscal year is from September 1 to August 31, then budget development for the new fiscal year will begin sometime in early summer—or perhaps even earlier depending on the size and complexity of the organization. Because of the number of approval layers, large health systems usually begin the budget process much earlier than smaller systems or single facilities.

Health care organizations usually have a defined procedure in place for budget development. This defined procedure tells managers whether the budget development will use the incremental method, zero-based method, or some other method defined by the organization. Organizations may also define whether they use a "top-down," "participatory," or "iterative" approach to budgeting. In the top-down approach, upper management sets budget goals and imposes those goals on the rest of the organization. In the participatory approach, the people responsible for achieving the budget goals are included in goal setting. The iterative approach is a combination of the top-down and the participatory approach, with upper management defining strategic goals and then unit leaders developing their operating budgets to incorporate their individual goals in conjunction with the organization's strategic goals.

One key to understanding budgets is to know the *unit-of-service* on which costs and revenues are based. "Patient-days" is the common unit-of-service for inpatient facilities; patient visits or visits by categories (short, intermediate, long) are the units-of-service for ambulatory clinics and home health agencies. Budgets are then developed on the basis of the units-of-service predicted for a given period. For example, the nurse manager in a hospital intensive care unit bases his or her budget on the average number of days that patients are expected be on the unit over the course of 12 months. The director of the home health agency bases his or her budget on the number of home visits that will be made during a 12-month period. The unit-of-service may vary depending on the organization, setting, and financial policies; thus it is essential that the nurse understands the unit-of-service in the area in which he or she is employed.

Following are the basic steps for developing a budget:

1. Review the strategic plan to identify goals and objectives; the budget is developed to accomplish these goals and objectives.
2. Set budget assumptions on which to base budgeting decisions. Budget assumptions deal with issues that affect the future performance of the organization and address questions such as: Are supply prices likely to increase or decrease, and by what percentage? What salary range will ensure that the organization is able to recruit and retain quality employees? What will the cost of the health insurance plan be in the coming year? What are the competitors offering in terms of new services? Is the patient census likely to increase or decrease over the next year? Budget assumptions should be developed by a team of managers from different departments and areas of expertise to make certain that consideration is given to all issues that will affect the budget.
3. Gather information about past results, and use the information in combination with budget assumptions to set reasonable expectations about future performance.
4. Predict the units-of-service that will be provided during the budget period.
5. Project expected revenues on the basis of the units-of-service.
6. Project expenses on the basis of the units-of-service. Determine expenses for the labor budget first, based on the predicted units-of-service and the number of **full-time equivalents** (FTEs) needed to provide the predicted service volume. Each full-time employee is considered one **FTE**, or 2080 hours per year (40 hours per week). In some organizations, nurses are scheduled for three 12-hour shifts each week, 36 hours per week or 1872 hours per year, and each is considered 0.9 FTE. After determining units of service and related FTEs, other expenses are fairly straightforward to project.

Developing the budget is generally a process that involves many discussions among many different managers, from finance to nursing. It is important that nurses have a strong and knowledgeable voice in the budget process so that nursing and patient care needs are appropriately addressed. Box 18.3 lists hints to improve your budgeting skills.

BOX 18.3   Hints to Improve Your Budgeting Skills

- Understand your organization's budgeting process. What guidelines do you need to follow? What is the timing of the budget process? What key managers can serve as a resource to help you understand the budget process?
- Learn your department's *unit-of-service* and exactly how it is defined.
- Build a relationship with a finance person in the organization, and collaborate routinely on improvement projects; invite finance staff to your unit meetings, and ask to participate in theirs; communicate regularly.
- Review financial reports with the finance person to make sure you are correctly interpreting the reports.
- Understand each line in your budget. If you do not know what something means or where a number comes from, find out.
- Have ongoing discussions with your management team throughout the budgeting process. The more you participate in the planning process, the better you will understand the budget and your responsibilities related to it.
- Learn your organization's capital budgeting process and what qualifies a purchase as a capital expenditure.

VARIANCE ANALYSIS

One primary use of a budget is to evaluate the financial progress of the department or unit. **Variance analysis** is the process by which deviations from budgeted amounts are examined through comparison of actual financial performance results against expected, or budgeted, performance. Through this process, variances are evaluated on quantitative and qualitative bases. Quantitative analysis focuses on numerical variances to the budget. In other words, are you over or under budget for labor (employee salaries), supply usage, or revenue generated? See Table 18.1 for a sample budget and variance report.

Qualitative analysis of budget variances focuses on reconciling the underlying assumptions on which the budget was based with current conditions. In many cases, the daily operations for a department or unit changes in ways that render the budget assumptions invalid. For example, a unit may be budgeted for nurse staffing at 5 hours per patient-day based on a given patient acuity level. Then the hospital's admission patterns change and a larger number of patients with significantly higher acuity levels are admitted to this unit. The labor used increases to 7 hours per patient-day based on the new acuity level. This sort of qualitative change can make budgets difficult, if not impossible, to adhere to without modification. Nurse leaders in the clinical department or unit are best positioned to determine why variances have occurred because variances are almost always related to a clinical issue such as the one just described.

Variance information is presented by means of certain standard reports. Through such reports, nurse managers are able to compare the budgeted amounts for expense items such as nurse salaries and patient supplies with what was actually spent for the items. From there the nurse manager can consider what is occurring in the clinical setting to explain the variances in budgeted and actual expenditures. Nurses are encouraged to examine variance analysis reports and seek guidance from other managers or supervisors to learn more about reading the reports and becoming more comfortable with variance analysis.

COST CONCEPTS RELATED TO BUDGETING

When considering the budget, one must have a basic understanding of how much health care services cost and how to predict changes in costs. Consider this question: How much does it cost to provide nursing care to one patient for one 12-hour shift? Unfortunately, the answer is not simple because many factors affect how much something costs. An important step to understanding costs is to review the primary types of costs that accountants consider when determining the cost of services in a health care setting; they are as follows:

- *Service unit or unit-of-service:* The basic measure of the product or service being produced. The unit-of-service varies with the health care setting and type of service being provided. Examples include patient-days (hospital), home care visits (home health agency), patient visits (outpatient clinic), and operating room time (outpatient surgical center).
- *Direct costs:* Costs that can be traced directly to the production of the unit-of-service. Examples include

TABLE 18.1 Sample Budget and Variance Report:

Hometown General Hospital: Department Performance Analysis—Med-Surg for Period Ending 09/20/2018

	Prior Year Actual 9/17	CURRENT MTD (MONTH)		MTD Var (Variance) 9/18	CURRENT YTD (YEAR-TO-DATE)			PRIOR YEAR	
		Actual 9/18	Budget 9/18		Actual 9/18	Budget 9/18	YTD Variance 9/18	Prior Year 9/17	Prior Year Variance
Gross Revenue									
Inpatient revenue	1,276,525	1,300,122	1,322,904	−22,782	11,087,012	12,575,946	−1,488,934	12,733,822	−1,646,810
Outpatient revenue	0	0	0	0	0	0	0	0	0
Other revenue	0	0	0	0	0	0	0	0	0
Total gross revenue	1,276,525	1,300,122	1,322,904	−22,782	11,087,012	12,575,946	−1,488,934	12,733,822	−1,646,810
Operating Expenses									
Total productive labor	241,270	293,541	257,954	35,587	2,375,340	2,419,097	−43,757	2,376,009	−669
Total nonproductive labor	29,012	40,031	37,352	2679	359,759	359,453	306	328,128	31,631
Employee benefits and taxes	40,372	38,483	41,133	−2650	366,203	401,616	−35,413	398,766	−32,563
Total SWB (salaries, wages, and benefits)	310,653	372,055	336,439	35,616	3,101,302	3,180,166	−78,864	3,102,903	−1601
Supplies	25,687	20,506	22,628	−2123	193,223	213,853	−20,630	219,267	−26,044
Medical and clinical fees	0	0	0	0	0	0	0	0	0
Contracted department and other fees	298	0	41	−41	506	371	135	929	−424

Repairs and maintenance	0	0	20	−20	0	184	−184	242	−242
Utilities and telephone	0	0	0	0	0	0	0	0	0
Rent, lease, and equipment rental	0	0	0	0	1485	0	1485	0	1485
Other controllable expenses	883	1232	953	279	8617	8,741	−124	14,041	−5424
Other noncontrollable expenses	0	0	0	0	0	0	0	0	0
Total operating expenses	337,520	393,792	360,081	33,711	3,305,132	3,403,315	−98,183	3,337,382	−32,249
Gross margin	939,005	906,330	962,823	−56,493	7,781,880	9,172,631	−1,390,751	9,396,440	−1,614,561
Gross margin percentage	73.56	69.71	72.78	−3.07	70.19	72.94	−2.75	73.79	−3.6
Department patient-days	841	853	871	−18	7283	8280	−997	8384	−1101
Average daily census	28	28	29	−1	27	30	−4	31	−4
Observation days	1.67	3.5	5.5	−2	41.54	49.38	−7.83	48.17	−6.63
Total department patient-days	842.67	856.5	876.5	−20	7324.54	8329.38	−1,004.83	8432.17	−1,107.62

The budget report shows dollar performance, comparing actual revenues and expenses with budgeted revenues and expenses for the same month of the prior year, current month, and current YTD, and the annual totals and variances for the prior year. YTD is the totals for the prior months plus the current month in the fiscal year. The department has spent $33,711 (shaded in *green*) more than budgeted for expenses for the current month, but for the current YTD, the department has spent $98,183 (shaded in *yellow*) less than budgeted for expenses.

nursing care and supplies to provide direct patient care. The important concept to remember about direct costs is that they vary with the volume of services. As the patient census rises, the need for additional nursing care and supplies increases.

- *Indirect costs:* Costs that are incurred as a result of the organization's operating expenses but are not directly related to providing the unit-of-service. Examples include salaries for administrative personnel and expenses for security, housekeeping, utilities, and building maintenance. Indirect costs are sometimes referred to as "overhead."
- *Full cost:* The total of all costs associated with a unit-of-service; it includes direct and indirect costs.
- *Fixed costs:* Costs that do not change as the unit-of-service volume changes. For example, administrative salaries do not change regardless of the patient census on the nursing units. The important point to remember about fixed cost is that they remain steady regardless of the change in units-of-service (e.g., patient-days). As the units-of-service increase, the greater the number to share fixed costs. Conversely, as the units-of-service decrease, the fewer the number to share fixed costs. An organization's finance leaders are always interested in increasing volume to provide additional revenue to help cover fixed costs.
- *Variable costs:* Costs that vary directly with changes in the volume of units-of-service. For example, in an ambulatory clinic, the cost of immunizations varies directly with the number of patients who receive immunizations.

This list provides only a basic introduction to cost terminology; it does not provide a comprehensive range of cost accounting terminology and concepts. However, it does demonstrate the complexity of assessing and managing costs.

IMPROVING THE COST AND QUALITY OF CLINICAL CARE

Nurses face challenging situations given the nursing shortage, the focus on cost reductions and improved quality and safety, and the increasing acuity of patients in all settings from hospitals to home health agencies to nursing homes. At the same time, organizational leaders are faced with challenging economic times, declining reimbursements, and increasing costs in all areas. Changes to improve quality and reduce costs must be made! How can nurses collaborate with organizational leaders and financial managers to make a difference? Nurses are at the front lines of health care and are key to enhancing the *value* of health care, with value being the combination of quality and cost. Nurses can truly affect the quality and cost of care in significant ways:

- As patient advocates, nurses can ensure appropriate care planning and proper follow-up—especially for people with one or more chronic conditions such as congestive heart failure and diabetes—to help them have the resources needed to stay as healthy as possible and stay out of the hospital (Rambur & Nickitas, 2015).
- As advocates for evidence-based practice, nurses can engage in robust evidence-based quality improvement projects that will lead to better patient outcomes and significantly lower costs by reducing the occurrence of complications such as pressure ulcers, falls, and central-line infections (Goetz et al, 2011).
- As advocates for efficient operations, nurses should understand the staffing budget and how it relates to patient acuity to ensure that appropriate nursing resources are available to meet patient care needs (Kolakowski, 2016).
- As advocates for appropriate supply usage, nurses can identify the most cost-effective patient care supplies to replace more expensive products as well as identify ways to reduce waste and use supplies more efficiently (Johnson et al, 2012).

As nurses step up to the challenge of enhancing the value of health care—improved quality and lower costs—they must be able to measure and document their contributions. Only by understanding the basics of budgeting and costs can nurses demonstrate their contributions to reduced readmissions, lower complication rates, fewer never events, shorter length of stay, improvements in supply use costs, and overall lower costs per patient combined with increased quality.

SUMMARY

The financial well-being of health care organizations—and the value of health care—rests largely in the hands of the clinical team, with the budget serving as the financial guideline that enables the clinical team to provide quality patient care and achieve strategic goals. This chapter has reviewed the four major functions of the organization's budget: planning, communicating and coordinating, monitoring progress, and evaluating performance. Elements of the three basic types of budgets—operational, labor, and capital—have been described along with the two primary approaches to budgeting—incremental and zero-based. The nurse's role in affecting the organization's financial performance by being an advocate for proper patient care planning and follow-up, evidence-based practice, efficient operations, appropriate supply use, and prevention of complications and hospital-acquired conditions is also reviewed.

The reader is cautioned that this chapter merely provides a general overview of budgeting basics to serve as a framework on which nurses can continue to build their knowledge of health care finance and budgeting. As nurses advance into supervisory and management positions, it is essential that they further develop their skills and knowledge in budgeting through personal study, working with mentors, attending classes, reading books and journals, and joining professional organizations that promote health care finance and budget knowledge.

REFERENCES

Goetz, K., Janney, M., & Ramsey, K. (2011). When nursing takes ownership of financial outcomes: achieving exceptional financial performance through leadership, strategy and execution. *Nursing Economic$*, *29*(4), 173–182.

Johnson, D., Bell, B., Elgendy, J., McDonald, E., West, F., Wenzel, L., et al. (2012, August). Don't waste green! Launching a budget awareness campaign. *Nursing Management*, *43*(8), 51–54.

Kolakowski, D. (2016, February). Constructing a nursing budget using a patient classification system. *Nursing Management*, *47*(2), 14–16.

Rambur, B., & Nickitas, D. M. (2015, May-June). Understanding health and payment reform – essential for the new world of nursing: an interview with Betty Rambur. *Nursing Economic$*, *33*(3), 155–160.

Talley, L. B., Thorgrimson, D. H., & Robinson, N. C. (2013). Financial literacy as an essential element in nursing management practice. *Nursing Economic$*, *31*(2), 77–82.

19

Effective Communication and Conflict Resolution

Anna Marie Sallee, PhD, MSN, RN

How is your message being received?

Ⓔ Additional resources are available online at: *http://evolve.elsevier.com/Cherry/*

> *"The greatest problem of communication is the illusion that it has been accomplished."*
> **George Bernard Shaw**

LEARNING OUTCOMES

After studying this chapter, the reader will be able to:

1. Outline factors that can influence the communication process.
2. Communicate effectively with diverse intergenerational and interdisciplinary team members.
3. Apply positive communication techniques in diverse situations.
4. Recognize negative communication techniques.
5. Evaluate conflicting verbal and nonverbal communication cues.
6. Examine constructive methods of communicating in conflict situations.
7. Respond to inappropriate use of logical fallacies in communication.
8. Develop professional social media interaction behaviors.

KEY TERMS

Active listening The process of hearing what others are saying with a sense of seriousness and discrimination.

Conflict An experience in which there is simultaneous arousal of two or more incompatible motives.

Filtration Unconscious exclusion of extraneous stimuli.

Information The data that are meaningful and alter the receiver's understanding.

Interpretation Receiver's understanding of the meaning of the communication.

Negative communication Behaviors that block or impair effective communication.

Perception The manner in which one sees reality.

Positive communication Behaviors that enhance effective communication.

PROFESSIONAL/ETHICAL ISSUE

Altah is a recent registered nurse (RN) graduate who works on an active medical-surgical floor in a large hospital in a university town. She has observed a colleague using the computer system to look up information on acquaintances who have been hospitalized at the facility—even from previous years. One night she observes the RN looking up personal health information on a hospitalized athlete who plays at the university and is a local/regional celebrity. Altah knows the nurse's actions are unethical and illegal. However, she recognizes the nurse is well liked by both their coworkers and the administrative personnel at the hospital. She is vibrant and friendly and has many years of experience. Altah, however, is new to nursing and still on a high learning curve. As a single mother of two, she struggled to finish nursing school and support her family, accruing significant educational loans in the process. She is fearful that if the hospital administration feels forced to make a choice, she may lose her job. She struggles with whether to report the nurse or stay silent and hope that someone else will take action.

What ethical principles are in conflict here? Do you believe Altah's fears regarding her job security are legitimate? What communication techniques will be important for Altah to use in this situation? Discuss possible options for Altah.

VIGNETTE

Stacy Shannon, RN, the charge nurse on 4-East, receives a telephone call from the secretary in the emergency department (ED) to inform Stacy that a patient is ready for transfer. Stacy was expecting this patient but had not anticipated the transfer would occur so soon and had not yet informed the nurse who would be assigned to the patient. The ED secretary explains that there are many patients waiting to be seen in the ED and it is becoming increasingly chaotic. Stacy replies that she will locate the nurse who will be assigned to the patient and facilitate the transfer as soon as possible. As Stacy goes down the hallway to locate this particular nurse, she learns that the nurse has left the unit on a short break and is expected back within 10 minutes.

Stacy calls the ED secretary to arrange for the transfer to occur in 20 minutes. To her surprise, she finds out that the patient has left the department and is being brought to 4-East immediately. Within a few moments, the patient and ED nurse arrive. The ED nurse states that he wants to give report on this patient quickly because he needs to return to the ED right away. Stacy assists him in transferring the patient to a bed and making the patient as comfortable as possible.

As Stacy completes this process, the nurse who was on break returns to the unit, learns that she has a new patient she did not expect, and immediately has to receive report from the ED nurse. Stacy notes through both body language and tone of voice that the interaction between the two nurses is less than cordial.

Within 10 minutes Stacy receives a telephone call from the ED charge nurse, who wants to discuss this incident. Negative comments are made about the 4-East nurse who left the unit "unannounced" and that "there is a concern for patient safety." How can Stacy best facilitate a positive outcome in this situation?

Questions to Consider While Reading This Chapter:

1. What communication strategies should Stacy use to respond to the accusations being made by the ED charge nurse and resolve the conflict?
2. What strategies can Stacy use to build a trusting relationship between her and the ED charge nurse?
3. What positive communication techniques could have prevented this situation from occurring?
4. What nonverbal cues might Stacy have observed between the two nurses during the report exchange?
5. Should Stacy have intervened when she observed the interaction between the two nurses? If so, how?
6. What strategies can Stacy implement to improve the communication skills of her staff?

CHAPTER OVERVIEW

Effective communication is a foundational component of professional nursing practice. The development of effective communication skills can only enhance each nurse's professional image while building strong relationships with both patients and colleagues. Understanding communication processes and principles is required for nurses to interact professionally with patients, families and significant others, nursing peers, managers, student nurses, physicians, other members of the interdisciplinary team, and the public. Nurses communicate through a variety of media, including the spoken and written word, demonstration, role modeling, and, on occasion, public appearances. The exchange of ideas and feelings is hardly limited to verbal communication. Many types of nonverbal communication are often as meaningful as, and in many instances more meaningful than, audible expression. Because communication is such a complex process, there are infinite opportunities for sending or receiving incorrect messages. All too frequently, communication is faulty, resulting in misperceptions and misunderstandings. This chapter reviews the communication process and its components, communication styles, and principles of effective communication in professional nursing, including special communication issues.

OUR PROFESSION SPEAKS

Nurses must be as proficient in communication skills as they are in clinical skills.

American Association of Critical Care Nurses, Standard 1, in Standards for Establishing and Sustaining Health Work Environments (2016)

Open and candid communication with patients and their families is a key component of safe and effective health care.

The Joint Commission (2016)

THE COMMUNICATION PROCESS

The human voice is the most beautiful instrument of all, but it is the most difficult to play.

Richard Strauss

Communication is a process requiring certain components. There must be a sender, a receiver, and a message. Effective communication is a dynamic process: With a response (feedback), the sender becomes the receiver, the receiver becomes the sender, and the message changes. The method of delivery influences the effectiveness of communication. In addition, communication is affected by many subcomponents, both environmental and in the minds of the communicators. When communication with another person occurs, verbally or nonverbally, a typical pattern develops that includes the actual message being sent, the receiver's belief or interpretation of that message, and the reaction to the message.

Think about the communication activities that occur in the health care setting. There is often much to communicate in a limited time and sometimes during very high stress situations. In addition to the actual message, personal goals or hidden agendas can influence the way a message is delivered and/or received. For this reason, it is very important to understand the many elements that influence the communication process.

Interpretation

Interpretation of information can be influenced by such factors as context, environment, precipitating event, preconceived ideas, personal perceptions, style of transmission, and past experiences. Because of the interaction of these factors, the sender's message may mean to the receiver something that was entirely unplanned or unexpected by the sender (Fig. 19.1).

Context and Environment. *Context* refers to the entire situation relevant to the communication, such as the environment, the background, and the particular circumstances that lead to the discussion. *Environment* can denote physical surroundings and happenings and the emotional conditions involved in the communication.

Precipitating Event. *Precipitating event* refers specifically to the event or situation that prompted the communication. Precipitating event is a specific single event, whereas context describes the whole ambiance of the situation with the inclusion of multiple circumstances that have led to the precipitating event.

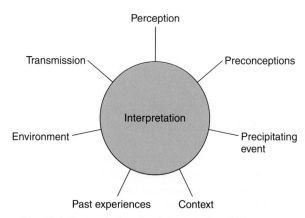

Fig. 19.1 Factors Influencing Interpretation of Messages.

Preconceived Ideas. *Preconceived ideas* are conceptions, opinions, or thoughts that the receiver has developed before the encounter. Such ideas can dramatically affect the receiver's acceptance and understanding of the message.

Style of Transmission. *Style of transmission* involves many aspects of the manner of conveyance of the message. Transmission styles include aspects such as open and closed statements and questions, body language, method of organizing the message, degree of attention to the topic and to the receiver, vocabulary chosen (professional jargon versus language a layperson could easily understand), and intonation.

Past Experiences. Each person comes to any type of communication, whether it is friendly conversation, informational lecture, staff meeting, performance evaluation, or any other possible scenario, with "baggage" in terms of past experiences. Because past experiences are a variety of positive, neutral, and negative events, the influence that the experiences can and will have on communication may be positive, neutral, or negative. *The importance of recognizing that any reaction from the receiver may be biased by previous experiences cannot be overstated.* An astute sender begins to investigate such a possibility if the receiver reacts in an unexpected or inappropriate manner to information that was not expected to produce such a response, which may range from nonresponse to overly vehement response.

Personal Perceptions. Personal perceptions can have a profound effect on the quality of communication. **Perception** is awareness through the excitation of all the senses. Perception can be described as all that the person knows about a situation or circumstance based on what each of the senses—taste, smell, sight, sound, touch, and intuition—discover and interpret.

Filtration

The most concise delivery of information is subject to some amount of filtration. Think of the process as similar to washing vegetables in a colander. A large amount of water is poured over the produce. Some of the water comes quickly through the colander holes; some water drips through more slowly; and some water hangs on the contents or settles in the solid portions of the colander and never filters through. If people were

not able to filter out a portion of the stimuli that bombard them daily, the clutter would be unmanageable! At the same time, however, it is possible to filter out some part of intended communication that is essential to understanding the communication.

Feedback

Feedback, simply put, is the response from the receiver. However, as with all communication, feedback is a dynamic process. As the receiver interprets and responds to the original message, the sender begins the same process of feedback to the receiver. Because of this circular property, the process frequently is referred to as the *feedback loop* (van Servellen, 1997). As with the original message, feedback is not confined to verbal responses alone. Both communicants constantly assess nonverbal communication as well. Feedback is formed on the basis of all the components of interpretation and filtration.

VERBAL VERSUS NONVERBAL COMMUNICATION

What you do speaks so loud that I cannot hear what you say.

Ralph Waldo Emerson

The most important thing in communication is hearing what isn't said.

Peter F. Drucker

Verbal Communication

Verbal communication, the most common form of interpersonal communication, involves talking and listening. Important clues to verbal communication are the tone or inflection with which the words are spoken and the general attitude the speaker uses. Suzette Haden Elgin refers to the "tune the words are set to" (1993). The key to the true meaning of a statement may be contained in the emphasis placed on a specific word. Consider how differently the following phrase could be perceived according to the inflection, or the emphasis on the wording:

- You are going to *bed*.
- *You* are going to bed.
- You *are going* to bed.

With an emphasis on *bed,* the first phrase most likely will be perceived as an inquiry. The second phrase might imply that you are going to bed, but no one else is. The last phrase, an imperative (or command), gives the impression of increased emotion, such as anger or frustration.

Another element central to verbal interaction is the concept of attitude. Being aware of and learning to understand the concept of attitude is key to effective communication. Attitude involves a predisposition or tendency to respond in one way or another. Often the attitude that accompanies a verbal interaction, which can be positive or negative, is much more meaningful than the actual words spoken. Although we may hear "attitude" in a person's tone of voice, it is most often communicated "loud and clear" through nonverbal communication.

Nonverbal Communication

Oops! Did I just roll my eyes out loud?

Facebook Posting

Nonverbal communication involves many factors that either confirm or deny the spoken word. Facial expression, the presence or absence of eye contact, posture, and body movement all project a direct message. Indirect nonverbal messages might include dressing style, lifestyle, or material possessions. Never presume that external trappings and physical presentation do not influence the quality of communication. Preconceived ideas and expectations interpret input from all such sources, often on an almost subconscious level.

Consider the following scenario: Rhonda, a young wife and mother, was admitted to the ED with significant abdominal pain. As the nurse inquires about her symptoms, Rhonda repeatedly glances at her husband, Tommy, before she answers. Although she denies any pain at this time, you observe that she guards her stomach, has a "clenched" jawline, and does not make eye contact with you. As you assess and question Rhonda, Tommy often interrupts with comments such as, "She's just fine. It was only a stomachache, and it's gone this morning, isn't it, dear?" Which message seems more likely to be true—the verbal or the nonverbal? How will you address the nonverbal cues? As you read the remainder of this chapter, consider strategies that you can use to enhance communication between this husband and wife.

The avoidance of eye contact may be construed to mean that the speaker is shy, scared, or not telling the truth. The judgment as to which condition is correct is based on all the factors that feed into the receiver's interpretation—perception, preconceptions, precipitating event, context, past experiences, environment, and transmission. Faced with the many opportunities for incorrect interpretation, is it any wonder that misunderstandings occur?

An important concept to remember is that when the verbal and nonverbal messages do not agree, the receiver is more likely to believe the nonverbal message. In 1971, Albert Mehrabian (1981) conducted a seminal study on nonverbal communication in which he found that most communication is 55% nonverbal, 38% vocal signals (such as tone, pitch, and pace), and *only 7% the actual words we say.* Mehrabian's study has significantly influenced our understanding of the "silent messages" we send. In fact, body language is often the most trusted indicator for conveying feelings, attitudes, and emotions (Borg, 2011) because it so often comes from our subconscious—which is much less likely to deceive! Nonverbal language includes such things as dress, posture, facial expression, eye contact, body movements, body tension, spatial distance, touch, and voice. For nurses, body positioning toward the patient, a relaxed stance, a gentle touch, and an open face signal total presence.

An understanding of the importance ascribed to body language and other nonverbal clues to the intent of the message explains the advantage of face-to-face communication whenever possible. Although a telephone conversation supplies verbal messages, intonation, and feedback, other signals are missing, such as facial expression, body position, and environmental clues. The perils inherent in written and electronic communication are discussed later in this chapter.

POSITIVE COMMUNICATION TECHNIQUES

Effective communication involves a positive exchange of ideas between or among individuals. The successful communicator strives to demonstrate openness, availability, and acceptance both verbally and nonverbally. Following are some of the many techniques that help achieve positive communication style.

Developing Trust

Trust between the nurse and the patient is essential to good communication and often must be cultivated.

Factors that enhance the development of trust include openness on the part of the nurse, honesty, integrity, and dependability. The nurse can demonstrate these factors by:

- Communicating clearly in language that laypersons can understand.
- Keeping promises.
- Protecting confidentiality.
- Avoiding negative communication techniques such as blocking and false reassurance.
- Being available to the patient.

The need for trust in the health care setting is not limited to the nurse-patient relationship but, rather, pervades all working relationships. Care is more effective when the nursing team and the interprofessional team share the essential element of trust.

Using "I" Messages

The use of "I" messages is a fundamental component in acceptable communication. Consider the following exchange.

Laura: "You make me so mad, Donald."

Donald: "I don't mean to make you mad."

Laura: "Well, you do. You never think about how I feel. You know I hate it when you leave a patient's room as cluttered as 103."

Donald: "You don't have the vaguest idea what went on here last night! That's what I hate about you—always so quick to judge. You are so critical. You must think that you are perfect!"

When a comment starts with "you," most commonly the receiver's defenses promptly go on alert. The use of "you" in such a context sounds—and most probably is meant to be—accusatory. Notice how the emotions quickly escalate to anger. Also notice that although the receiver initially tries to sound conciliatory, he soon begins to respond in a similar accusatory form. Instead of using accusatory and defensive language, the sender should frame the comment in terms of how it makes her or him feel. Consider this alternative:

Laura: "Donald, I feel so upset when I find a cluttered room like 103 at the beginning of my shift. I feel as if I am behind when I start."

The difference is obvious. When "I" messages are used, they are less likely to sound accusatory. By using such an opening, the sender allows the receiver to respond to the true message rather than start to mount a defense. It allows for more effective communication

because the receiver is more likely to offer an explanation such as the following:

Donald: "I'm really sorry about room 103, Laura. I guess the wheel that doesn't squeak doesn't get oiled, as they say. Our shift started last night with a patient coding right after he arrived from the emergency room. There was no family here. It took forever to find them and then to support them through the shock. About the time things settled down, the patient in room 110 coded. It was quite a night."

In this instance, the "I" message enhances communication by giving Donald the opportunity to address the real concern. In addition, if Laura is truly astute, she has a wonderful opportunity to support her colleague by voicing appreciation for the working circumstances of his shift. Most people respond gratefully to recognition and commiseration. The exchange could build collegiality between the two coworkers and perhaps between the two shifts.

Establishing Eye Contact

As mentioned previously, the avoidance of eye contact can be interpreted in a number of different ways. A person who does not make eye contact may be thought to be shy, scared, insecure, preoccupied, unprepared, or dishonest—the list could go on and on. None of these qualities is likely to be appreciated in a primary caregiver. By making direct eye contact, the nurse gives undivided attention to the patient, and the patient is likely to feel valued and understood by the nurse. Eye contact in essence says, "I am wholly available to you. What you are saying is important to me."

Eye contact is equally important in communication with coworkers and other members of the interprofessional team. This quality is lost in telephone conversations or written communications.

Keep in mind, however, that the use of direct eye contact is a Western value. In some cultures, avoidance of eye contact is considered more appropriate social behavior. By careful observation, the nurse will quickly recognize whether direct eye contact is interpreted as inappropriate or disrespectful. Nurses must make every effort to be sensitive to the cultural values of clients and their coworkers to enhance effective communication.

Keeping Promises

Little else can destroy the fragile trust developing in any interpersonal relationship as quickly as making and then breaking promises. Inherent in the concept of promise keeping are the qualities of honesty and integrity. Once a commitment is made, every effort must be expended to fulfill the expectation. Sometimes the request is impossible to satisfy. If this happens, the nurse must explain the situation or circumstances. The fact that the patient understands that the nurse has made an effort to meet his or her needs or desires is often more important than whether the goal is accomplished. If the nurse responds, "I'll check on that," and then finds the request impossible to fulfill but never returns with an explanation, the lack of dependability perceived by the patient (or colleague) will surely drive a wedge into the relationship.

Expressing Empathy

Empathy is the ability to mentally place oneself in another person's situation to better understand the person and to share the emotions or feelings of that person. Empathy is not feeling sorry for another; rather, it is understanding the experiences of the other person, and it is integral to the therapeutic relationship. The nurse is able to perceive and address the needs of the patient without becoming so emotionally involved as to become inappropriately immersed in the situation.

Using Open Communication

Certain styles of phrasing questions and statements lend themselves to obtaining more information. For example, suppose Chris asks Mr. Barrow, "Do you know where you are?" and Mr. Barrow responds, "Yes." Can Chris assume that Mr. Barrow knows he is in the hospital? Not necessarily. Chris may be surprised to hear a completely unexpected response if he rephrases the inquiry:

Chris: "Mr. Barrow, tell me where you are."

Mr. Barrow: "Why, I'm in the honeymoon cabin of the Titanic, of course. Have you seen my lovely bride?"

Using open-ended questions or statements that require more information than "yes" or "no" responses can help gather enough facts to build a more complete picture of the circumstances. Questions or statements that are phrased to require only one- or two-word responses may miss the mark entirely.

Clarifying Information

Both communicants have a responsibility to clarify anything not understood. The sender should ask for feedback to be certain the receiver is correctly interpreting what is being said. The receiver should stop the sender anytime the message becomes unclear and should provide feedback regularly so that misinterpretation can be identified quickly. Such phrases as "What I hear you saying is . . ." and "I understand you to mean . . ." help communicate to the sender what is being perceived. Other techniques of clarification include using easily understood language, giving examples, drawing a picture, making a list, and finding ways to stimulate all the senses to enhance the ability to understand.

Being Aware of Body Language

Body positioning and movement send loud messages to others. The nurse can imply openness that facilitates effective communication through awareness of body position and movement. In addition to eye contact, effective communication is enriched through an open stance, such as holding one's arms at the sides or out toward the patient, rather than crossed, or leaning toward the patient as if to hear more clearly, rather than away from the patient.

Using Touch

Most people have a fairly well-defined personal space. It is important for the nurse to be sensitive to each patient's personal preference and cultural differences in terms of touch. However, for many people, a gentle touch can scale mountains in terms of demonstrating genuine interest and concern. A pat on the back, a hand held, a touch on the shoulder—these are all behaviors that indicate availability and accessibility on the part of the nurse.

NEGATIVE COMMUNICATION TECHNIQUES

Several negative communication techniques have been alluded to in the previous discussion. Closed communication styles, such as asking yes-or-no questions and making inquiries or statements that require other single-word answers, potentially limit the response of the person and may prevent the discovery of pertinent facts. Closed body language can also hinder effective communication. Crossed arms, hands on the hips, avoidance of eye contact, turning away from the person, and moving away from the person all impose a sense of distance in the relationship. Three other techniques that are detrimental to good communication are termed *blocking, false assurances,* and *conflicting messages.*

Blocking

Blocking occurs when the nurse responds with non-committal or generalized answers. For example:

"Nurse, I've never had surgery before. I'm afraid I might not ever wake up." Mr. Clayton is twisting the bed sheet as he speaks.

"Oh, Mr. Clayton, many people feel that way. It'll be okay." Makayla Butler, RN, smiles brightly, pats his hand, picks up the dirty linen bag, and bounces out of the room.

Does Mr. Clayton feel reassured? Not likely. Will he be inclined to broach the subject with Makayla again? Probably not. Makayla has incorporated some important aspects of positive communication into her response—cheerfulness and touch—but she has not truly communicated. She has effectively blocked Mr. Clayton's attempt to get the reassurance he wanted from her. He may be too intimidated to ask anyone else, assuming that his fear is invalid.

By generalizing in this way, Makayla has trivialized Mr. Clayton's concerns. He is not "many people." He needs to be validated as an individual experiencing a legitimate feeling. Makayla can validate his fear and put it into perspective at the same time with a different approach:

Makayla: "What makes you think you might not wake up, Mr. Clayton?"

Mr. Clayton: "Well, my wife's cousin's husband had surgery about 25 years ago, and he never woke up."

Makayla: "What kind of surgery did he have?"

Mr. Clayton: "Uh, it was some kind of heart surgery, and he had another heart attack on the table and died right there."

Makayla: "It sounds like his condition was critical going into surgery."

Mr. Clayton: "Yes, ma'am. He'd been sick for a long time."

Makayla: "It's not uncommon to feel afraid of having anesthesia, especially if you have never had surgery before. There are rare cases in which complications do occur during surgery. That's why we put the disclosures on the consent form, so that you will know just what the risks are. Thankfully, though, most surgeries are without such drastic problems. Although your gallbladder certainly has made you uncomfortable, you are otherwise in good health. The tests that were done before surgery, like the chest radiograph and the laboratory work, show that you are healthy and should do well with the anesthesia. That drastically decreases the chance for complications in your case. I will be glad to answer any other questions you have or to ask the anesthetist to come and talk with you some more."

Makayla has validated Mr. Clayton's feeling as legitimate, provided an explanation with reasonable reassurances, and offered to explore the issue with him further or to have someone else talk with him.

Some things are difficult to talk about with another person. The dying patient may want to talk about how he or she feels, ask questions, or perform a life review. A nurse who is uncomfortable with such topics may consciously or unconsciously block communication about them through generalizations or closed responses. Avoidance of the blocking technique requires a good understanding of oneself. If unable to provide the open communication the patient obviously needs, the nurse should access other personnel who are more comfortable in the situation.

False Assurances

False assurances are similar to blocking and have about the same effect. When someone is trying to get real answers or express serious concerns, an answer such as "Don't worry" or "It'll be okay" sends several unintended messages. Such answers can be interpreted by the patient as placating or showing a lack of concern or a lack of knowledge of the situation. The patient might even conclude that the nurse is being neglectful through trivialization of an issue that is important to him or her. At the very least, the nurse has neither recognized the need the patient has expressed nor provided validation.

Conflicting Messages

Conflicting messages also have been alluded to in the previous discussion. If a person professes pleasure at seeing someone but draws back when that person extends a hand of greeting, the nonverbal message speaks more loudly than the words spoken. If a nurse enters a room and goes through the routine greeting by rote (even with a smiling face and a bouncing step), a patient can quickly perceive this and consider the nurse less approachable.

The nurse's statement that the patient's condition is important to the nurse followed by failing to answer the call bell in a timely manner or by forgetting to bring items promised to the patient sends a double message. Such behavior can leave the patient confused, frustrated, or angry. Carrying through with a commitment, no matter how unimportant it may seem, is a premier method of saying to the person, "You are important to me."

Logical Fallacies

Logical fallacies are related to an individual's culture, gender, background, and personal experiences and are barriers to meaningful communication. Individuals often cannot separate moods, thoughts, and perceptions, for they become interconnected in one continuous evaluation process, involving feeling, thinking, and responding. In times of increased stress, as is common in health care settings, it is more likely that people will employ faulty thinking that affects the communication process. Recognition of distortions and faulty logic will promote effective communication and reduce confusion or even prevent conflict. Following are examples of logical fallacies that are frequently encountered.

Ad Hominem Abusive. *Ad hominem abusive* is an argument that attacks the person instead of the issue. The speaker hopes to discredit the other person by calling attention to some irrelevant fact about that person. Perhaps a nurse has just had a disagreement with a physician about lab results that were not properly reported. The nurse makes the following comment to colleagues: "She thinks she's so smart just because she's a doctor." What does that have to do with the disagreement? Nothing. It is an unwarranted attack on the doctor. Does it accomplish the purpose? Very likely, the group will be influenced by the disparaging comment. They may also become angry at the physician, who had legitimate cause to be upset about not receiving lab results. Ultimately, the issue of unreported lab values is lost in the personal attack against the physician.

Appeal to Emotion. Appeal to emotion is an attempt to manipulate other people's emotions in order to avoid the real issue. For example, consider Deb Engles, RN, who has repeatedly failed to document patient care properly. She has been called into the nurse manager's office to discuss the incident and receives a written warning. She comes out tearful. It is obvious to her colleagues that she has been reprimanded. She begins to discuss the problem and makes the following statements: "I am the first person in my family to even go to college. I'm a single parent, and I've worked so hard to get where I am. Our manager doesn't care anything about that. She just wants to pass out written warnings to cover herself. She doesn't care about us as individuals." After a bit of this type of talk, the entire staff is probably becoming angry with the nurse manager—who may feel bad that she had to give the written warning because she does indeed care about her staff. However, Deb has successfully deflected the attention away from the real issue, failure to document properly, which was legitimately addressed.

Red Herring. Red herring is the introduction of an irrelevant topic in order to divert attention away from the real issue. Two nurses, Brian and Nikoah, are having an argument regarding Brian's failure to complete his assigned tasks. Brian states, "It's not my work that you're really mad about. It's that I'm a guy. You just don't like male nurses." Nikoah then begins to defend herself, denying any prejudice against male nurses. The focus of the argument has been turned from the real issue, Brian's failure to complete his assigned tasks, to a situation in which Nikoah is on the defensive about her opinion of male nurses.

LISTENING

Nature has given men one tongue and two ears, in token that we should listen twice as much as we speak.

Epictetus

Listening certainly is as important an element in clear and effective communication as any other component. Many distracters contribute to poor listening habits. Framing an answer while the other person is still talking interferes with receiving the entire message. Environmental disturbances can provide major disruption. A crying baby, a call light buzzing, and multiple concurrent conversations in a busy nurses' station are a few of the interruptions that jumble the simplest of instructions. Preexisting concerns or worries can block absorption of conversation because of the preoccupation. Attempts to continue work in progress leads to inattention. Ineffective engagement or peculiar mannerisms on the part of the speaker can be distracting. A person who does not make eye contact, shuffles through papers while talking, or over-uses hand movements actually can deter communication. Active listening involves three steps: (1) listening carefully to know what was said; (2) processing the information you heard; and (3) making a decision about what you heard. Does it make sense? Do you believe it? How can you respond appropriately?

As the receiver, you can use a number of techniques to facilitate the ability to listen:

- Give undivided attention to the sender by moving to a quieter area to avoid distractions and stopping the speaker to clarify any points you haven't understood.
- Provide feedback in terms of the perceived meaning of the message by rephrasing in your own words.
- Give attention to positioning so you are facing the sender and making eye contact.
- Note nonverbal messages, such as body language, and respond to them.
- Finish listening before you begin to speak.

If you have accomplished each of these steps, you have engaged in active listening. Active listening dramatically improves the likelihood of receiving the correct message. Equally important, active listening implies a respect for the speaker and communicates a regard for what the speaker has to offer. The nonverbal message that active listening delivers is, "I value you, and what you have to say is important to me."

WRITTEN AND ELECTRONIC COMMUNICATION

Clear, accurate, and accessible documentation is an essential element of safe, quality, evidence-based nursing practice.

American Nurses Association (2010)

I admire machinery as much as any man, and am as thankful to it as any man can be for what it does for us. But, it will never be a substitute for the face of a man, with his soul in it, encouraging another man to be brave and true.

Charles Dickens

Charles Dickens referred to the brand-new telegraph when he admired machinery. Little could he imagine the advances of electronic communication over the decades. But his message is as appropriate today as in the late 1800s. Nothing quite replaces face-to-face communication and the accompanying nonverbal cues. However, written and electronic communications do open valuable new levels of connection and information exchange.

Health care in the United States is rapidly moving to the computer-based electronic health records (EHR) to effect higher-quality patient care, with most hospitals and health care organizations using some type of EHR. Unique issues impact the transition to the EHR. Perhaps the most positive aspect is in improved communication among health care providers within the institution as well as between geographically distant sites, which results in prompt and knowledgeable care for individual patients. On the negative side is concern about maintaining patient confidentiality and privacy, an expectation that must be met with diligent attention to appropriate system management and careful individual protection of information, passwords, and other access sources for the EHR.

As communication moves into the cyber environment with the use of the EHR, e-mail and attachments, intranets, chat rooms for clinical discussions/meetings, and further into the realm of social media (see later discussion in this chapter), the style of health care recording is changing. Nurses' electronic clinical notes often comprise detailed checklists, which are designed to address a myriad of potential findings and streamline time spent charting. However, most checklist pages include a box for additional comments/explanations, and charting programs include some vehicle for a narrative entry. The following discussion is just as applicable to electronic charting as to pen-and-paper charting—perhaps even more so. By their very nature, checklists do not allow for the unexpected or aberrant event. As tempting as it may be to confine the nursing record to the checklists, some occurrences simply cannot be adequately described without a narrative entry.

Accuracy

Absolute accuracy is paramount in recording legal documentation. For the nurse, this statement most specifically applies to the nursing notes and any other entry the nurse makes in the patient's chart. Every effort should be made to report concisely, descriptively, and truthfully. To write "Patient walked today" is not adequate. A more concise and descriptive entry reads, "Patient walked to the nurses' station and back three times this shift, a total distance of 96 yards." (Many hospitals have distance measures marked in the hallway for this purpose.)

Consider the following situation: Cody Johnson, RN, entered the patient's room and found her agitated and speaking loudly into the telephone as she twisted her hair with her free hand. She was crying and periodically pounded the bedside table with her fist. Later, the patient told Cody that she had been talking with her mother. Would it be appropriate for Cody to chart, "Patient became very angry with her mother while talking on the telephone"? No. The nurse must be diligent not to include personal judgments or quantify the patient's emotional state in such terms.

More accurately, Cody could chart, "Patient found crying while talking on the telephone in a loud tone to her mother. Patient was twisting her hair and hitting bedside table with her fist." The information is descriptive and states exactly what Cody observed factually without any judgmental conclusions. If, however, the patient had said, "My mother makes me so mad," Cody could have charted the statement as a direct quote (enclosed in quotation marks).

Attention to Detail

In addition to absolute accuracy, written documents should be descriptive. As mentioned previously, information should be quantified whenever possible. How many feet did the patient walk? How many times was the patient out of bed? How many cubic centimeters of fluid did the patient drink? Precisely what did the patient say?

Words can be used to depict a verbal picture of a wound, rash, bruise, or any type of injury or situation. Illustrative terms can create a mental image for the person reading the notes, memo, or other communication. Descriptive categories can include measurement, color, position, location, drainage, or condition when speaking of a physical condition; time, setting, people present, issues, or goals when reporting a discussion; and direct quotes when describing a meeting, conference, evaluation, or other interchange. Consider the differences between the following written communications:

- "1000: Dressing change completed. Site healthy."
- "1000: Dressing change completed. Edges of 4-inch surgical wound approximated, no drainage noted. Skin pink without any redness or edema."

BOX 19.1   Incomplete E-Mail Message
Date: 12/18/2015
To: Bonnie Thompson, RN, BSN, Nurse Manager From: Jessica Lindsay, RN, BSN, Charge Nurse Subject: Student precepting
I have had lots of complaints about Lucas Alfred's treatment of students. I do not think he should be assigned as a preceptor anymore and do not plan to do so from now on.

The second entry allows the reader to "see" the wound mentally and follow the progress of healing, even when unable to be present at the time of the dressing change. A good rule when describing any kind of break in skin integrity—from a stabbing, a surgical wound, an intravenous line, and so on—is to describe color, drainage, and presence or absence of edema.

Consider the written communication in Box 19.1. What does this message really tell the nurse manager? Not much—only that there is some kind of perceived problem between Lucas and the students. The nurse manager cannot tell, from the information provided, whether the problem is "real," is based on a bias of Jessica's or a student, or has occurred more than once; whether an interpersonal communication problem or misunderstanding exists; or whether obvious mistreatment of a student or students has occurred.

Now consider the written communication in Box 19.2. Carefully constructing a factual message of this length is more time-consuming initially, but it will save a lot of frustration in the long run. The nurse manager now has a clear picture of what has occurred and knows that an ongoing problem exists. Most appropriately, Jessica will speak to Bonnie about the problem, even if only briefly. However, a written account of the incident must be submitted and should be composed promptly while the facts are freshly remembered. Additionally, written communication often is the first source of contact because the nurse manager is not likely to be immediately available on all shifts.

The skill of writing concisely yet descriptively must be developed. Over some time, nurses build a repertoire of phrases and illustrative terminology that are useful and effective. Often, when a nurse is stumped as to how to express a situation, she or he will ask a colleague, "How would you write . . .?" Accessing the experience and expertise of nursing peers is productive in terms of

BOX 19.2 Descriptive, Thorough E-Mail Message

Date: 12/18/2015

To: Bonnie Thompson, RN, BSN, Nurse Manager
From: Jessica Lindsay, RN, BSN, Charge Nurse
Subject: Student precepting

Today (Monday, August 18) at 0710 I observed what appeared to be an animated conversation between Lucas Alfred, RN, and John Roberts, a student nurse from North Hills University. As I moved toward them, I heard Lucas say loudly, "Well, you better stay with me because I am not going to come looking for you all day. I know how lazy students are." I asked Lucas, "Is there a problem?" He replied, "Oh, no problem. I just hate having students, that's all. They're more trouble than they're worth." I asked Lucas, "Would you prefer that I reassign the student?" He shrugged his shoulders and walked away. I suggested to the student that I assign him to another nurse for the day. He responded, "I'd really appreciate that. Mr. Alfred has let me know since I arrived that he didn't want to work with me."

Because this group of students has been on the unit 2 days per week for the past 3 weeks, I spoke to the other students who had worked with Lucas and asked them how things had gone. The other three students who have worked with him reported similar experiences.

I would like to arrange a time to meet with you and Lucas to address this problem.

BOX 19.3 Unclear, Rambling E-Mail Message

Date: 12/18/2015

To: Bonnie Thompson, RN, BSN, Nurse Manager
From: Jessica Lindsay, RN, BSN, Charge Nurse
Subject: Student precepting

Today at about 0730 (it may have been earlier because I don't remember whether the breakfast trays had been served or not), I observed what appeared to be an animated conversation between Lucas Alfred, RN, and John Roberts, SN, a student nurse from North Hills University. I thought they might be arguing, but I couldn't tell for sure, so I decided to go over and see what the conversation was about. It really seemed like Lucas was angry because he was talking loudly and not smiling and neither was the student smiling, and I heard Lucas say, "Well, you better stay with me because I am not going to come looking for you all day. I know how lazy students are." Well I could just imagine how that made the student feel, so I asked, "Is there a problem?" even though it was pretty obvious that something was wrong. Lucas said, "Oh, no problem. I just hate having students, that's all. They're more trouble than they're worth." I asked Lucas, "Would you prefer that I reassign the student?" He shrugged his shoulders and walked away. Well I don't know for sure about the student, but I really thought that was rude. I suggested to the student that I assign him to another nurse for the day. He responded, "I'd really appreciate that. He has let me know since I arrived that he didn't want to work with me." Well I know how that would make me feel—to be a student and be treated that way.

The same group of students has been on the unit 2 days a week for the past 3 weeks (maybe a month, I'm not sure, and some of them may have been here on makeup days too), so I talked to other students who had worked with Lucas and asked them how things had been going. They said he'd acted the same way to them. We need to talk to him.

problem solving while also demonstrating respect for the colleague.

Thoroughness

The message examples in the previous section also illustrate the need for thoroughness. In addition to being descriptive in terms of the incident, Jessica's message in Box 19.2 reported her interview with other nursing students. By doing so, Jessica is thorough in describing and reporting the extent of the problem she has discovered. Providing such completeness of information helps prevent communication breakdown. Anticipating and answering relevant questions before they are asked exemplifies thoroughness and clarifies communication.

Conciseness

Written communication must be concise. The message must state the necessary information as clearly and as briefly as possible. Consider the message written in Box 19.3. Whew! Extraneous details tend to confuse more than clarify. An inherent dilemma often develops as the nurse attempts to determine how to be descriptive and concise at the same time. One must determine what facts are pertinent to enable the reader to understand the true message. When in doubt and when appropriate, the writer can ask another party to read the message and provide feedback as to what the reader believes the message means. However, the right to confidentiality and privacy of the people involved must be observed. This basic principle applies to patients, families, students, members of the health care team—to all persons. Consequently, the nurse must be as judicious in handling written material in a confidential matter as with any other form of communication.

Electronic Communication

When speaking aloud you punctuate constantly—with body language. Your listener hears commas, dashes, question marks, exclamation points, [and] quotation marks as you shout, whisper, pause, wave your arms, roll your eyes, wrinkle your brow. In writing, punctuation plays the role of body language. It helps the readers hear the way you want to be heard.

Russell Baker

More and more communication is computer-based, using e-mail, text messages, chat rooms, file attachments, and other electronic modes. The computer-based written record can be somewhat more transient than other written documents. For example, e-mails are often read and then deleted. However, remember that communication via the computer can be saved and is often retrievable even after deletion. As with any form of written communication, computer-based interaction loses nonverbal cues. Therefore, it is important for the sender to elicit feedback and/or for the receiver to ask for clarification if the meaning of the communication is not clear.

HANDOFF REPORT

A handoff is a transfer and acceptance of patient care responsibility achieved through effective communication.

The Joint Commission (2017)

A handoff report occurs any time the primary care of a patient is transferred from one health care provider to another. Examples include end of shift, relocation to another facility or unit within the current facility, and transfer to the operating room, radiology, dialysis, or other areas for testing or shorter periods of care. Every time patient care is transferred represents a potential for patient harm related to lack of

adequate information about the patient and his or her care needs. Information can be insufficient, inaccurate, untimely, misinterpreted, or undergo any number of other missteps that result in minor to severe harm to the patient. Once again, the sender-receiver dichotomy with all the associated communication skills is of primary importance.

The Joint Commission (2017) recognized the inherent danger of inadequate handoff reporting by issuing a *Sentinel Event Alert* (PC.02.02.01 EP2) identifying the associated risks and frequent underlying causes as well as suggestions for improvement. Attention to handoff reporting is particularly important because of the high number of handoffs that occur in health care and the severity of errors that can result.

Perhaps the most important condition of handoff reporting is that it must be real-time, face-to-face. Recording the report or providing it in written or electronic form leaves too many opportunities for missed data and misunderstanding. Give and take between the sender and receiver must occur so that clarification and feedback are possible. Certainly, written reinforcement of a verbal face-to-face report is essential. Reports should also be given in situations free from interruptions.

Many facilities use a standardized format or mnemonic for a systematic approach to end-of-shift and other handoff reports. In the absence of formal report formatting, individuals can certainly develop their own style of reporting that covers all aspects of the patient's condition and care. Following a systematic approach every time enhances the quality of the report, thereby protecting the patient.

Essentials of an effective report include the basic SBAR: situation, background, assessment, and recommendation (The Joint Commission, 2017) as well as pertinent information regarding patient events during your shift. Information should promote continuity of care. Consider:

- What events from the last shift continued on your shift and are likely to continue into the next shift? Providing a picture of ongoing care needs and patient responses prepares the accepting provider (receiver) for effective continuation of care.
- When addressing standard criteria, report what happened with the patient on your shift. For example:
  Diet: Regular, patient ate about 60% of meals today but takes fluids easily; offered liquid nutrition drink between meals.

Activity: Up ad lib, patient gets up in the room without difficulty; he walked from his room to the unit entry door twice today, requires accompanying staff because he becomes weak when walking longer distances.

- Offer a brief head-to-toe assessment with a focus on the systems of concern.

Always give the receiver an opportunity to ask questions and clarify information. If a question or problem requires further exploration, work with the receiver to determine the appropriate action. Consistently be aware that it is the sender's responsibility to relay sufficient information to move the provision of quality care forward.

COMMUNICATION STYLES

Communication is influenced by a myriad of individual characteristics learned over a lifetime. However, communication specialists generally recognize four basic communication styles: (1) assertive, (2) aggressive, (3) passive, and (4) passive-aggressive.

Assertive Communication

The healthiest form of communication is the assertive style. Assertive individuals pronounce their basic rights without violating the rights of others. Assertive communicators are honest and direct while valuing and respecting other individuals' views and seeking a win-win solution without the use of manipulation or game playing. Assertiveness includes active listening and reflective feedback so that other individuals recognize that their opinions are valued as the assertive communicator seeks to find an acceptable solution without compromising his or her own needs.

Assertive communication requires self-confidence and the ability to set limits rather than to succumb to pressure to avoid disappointing or hurting others at the expense of one's own needs and expectations. Although it is the most effective style of communication, healthy assertiveness is difficult for many people to develop. Therefore, assertive communication is typically the style most people use least.

Aggressive Communication

Aggressive communicators make decisions for themselves and others with the intent of always coming out "the winner." Aggressive individuals want their needs met exclusively and immediately, using guilt, hurt, anger, and a repertoire of other manipulation tools. Aggressiveness may use honesty but in a hurtful, manipulative way. Aggressive individuals commonly feel superior to others and behave in very controlling ways. Persons with whom they communicate often feel humiliated, defensive, resentful, and hurt. Aggressive behavior often leads to and certainly escalates conflict.

Passive Communication

Passive communicators are the polar opposite of aggressive communicators. They allow others to make decisions for them in the hope of avoiding confrontation or difficult situations. Passive communicators are typically inhibited, indirect, and self-denying because they feel those characteristics make for the safe route. If they win in a situation, it is purely by chance, typically because they happen to share the opinion of the more aggressive person in the exchange. Passive individuals are dishonest because they would rather succumb than state their true feelings or needs.

Passive-Aggressive Communication

Passive-aggressive communicators combine the worst of both styles. These individuals avoid direct confrontation while manipulating others in order to achieve their personal goals. They appear to be honest but "come in the back door" by undermining other individuals through gossip, pouting, playing the victim, and other manipulative behaviors that create or escalate conflict. They win in situations by making other individuals look bad.

SPECIAL INFLUENCES ON COMMUNICATION

Development of truly effective communication necessitates understanding various circumstances that influence communication. In addition to the concepts discussed up to this point, characteristics exist that might impede efficacious exchange of information. Issues such as gender differences, generational differences, cultural diversity, and dissimilarities in the professional approach of the various health care disciplines all contribute to disparate understandings and interpretations.

Communication and Gender Differences

A significant clarification must be made regarding communication between men and women. The information about gender differences resulting from socialization (although based on research and many years of observations and writings) consists of generalizations and should be viewed from that perspective. Attributes described do not necessarily apply to all persons or all the time. Nevertheless, a plethora of observations indicate that men and women solve problems, make decisions, and communicate from different perspectives on the basis of socialization that begins shortly after birth. Typically, boys are taught to be tough and competitive; girls are taught to be nice and avoid conflict. Dr. Pat Heim (1995) suggests, "Playing team sports, boys learn to compete, be aggressive, play to win, strategize, take risks, mask emotions, and focus on the goal line." Regarding girls' play, Dr. Heim comments, "Relationships are central in girls' culture and therefore they learn to negotiate differences, seek win-win solutions, and focus on what is fair for all instead of winning."

For the most part, women work toward compromise, even when it means relinquishing some of the original goal. Often, women use indirect channels such as questions to guide a conversation toward the point they want to make. Preserving relationships is usually of paramount importance to women. The role of peacemaker and nurturer has been a traditional expectation of women throughout the ages.

Generally, men work toward winning. Traditional role expectations of men have included provider and protector. Men learn early in life how to focus on goals and move aggressively toward accomplishment. Team sports teach men that relationships are not destroyed in the "battle" (Heim, 1995). Consequently, men have been socialized to behave assertively when such performance is needed in pursuit of the goal and then move on without loss of friendships. Women have been socialized to believe that assertive behavior will endanger relationships and that conflict should be avoided to preserve friendships.

Men typically use communication as a tool to deliver information, whereas women value the process of communication itself as an important part of the relationship. Therefore, in an effort to improve communication, men might try spending more time in discussion, and women might try to phrase comments more succinctly.

Progress has been made over the years as women move into more lateral working situations, but the problem of gender communication style differences persists. Booher (2017) echoes these thoughts in light of today's work environment: "Little did we know that the communication differences we experienced as children on the playground would move from the classroom to the boardroom. Neither men nor women are better communicators. They're just different." Awareness of this difference supports effective communication in the health care environment, where effective transfer of information is essential.

Communication and Generational Differences

In recent years, much attention has been focused on the fact that our society has at least four distinct generational groups. They are variously described as follows:

- Silents/Traditionalists/Veterans—born before the mid-1940s
- Baby Boomers—born between the mid-1940s and the mid-1960s
- Generation X (Gen Xers)—born between the mid-1960s and 1980
- Generation Y/Millennials—born between 1981 and 2000
- Homeland Generation or Homelanders—variously described as born since 9/11/01 or 2000 (CBS News, 2010; Nurse Educator, 2009).

Awareness of generational differences and the accompanying differences in communication styles is important to nurses from two perspectives—communication with the patients/families and communication with one another.

Traditionalists. Members of this oldest surviving generation follow the rules, valuing authority, formality, and the chain-of-command. They take pride in accomplishment, are strong decision makers, and have a good sense of self. Tradition is important to them, making them more likely to make decisions according to what has or has not worked in the past. Appearance and respect are important to them. Therefore, they appreciate communication in a more formal style, appropriate dress, and displays of respect. They may be put off by multiple tattoos, earrings, and various styles of scrubs or other health care attire. They are more likely to respond to formal communication than to the casual or direct approach in a spontaneous setting.

Baby Boomers. Baby Boomers grew up in an era of prosperity that formed their worldview, values, and work ethic. Although they questioned political policy, authority, and social mores, they ultimately embraced work as a definition of self-worth, adopting a strong work ethic, becoming goal-directed, and experiencing the accompanying struggle with work–personal life balance. These attributes lead to an expectation of similar commitment from younger generations. Effective communication with Baby Boomers includes direct information in a personable approach, a formal plan, and acknowledgment of value, purpose, and respect.

Generation X. The milieu that Gen Xers experienced during their formative years was fraught with insecurity. The breakdown in many of the traditional security sources previous generations enjoyed helped create a generation of independent problem solvers. The increase in divorces; the prevalence of acquired immunodeficiency syndrome, gangs, and abortions; and the exposure of corrupt government officials and policies created an unstable societal environment in which individuals who could meet challenges, recognize and respond to opportunity, and become comfortable with diversity excelled. Xers value autonomy in their work, decision making, and life choices, but at the same time value the team and teamwork. Although they may appear to move too quickly and to be insensitive, having grown up in a technology-based society, they are capable of fierce commitment to tasks they value. These individuals should be allowed to be highly involved in decision making about health care—whether they are the providers or the recipients.

Millennials. Millenials are the most diverse and most globally thinking generation in the workforce, in large part because of technology, which provides unfettered access to global issues and occurrences. Many come from or are close to "nontraditional" families and have witnessed unparalleled violence within the borders of our country. Their comfort with technology and diversity are hallmark characteristics. They value inclusion, team effort, and collective action, and they are quite adaptable to rapid change. Because they are focused on cohesiveness and peer orientation, they value immediate feedback. Such activities as "huddles"—periodic and end-of-shift briefings that allow the team to "stay informed, review work, make plans, and move ahead rapidly" (Institute for Healthcare Improvement, 2014)—work particularly well with this group of communicators.

Homelanders. The line between Millennials and Homelanders is blurry, starting with the choice of years for transition from one to the other. Influences on Homelanders include the cascade of occurrences within our borders starting with 9/11 as well as continuously burgeoning technology. The year 2008, with "the recession and the election of the nation's first black president" (CBS News, 2010) is heralded as a seminal year in the development of this group, which is not quite at working age but approaching it quickly. Like Traditionalists, this generational group is growing up in a time of financial and political insecurity at home and globally. They are comfortable with multitasking, diversity, and technology like no one before them. Homelanders are expected to pursue college education as a matter of necessity as the gap between those who are financially sound and those who are not continues to widen. It remains to be seen how they will relate in the workplace or in the role of health care recipient, but we can expect articulate, motivated, tech-savvy individuals coming of age in the near future.

Communication and Cultural Diversity

Although Chapter 10 is devoted to cultural and social issues, it is important to highlight cultural issues specific to communication. Sensitivity to cultural differences is an integral part of the nurse's responsibility. Many cultural beliefs are tightly interwoven with strong religious convictions. Societies throughout the world depend on a variety of alternative healing sources as strongly as or even more strongly than on medical science. Some people rarely have an opportunity to interface with medical science as it is known in developed countries.

The obvious difficulty is a potential language barrier. Even if the person speaks English as a second language, the preponderance of slang terms and colloquialisms can confound a literal translation. Additionally, the stress associated with illness and possibly hospitalization only adds to the potential for misunderstanding and frustration. Fortunately, most communities have interpreters willing to translate in the health care setting. The variety of language interpreters (including sign language for the deaf) available even in smaller communities is surprising.

Many forms of communication do not carry the same meanings in various cultures. In some instances, direct eye contact is to be avoided if possible. Touch, also considered a positive communication technique in Western culture, may be perceived as a serious invasion of privacy. Some gestures considered innocuous in one culture may represent vulgarity in another. Some cultures strictly adhere to paternalism; unless the male head of the family agrees to a procedure or treatment, the family member will refuse under any circumstance. Although many people share a sense of modesty, some cultures experience a greater feeling of violation at having to expose certain body parts than do others. The consumption of certain foods, the use of blood or blood products—the possibilities of culturally diverse practices are endless. The prudent nurse must become knowledgeable about the specific cultural practices in the region of her or his employment. (See Chapter 10 for further discussion of communication issues related to culture.)

Interprofessional Team Communication

The *interprofessional team* is composed of people from a variety of disciplines who approach health care from the unique perspectives of the theories and therapies of their individual professions. Consider the variety represented by nurses, physicians, dietitians, respiratory therapists, pharmacists, occupational therapists, physical therapists, psychologists, and social workers. Then add to the mosaic the sublevel of specialists: cardiologists, endocrinologists, oncologists, orthopedists, clinical nurse specialists, recreational therapists, nurse anesthetists, nurse practitioners, and nurse scientists. RNs with varied educational backgrounds (diploma, associate degree, Bachelor or Master of Science in nursing) and licensed vocational nurses are often found in the same unit with similar assignments. Now add managers, administrators, unlicensed assistive personnel, clerical staff, accountants, and housekeeping, to name a few. Also consider cultural and generational differences among health care professionals and workers. Is it any wonder that communication disasters occur?

All of the positive communication techniques previously discussed must be used to clearly understand another's perception. Listening is an essential tool for determination of the intended message as seen from the unique perspective of the other discipline. Frequent clarification and a sense of "safety" are paramount as people explore the meanings that each person attributes to the situation and the discipline-specific suggested solutions. Realization that the fundamental goal of all health care professionals and of ancillary staff is to provide quality patient care should facilitate positive communication.

Confidentiality and Privacy

No discussion of communication is complete without reference to issues of confidentiality and privacy. Breach of confidentiality and the patient's right to privacy through careless gossip has ethical and legal ramifications. Thoughtless conversation in the elevator, the cafeteria, the parking lot, or any other public place has created heartache for the patient and the health care provider alike.

Other sites where communication about confidential or personal patient issues needs to be controlled include the nurses' station, any desks or tables along the halls, and the utility rooms. Such locations are not often viewed as "public" places, but many people pass by these areas and overhear information. Exchange of patient information should occur only between persons with the need and right to know and should take place in private areas.

SOCIAL MEDIA—WARNING! WARNING! WARNING!

. . . the inherent nature of social networking invites the sharing of personal information or work experiences that may reflect poorly on a nurse's professionalism.
American Nurses Association, Principles for Social Networking and the Nurse, 2011

Social Media: Good and Bad

Social media sites have burgeoned in the last decade, connecting health care professionals across the country and globally. Health care–related sites, chat rooms, blogs, forums, and video sites provide an unparalleled opportunity to network, share, and problem-solve health care issues.

Nurses can positively use electronic media to share workplace experiences, particularly those events that are challenging or emotionally charged.
National Council of State Boards of Nursing [NCSBN], 2011

The professional value of social media comes with a very serious caveat. The patient retains his or her right to confidentiality and privacy in every medium. Not only must nurses be very careful in not using a patient's name, but they must be thorough in avoiding any other type of identifying information. Such information may include geographical location, facility name, room number, or the patient's age, gender, and diagnosis combined with any of these data.

Nurses, like most of our society, are connected in their personal lives to multiple online social media sources such as Facebook, Twitter, and various blogs. Sitting at home alone with a computer may create a sense of privacy, but nothing could be further from the truth. Postings intended for immediate family or friends and protected by the site's privacy policy are not infallible. Anything posted online exists forever on a server somewhere, even if it is deleted from the site. This information is forever discoverable in a court of law and can be used in a trial (NCSBN, 2011). Friends might find your story so touching or endearing that they repost to their friends, and the story takes on a life of its own with no available control of dissemination on your part.

A good example of the unintended outcome of a moment's misjudgment is presented in NCSBN's (2011) social media guidelines. A nursing student took a picture of a minor child (with permission) and posted it to her Facebook page with a comment about his bravery during his illness and how much she loved her chosen profession. Although she did not identify the patient by name, the patient's room number was visible in the photo. The patient and his hospital were identified by others viewing the post. Ultimately, the hospital was charged with a violation of the Health Information Portability and Accountability Act (HIPAA), the nursing program was barred from the clinical site, and the student was expelled. Nursing board actions against a student who makes inappropriate disclosures on a social media site could include the following:

- Unprofessional conduct
- Unethical conduct
- Moral turpitude
- Mismanagement of patient records
- Revealing a privileged communication
- Breach of confidentiality (NCSBN, 2011)

The nursing student's actions in this example also violated state and federal law, putting her at jeopardy of "both criminal and civil penalties, including fines and possible jail time" (NCSBN, 2011).

Certainly it was never the student's intent to behave unethically, but her actions created this cascade of events. As a profession, we are held to a very high ethical standard to protect our clients' confidentiality. We must be very attentive to our actions.

Another issue that has appeared is the use of texting for communication of patient information among health care providers. Concerns about texting are that the receiving individual is not able to unequivocally verify the identity of the person sending the text and there is no way to make a copy of the original message to place in the permanent record. Anything that is sent electronically has the potential to be inadvertently misdirected and/or intercepted. The use of secure texting may become a reality in the future as technology advances; nurses are encouraged to learn about and understand policies regarding texting in the health care organizations where they practice.

Proper use of social media can open venues of learning, career advancement, mentoring, and networking, enhancing the global perspective in your nursing career. Use this opportunity wisely and with consideration of the permanence, wide visibility (beyond anything you may intend), and potential impact of your postings.

Online Etiquette

Interactions online are guided by the same sense of decency that any other style of communication dictates. Here are some simple rules:

- Be nice. Be ethical. Don't say anything to someone online that you wouldn't say in a face-to-face conversation, and certainly don't fan the flame of conflict or anger.
- Remember the TMI (too much information) concept. Don't give more personal information than others want to hear.
- Write with clarity. Reread what you've written to determine whether it is clear or whether it might be interpreted differently from what you intended.
- Respect others, including their privacy.
- Use discretion. Online postings live forevermore in cyberspace.
- Obey copyright laws.

UNDERSTANDING AND MANAGING CONFLICT

Nurses maintain professional, respectful, and caring relationships with colleagues and are committed to fair treatment, transparency, integrity-preserving compromise, and the best resolution of conflicts.

American Nurses Association, Code of Ethics for Nurses with Interpretive Statements

The Nature of Conflict

A major goal of communication is to establish understanding and cooperation with others. However, much of our social environment is characterized by interactions that involve conflict, misunderstanding, and a failure to communicate. When more than one person is involved in the interaction, a potential exists for disagreement and misunderstanding. When the interaction becomes stressful, taking on a competitive, hostile, or oppositional nature, it can be classified as conflict (Mayer, 2000). Conflicts stemming from differences in goals or desires are not good or bad. The two fundamental bases for conflict are information (one person has information that another does not have, or two individuals have different sets of information) and perception (people see things differently on the basis of their unique belief systems). Despite the discomfort, disparate points of view can result in constructive behavior and positive outcomes.

Conflict, like stress, can have both beneficial and detrimental consequences to an individual. Some of the benefits that may arise from conflict include: (1) recognize talents and innovative abilities; (2) identify an outlet for expression of aggressive urges; (3) introduce innovation and change; (4) diagnose problems or areas of concern; and (5) establish unity (Mayer, 2000). Harmful consequences of prolonged conflict include a negative effect on emotional and physical well-being, an emphasis on one's own welfare over that of the group, a diversion of time and energy from important goals, financial and emotional costs, and personal fatigue.

Most of us experience abundant opportunities for conflict, which may be related to the fact that we bring to our relationships an accumulation of attitudes, beliefs, opinions, and habits. Thus conflict is normal and is not necessarily something to avoid. Although uncomfortable, conflict signals the presence of diverse points of view, which can spark creativity, nourish growth, and strengthen relationships. Maintaining an environment supportive of professional, clear, and sensitive communication enables individuals to fight more productively, with less hurt, and with a greater chance of resolving differences and disagreements. Characteristics of environments that support professional communication are (Gibb, 1961):

- *Empathy:* Involves feeling what the other person is feeling and seeing the situation as they see it; entails believing that the other person's feelings are valid, legitimate, and justified.
- *Equality:* Holds that all participants in the process are equal; respect for individual differences is apparent, and people are comfortable expressing themselves freely and openly.
- *Openness:* Requires that feelings and thoughts are stated directly and honestly; no attempt is made to hide or disguise the real object of disagreement.
- *Positivity:* Entails capitalizing on agreements and using them as a basis for approaching disagreements and impasses; conflict is viewed as positive, and individuals involved express positive feelings for one another and the relationship.
- *Supportiveness:* Allows feelings to be expressed with spontaneity rather than with strategy; requires flexibility and a willingness to change personal opinions and positions.

Adopting these communication attitudes and using the positive communication strategies previously discussed can prevent most episodes of conflict in the workplace. However, situations are bound to arise in which the nurse will need to know how to handle a conflict situation and achieve a positive resolution.

Conflict Resolution

People's ability to connect with one another, especially during times of conflict, depends on their capacity to tune into the subtle messages that reveal how a message is actually being received. We seldom create conflict intentionally. Rather, it occurs because we may not be aware of how our own behavior contributes to interpersonal problems. Because interpersonal communication is fragile, there may be barriers to an effectual and meaningful process. Successful resolution to conflict begins to occur when people are aware of their own and others' feelings and emotions and believe that these concerns are relevant and respected.

The first step in conflict resolution is to recognize how individuals manage conflict. The most common conflict resolution styles are:

- *Avoidance:* One person uses passive behaviors and withdraws from the conflict; neither person is able to pursue goals.
- *Accommodation:* One person puts aside his or her goals to satisfy the other person's desires.
- *Force:* One person achieves his or her own goals at the expense of the other person.
- *Compromise:* Both people give up something to get partial goal attainment.
- *Collaboration:* Both people actively try to find solutions that will satisfy them both.

Awareness of one's usual conflict resolution style will go far in understanding how one's own behavior contributes to disagreements. For example, if an individual nurse recognizes avoidance as his or her common style of dealing with conflict, then it would be important for that nurse to review the communication strategies presented in this chapter to identify specific techniques that can be used to develop a more collaborative style of conflict resolution.

Important points to remember: Don't make it personal or take it personally. Use "I" rather than "you" messages to avoid defensive responses. Keep the focus on the issue, not personalities. Do not create an environment in which other individuals respond defensively in order to protect themselves. Do not respond to a conflictive situation as a personal attack—even if it feels like one. Focus and refocus on the issue or behavior rather than the individual.

Another—and very important—step in conflict resolution is active listening (Axelrod and Johnson, 2003). Many of us are apprehensive or reticent when communicating during times of conflict, but active listening can reduce the emotional charge from the situation so that both parties can deal with their differences and assist in resolving the conflict. Some excellent active listening techniques and examples are provided in Table 19.1.

Finally, the principle that underscores all successful conflict resolution is that all people involved must view their conflict as a problem to be solved mutually so that each has a sense of winning or discovering options that are acceptable to all. Although this is an easy principle to understand, it can be challenging to put into practice. If both people can remain open, honest, and respectful of each other's positions, feelings of resentment may be minimized. Box 19.4

TABLE 19.1	**Active Listening Techniques**		
Technique	**Why Done**	**How Done**	**Example**
Paraphrasing the content of the message	Shows that you are listening, checking meaning, and interpreting the content	Restate the basic ideas and facts in your own words	"What I hear you saying is that you weren't consulted" or "So, you weren't consulted about this?"
Reflecting the emotion of the message	Shows understanding of how the person feels; reflects what is observed rather than what is heard; helps the other person evaluate his or her own feelings after hearing them expressed by someone else	Listen to voice tone, and watch for nonverbal cues that indicate feelings; listen to what the person tells you he or she is feeling; state back how you perceive the feeling	"So you are angry about what happened?"
Open questioning	Obtains more information and avoids any assumptions about what the other person is thinking; encourages the other person to talk	Ask questions that begin with "what," "how," "when," and "where"; use questions that begin with "why" cautiously	"What happened after you spoke with her?"
Acknowledging	Conveys that you appreciate the other person's perspective; recognizes his or her worth and actions	Acknowledge the value of the person's issues and feelings (shows appreciation for his or her efforts and actions)	"That must be very frustrating."

Continued

TABLE 19.1	Active Listening Techniques—cont'd		
Technique	Why Done	How Done	Example
Summarizing	Reviews progress; pulls together important ideas and information; establishes a foundation for further discussion	Restate the central ideas and feelings you have heard	"So basically what is most important to you is . . . ."
Framing	Communicates your message in a way the other person will be more open to hearing; increases the opportunity of meeting his or her goals	Present your message in a hopeful, nonjudgmental, and open-ended way; point to common ground and away from differences	"I think it would be best to speak to your supervisor directly about these issues, because she is more directly involved with implementation than I am; what do you think about this idea?"
Reframing	Helps others see their concerns in a new light; broadens the meaning of an issue to identify needs or interests; diffuses negative feelings; establishes a focus for resolution	Recognize underlying needs; reword concerns from negative to neutral or positive, past to future, problem to opportunity	"It sounds as if you would like more direct communication to resolve concerns."

From Axelrod, L., and Johnson, R. (2003). *Successful resolution.* Vancouver, BC: The Neutral Zone. Used with permission from The Neutral Zone, Vancouver, BC.

BOX 19.4   Professional Response to Verbal Conflict

1. Maintain an open and empathetic tone of voice.
2. Maintain eye contact (keeping cultural differences in mind). This may be difficult, but it conveys to the other party that you are confident and competent.
3. Maintain an open body stance with your hands at your sides or open toward the person (but not invading the other person's space). Do not cross your arms, tap your foot, wag your finger, or perform any body language that is commonly associated with anger.
4. Do not physically back away unless you perceive you actually are in physical danger. By standing your ground, your will convey the message of assurance through your carriage.
5. Be aware of your own values, beliefs, and cultural perspectives.
6. When a conversation is obviously escalating, move to a more private location.
7. Listen actively and carefully without criticizing or being defensive.
8. Focus on the problem or issue, not the person(s) involved.
9. Use "I" messages that state your thoughts, feelings, and beliefs in an open and clear manner.
10. Use nonjudgmental, noninflammatory language, such as "It seems to me . . . ."
11. Establish ground rules to maintain a safe environment for dialogue, such as that only one person speaks at a time while the other listens.
12. Offer explanations, but do not make excuses.
13. Be redundant, summarize, and convey the same idea in more than one way.
14. Try to understand the intended meaning of what other people are saying.
15. Identify ideas that clarify your own issues and concerns, and that are helpful to find solutions.
16. Avoid unhelpful responses to conflict, such as arguing, sarcasm, moralizing, disbelief, contradiction, criticism, ridicule, and threats.
17. Use metaphors and analogies as gentle ways to create and maintain rapport.
18. Maintain a positive context by stating what you want, and avoid stating what you do not want.
19. Repeat, or play back, what you believe you are hearing.
20. If you say you will take care of something, report something, or change something, do it. Then seek out the person to whom you made the commitment and report your action and the result. Little else goes as far as demonstrating that you are dependable and want to work toward a solution.
21. In more difficult situations, consider using a neutral facilitator who understands his or her role.

presents some basic strategies that can augment a professional response to conflict. The principles listed are remarkably effective in cases of conflict and will help the nurse present herself or himself as a confident and competent professional who will not react to inappropriate behavior in like form but also will not withdraw from the issues. As always, the focus should be kept on quality patient care.

SUMMARY

In today's health care environment, where high stress levels are all too common and patient safety, quality care, and financial constraints are everyday concerns, nurses play a vital role in promoting a productive work environment in which trust and rapport among the health care team is common and all are working toward the same goal—delivery of safe, timely, efficient, effective, and patient-centered health care. Professional, clear, and sensitive communication provides the foundation for creating such supportive, effective care environments.

The first step toward developing a professional communication style is understanding the many complex and varied factors that influence the communication process, such as gender, cultural, generational, and interdisciplinary differences, each of which presents many challenges for the nurse who must strive to understand and to be understood. The second step is adopting positive communication techniques, which include developing trust, using "I" messages, establishing eye contact, keeping promises, feeling empathy, using an open communication style, clarifying information, and being aware of body language. The third step is for each nurse to reflect on his or her use of negative communication techniques, such as blocking, false assurances, conflicting messages, logical fallacies, and cognitive distortions, that may interfere with effective relationships with patients and coworkers. Recognizing—then avoiding—the use of these negative communication techniques is essential if the nurse is to move toward a more professional communication style. The next step in developing a professional communication style is learning to address and resolve conflict in a positive way. Role playing with trusted colleagues using the conflict resolution techniques discussed in this chapter can help the nurse become more adept at managing conflict.

Demonstrating a professional, clear, and sensitive communication style is an essential component of the professional nursing skill set. As the foundation for effective, supportive work environments and excellent patient care, professional communication must be one goal every nurse strives to achieve.

REFERENCES

American Association of Critical Care Nurses. (2016). *Standards for establishing and sustaining healthy work environments.* Retrieved from https://www.aacn.org/~/media/aacn-website/nursing-excellence/healthy-work-environment/execsum.pdf?la=en.

American Nurses Association. (2010). *Principles for nursing documentation.* Silver Spring, MD: Nursesbooks. Retrieved from http://nursesbooks.org/Main-Menu/eBooks/Principles/eBook-Principles-for-Nursing-Documentation.aspx.

American Nurses Association. (2011). *Principles for social networking and the nurse.* Retrieved from https://www.nursingworld.org/~4af4f2/globalassets/docs/ana/ethics/social-networking.pdf.

American Nurses Association. (2015). *Code of ethics for nurses with interpretive statements.* Retrieved from http://nursingworld.org/DocumentVault/Ethics-1/Code-of-Ethics-for-Nurses.html.

Axelrod, L., & Johnson, R. (2003). *Successful resolution.* Vancouver, BC: The Neutral Zone.

Booher, D. (2017). *Gender benders: Gender negotiation communication style differences: Women.* Retrieved from https://www.negotiations.com/articles/gender-bender/.

Borg, J. (2011). *Body language: How to know what's really being said.* Dorchester, Dorset, UK: Dorset Press.

CBS News. (2010). *Generation X (and Y) are history: What's next?* Retrieved from http://www.cbsnews.com/stories/2010/06/10/business/main6568258.shtml.

Elgin, S. H. (1993). *Genderspeak: Men, women, and the gentle art of verbal self-defense.* New York: John Wiley & Sons.

Gibb, J. (1961). Defensive communication. *Journal of communication, 11,* 141–148.

Heim, P. (1995). Getting beyond "she said, he said". *Nursing administration quarterly*, *19*(2), 6–18.

Institute for Healthcare Improvement. (2014). *Huddles.* Retrieved from http://www.ihi.org/knowledge/Pages/Tools/Huddles.aspx.

Mayer, B. (2000). *The dynamics of conflict resolution.* San Francisco: Jossey-Bass.

Mehrabian, A. (1981). *Silent messages: Implicit communication of emotions and attitudes.* Beverly, MA: Wadsworth.

National Council of State Boards of Nursing. (2011). *A nurse's guide to the use of social media.* Retrieved from https://www.ncsbn.org/NCSBN_SocialMedia.pdf.

Nurse Educator. (2009). *Generational conflict in nursing: How to relate to colleagues from multiple generations.* Retrieved from http://journals.lww.com/nurseeducatoronline/Fulltext/2009/01000/Generational_Conflict_in_Nursing__How_to_Relate_to.12.aspx.

The Joint Commission. (2017). *Sentinel event alert: Inadequate hand-of communication.* https://www.jointcommission.org/assets/1/18/SEA_58_Hand_off_Comms_9_6_17_FINAL_(1).pdf.

The Joint Commission. (2016). *Busting the myths about engaging patients and families in patient safety*. Retrieved from https://www.jointcommission.org/busting_the_myths_about_engaging_patients_and_families_in_patient_safety/.

The Joint Commission. (2013). *SBAR - A powerful tool to help Improve communication!* Retrieved from https://www.jointcommission.org/at_home_with_the_joint_commission/sbar_%e2%80%93_a_powerful_tool_to_help_improve_communication/.

van Servellen, G. (1997). *Communication skills for the health Care professional: Concepts and techniques.* Gaithersburg, MD: Aspen.

20

Delegation—linking together for better care.

Effective Delegation and Supervision

Barbara Cherry, DNSc, MBA, RN, NEA-BC,
Margaret Elizabeth Strong, DNP, RN, NE-BC

ⓔ Additional resources are available online at: *http://evolve.elsevier.com/Cherry/*

LEARNING OUTCOMES

After studying this chapter, the reader will be able to:

1. Evaluate the effect of changes in the current health care system on nurse staffing patterns and responsibilities.
2. Outline six topic areas that the professional nurse should consider when making delegation decisions.
3. List nine essential requirements for safe and effective delegation.
4. Incorporate principles of delegation and supervision into professional nursing practice to ensure safe and legal patient care.

KEY TERMS

Accountability "To be answerable to oneself and others for one's own choices, decisions and actions" (American Nurses Association [ANA], 2015a).

Assignment The distribution of work that each staff member is responsible for during a given work period; includes routine care, activities, and procedures that are within the staff member's authorized scope of practice and/or job description (National Council of State Boards of Nursing [NCSBN], 2016; ANA and NCSBN, 2014).

Competency The ability of an individual to perform defined behaviors proficiently by demonstrating the appropriate knowledge, skills, attitudes, and professional judgment required for a specific role or setting.

Delegation Transferring to a competent staff member the authority and responsibility to perform a selected nursing task that the staff member would not normally be allowed to perform; the RN retains accountability for the delegated task (ANA and NCSBN, 2014).

Supervision The active process of directing, guiding, and influencing the outcome of an individual's performance of an activity or task (ANA, 2012).

Unlicensed assistive personnel (UAP) Individuals who have not received practice licenses but who are trained to function in an assistive role to the RN by performing patient care activities as delegated by the nurse; may include nursing assistants, clinical assistants, orderlies, health aides, and those with other titles designated within the work setting (NCSBN, 2016).

PROFESSIONAL/ETHICAL ISSUE

Nicole Adams, Registered Nurse (RN), has taken a position as the new charge nurse for a 24-bed medical-surgical unit at a long-term acute care and rehabilitation hospital. Nicole is excited about this new opportunity but is apprehensive because this is her first position as a charge nurse. After completing the hospital's orientation program, Nicole reports to her unit for her first official day as charge nurse. She is immediately approached by a licensed practical nurse (LPN), who says, "I've worked here for 8 years and I always can take care of everything. I'll complete all patient assessments and let you know about anything you might need to follow up with." Nicole is alarmed about this statement but knows she must handle the situation carefully to ensure she follows safe delegation practices while also developing a good working relationship with the LPN. Discuss what elements of delegation Nicole should consider in this situation and what the best approach with the LPN might be.

VIGNETTE

Glenda Miller, BSN (Bachelor of Science in Nursing), RN, is the charge nurse on a medical-surgical floor of a hospital. She has just received report from the 7 PM to 7 AM shift and is about to make assignments for the 7 AM to 7 PM shift. The philosophy of the unit is that the RN coordinates all patient care. Today on this 12-bed unit there are eight patients and four empty beds. The nursing staff consists of Ms. Miller, one RN, one LPN, one nursing assistant, and one unit secretary. The following interprofessional team members are available for specific patient care needs: respiratory therapist, physical therapist, occupational therapist, speech therapist, medical social worker, and chaplain. The patients are medically complex with extensive nursing care needs, including psychosocial and emotional support. The patients are described to Ms. Miller as follows:

502: Mr. A. is ventilator dependent with an infection that requires intravenous (IV) antibiotics every 12 hours. He needs to be out of bed in a chair twice a day. He has a stage I sacral decubitus ulcer and a percutaneous endoscopic gastrostomy (PEG) tube with bolus feedings. He is very hard of hearing, tries to speak, and becomes very frustrated and uncooperative.

503: Mrs. B., age 77, is on day 2 of 40 days of antibiotics for osteomyelitis. She is dehydrated with a central line in her right subclavian and on total parenteral nutrition (TPN). She needs to be out of bed and ambulated in the room. She receives a respiratory treatment every 4 hours and needs assistance with AM care. Her daughter is at her bedside and is very upset that her mother may need to go to a nursing home.

504: Mr. C., age 52, is to be discharged to a rehabilitation hospital today. Discharge records need to be prepared for the transfer. The family is at his bedside and is extremely anxious.

507: Mr. D., age 64, has TPN infusing into a left subclavian catheter and is on multiple antibiotics. He has vancomycin-resistant *Enterococcus* in his urine and a stasis ulcer on his left leg that requires Pulsavac treatment every day.

508: Mr. E., age 72, is a ventilator-dependent patient who will start weaning this AM. He is on continuous tube feedings and IV antibiotics and needs to be assessed for a peripherally inserted central catheter (PICC) line. He is to begin ambulation in the hall twice a day per physician's orders. He also needs to have a pharyngeal speech evaluation scheduled.

509: Mrs. F., age 66, is 3 days post cerebrovascular accident (CVA) and unable to move her right extremities. She has an IV infusing via her left arm. Her blood pressure is 170/100. She needs total care with personal hygiene and feeding. The physician just ordered range-of-motion exercises every day. Her husband is at her bedside crying continually and asking, "What am I going to do now?"

510: Mr. G., age 52, has been off the ventilator for the past 24 hours and is doing very well. He continues on respiratory treatments every 4 hours. His TPN is being decreased, and his PEG feedings are increasing. Glucose monitoring has been ordered every 4 hours and IV antibiotics every 12 hours. He has an indwelling urinary catheter to gravity drainage. He needs to be out of bed, ambulating in the hall with assistance. If he stays off the ventilator, he will be discharged in 5 days. The family needs to find a nursing home for him; however, the family has not visited Mr. G. since his admission 18 days ago.

511: Mr. H., age 49, is a new admission who will be coming from the intensive care unit (ICU) sometime during the shift.

In addition to the tasks mentioned, routine activities of taking vital signs, giving scheduled medications, updating care plans, and answering call lights must be assigned.

When reviewing the tasks to be accomplished, Ms. Miller must consider several issues to make safe and effective assignment and delegation decisions.

Questions to Consider While Reading This Chapter:

1. Which of the tasks listed in the vignette must the RN perform as required by your state's nurse practice act?
2. Which of these tasks can be delegated to the nursing assistant?
3. How can the training, skills, and competencies of the LPN or licensed vocational nurse (LVN) and nursing assistant be determined?
4. How can other members of the interprofessional health care team contribute most effectively to meet patients' needs?

CHAPTER OVERVIEW

The safe and effective delivery of patient care is the fundamental goal of every health care organization. To accomplish this goal cost effectively, teams of diverse professionals and assistants are used to deliver care. Because the RN is most often responsible for coordinating care provided by the various team members, he or she must clearly understand and be able to effectively use the management processes of delegation and supervision to ensure high-quality, safe patient care. This chapter highlights issues that influence staffing patterns and the delegation and supervision processes. The chapter also discusses the RN's role and responsibility in delegating to and supervising staff members, including unlicensed assistive personnel (UAP) and LPNs or LVNs, and provides useful guidelines for establishing a safe and effective delegation and supervision practice.

DELEGATION AND SUPERVISION IN THE HEALTH CARE SYSTEM

In today's complex health care environment, nursing must be knowledge-based, not task-based. Nurses are accountable to provide "culturally sensitive, safe, timely, efficient, patient-centered, equitable, and effective nursing care for consumers in a variety of settings across the continuum of health care" (ANA, 2012). Several factors influence staffing patterns and the provision of patient care across multiple health care settings from hospitals to home health. First, reduced reimbursement from Medicare, Medicaid, and private insurance companies has led to cost-cutting measures. Second, the Patient Protection and Affordable Care Act has allowed more people to have health insurance, so more people are seeking health care. Third, the consumer is now paying a higher co-pay for care and is demanding that care be provided in an effective and efficient manner. Fourth, the strong focus on safety and quality is requiring health care systems to make rapid changes for continual improvement. Fifth, advances in medical technology are causing a sharp increase in the cost of providing care. Finally, an increase in patient acuity (severity of illness) and complex treatments contribute to health care environments struggling to address multiple complex priorities with dwindling resources. Using unlicensed assistive personnel (UAP), such as nursing assistants and patient care technicians, is one strategy to increase the cost-effectiveness of providing patient care.

As the use of UAP increases, the RN is obligated to delegate more tasks to people who do not have clearly defined parameters for education, training, job responsibilities, and role limitations. The RN must know that the profession defines the scope and standards of practice, and that the state nurse practice acts define the legal parameters for nursing practice (NCSBN, 2016). It is important that the RN work closely with nonclinical administrators and managers to make sure they understand that the nursing process cannot be delegated to anybody other than the RN.

In support of the role of UAP in delivering patient care, the *Joint Statement on Delegation* (ANA and NCSBN, 2014) states, "There is a need and a place for competent, appropriately supervised, unlicensed assistive personnel in the delivery of affordable, quality health care." As health care facilities continue to seek more cost-effective ways to provide care, RNs must learn new ways of managing care and delegating tasks.

WHAT IS DELEGATION?

Delegation is a legal and management concept that involves assessment, planning, intervention, and evaluation. Delegation, as defined by the American Nurses Association (ANA, 2015b), is "the transfer of responsibility for the performance of an activity from one individual to another while retaining accountability for the outcome." Although RNs can transfer the responsibility and authority for the performance of an activity, they remain accountable for the overall nursing care. When delegating tasks, the nurse should understand the delegatee's competencies, communicate succinctly, offer clear guidelines in advance, monitor progress, and remain accountable for the final outcomes of care.

Delegation is a two-way process in which the RN requests that a qualified staff member perform a specific task. When delegating, the RN delegator is accountable for (NCSBN, 2016):

- Determining patient needs and when to delegate.
- Being available to the delegatee.
- Assessment and follow-up evaluation.
- Any intervention or corrective actions that may be required to ensure safe and effective care.
  The delegatee is accountable for:
- His or her own actions.
- Accepting delegation within the parameters of his or her competency level.
- Communicating the appropriate information to the delegator.
- Completing the task.

Delegation is a management strategy that when used appropriately can ensure the accomplishment of safe and effective patient care. "All decisions related to delegation and assignment are based on the fundamental principles of protection of the health, safety, and welfare of the public" (Duffy and McCoy, 2014).

WHAT SHOULD AND SHOULD NOT BE DELEGATED?

Unfortunately, there is no easy answer to the question of what can and cannot be delegated. The answer varies depending on the (1) nurse practice acts and other applicable state laws, (2) patient needs, (3) job descriptions and competencies of staff members, (4) policies and procedures of the health care organization, (5) the clinical situation, and (6) professional standards of nursing practice. To establish a safe, effective delegation practice, the RN must seek guidance and integrate information regarding each of these areas as discussed in the following paragraphs.

State Nurse Practice Acts

Each state's nurse practice act provides the legal authority for nursing practice, including delegation. However, each state's nurse practice act expresses delegation criteria differently, and the criteria often are not clearly spelled out in the act, or they may be presented in various parts of the act. It is absolutely essential that every RN be familiar with his or her state nurse practice act and know the delegation criteria contained within it (NCSBN, 2016). Box 20.1 presents policies common to many nurse practice acts.

If the nurse practice act does not provide clear direction regarding delegation, the state board of nursing may be able to offer guidance. The board of nursing may have developed definitions, rulings, advisory opinions, or interpretations of the law to provide guidance regarding delegation activities. Many state boards of nursing may also have practical tools available, such as delegation decision trees or delegation checklists. Figure 20.1 shows a delegation decision tree recommended by the NCSBN that provides an excellent framework for the four steps in the delegation process—assessment and planning,

---

BOX 20.1   Policies Common to Many State Nurse Practice Acts

- Only nursing tasks can be delegated, not nursing practice.
- The RN must perform the patient assessment to determine what can be delegated.
- The LPN or LVN and UAP do not practice professional nursing.
- The RN can delegate only what is within the scope of nursing practice.
- The LPN or LVN works under the direction and supervision of the RN.
- The RN delegates based on the knowledge and skill of the person selected to perform the delegated tasks.
- The RN determines the competency of the person to whom he or she delegates.
- The RN cannot delegate an activity that requires the RN's professional skill and knowledge.
- The RN is accountable and responsible for the delegated task.
- The RN must evaluate patient outcomes resulting from the delegated activity.
- Health care facilities can develop specific delegation protocols, provided they meet the state board delegation guidelines.
- Delegation requires critical thinking by the RN.

LPN, licensed practical nurse; *LVN,* licensed vocational nurse; *RN,* registered nurse; *UAP,* unlicensed assistive personnel. From Johnson, S H. (1996). Teaching nursing delegation: analyzing nurse practice acts. *J Contin Educ Nurs, 27*(2), 52-58.

Fig. 20.1 Decision Tree for Delegating to Nursing Assistive Personnel. (From the Joint Statement on Delegation, American Nurses Association and National Council of State Boards of Nursing. Available online at https://www.ncsbn.org/Delegation_joint_statement_NCSBN-ANA.pdf. Used with permission from the American Nurses Association and the National Council of State Boards of Nursing, 2006.)

communication, surveillance and supervision, and evaluation and feedback.

Most states also have a practice act to govern practice by LPNs or LVNs. Because the practice of LPNs or LVNs varies significantly from state to state, RNs should know the LPN or LVN practice act in the state in which they practice and understand the LPN's or LVN's legal scope of practice. The delegation decision tree presented in Figure 20.1 is also applicable to delegation to LPNs and LVNs. State law generally does not define practice by UAP, although such practice should be governed by the health care organization's policies.

Patient Needs

When deciding to delegate, the RN must remember that tasks can be delegated but nursing practice cannot. The functions of assessment, evaluation, and nursing judgment cannot be delegated. In general, the more stable the patient, the more likely delegation is to be safe. However, it also is important to remember that many tasks that can be delegated may also carry with them a nursing responsibility. Taking vital signs on a physiologically stable patient after a CVA could be delegated to the UAP, but the task presents an opportunity for the RN to assess the patient's cognitive functioning. In the vignette presented at the opening of this chapter, Ms. Miller should not delegate any care for the newly admitted patient until the nursing assessment is complete.

Job Descriptions and Competencies

The RN who is delegating has the responsibility of knowing the background, skill level, training received, and job requirements of each person to whom tasks are delegated. The job description provides important information about what a staff member is allowed to do and delineates the specific tasks, duties, and responsibilities required of the person as a condition of employment. Job descriptions generally comply with state laws and the health care organization's standards of care. However, in all cases, legal requirements related to delegation supersede any organizational requirement or policy.

The RN should be aware of what type of education and training the person received to function as described in the job description. The RN should also know what kind of orientation is provided to new employees. In the opening vignette, the LPN's job description most likely would include duties such as "perform dressing changes" and "administer oral medications," but Ms. Miller also should know the LPN's knowledge and skill level for the population of patients on the unit.

In addition to requiring job descriptions for care providers, health care organizations also require employees to demonstrate that they are competent to perform certain technical procedures and to apply specific knowledge to safely care for patients. Written documentation of those skills and knowledge for which the employee has demonstrated competency is maintained in the employee's personnel file. Most health care organizations require employees to undergo annual competency training for aspects of care unique to the population of patients generally being cared for in the nursing unit. Box 20.2 provides an example of annual competencies to be demonstrated by nurses in a family practice ambulatory care clinic. Various regulatory and accrediting agencies, such as The Joint Commission (TJC), require written documentation of staff competencies.

Organizational Policies and Procedures

When delegating, the RN should comply with the specific skill requirements designated in the organization's written policies and procedures, which usually describe the supervision required for a specific task and how problems or incidents should be reported and documented. Again, it is important for the nurse to remember that the legal requirements related to delegation supersede any organizational requirement or policy. The RN should also know the organization's general standards of

---

BOX 20.2   Annual Competencies to Be Demonstrated by Registered Nurses and Licensed Vocational Nurses in a Family Practice Ambulatory Care Clinic

- Safety rules and regulations
- Health Insurance Portability and Accountability Act (HIPAA) policies and procedures
- Patient safety goals
- Infection control
- Telephone triage
- Glucose testing
- Patient education and health literacy
- Medication management
- Reporting abuse and neglect
- Documentation in the medical record
- Handling emergencies in the outpatient setting

care, such as infection control, and should ensure that the delegatee has the necessary knowledge and skills to comply with the standards. In the opening vignette, Ms. Miller should be aware of the hospital's policy regarding the orientation process. All clinical staff members should have received training about the unit's infection control, emergency, and safety procedures.

Clinical Situation

Each delegation opportunity presents the RN with a variety of considerations, including the delegatee's current workload and the complexity of the task in relationship to the patient. Does the staff member realistically have time to accomplish the task? Is the staff member familiar with characteristics of the patient population (e.g., pediatric or geriatric) and with the task to be performed? Is the RN able to provide the appropriate level of supervision? Other considerations include the availability of resources, such as supplies and equipment.

Professional Standards of Nursing Practice

Professional standards of nursing practice, as established by professional nursing organizations, exist to guide the RN in providing patient care. According to the ANA (2015b), "The Standards of Professional Nursing Practice are authoritative statements of the duties that all registered nurses, regardless of role, population, or specialty, are expected to perform competently. The standards are subject to change with the dynamics of the nursing profession, as new patterns of professional practice are developed and accepted by the nursing profession and the public." To practice safe delegation, the RN should be familiar with the standards of practice outlined in the ANA's *Nursing: Scope and Standards of Practice* (2015b) and with the standards for any specialty area in which the RN practices (e.g., geriatric, pediatric, nursing administration, public health).

As an accepted standard of care, the RN should use professional judgment to determine activities that are appropriate to delegate on the basis of the concept of providing safe and effective patient care and protecting the public. In delegation, the RN considers the following:
- Assessment of patient condition
- Capabilities of the nursing and assistive staff
- Complexity of the task to be delegated
- Amount of clinical oversight (supervision) the RN will be able to provide

- Staff workload

Responsibilities related to making nursing judgments cannot be delegated except to another qualified registered nurse. Examples of responsibilities that cannot be delegated include:
- Initial nursing assessment and any subsequent assessment that requires professional nursing knowledge, judgment, and skill
- Determination of nursing diagnoses, establishment of nursing care goals, development of the patient plan of care, and evaluation of the patient's progress with the plan of care
- Any nursing intervention that requires professional knowledge, judgment, and skill

Box 20.3 presents a list of questions to assist the nurse in making delegation decisions.

DEVELOPING SAFE DELEGATION PRACTICES

For the RN to make safe, effective delegation decisions, a good understanding of what should and should not be delegated on the basis of the previous discussion is required. However, safe delegation decisions require more! The RN also must know the patient, the staff members to whom he or she is delegating, and the tasks to be performed. The RN must provide for effective outcomes by clearly communicating expectations, supporting and appropriately supervising the delegatee, evaluating the outcomes, and reassessing the patient after the delegated task is completed. Following is a brief discussion of these essential requirements for safe and effective delegation.

Know the Patient

A nursing assessment must be completed before delegation—the RN must know the level of care required by the patient, considering his or her clinical, physiologic, emotional, cognitive, and spiritual status. Is the patient's condition considered stable? Generally, the more stable the patient the more likely delegation of care is to be safe. What is the potential for change in the patient's condition as a result of the delegated task? If there is moderate to high risk that the task will result in a change in the patient's condition, delegation should not be considered. Can the patient's safety be maintained with delegated care? The answer to this question must be a firm "yes" for delegation to be considered.

BOX 20.3 Questions to Guide Decision-Making in Delegation

A. State nurse practice act:
1. Is the task within the RN's scope of practice?
2. Does the nurse practice act address delegation of the task?
3. Does the task to be delegated require the exercising of nursing judgment?
4. Is the RN delegator willing to accept accountability for the performance of the delegated task?

B. Job description and competencies:
1. Does the RN delegator understand the nature of the task and have the knowledge, skills, and competency required to perform the task?
2. Does the delegatee have the appropriate education, training, skills, and experience to perform the task?
3. Is there documented or demonstrated evidence that the delegatee is competent to perform the task?
4. Does the delegatee perform the task on a routine basis?
5. Is the delegatee familiar with the patient population?

C. Organizational policies and procedures:
1. What skill level and level of supervision are required for the task as stated in the organization's policy/procedure manual?
2. What is the policy or procedure for documenting tasks and reporting results, observations, problems, or unusual incidents?
3. Does the delegatee have the necessary knowledge and skills to comply with general standards of care, such as infection control?

D. Clinical situation and task:
1. Is adequate supervision by the delegator available?
2. Are adequate resources available, including supplies and equipment, to the delegatee?
3. What is the delegatee's current workload? Does the person realistically have time to perform the task?
4. How complex is the task? Does it frequently recur in the daily care of patients? Does it follow a standard and unchanging procedure?

E. Patient needs:
1. Has the nursing assessment and plan of care been completed by the RN?
2. What is the patient's clinical, physiologic, emotional, cognitive, and spiritual status?
3. Is the patient's condition considered stable?
4. What is the potential for change in the patient's condition as a result of the delegated task?
5. Can the patient's safety be maintained with delegated care?

F. Professional standards of nursing practice:
1. What specific standards of nursing practice apply to the specific situation?
2. Does the delegated task include health counseling, teaching, or other activities that require specialized nursing knowledge, skill, or judgment?

Know the Staff Member

Before the task is delegated, the delegatee must have the skills and knowledge necessary to perform the task, as evidenced by the person's job description, training program, and documented competencies. Experience and past job performance should also be taken into account. Is the staff member knowledgeable about and trained to perform the task? Does the staff member perform the task routinely? The right person must be selected for the right task. It is very helpful for the RN to be involved in development of job descriptions, training programs, and competency documentation for staff members.

Know the Task(s) to Be Delegated

The RN delegator must be competent and skilled in performing any task he or she is considering delegating,

and the task must be within the RN's scope of practice. Routine, standardized tasks that are performed according to a standard and unchanging procedure and have predictable outcomes are the safest to delegate. These routine tasks are most likely to have been documented in the staff member's competencies and may require fewer directions and less supervision. Complex tasks or activities that pose a high risk for patient complications or unpredictable outcomes should be examined closely before delegation is considered.

Explain the Task and Expected Outcomes

The RN should explain the delegated task, what must be done, and the expected outcomes. If necessary, the task is outlined in writing. Failure to effectively communicate what is expected may result in unsatisfactory performance, errors, and possible harm to the patient.

Directions should be provided clearly and concisely. Demonstration and return demonstration by the delegatee or other in-service education may be required. Delegation of the task is acceptable only if the staff member understands the task and is adequately prepared to carry it out.

Expect Responsible Action from the Delegatee

When the staff member accepts and understands the task, he or she should then be allowed to perform the task. The staff member becomes responsible for his or her own actions and is obligated to complete the task as mutually agreed. It is important to note that the delegatee cannot delegate the task to another person; for example, if the RN delegates a task to a nursing assistant, that nursing assistant cannot ask another nursing assistant to perform the task. The RN should provide appropriate supervision but should not intervene in task performance unless assistance is requested or an unsafe situation is recognized. Interfering with the delegatee's task will negate his or her responsibility and obligation. The RN should expect responsible actions, give authority, and retain accountability.

Assess and Supervise Job Performance

Supervising job performance provides a mechanism for feedback and control. The RN assesses job performance by making frequent rounds, observing, and communicating (e.g., asking about progress, and determining whether there are any questions or concerns). The appropriate level of supervision should be determined. The RN should be available to the delegatee in case there are any questions or unexpected problems. Supervision should be performed in a positive and supportive manner to reassure the staff member that his or her work is important and appreciated. The RN should intervene immediately if the task is not being performed in a safe and appropriate manner. Poor performance must be documented and reported to the nurse manager. Poor performance should never be ignored. When a mistake is made, it should be used as a learning opportunity for all staff involved.

Evaluate and Follow-Up

Once the task is complete, the RN should evaluate the staff member's performance and reassess the patient to ensure that the expected outcomes were achieved. If the patient's care outcomes or the delegatee's job performance necessitate it, the RN should follow up with required interventions. Appropriate evaluation and follow-up will ensure a positive outcome for both patient and staff member. Box 20.4 presents some important steps to remember after the decision to delegate has been made.

Understand High-Risk Delegation

The RN often expresses concern about legal liability—"putting my license on the line"—when delegating to unlicensed staff members. How does the RN know whether he or she might be at risk when delegating? In ANA's *Principles for Delegation* (2012), eleven principles provide guidance and help inform the RN's decision-making regarding delegation:

1. The nursing profession determines scope and standards of practice.
2. The RN is responsible and accountable for the provision of nursing practice.

BOX 20.4 From Deciding to Delegate to Actual Delegation: Steps to Remember

A. Communicate effectively.
 1. The delegatee accepts the delegation and accountability for carrying out the task correctly.
 2. The RN delegator provides clear directions to the delegatee, including what specific task is to be performed, for whom the task is to be done, when the task is to be done, how the task is to be performed, what data are to be collected, and any patient-specific instructions.
 3. The RN delegator clearly communicates expected outcomes and time lines for reporting results.
B. Provide appropriate supervision.
 1. Monitor performance to ensure compliance with established standards of practice and organizational policies and procedures.
 2. Obtain and provide feedback.
 3. Intervene if necessary.
 4. Ensure proper documentation.
C. Evaluate and reassess.
 1. Reassess the patient.
 2. Evaluate the performance of the task and the delegatee's experience.
 3. Reassess and adjust the overall plan of care as needed.

3. The RN directs care and determines the appropriate utilization of resources when providing care.
4. The RN may delegate the task but not the nursing process itself.
5. The RN must consider the policies and procedures of the agency as well as the knowledge and skills, training, diversity awareness, and experience of person being delegated to.
6. The RN decision to delegate is based on the RN's judgment related to the complexity of care, the availability and competence of the person accepting the delegation, and the type and intensity of supervision required.
7. The RN acknowledges that delegation involves the concept of mutual respect.
8. Nurse leaders are accountable for systems to access, monitor, verify, and communicate ongoing competency requirements in areas related to delegation.
9. The agency is accountable to provide sufficient resources to enable appropriate delegation.
10. The agency is accountable for ensuring that the RN has access to documented competency information for the staff to whom the RN will be delegating tasks.
11. Agency policies regarding delegation are developed with active participation of RNs.

One method to avoid high-risk delegation and simplify the delegation process is referred to as the Five Rights of Delegation (ANA and NCSBN, 2014):

1. *The right task:* Ensure that delegated tasks conform to the established guidelines.
2. *The right circumstances:* Delegate tasks that do not require independent nursing judgment.
3. *The right person:* Delegate to someone who is qualified and competent.
4. *The right direction and communication:* Give clear explanation about the task and expected outcomes, and indicate when the delegatee should report back to the RN.
5. *The right supervision and evaluation:* Invite feedback to assess how the process is working and how to improve the process. Also evaluate the patient's outcomes and results of the tasks.

RNs can prevent being placed into unsafe, risky delegation situations by adhering to the safe delegation practices recommended in this chapter. Consider the legal case in which an elderly patient was admitted to the hospital and died shortly after admission by aspiration of food after the nursing assistant left a turkey sandwich on the table for the patient to eat (Legal Eagle Eye, 2010). The patient's family sued the hospital for wrongful death, the nurse was ruled negligent, and the family won the case. In this situation, the nurse was informed by the admitting physician that the patient had dysphagia, a swallowing disorder, and needed to be supervised while eating. Unfortunately, the nurse failed to meet the standards of nursing care by not supervising the patient's eating herself or ensuring that the nursing assistant clearly understood the risk involved for a patient with dysphagia and had the skills necessary to respond to an emergency. This legal case could have been prevented had the nurse practiced the principles and strategies for safe delegation presented in this chapter. For an example demonstrating excellence in delegation practice in a home health care setting, see Case Study 20.1.

SUPERVISION

Supervision is defined by the ANA (2012) as "the active process of directing, guiding and influencing the outcome of an individual's performance of a task." Supervision may be categorized as on-site, in which the nurse is physically present or immediately available while the activity is being performed, or off-site, in which the nurse has the ability to provide direction through various means of written, verbal, and electronic communication (Duffy and McCoy, 2014). On-site supervision generally occurs in the acute care or ambulatory care settings where the RN is immediately available. Off-site supervision may occur in home health care practice, community settings, and long-term care facilities.

Various levels of supervision may be required on the basis of the task delegated and the education, experience, competency, and working relationship of the people involved (Hansten and Jackson, 2009):

- *Unsupervised:* One RN is working with another RN in a collegial relationship, and neither RN is in the position of supervising the other. Each RN is responsible and accountable for his or her own practice. However, the RN in a supervisory or management position (e.g., team leader, charge nurse, nurse manager), as defined by the health care organization, will be in a position to supervise other RNs.
- *Initial direction and/or periodic inspection:* The RN supervises a licensed or unlicensed caregiver, knows the person's training and competencies, and has

---

CASE STUDY 20.1 Excellence In Delegation Practice

Amy Laurence, RN, works for a home health care agency. Ms. Laurence manages a caseload of 35 patients and makes between 6 and 8 skilled nursing visits a day. Several of Ms. Laurence's patients need assistance with activities of daily living, such as personal hygiene and mobility. Ms. Laurence assigns these tasks to the home health aides (HHAs) with whom she has worked with over the past 6 to 12 months. From her ongoing evaluation of patient outcomes and supervision of these aides, she knows they are skilled and proficient in performing their assigned tasks.

Five of Ms. Laurence's patients are newly diagnosed with diabetes and need extensive assistance with monitoring blood glucose levels and administering insulin. The home health care agency where Ms. Laurence works has recently adopted a diabetic delegation policy. This policy allows HHAs that have been specifically trained and certified to perform glucose testing and give insulin from prefilled, labeled syringes. Ms. Laurence actively participates in the training classes to certify HHAs in diabetic care.

In caring for her patients with diabetes, Ms. Laurence does extensive diabetic teaching with each of her patients and sees them weekly to assess their learning, monitor their physiologic status, evaluate and adjust their individualized plans of care, and provide ongoing education and support as needed. During the weekly visits, Ms. Laurence fills and labels the exact number of insulin syringes with the correct doses of insulin to last the week. Ms. Laurence is

then able to delegate the daily insulin administration and glucose monitoring to the HHAs certified in diabetic care. During the initial delegation process, Ms. Laurence makes supervisory visits to each patient's home to ensure that the HHA is performing the tasks correctly and has been carrying them out according to the patient's plan of care. To provide appropriate supervision of these delegated tasks, Ms. Laurence plans her weekly skilled nursing visits to coincide with the HHAs' daily visits. During these visits, Ms. Laurence observes each HHA perform the glucose testing and insulin administration and reinforces any specific training needed. Following these supervisory visits, Ms. Laurence is confident that the HHAs are competent to perform the delegated tasks.

In this case, Ms. Laurence is following all of the criteria essential for safe delegation in her state. She is adhering to the agency's policy, which also is in line with the state board of nursing rules for delegation in a home health care setting. She has actively participated in the training programs for the HHAs and provided clear direction during the initial delegation process. Ms. Laurence provides ongoing patient assessment, care evaluation, and supervision of the HHAs. In performing appropriate delegation, Ms. Laurence is able to focus her energy on skilled nursing services, such as providing patient education, assessing and monitoring patients' physiologic condition, and coordinating the care for the interprofessional home health care team.

---

developed a working relationship with the staff member. For example, the RN has been working with the nursing assistant for 6 months and is comfortable in giving initial directions for a delegated task and following up with the assistant once during the shift.

- *Continuous supervision:* The RN has determined that the delegatee needs frequent to continual support and assistance. This level of supervision is required when the working relationship is new, the task is complex, or the delegatee is inexperienced or has not demonstrated an acceptable level of competence.

ASSIGNING VERSUS DELEGATING

Assigning tasks is not the same as delegating tasks. *Assignment,* as defined by the ANA (2012), is "the distribution of work that each staff member is responsible for

during a given work period." An assignment designates those activities that a staff member is responsible for performing as a condition of employment and is consistent with the staff member's job position and description, legal scope of practice, and training and educational background. The staff member assumes responsibility and is accountable for completing the assignment.

Assignment Considerations

Assigning groups of patients to various care providers, including UAP and LPNs or LVNs, is not appropriate. For example, UAP cannot be assigned to a patient or group of patients, but rather should be assigned to an RN. Typical assignments for UAP include passing trays, assisting patients with activities of daily living, transporting patients, stocking supplies, and completing delegated tasks for the RN. The LPN or LVN may be assigned specific patients for whom to perform care, but the RN remains responsible for all nursing practice activities, including patient assessment, care planning, and patient teaching.

The RN is also responsible for assignments made to personnel in the clinical setting. Several factors should be considered when making assignments:

- *Patient's physiologic status and complexity of care:* Are vital signs unstable? Is the patient's condition changing rapidly? Does the patient have multisystem involvement? Does the patient need extensive health education? Does the patient need extensive emotional support? What technology is involved in the care (e.g., cardiac monitor, intravenous pump, patient-controlled analgesia pump)? Patients with more unstable physiologic status or complex care requirements need a higher level of skilled care.
- *Infection control:* To what extent are isolation procedures required? Which patients could be adversely affected as a result of cross-contamination? For example, a new patient is admitted with a history of night sweats and chronic cough. The results of a sputum culture are pending. Another patient on the unit was admitted with complications resulting from chemotherapy. The same caregiver should not be assigned to a potentially infectious patient and an immunosuppressed patient.
- *Degree of supervision:* What level of supervision, direct or indirect, is required on the basis of staff members' education, experience, skill level, and competence? Is the appropriate supervision available? The on-call RN who works an occasional weekend may require more supervision than the LPN who has worked in the unit full time and has demonstrated competence in caring for the patient population on the unit.

Note that the most experienced skilled staff members should not be exclusively assigned to the most complex, difficult cases. Assignments should be used as a staff development tool. Assigning a less experienced nurse to a more complex patient, but at the same time increasing the level of supervision, increases that nurse's skill level, competence, and confidence while maintaining safe, effective patient care.

Working with Interprofessional Health Care Team Members

Other health professionals, including respiratory therapists, physical therapists, occupational therapists, speech therapists, nutritionists, medical social workers, and chaplains, are very valuable in helping meet patient care needs. In the vignette for this chapter, Ms. Miller will need to coordinate the efforts of each of the interprofessional team members available to her unit to accomplish the many and varied tasks needed by the patients for whom she is responsible and accountable. For example, the respiratory therapist monitors all patients on ventilators and assists in the weaning process. The medical social worker provides valuable assistance to identify family support and assists with nursing home placement for Mr. G. The speech therapist can work on communication techniques with Mr. A., the ventilator-dependent patient who becomes very frustrated when he tries to speak.

BUILDING DELEGATION AND SUPERVISION SKILLS

Effective delegation and supervision are underlying qualities for the success of working with others efficiently and being able to provide safe, cost-effective care to patients. Delegating can be very difficult, especially for the novice nurse. Some of the struggles the nurse has are the fear of being disliked, fear of making a mistake, inexperience in working with UAP, LPNs, or LVNs, lack of confidence, and lack of knowledge of the delegation process itself. Because delegation and supervision involve interactions between two people, the RN needs to develop strong interpersonal skills and a supportive work environment to guarantee effective delegation and supervision situations. Following are management skills RNs need to develop to become proficient at delegation and supervision.

Communicate Effectively

Clear communication is the key to successful delegation and supervision. The first step toward effective communication is for the RN to know exactly what needs to be done and what outcomes are expected. What is the specific task to be done? For whom is the task to be done? When is the task to be done? How is the task to be performed? What is the expected outcome? What feedback is expected? Why does the task need to be done in a certain way?

Maintaining self-control and confidence is an important communication skill. New RNs often have expressed concern about delegating to more seasoned

LPNs or LVNs or UAP. "I have been working here for 12 years, and I do not need you telling me what to do" might be a typical response directed to the new RN. The RN's correct response is to maintain composure and confidence and remain positive. "I really appreciate your experience and knowledge, and I need you to help our team and patients by . . . [describe the task clearly]."

It also is important to listen carefully to the delegatee's response. Did the delegatee appear to listen and understand the directions? Did he or she appear hesitant to accept the task? Angry? Uninterested? Frustrated? If a delegation action elicits a negative response from the delegatee, the RN should ask for feedback using open-ended, nonthreatening statements, such as "You seem unsure about performing this task." The RN should always provide an opportunity for the delegatee to ask questions. The positive communication techniques discussed in Chapter 19 provide additional guidelines to enhance delegation skills.

Create an Environment of Trust and Cooperation

Staff members will report problems more quickly if they know that the reaction from the supervisor will be nonthreatening and nonjudgmental. When mistakes occur, the person making it should not be blamed or criticized; rather, the supervisor should look for root causes and system issues, such as inadequate training or an excessive workload. Encouraging staff members to report and discuss problems is an excellent method of improving patient care and maintaining a helpful, supportive attitude. Just as the RN establishes trust and rapport with patients, he or she should strive for the same type of supportive relationships with staff members.

Provide Feedback and Follow-Up Evaluation

The delegation process is not complete until the RN reassesses the patient and adjusts the plan of care as indicated. The RN should also provide honest feedback to the delegatee about his or her performance. An easy, although often overlooked, delegation skill is to praise good performance. Often more difficult for the RN, and sometimes ignored, is the duty to address poor job performance.

The RN should tell the staff member about mistakes in a supportive manner—in private—with a focus on "learning from mistakes." However, if the staff member performs in an inappropriate, unsafe, or incompetent manner, the RN must intervene immediately and stop the unsafe activity, document the facts of the performance, and report to the supervisor. In addition, the RN should request additional training or other appropriate action for the staff member to ensure that patient safety is protected. The RN has a professional responsibility to intervene appropriately when poor performance is observed.

SUMMARY

Effective delegation and supervision are essential skills for the professional nurse in any practice role or setting, especially with the increased use of UAP to provide health care services. Although there is no definitive list of what can and cannot be delegated, the RN is guided to safe, effective delegation and supervision through an assessment of (1) the clinical situation; (2) patient needs; (3) the job descriptions and competencies of the assistive and vocational or practical nursing personnel; (4) the health care organization's policies and procedures; (5) nurse practice acts and other regulations and applicable state laws; and (6) professional standards of nursing practice. This chapter presents information to assist the RN with delegation decisions and also discusses effective delegation and supervision skills, including communicating effectively, creating an environment of trust and cooperation, and providing feedback and follow-up evaluation. These activities and skills provide the tools the RN needs to provide safe and legal delegation in practice.

REFERENCES

American Nurses Association. (2015a). *Code of ethics for nurses with interpretive statements*. Silver Spring, MD: American Nurses Association.

American Nurses Association. (2012). *Principles for delegation*. Silver Spring, MD: American Nurses Association.

American Nurses Association. (2015b). *Nursing: Scope and standards of practice*. Washington, DC: American Nurses

Association. Retrieved from http://www.nursesbooks.org/ebooks/download/Nursing-Scope&Standards-3E.pdf.

American Nurses Association and National Council of State Boards of Nursing. (2014). *Joint statement on delegation*. Retrieved from https://www.ncsbn.org/Delegation_joint_statement_NCSBN-ANA.pdf.

Duffy, M., & McCoy, S. F. (2014). *Delegation and you*. Silver Spring, MD: American Nurses Association, Nursebooks.org.

Hansten, R. I., & Jackson, M. (2009). *Clinical delegation skills: A handbook for professional practice* (4th ed.). Sudbury, MA: Jones and Bartlett.

Johnson, S. H. (1996). Teaching nursing delegation: analyzing nurse practice acts. *Journal of Continuing Education in Nursing, 27*(2), 52–58.

Legal Eagle Eye: Newsletter for the Nursing Profession. (2010). *Patient chokes, dies: Nurse ruled negligent, delegated supervision of patient to aide. 18*(1). Retrieved from http://www.nursinglaw.com/jan10ang7.pdf.

National Council of State Boards of Nursing. (2016). *National guidelines for nursing delegation*. Retrieved from https://www.ncsbn.org/NCSBN_Delegation_Guidelines.pdf.

21

Staffing and Nursing Care Delivery Models

Barbara Cherry, DNSc, MBA, RN, NEA-BC

Staffing and assigning work are two important and challenging roles for nurses.

ⓔ Additional resources are available online at: *http://evolve.elsevier.com/Cherry/*

LEARNING OUTCOMES

After studying this chapter, the reader will be able to:

1. Outline key issues surrounding staffing for a health care organization.
2. Evaluate lines of responsibility and accountability associated with various types of nursing care delivery models.
3. Analyze the advantages and disadvantages of nursing care delivery models in relation to patient care in various settings.
4. Differentiate among several nursing care delivery models by evaluating their defining characteristics.
5. Explain the purpose and components of nursing case management.
6. Summarize criteria to be considered in developing future models of nursing care delivery.

KEY TERMS

Clinical pathway Clinical management plans that specify the optimal timing and sequencing of major patient care activities and interventions by the interprofessional team for a particular diagnosis, procedure, or health condition and that are designed to standardize care delivery (Coffey et al, 2005); clinical pathways may also be called critical paths, practice protocols, or care maps.

Clinical practice guidelines (CPGs) Recommendations for appropriate treatment and care for specific clinical circumstances; guidelines are developed through a systematic process to integrate the best evidence for treating specific medical conditions and assist health care providers to make decisions about appropriate treatment (Institute of Medicine et al, 1990).

Nursing care delivery model Also called care delivery system or patient care delivery model; details the

way work assignments, responsibility, and authority are structured to accomplish patient care; depicts which health care worker is going to perform what tasks, who is responsible, and who has the authority to make decisions.

Patient acuity Indication of the severity of the patient's illness and the amount and complexity of nursing care required; high acuity indicates a need for more intense, complex nursing care, and lower acuity indicates a need for moderate, less complex nursing care.

Patient classification system Method used to group or categorize patients according to specific criteria and care requirements and thus help quantify the patient acuity, or amount and level of nursing care needed.

Patient outcome A measurable condition that results from interventions by the health care team; a change in a person's health after treatment; outcomes may be positive, such as better mobility or improved laboratory values, or negative, such as infection, fall, or death.

Staff mix Combination of categories of workers employed to provide patient care (e.g., RNs, LPNs or LVNs, and UAP).

Staffing Ensuring that an adequate number and mix of health care team members (e.g., RNs, LPNs or LVNs, UAP, clerical support) are available to provide safe, quality patient care.

Unlicensed assistive personnel (UAP) Individuals who have not received practice licenses to practice but who are trained to function in an assistive role to the RN by performing patient care activities as delegated by the nurse; may include nursing assistants, clinical assistants, orderlies, health aides, and other titles designated within the work setting (NCSBN, 2016).

PROFESSIONAL/ETHICAL ISSUE

LaMicha Hopkins, Registered Nurse (RN), staff nurse in a pediatric unit, is becoming concerned about quality of care issues on her unit. When she first came to work in this unit 18 months ago, she was very impressed with the quality of care the patients received and the camaraderie among the nurses. Team nursing was fully implemented and all nurses supported one another and the families to ensure that the pediatric patients received the best care possible. She was thrilled to have become part of such a great team and to be able to provide excellent care to her patients. Over the last few months, patient acuity and patient census have increased but the number of nurses on the unit has not changed. In response to the higher workload, charge nurses have started making patient care assignments on the basis of tasks rather than the team nursing model, explaining to the staff nurses that assignments by task is a more efficient way to get the work done. Some of LaMicha's colleagues have expressed dissatisfaction with their ability to provide good nursing care, and they are also noticing more complaints from family members. LaMicha believes that the shift away from the team nursing model, along with the higher patient volume and acuity, has led to fragmented care and a loss of the team spirit once so prevalent among the nurses.

What can LaMicha do as a staff nurse to help find a resolution to the staffing concerns? What data might be available to staff nurses to help them assess patient outcomes and patient and nurse satisfaction for a quantifiable analysis of the staffing situation? Who should be involved in evaluating and making decisions about staffing and nursing care delivery models? How can LaMicha approach the charge nurses and/or the nurse manager to help address the situation?

VIGNETTE

As a student nurse, John Knox noticed during rotations through the different clinical areas that the RNs had various types of responsibilities and duties. On the medical-surgical units, RNs supervised a group of licensed practical nurses (LPNs) and nursing assistants who provided direct patient care, and the RNs performed patient assessments, care planning, and education. In the critical care unit, RNs provided all the care required by the patient with little help from any other caregivers. In the obstetric unit, two RNs worked as a team to provide care to laboring mothers. In the outpatient health clinic, each RN was assigned to perform specific tasks; one nurse was assigned to do all diabetic teaching, and another was assigned to triage all telephone calls from patients. Some of the clinical areas used a mostly RN staff, whereas other clinical units had a variety of staff, from RNs to nursing assistants. John had many questions about why care delivery was very different in the different clinical sites.

Questions to Consider While Reading This Chapter:

1. Why is the RN's work assignment different in different units—obstetrics, critical care, medical-surgical, and the outpatient clinic?
2. Who decides how many nurses and other personnel are needed to staff a clinical site?
3. How do nurse managers on nursing units decide how assignments will be made?

4. Who has responsibility and authority for making patient care assignments?

CHAPTER OVERVIEW

Of all the nurse's varied and complex roles, staffing and assigning work are probably the most challenging and certainly the most important to the delivery of safe, quality patient care. Charge nurses spend a significant amount of time on staffing issues. *Staffing* ensures that an appropriate number and level of staff members are available to provide care; *assigning* is the method used to divide work tasks among the various staff members. This chapter presents a brief introduction to staffing and its surrounding issues, such as acuity levels and staff satisfaction. A description follows of various nursing care delivery models, which detail how work assignments are structured. Also discussed are telehealth and case management as nursing care delivery models, in addition to the use of clinical pathways and clinical practice guidelines.

STAFFING

Staffing can be defined as the activities required to ensure that an adequate number and mix of health care team members (e.g., RNs, licensed vocational nurses [LVNs] or LPNs, unlicensed assistive personnel [UAP], clerical support) are available to meet patient needs and provide safe, quality care. Important research is validating the contribution and value of RNs to improving patient outcomes, reducing rates of complications and length of hospital stays, and preventing premature mortality (Ball et al, 2017; Driscoll et al, 2018). Two landmark reports—*Keeping Patients Safe: Transforming the Work Environment of Nurses* (Institute of Medicine [IOM], 2004) and *The Future of Nursing: Leading Change, Advancing Health* (IOM, 2011)—have strongly affirmed nurses' essential roles in achieving quality patient care and safety. For nurses to have the greatest opportunity to achieve safe, quality care, staffing systems must (1) address individual and aggregate patient care needs; (2) incorporate clinical competencies of nurses and other team members to provide care to specified patient populations; (3) reflect the value of RNs as vitally important to the organization; and (4) provide nurses time to exercise professional judgment and acknowledge that patient needs can change from moment to moment (American Nurses Association

[ANA], 2012). While healthcare leaders appreciate the overall value of the RN in providing patient care, they must consider specific staffing issues related to (1) patient needs, (2) nursing characteristics, and (3) organizational needs.

Staffing and Patient Needs

Primary considerations for staffing a specific nursing unit are the number of patients; the level of intensity of care required by those patients (commonly referred to as patient acuity); contextual issues, such as the architecture and geography of the environment and the available technology; level of preparation and experience of the staff members providing the care; and the quality of the nurses' work life (ANA, 2012). Using only the number of patients who require care is an ineffective way to plan staffing because of the wide range of care requirements needed by individual patients. To account for the diverse care needs and quantify the intensity of care required by a group of patients, nurses use various patient classification systems.

Patient Classification Systems. Patient classification systems group or categorize patients according to specific criteria and care needs and thus help quantify the amount and level of care needed, referred to as the *acuity level*. The higher the acuity level, the more intense and complex the patient's nursing care needs. For example, patients may be grouped in such categories as "uncomplicated postpartum" or "ventilator dependent." These two groups of patients require very different levels and amounts of care and therefore are categorized at different acuity levels. Imagine the many different kinds of patients treated by a health care facility, and you can begin to picture the complexity of patient classification systems. Electronic patient classification systems that extract data from the electronic health record and determine patient acuity scores are now available to streamline the method of managing patient acuity.

Because of this complexity and the differences in patient populations across different health care facilities, patient classification systems vary from organization to organization. However, the ANA (2012) has recommended that the following physical and psychosocial factors be considered in the determination of the intensity of care required for any group of patients:

- Age and functional ability
- Complexity of care needs

- Communication skills
- Cultural and linguistic diversities
- Severity and urgency of the admitting condition
- Scheduled procedures
- Ability to meet health care requisites
- Psychosocial support needs
- Other specific needs identified by the patient and by the RN

Understanding the intensity of care required by individual patients and groups of patients on the basis of these factors is the first step in developing effective patient classification systems and planning for appropriate staffing levels. The second step is knowing the level of preparation, skill, and experience of the staff members who are available to provide patient care.

Staffing and Nursing Characteristics

It is of critical importance that the staff members available to provide patient care have the educational preparation, skill, clinical judgment, and experience necessary to meet patient care needs. Another consideration in staffing is the clinical competencies that are required to care for the population being served as well as the nurse's competency with technology and clinical interventions (ANA, 2012). In recognition of the importance of nurse competencies in staffing, the American Association of Critical Care Nurses (AACN) recommends the *AACN Synergy Model for Patient Care* (AACN, 2014). Staffing systems based on the Synergy Model match patient needs and nurse characteristics to achieve ideal patient outcomes. The nurse who is responsible for making staffing decisions must be aware of each staff member's educational level, competencies, experience, skill, and training. Ideally, clinical support from experienced RNs should be available to support and advance the skills of those RNs and other staff members with less experience.

Nursing Satisfaction. Nurses who are satisfied with their work generally provide higher quality, more cost-effective care. Staffing systems should address the quality of work life for the nursing staff as equal in importance to the quality of patient outcomes. Attention to staff schedules is a major responsibility for the nurse manager, especially in light of the 24-hour/day, 365-day/year staffing needs in many health care facilities. Creative staffing options are available to meet the varied needs of staff members, including the following:

- 9- or 10-hour shifts, 4 days per week
- 12-hour shifts, 3 days per week
- Combination of 8-hour and 12-hour shifts
- Premium pay or part-time staff for weekend work
- Job sharing, flextime, and/or staff self-scheduling.

Each of these options has various advantages and disadvantages. For example, long shifts over consecutive days may result in clinical errors when nurses become fatigued. Self-scheduling is a popular staffing technique in which the responsibility for staffing the unit is delegated to the employees on the unit who work collectively to design the schedule according to pre-established staffing criteria and some guidance from the manager. No one scheduling system has proven to be best overall for staff satisfaction. However, staffing methods that allow nurses to be involved in the design of their work schedules is key to staff satisfaction and nurse retention (Shimp, 2017).

Staffing and Organizational Needs

The three basic organizational needs that are significantly affected by staffing are: (1) financial resources, (2) licensing regulations and The Joint Commission (TJC) or other accreditation standards, and (3) customer satisfaction.

Financial Resources. Productivity, the ratio of the amount of outputs produced (e.g., home visits) to the specific amount of input (nursing hours worked), is the measure of staffing efficiency. Because staff salaries are by far the largest expense for any health care organization, productivity—or the efficient use of staff—has a direct effect on the organization's bottom line. Fortunately, even though RNs typically represent the highest-paid staff in a facility, they are also the key to improved quality outcomes and reduced costs, thus representing a very good investment for the health care organization (ANA, 2018). It is important to remember that most health care organizations continue to function under tight financial constraints, making efficient management of staff essential to ensure the organizations' financial solvency. The nurse manager is accountable for appropriately managing staffing to stay within budgetary guidelines for the following:

- Numbers of staff working at any given time to provide care to a given number of patients

- **Staff mix**, the combination of types of workers present to provide patient care (e.g., RNs, LVNs or LPNs, and UAP)

Licensing Regulations and Accreditation. Health care facility licensing agencies, such as a state health department, and accreditation agencies, such as TJC, address minimum staffing levels. However, TJC and most state licensing agencies do not impose mandatory staffing ratios. These agencies do look for evidence that patients receive adequate care, which can occur only with adequate staffing. They also require documentation of staff training and competency to care for the organization's specific patient population. Licensing regulations for long-term care facilities stipulate minimum RN coverage for the unit but do not mandate specific nurse-to-patient ratios.

State legislative bodies and professional organizations have addressed staffing in various ways. In 1999, California became the first state to enact legislation requiring hospitals to meet minimal staffing standards. Rather than mandating staffing ratios, the ANA recommends staffing committees that develop unit-specific staffing plans with input from direct-care RNs and on the basis of various factors, including nurse experience and education, patient numbers, patient acuity, and patient outcomes. Recommendations for effective staffing committees are as follows (Dawson, 2014):

- Staff nurses must be involved in creating work schedules.
- Work schedules must be predictable so that nurses can plan for family and personal responsibilities.
- Work hours should be limited to 40 hours within 7 days with work shifts no longer than 12 hours.
- Nurses should have 10 consecutive hours off duty to allow for 7 to 9 hours of sleep.
- Uninterrupted rest breaks must be provided during the work shift.
- Nurse-sensitive patient outcome data should be used to support appropriate staffing.

The National Database of Nursing Quality Indicators (NDNQI) serves as a resource for data on nurse-sensitive outcomes, including patient falls, catheter-associated urinary tract infections, and nurse turnover and job satisfaction. Such data can serve as a powerful influence for nurses to advocate for safe staffing.

Customer Satisfaction. Perhaps most critical to an organization's success in a competitive health care environment is customer (patient) satisfaction. The key to customer satisfaction is the patient's personal interaction with the organization's employees. Positive and therapeutic interactions between clinicians and their patients and families can play a very significant role in improving patient health and clinical outcomes. With the advent of health care reform, patient satisfaction is now tied directly to financial rewards for hospitals. Medicare reimbursement rewards inpatient hospitals for providing quality care to include patient satisfaction. Appropriate staffing with well-trained, competent, professional nurses is essential to ensure patient satisfaction and allow hospitals to gain the financial rewards of high patient satisfaction.

Further Study of Staffing

This section has provided the reader with a brief introduction to staffing issues, such as scheduling options, patient classification systems, productivity and staff mix, and the RN's contribution to improved patient outcomes. These issues related to staffing in a health care organization are much more complex than may appear from this introduction. The reader, especially the person interested in entering nursing management, is encouraged to learn more about staffing and these related issues.

NURSING CARE DELIVERY MODELS

Nursing care delivery models, also called *care delivery systems* and *patient care delivery models*, detail the way task assignments, responsibility, and authority are structured to accomplish patient care. The nursing care delivery model describes which health care worker is going to perform what tasks, who is responsible, and who has the authority to make decisions. The basic premise of nursing care delivery models is that the number and type of caregivers are closely matched to patient care needs to provide safe, quality care in the most cost-effective manner possible.

The four classic nursing care delivery models used during the past six decades are: (1) total patient care, (2) functional nursing, (3) team nursing, and (4) primary nursing. Efforts to continually improve both the quality and cost-effectiveness of patient care have resulted in variations to these four classic models. Examples of variations include modular nursing and the partnership model (or co-primary nursing). Other types of nursing care models include patient-centered care, telehealth nursing, and case management. As the health care system continues to evolve in the twenty-first century with a focus on rapid patient turnover in acute care settings, growing use of outpatient and community-based settings, and evidence of the RN's valuable role in patient safety and improved outcomes, new models of nursing care delivery are continually emerging. Thus, considerations for future care delivery models are also presented.

Total Patient Care

The oldest method of organizing patient care is total patient care, sometimes referred to as *case nursing*. In total patient care, nurses are responsible for planning, organizing, and performing all care, including personal hygiene, medications, treatments, emotional support, and education, required for their assigned group of patients during the assigned shift. A diagram of the total patient care model is shown in Figure 21.1.

Advantages of the total patient care model are as follows:
- The patient receives holistic, unfragmented care by only one nurse per shift.
- At shift change, the RN who has provided care and the RN assuming care can easily communicate about the patient's condition and collaborate about the plan of care.
- The nurse maintains a high degree of practice autonomy.
- Lines of responsibility and accountability are clear.

Disadvantages of the total patient care model are as follows:
- The number of RNs required to provide total patient care may simply not be available because of nursing shortages or financial constraints.
- The RN performs many tasks that could be performed by a caregiver with less training at a lower cost.

Today the total patient care method is commonly used in the hospital's critical care areas, such as intensive care units and postanesthesia care units, where continuous assessment and a high degree of clinical expertise are required at all times. This method is less widely used in other patient care settings as health care organizations move to more efficient, interprofessional team approaches to patient care, allowing RNs to concentrate on aspects of care essential to good patient outcomes, such as providing patient teaching and evaluating the patient's response to the plan of care.

Functional Nursing

In the functional nursing method of patient care delivery, staff members are assigned to complete certain tasks for a group of patients rather than care for specific patients. For example, the RN performs all assessments and care planning, and administers all intravenous medications; the LVN or LPN gives all oral medications; and the assistant performs hygiene tasks and takes vital signs. An RN makes the assignments and coordinates the care. A diagram of the functional nursing care model is shown in Figure 21.2.

Advantages of the functional nursing model are as follows:
- Patient care is provided in an economic and efficient manner because less skilled, lower-cost workers are used in areas where task completion is the focus.
- A minimum number of RNs is required to supervise and to perform strictly nursing duties.
- Tasks are completed quickly, and there is little confusion about job responsibilities.

Disadvantages of the functional nursing model are as follows:
- Care may be fragmented, and the possibility of overlooking priority patient needs exists because several

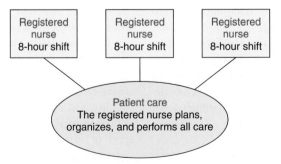

Fig. 21.1 The Total Patient Care (case method) Delivery Model.

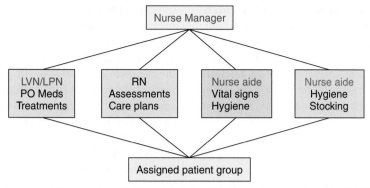

Fig. 21.2 The Functional Nursing Care Delivery Model. *LPN,* licensed practical nurse; *LVN,* licensed vocational nurse; *PO,* oral; *RN,* registered nurse.

different workers focus only on performing specific patient care tasks.
- The patient may feel confused because of the many different individuals providing different aspects of care.
- Caregivers may feel unchallenged and unmotivated when performing repetitive functions.

Although the functional nursing model is considered efficient and economical, the patient is treated by many caregivers who are not able to give personalized care because they are focused on performing a task, not on meeting patient needs. This model may not fit well in the new health care system, which emphasizes customer service. However, functional nursing care delivery is still appropriate in some care settings, such as the operating room.

Team Nursing

In team nursing, the RN functions as a team leader and coordinates a small group (generally no more than four or five) of ancillary personnel to provide care to a small group of patients. As coordinator of the team, the RN must know the condition and needs of all the patients assigned to the team and must plan for individualized care for each patient. The team leader is also responsible for encouraging a cooperative environment and maintaining clear communication among all team members. The team leader's duties include assessing patients and planning care, assigning duties, directing and assisting team members, giving direct patient care, teaching, and coordinating patient activities. A diagram of the team nursing model is shown in Figure 21.3.

Advantages of the team nursing model are as follows:
- High-quality, safe, and effective care can be provided with a relatively high proportion of support staff and/or UAP.
- Each team member participates in decision making and contributes his or her own special expertise in caring for patients.

Disadvantages of the team nursing model are as follows:
- Continuity of care may suffer if the daily team assignments vary and the patient is confronted with many different caregivers.
- The team leader may not have the leadership skills required to effectively direct the team and create a "team spirit."

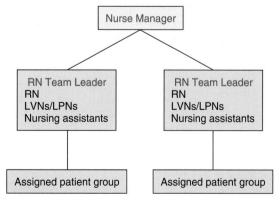

Fig. 21.3 The Team Nursing Model. *LPNs,* licensed practical nurses; *LVNs,* licensed vocational nurses; *RN,* registered nurse.

- Insufficient time for care planning and communication may lead to unclear goals and fragmented care.

Team nursing is an effective, efficient method of patient care delivery and has been used in most inpatient and outpatient health care settings. However, for team nursing to succeed, the team leader must have strong clinical skills, good communication skills, delegation ability, decision-making ability, and the ability to create a cooperative working environment. In an attempt to overcome some of its disadvantages, the team nursing design has been modified many times since its original inception, and variations of the model are evident in other methods of nursing care delivery, such as modular nursing.

Modular Nursing. *Modular nursing*, sometimes referred to as *pod nursing* (Friese et al, 2014), is a modification of team nursing that focuses on a smaller team assigned to a geographic location in the nursing unit. The nursing unit is divided into modules or districts, and the same team of caregivers is assigned consistently to the same geographic location. The concept of modular nursing calls for a smaller group of staff to provide care for a smaller group of patients than with team nursing. The goal is to increase the involvement of the RN in planning and coordinating care. To maximize efficiency, each designated module should contain all the supplies needed by the staff to perform patient care.

Primary Nursing

In primary nursing, the RN, or "primary" nurse, assumes 24-hour responsibility for planning, directing, and evaluating the patient's care from admission through discharge. This model differs significantly from the total patient care model in that the "primary nurse" assumes 24-hour responsibility for directing the patient's plan of care. While on duty, the primary nurse may provide total patient care or may delegate some patient care tasks to LPNs or LVNs or UAP. When the primary nurse is off duty, care is provided by an associate nurse who follows the care plan established by the primary nurse. The primary nurse, who has 24-hour responsibility, is notified if any problems or complications develop and directs alterations in the plan of care. A fundamental responsibility for the nurse in the primary nursing model is to maintain clear communication among all members of the health care team, including the patient, family, physician, associate nurses, and any other members of the health care team. A diagram of the primary nursing model is shown in Figure 21.4.

Advantages of the primary nursing model are as follows:
- One-to-one relationships between nurse and patient support relationship-based care.
- Nurses are able to practice with a high degree of autonomy and to feel challenged and rewarded.

Disadvantages of the primary nursing model are as follows:
- Implementation may be difficult because the primary nurse is required to practice with a high degree of responsibility and autonomy.
- The primary nurse must have high levels of clinical judgment and critical thinking to address clinical problems and to communicate effectively with the health care team.
- The RN may not be willing to accept the 24-hour responsibility required in primary nursing.
- The number of nurses required for this method of care may be difficult to recruit and may prove to be more costly for the organization.

The primary care nursing model lends itself well to home health nursing, hospice nursing, oncology nursing,

Fig. 21.4 The Primary Nursing Model.

and long-term care settings in which the patient requires nursing care for an extended period. Primary nursing may be more difficult to provide in acute care settings, where stays are short and the nurse may see each patient for only 1 or 2 days. Because the concept of primary nursing is sound, some organizations have modified this nursing care model and implemented partnership models that use a wider staff mix.

Partnership Model. The partnership model, sometimes referred to as *coprimary nursing,* is a modification of primary nursing. This model was designed to make more efficient use of the RN, who delegates nonprofessional tasks to the partner, thus providing more time for the RN to address professional demands, such as assessment and patient education. In the partnership model, the RN is partnered with an LVN, LPN, or member of the UAP, and the pair work together consistently to care for an assigned group of patients.

Advantages of the partnership model are as follows:
- The model is more cost-effective than the true primary care nursing system because fewer RNs are needed.
- The RN can encourage the training and growth of his or her partner.
- The RN can perform the nursing duties, and the partner can perform the nonnursing tasks.

Disadvantages of the partnership model are as follows:
- The RN may have difficulty delegating to the partner.
- Consistent partnerships are difficult to maintain because of varied staff schedules.

PATIENT-CENTERED CARE

Patient-centered care has been a core nursing value since the beginning of professional nursing; however, it is receiving renewed attention for all health professionals as a result of the IOM's focus on safety and quality in health care. The IOM (2001) defines *patient-centered care* as "providing care that is respectful of and responsive to individual patient preferences, needs, and values and ensuring that patient values guide all clinical decisions." Delivering patient-centered care means that nurses, physicians, and other health professionals partner with patients and families to ensure that health care decisions respect patients' wants, needs, and preferences and that patients have the education and support they need to make decisions about and participate in their own care. To give patient-centered care means to support patients to live their best possible lives within their own unique experiences.

Patient-centered care is more a philosophy of care than a typical nursing care delivery model as discussed in the previous sections. However, because patient-centered care has become a core focus in today's health care organizations, it must be incorporated as an essential component of any nursing care delivery model. Practical methods for engaging in patient-centered care are to include patients, families, and significant others in:
- Developing care plans and discharge plans that address the uniqueness of the individual and his or her life and family circumstances.
- Participating in shift-change or other handoff reports.
- Receiving education when and how the individual needs it to make informed decisions.

Many health care organizations are now establishing family or consumer advisory councils to engage former patients and families to advise organizational leaders in ways to involve patients and families in decision making and care improvements.

The nurse, as coordinator of the interprofessional team, is responsible for making the patient and family an integral part of the team, keeping the patient involved in decision making, and promoting an environment respectful of the patient's wants, needs, and preferences.

CASE MANAGEMENT

Case management is a model of care in which an RN case manager coordinates patient care with the goal of focusing attention on the quality, outcomes, and cost of care throughout an episode of illness and helping the patient move through the continuum of care. Case managers may be employed by health insurance companies to guide care for health plan members or they may be employed by hospitals to coordinate individual patients' care throughout the course of illnesses. Hospital nurse case managers manage a caseload of patients from preadmission (or onset of illness) to discharge (or resolution of illness). Although case managers generally do not perform direct-care duties, they assume a planning and evaluative role and collaborate with the interprofessional health care team to ensure that goals are met, quality is maintained, and progress toward discharge is made. For example, the nurse case manager coordinates arrangements to move the patient from acute care to rehabilitation to home health to independent living, as determined by patient needs. See Case Study 21.1 for an example of case management.

Case Management Related to Other Nursing Care Delivery Models

Nursing case management in a health care facility supplements nursing care and does not take the place of the nursing care delivery model in place to provide direct patient care. For example, if a hospital's medical-surgical unit uses a team nursing approach to patient care, a system of case management might also be in place to assist with coordinating the patient's total care through discharge. Case management is not needed for every patient in a health care facility and generally is reserved for chronically ill, seriously ill or injured, and long-term, high-cost patients.

Newer Models of Case Management

As health care reform focuses on moving care from expensive acute care settings to less costly community and home settings, newer care models with a foundation in case management are emerging. The first such model is the use of *patient navigators*. First conceptualized in cancer treatment, patient navigators help patients maneuver through the maze of medical appointments, treatments and procedures, insurance and payment systems, patient-support services, educational resources, and the multiple other components of the health care system. The use of patient navigators has been expanded to better manage patients with chronic diseases such as diabetes and hypertension. Patient navigator responsibilities include helping patients access resources such the community food bank and free medication programs, making home visits to assess the home environment and implications for chronic disease management, and communicating with other members of the health care team to support appropriate care decisions.

A second model, *transitional care*, has provided a new role for the RN. As patients with complex care needs move through different levels of care and between multiple providers, communication may be rushed and inadequate, resulting in medication errors, lack of follow-through on key referrals, duplicative testing, inconsistent patient monitoring, and overall poorer patient outcomes (National Transitions of Care Coalition, 2018). Health care systems are recognizing the value of

---

CASE STUDY 21.1 Functions of a Case Manager

The following is a case study demonstrating the functions of the nurse case manager:

Mr. Smith, 58 years of age, was diagnosed with lung cancer 1 year ago. He has been in Medical Center Hospital with multiple complications for more than 3 weeks. Debra Welch, RN, the case manager assigned to Mr. Smith's case, is working with the patient, family, physician, other members of the health care team, and the insurance company to determine a timely, cost-effective discharge plan. Debra has performed a comprehensive health assessment and understands the patient's condition and the available support systems. The physician, patient, family, and health care team agree that Mr. Smith's prognosis is grave and that the treatment plan should be for palliative care only. Pain management is most important at this stage of the disease. Mr. Smith has a strong desire to go home, and his wife and adult daughter are willing to share the responsibility for home care. Debra also has identified the family's need for emotional support to deal effectively with the terminal illness.

After contacting Mr. Smith's insurance company, Debra learns that the company does not provide home health care or hospice benefits but that the patient could be transferred to a subacute facility for continued care. Knowing Mr. Smith's strong desire to go home and the support systems in place, Debra identifies all the costs for home care (hospital bed, bedside commode, oxygen, wheelchair, and hospice support with pain management) and reports the comparative costs of home care and subacute care to the insurance company. By demonstrating that home care is less expensive than inpatient subacute care, Debra is able to successfully negotiate a payment for home care from Mr. Smith's insurance company.

Debra's next responsibilities as case manager are to coordinate Mr. Smith's discharge and to arrange for home services needed, including hospice care and medical equipment. The home plan of care is developed by the health care team. Debra communicates the plan of care to the home care providers to ensure unfragmented care. As a result of case management, Mr. Smith and his family are able to go home with continued support and a smooth transition of care.

nurses to facilitate safe and effective transitions for chronically ill patients to ensure good communication across settings and providers, appropriate follow-up, clear understanding of the prescribed medication regimen, assistance with referrals for needed resources such as transportation and medications, and, most important, encouraging patients and families to take an active role in their health care. Nurse case managers, patient navigators, and transitional care nurses all have similar goals—to work throughout the maze of health care entities to ensure that patients receive the best care possible at the lowest cost with the resources they need to be successful in managing their own care to the extent possible.

CLINICAL PATHWAYS

Clinical pathways, also called *critical paths, practice protocols, patient care protocols,* and *care maps,* are clinical management plans that specify major patient care activities, interprofessional interventions, and desired outcomes within a specified time for a particular diagnosis or health condition. The advantage of the clinical pathway is that it provides a means of standardizing care for patients with similar diagnoses and defines key processes and patient goals in the day-to-day management of care. A similar but different term, clinical practice guidelines (CPGs), guide broader decision making and focus on the decisions to perform a procedure or service. For example, a CPG would be used to determine whether, on the basis of his specific cancer diagnosis, age, and other comorbidities, a patient diagnosed with prostate cancer should undergo radiation treatment. The clinical pathway would guide the care provided to a cancer patient currently undergoing radiation therapy. Clinical pathways are usually developed within the health care facility and are based on broader CPGs. Because clinical pathways dictate the type and amount of care given, they have financial implications for the health care facility.

In essence, the clinical pathway can be viewed as a road map the patient and health care team should follow to guide the patient's care management and recovery. As the patient progresses along the path, specified goals should be accomplished. If a patient's progress deviates from the planned path, a variance has occurred, and the interprofessional team members must create an action plan to address the problem or issue. Clinical pathways were developed in response to the need to identify quality, cost-effective care plans to reduce the patient's length of stay in the hospital. Accreditation agencies such as TJC may stipulate that certain health care facilities use clinical pathways or CPGs to meet accreditation standards.

Components of Clinical Pathways

Components of a clinical pathway include physical assessment guidelines, laboratory and diagnostic tests, medications and procedures, safety and self-care activities, nutrition requirements, patient and family education, discharge planning, and milestones the patient should achieve through the progression of care. Many clinical pathways also address triggers, which are events that identify potential or actual variations in the patient's response to the planned interventions. Common uses for clinical pathways in acute care settings are for the treatment of community-acquired pneumonia, common surgical procedures such as total hip and knee replacements, and stroke or transient ischemic attack.

Clinical pathways may be developed by a team in the organization to include representatives from nursing, medicine, therapy, pharmacy, and dietary services. Professional medical and nursing associations and the Agency for Healthcare Research and Quality (AHRQ) (http://www.guidelines.gov) are excellent sources for currently recommended evidence-based CPGs.

CHOOSING A NURSING CARE DELIVERY MODEL

The nursing care delivery models presented in this chapter can be integrated into a variety of health care settings, including acute care, long-term care, ambulatory care, home care, and hospice. The organizational structure, patient needs, and staff availability influence which delivery system will be used.

Acute care settings may use different types of care delivery models for various patient care units. Emergency departments often use functional approaches to care because emphasis is on efficient assessment and immediate treatment. Team nursing is frequently used in medical-surgical units, whereas total patient care is common in critical care units.

In long-term care settings, such as nursing homes, skilled nursing facilities, and rehabilitation settings, patients remain in the care settings for extended periods. Therefore, the care delivery models may be structured differently from those in the acute setting. Because of its economy and efficiency, functional nursing may be used for daily care tasks, whereas a form of primary care nursing is used for assessment, care planning, and evaluation.

The variety of ambulatory care settings continues to grow as health care moves out of the more expensive inpatient settings to the less costly outpatient settings. Outpatient surgery centers, minor emergency clinics, outpatient cancer centers, outpatient dialysis units, outpatient birthing centers, health clinics, and physicians' offices are examples of ambulatory care settings. The nursing care delivery model used in ambulatory settings varies widely, depending on the type of patients being treated and their particular needs. For example, in outpatient dialysis units, a combination of functional and primary care nursing usually works well. Patient care technicians are assigned to perform specific patient care functions, such as dialysis machine setup and treatment initiation, whereas the RN is assigned primary nurse responsibilities for a group of patients to ensure effective assessment, care planning, and care coordination with the interprofessional team. Telephone nursing is becoming increasingly important as a method of care delivery in ambulatory settings.

Home health care agencies often use a variation of the primary care model. Although in home care the RN does not provide 24-hour care, he or she is responsible for the patient's needs for a 24-hour period and will coordinate intermittent care provided by others, including the home health aide and therapists involved in the patient's care. In the home health care setting, the RN may also function in the role of case manager for his or her assigned patients.

In every care setting, nurses should carefully evaluate the nursing care delivery model to ensure safe, efficient, and effective patient care. In the evaluation of any nursing care delivery model, the following questions should be asked:

- Is patient safety ensured while optimal patient satisfaction and patient outcomes are achieved in a timely, cost-effective manner?
- Is patient-centered care being provided with significant involvement of the patient and his or her family or significant other?
- Are nurses, physicians, and other health care team members satisfied with the safety and quality of care they are able to provide?
- Does the system allow for implementation of the nursing process in a timely and efficient manner?
- Does the system facilitate communication among all members of the health care team?

FUTURE NURSING CARE DELIVERY MODELS

Without a doubt, the ways in which nursing care is delivered over the next 20 years will change dramatically as a result of the following factors:

- Rapid technologic advances in medical care with less invasive procedures for disease treatments
- Fast-paced patient turnover in acute care settings; the rapid discharge and admission cycle is now referred to as "churning"
- Evidence of the RN's value in promoting patient safety and quality of care
- Strong focus on patient satisfaction, safety, and outcomes of care
- Consumers' demands for instant access to care and information
- Need to engage patients and families to become active partners to address their own health care needs

Because acute care settings now admit only the most seriously ill or injured individuals with a focus on stabilization and transition, the traditional models of nursing care may no longer apply. In the past, nurses provided care on the basis of comprehensive knowledge of the patients' needs, which were learned by caring for the patients over an extended period. Now nurses may have an entirely new group of patients to care for every shift or even more than once during a shift. Identifying effective models of care to support the rapid transition of patients from one setting to another will be a continuing challenge for nurses and health care organizations.

Nurses in outpatient and community-based settings are challenged with similar problems in attempting to address (1) patients' demands for instant access to care and information and (2) patients' needs for support and education to address lifestyle and personal choices that may affect their health.

Relationship-based care must also be considered part of the care delivery model in high-tech fast-paced environments where nurses struggle to provide care that is consistent with nursing values of compassion, caring, and healing. Therapeutic relationships to promote optimum health for our patients and communities are the essence of nursing practice and must be accepted as a primary responsibility by every RN. Without a doubt, new and innovative models of care must and will emerge to address the challenges of today's complex health care environment (Mensik, 2016).

SUMMARY

All nurses must be concerned that patient care is delivered in the most efficient and cost-effective method possible and that staffing is appropriate to ensure safe, high-quality care and contributes to staff satisfaction. For this reason, nursing care delivery models have undergone tremendous change throughout the past decade and will continue to evolve as organizations look for ways to improve patient safety and outcomes in complex health care systems that are challenged by the need to reduce costs, rapidly advancing technology, high patient turnover, and consumer demand for instant access and information. Regardless of changes that are certain to occur, the RN will retain responsibility for evaluating nursing care delivery models to ensure that patient care is delivered safely and efficiently, that caregivers are competent and legally qualified to perform the duties they have been assigned, and that high-quality, safe, patient-centered care and staff satisfaction are maintained.

REFERENCES

American Association of Critical Care Nurses. (2014). *The AACN Synergy Model for Patient Care.* Retrieved from https://www.aacn.org/nursing-excellence/aacn-standards/synergy-model.

American Nurses Association. (2012). *Principles for nurse staffing* (2nd ed.). Silver Spring, MD: American Nurses Association.

American Nurses Association. (2018). *Nurse staffing.* Retrieved from http://www.nursingworld.org/MainMenuCategories/ThePracticeofProfessionalNursing/Nurse-Staffing.

Ball, J. E., Bruyneel, L., Aiken, L. H., Sermeus, W., Sloane, D. M., Rafferty, A. M., et al. (2017). Post-operative mortality, missed care and nurse staffing in nine countries: a cross-sectional study. *International Journal of Nursing Studies,* doi:10.1016/j.ijnurstu.2017.08.004.

Coffey, R. J., Richards, J. S., Remmert, C. S., LeRoy, S. S., Schoville, R. R., & Baldwin, P. J. (2005). An introduction to critical paths. *Quality Management in Health Care, 14*(1), 46–55.

Dawson, J. M. (2014). Nursing practice and work environment. *American Nurse Today, 10*(1), 16.

Driscoll, A., Grant, M. J., Carroll, D., Dalton, S., Deaton, C., Jones, I., et al. (2018). The effect of nurse-to-patient ratios on nurse-sensitive patient outcomes in acute specialist units: a systematic review and meta-analysis. *European Journal of Cardiovascular Nursing, 17*(1), 6–22.

Friese, C. R., Grunawalt, J. C., Bhullar, S., Bihlmeyer, K., Chang, R., Wood, W. (2014). Pod nursing on a medical/surgical unit: Implementation and outcomes evaluation. *The Journal of Nursing Administration, 44*(4), 207–211.

Institute of Medicine, Field, M. J., Lohr, K. N. (Eds.), (1990). *Clinical practice guidelines: Directions for a new program.* Washington, DC: National Academies Press.

Institute of Medicine. (2001). *Crossing the quality chasm: A new health system for the 21st century.* Washington, DC: National Academies Press.

Institute of Medicine. (2004). *Keeping patients safe: transforming the work environments of nurses.* Washington, DC: National Academies Press.

Institute of Medicine. (2011). *The future of nursing: leading change, advancing health.* Washington, DC: National Academies Press.

Mensik, J. (2016). Searching for the holy grail of care delivery models. *Nursing economic$, 34*(2), 90–91.

National Council of State Boards of Nursing. (2016). *National guidelines for nursing delegation.* Retrieved from https://www.ncsbn.org/NCSBN_Delegation_Guidelines.pdf.

National Transitions of Care Coalition. (2018). *Improving care transitions for all.* Retrieved from http://www.ntocc.org/WhoWeServe/tabid/56/Default.aspx.

Shimp, K. M. (2017). Systematic review of turnover/retention and staff perception of staffing and resource adequacy related to staffing. *Nursing economic$, 35*(5), 239–258.

22

Quality Improvement and Patient Safety

Kathleen M. Werner, MS, BSN, RN, CPHQ

Nurses are building bridges to patient safety and quality care.

ⓔ Additional resources are available online at: *http://evolve.elsevier.com/Cherry/*

LEARNING OUTCOMES

After studying this chapter, the reader will be able to:

1. Apply principles of quality improvement to the role of the professional nurse.
2. Analyze the basis for the increasing emphasis on health care quality and medical errors.
3. Analyze the role of health care regulatory agencies and how they have embodied the principles of quality improvement.
4. Discuss the role that process improvement can play in ensuring patient safety and improving quality in the health care system.
5. Describe the tools and skills necessary for successful quality improvement activities.
6. Discuss the professional nurse's role in promoting patient safety.

KEY TERMS

Cause-and-effect diagram Tool that is used for identifying and organizing possible causes of a problem in a structured format. It is sometimes called a fishbone diagram because it looks like the skeleton of a fish.

Clinical indicators Measurable items that reflect the quality of care provided and demonstrate the degree to which desired clinical outcomes are accomplished.

Customer Individual or group who relies on an organization to provide a product or service to meet some need or expectation. It is these customer needs and expectations that determine quality.

Failure mode and effects analysis (FMEA) A systematic process for identifying potential design and process failures before they occur, with the intent to eliminate them or minimize the risk associated with them.

Flowchart Picture of the sequence of steps in a process. Different steps or actions are represented by boxes or other symbols.

Hospital-acquired condition (HAC) A term used to indicate an unintended and typically adverse patient-acquired condition occurring as a result of being cared for in a hospital.

Institute of Medicine (IOM) A nonprofit organization that is part of the National Academy of Sciences with a mission of advancing and disseminating scientific knowledge to improve human health. The institute provides objective, timely, authoritative information and advice concerning health and science policy to the government, the corporate sector, the professions, and the public.

Never events Serious adverse events during an inpatient stay that should never occur or are reasonably preventable through adherence to evidence-based guidelines. The Centers for Medicare and Medicaid Services, through revisions in coverage and payment policies, provide hospitals with financial incentives to reduce the occurrence of never events.

Pareto chart A graphic tool that helps break down a big problem into its parts and then identify which parts are the most important.

Process A series of linked steps necessary to accomplish work. A process turns inputs, such as information or raw materials, into outputs, such as products, services, and reports. Clinical processes are a series of linked steps necessary for the provision of patient care.

Process variation The differences in how the steps in a work process might be accomplished and/or the variables that may affect each step in the process. Variation results from the lack of perfect uniformity in the performance of any process. Understanding variation in a process is necessary to determine the direction that improvement efforts must take.

Quality improvement (QI) Framework for taking action to systematically make changes that lead to measurable improvements in health care services for patients, staff, and organizations; quality is determined by the needs, expectations, and desired health outcomes of individuals and populations.

Root cause analysis (RCA) Method of problem solving that helps to identify how and why an event occurred. RCA is defined by TJC (2017a) as a process for identifying the basic or causal factors underlying variation in performance, including the occurrence or possible occurrence of a sentinel event. A root cause analysis focuses primarily on a positive, preventive approach to system and process changes.

Run chart Graph of data in time order that helps identify any changes that occur over time; also called a *time plot*. A run chart that to which a centerline and statistical control limits have been added is known as a *control chart*.

Sentinel event Defined by TJC (2017a) as a patient safety event that reaches a patient and results in death, permanent harm, or severe temporary harm and intervention is required to sustain life. Such events are called "sentinel" because they signal the need for immediate investigation and response.

Standardization Approach to process improvement that involves developing and adhering to best-known methods and repeating key tasks in the same way, time and time again, until a better way is found, thereby creating exceptional service with maximal efficiency.

The Joint Commission (TJC) A national agency that conducts surveys of inpatient and ambulatory facilities and certifies their compliance with established quality standards.

PROFESSIONAL/ETHICAL ISSUE

Christine Hamilton, RN, works in the cardiac step-down unit at large teaching hospital. Christine graduated from nursing school 6 months ago. She has been managing her own patient assignment for the last few months, but she continues to work closely with her mentor, an experienced RN who has worked on the unit for 15 years. Recently, Christine has become concerned about a pattern on the unit in which the nurses ignore alarms on medical devices. She knows that the purpose of the alarms is to alert caregivers about changes in patient conditions, but she also knows that alarms that do not work correctly can be a nuisance and pull nurses away from other important work. Her greatest concern is that ignoring alarms might result in patient harm. To make the situation more complicated, Christine does not feel comfortable in discussing her concerns with her mentor because she has overheard her mentor tell other nurses that there are times when it is okay to ignore alarms. How should Christine begin to address this situation with her colleagues or supervisor? Discuss how this safety concern might be addressed through the quality improvement process.

VIGNETTE

It was the third postoperative day for Mrs. Slattery in room 918 on the general surgical unit of Metro Hospital. As she arrived for her day shift, Suzanne Harper, RN, was eager to care for this patient. Suzanne had been with Mrs. Slattery every day since her admission and was looking forward to helping her prepare for discharge. Suzanne carried out the routine morning care and did a thorough assessment of Mrs. Slattery. Much to Suzanne's dismay, Mrs. Slattery was not her usual, upbeat self and was less cooperative than normal, stating, "I just don't have much energy. I know I should get up and walk, but I just don't feel like it." Suzanne also noted that Mrs. Slattery's temperature was higher than normal, so she alerted the surgical house staff during rounds. Mrs. Slattery's blood was drawn for a complete blood count (CBC) and a urine sample was collected. Within the hour, the answer to Mrs. Slattery's sudden lack of energy and enthusiasm became known—she had a urinary tract infection (UTI), most likely as the result of the indwelling catheter that had been placed during surgery and still remained. Mrs. Slattery would not be going home until the catheter was removed and treatment of the infection was well under way. Suzanne experienced the wisdom of "hindsight" by noting that the catheter should have been removed by postoperative day two. Owing to the surgeon's failure to write an order to discontinue the indwelling catheter in a timely manner— as well as Suzanne's failure to bring this to the provider's attention—Mrs. Slattery was now experiencing a setback in her recovery.

Suzanne began to reflect on the number of times this may have occurred with other patients. She also began to consider the implications of the lack of a consistent and standardized way to track the dwell time of urinary catheters. As in Mrs. Slattery's situation, the development of a urinary tract infection could cost $12,000 to $20,000 in additional expenses for the hospital; it would mean additional care and treatment with an extended length of stay that would not be paid by the patient's insurance company because the catheter-associated UTI would be deemed an event that should have been prevented. Multiplying this cost by just ten additional patients makes catheter-associated UTIs a significant financial burden for the organization. More important, patients experience discomfort and increased fatigue and run the risk for development of even more complications because of their decreased willingness or ability to cooperate with their postoperative care.

The next week, Suzanne approached her nurse manager and expressed concern about the delays in discontinuing indwelling urinary catheters that create the potential for catheter-associated UTIs. Suzanne's nurse manager thanked her for the feedback and expressed similar interest in resolving this problem. Infection prevention staff members had already been in preliminary conversations with Suzanne's manager about the increased risk of infection and were willing to work collaboratively with the nursing staff and physicians to find a solution to this problem. Suzanne eagerly volunteered to participate in a quality improvement team that was charged with standardizing the care processes for discontinuation of urinary catheters to ensure compliance with removal by postoperative day two for 100% of all patients.

The team met regularly for several weeks and gained a clear understanding of why both physicians and nurses "lost track of time" with respect to removal of these catheters. This was accomplished through the creation of a detailed picture of what typically occurred in documentation of postoperative orders by the surgical staff and the routine care implemented by nursing personnel. Breakdowns in this process for ensuring completeness of all necessary orders were identified, and the team began working on constructive ways to prevent these breakdowns in the future. The team worked with information technology experts to incorporate the indwelling catheter discontinuation order in an electronic order set easily accessible for all physicians. Furthermore, if the discontinuation order was not documented, an electronic alert would be sent to the attending surgeon to remind him or her to either complete the order or document the rationale for not doing so. Likewise, nursing staff would receive an electronic "best practice alert" reminding them to check the orders for this purpose.

Over time, with ongoing monitoring of the ordering practices and the catheter-associated UTI rates, significant progress was made, to the point that infection rates are now nearly zero. Suzanne knows that the proper steps are in place to guarantee that this successful infection reduction effort will be sustained through the thoughtful process that was developed. When her patients are ready for discharge, there will be no setbacks caused by situations that could have been prevented. Suzanne feels that she is a vested part of this success.

Questions to Consider While Reading This Chapter:

1. What key principles of quality improvement are demonstrated in the vignette?
2. What quality improvement tools did Suzanne and the team most likely use to identify the causes for catheter-associated UTIs?
3. What resources are available to help Suzanne and others in her organization learn more about improving the quality of health care?

CHAPTER OVERVIEW

Although Suzanne Harper's story depicted in the vignette seems credible and would be a logical way for any organization to begin addressing customer concerns, far too often this has not been the case. Hospitals and other health care organizations have been slow to recognize the necessity of a true customer perspective and to emphasize quality and safety in a proactive manner. The intention of this chapter is to make the reader aware of the pressing nature of the nation's quality health care crisis and to address the following questions:

- What is quality in health care?
- Who determines the degree to which quality is evident in our health care system?
- How can work processes be redesigned to improve quality?
- What do the potential answers to the first three questions mean for professional nursing accountability?

The responses to these questions, particularly in relation to nursing's commitment to become involved with quality improvement and to participate in its implementation, provide the elements of hope for determining and implementing sustainable, positive improvements in the design and delivery of health care.

THE URGENT CASE FOR QUALITY IMPROVEMENT IN THE U.S. HEALTH CARE SYSTEM

In an alarming 2000 report by the Institute of Medicine (IOM), titled *To Err Is Human: Building a Safer Health System,* the writers extrapolated and summarized data from two major studies and concluded that up to 98,000 patients die each year from preventable medical errors, confirming that poor quality of care is a major problem in the United States (IOM, 2000). An updated estimate, developed from studies that were published from 2008 to 2011, validated these original IOM statistics (James, 2013). Contributing factors cited in the original IOM report include the following:

- Overuse of expensive invasive technology
- Underuse of inexpensive care services
- Error-prone implementation of care that could harm patients and waste money

Following this report, the IOM released *Crossing the Quality Chasm: A New Health System for the 21st Century*

(2001) to define a vision for improving the quality of our nation's health care. This report states: "The U.S. health care delivery system does not provide consistent, high quality medical care to all people. Americans should be able to count on receiving care that meets their needs and is based on the best scientific knowledge—yet this frequently is not the case. Health care harms too frequently and routinely fails to deliver its potential benefits. Indeed, between the health care that we now have and the health care that we could have lies not just a gap, but a chasm" (p. 1).

The Quality Chasm report details a number of factors that have contributed to this chasm, including the unprecedented advancement of science and technology, the growing complexity of health care, changing public health care needs, and a poorly organized and uncoordinated health care delivery system. Although one aim of the Patient Protection and Affordable Care Act of 2010 was to improve the quality and efficiency of U.S. medical care services for everyone, indicators from recent reports show that the quality chasm between what we know is good care and what is current practice still exists:

- On average, 30% of Americans failed to receive recommended care in 2010; later data show that the quality of health care improved overall from 2000 through 2014-2015 but that the pace of improvement varied by priority area, with health care quality and disparities differing widely across states and regions (Agency for Healthcare Research and Quality [AHRQ], 2014, 2017).
- On average, patients are subjected to at least one medication error each day, with extremely high costs to patients, families, health care professionals, hospitals, and insurance companies (IOM, 2007).

The Quality Chasm report also offers six guiding aims for improvement that should be adopted by every individual and group involved in the provision of health care, including health care professionals, public and private health care organizations, purchasers of health care, regulatory agencies and organizations, and state and federal policymakers. These six guiding aims are collectively referred to by the acronym STEEEP. Individually, these aims call for health care to be (IOM, 2001):

- *Safe:* Preventing injuries to patients from the care that is intended to help them
- *Timely:* Reducing waits and sometimes harmful delays for both those who receive and those who give care

- *Effective:* Providing services based on scientific knowledge to all who could benefit, and refraining from providing services to those not likely to benefit
- *Efficient:* Preventing waste, including waste of equipment, supplies, ideas, and energy
- *Equitable:* Providing care that does not vary in quality because of personal characteristics, such as gender, ethnicity, geographic location, and socioeconomic status
- *Patient centered:* Providing care that is respectful of and responsive to individual patient preferences, needs, and values and ensuring that patient values guide all clinical decisions

To help establish a framework for accomplishing the significant redesign of the health care system, the writers of the Quality Chasm report formulated a set of 10 simple rules to guide improvement initiatives. Professional nurses must serve as role models for all health care professionals, caregivers, and administrators in practicing the following 10 rules (IOM, 2001):

1. *Care is based on continuous healing relationships.* Patients should receive care whenever they need it and in many forms, including face-to-face visits, via the Internet, by telephone, and other means as needed.
2. *Care is customized according to patient needs and values.* The system should be designed to meet the most common needs but should also be responsive to individual choices and preferences.
3. *The patient is the source of control.* Patients should be given the necessary information and opportunity to exercise the degree of control they choose over health care decisions that affect them.
4. *Knowledge is shared, and information flows freely.* Patients should have unfettered access to their own medical information and to clinical knowledge, with clinicians communicating effectively and sharing information.
5. *Decision making is evidence based.* Patients should receive care based on the best available scientific knowledge, and care should not vary illogically from clinician to clinician or place to place.
6. *Safety is a system property.* Patients should be safe; reducing risk and ensuring safety require greater attention to systems that help prevent and mitigate errors.
7. *Transparency is necessary.* The system should make available to patients and families information that allows them to make informed decisions, including information describing the system's performance on safety, evidence-based practice, and patient satisfaction.

8. *Needs are anticipated.* The system should anticipate patient needs rather than simply react to events.
9. *Waste is continually decreased.* The system should not waste resources (e.g., supplies, health professionals' time and energy) or patient time.
10. *Cooperation among clinicians is a priority.* Clinicians should actively engage in collaboration and communication to ensure an appropriate exchange of information and coordination of care.

The remainder of this chapter provides the reader with a set of principles and skills necessary to implement improvements and move toward a system of health care that is safe, timely, effective, efficient, equitable, and patient centered.

PRINCIPLES OF QUALITY IMPROVEMENT

Many buzzwords describe activities associated with quality improvement (QI). The most prevalent are total quality management (TQM), continuous quality improvement (CQI), continuous process improvement, statistical process control, and performance improvement (PI). The terms themselves are not as important as the principles they embody: assessing and improving work processes while focusing on what customers want and need. In the example of Suzanne and her patient, the work process is completing postoperative orders that include timely removal of an indwelling urinary catheter. The customer in this situation would be Suzanne's patient, who wants to recover from surgery without complications so that she can go home as soon as possible. Essentially the cornerstones of QI are quality, scientific approach, and "all one team" (Joiner, 1994).

Quality

To provide a better appreciation of the importance of these three QI cornerstones, a customer's perspective of quality must be considered, including the personal interactions he or she experiences with an organization's personnel in addition to the products or services he or she receives. The products or services provided to the customer are not made up of just the physical items or a one-time experience that the customer encounters, but rather of all the services that go with it. Organizations actually provide a "bundle" of products and services to customers to satisfy some need. If the service and product or outcomes together are perceived as a good value, a loyal customer following will be established. Or, as in the case presented in the vignette, Suzanne's patient might view the entire hospital stay negatively because of the delay in discharge due to a preventable complication.

Scientific Approach

The scientific approach, the second cornerstone of QI, emphasizes that to make significant improvements in an organization's processes, decisions must be based on sound, valid data, and the people managing the processes must have a clear understanding of the nature of variation in processes. Remember that a process is a series of linked steps necessary to accomplish work. For example, the steps necessary to complete a new medication order, from the time the order is received until the medication is administered to a patient, is a process. Understanding process variation—the differences in how the steps in the process might be accomplished and/or the variables that may affect each step—is necessary to identify the direction that improvement efforts must take.

Two types of variation in processes can occur: common cause variation and special cause variation. Processes that demonstrate common cause variation are stable, predictable, and statistically in control. Processes that demonstrate both common cause and special cause variation are unstable, unpredictable, and not in statistical control. The actions that should be taken to implement improvements under each type of variation are significantly different.

The best way to understand common cause and special cause variations is to use Suzanne's example again. Suzanne's team members collected data over time regarding the number of times patients' surgeons failed to write postoperative orders that included discontinuation of urinary catheters. Overall, the number of missed orders showed variability because of numerous factors associated with this process, one example being the total number of patients with postoperative orders on any given day. The team recognized the total number of postoperative patients as common cause variation and realized that to decrease the occurrence of missing elements within these orders, the overall process would need to be studied to determine the best ways to change the postoperative care processes, regardless of the total volume of patients.

The team was also aware of a significant physician learning curve associated with the automation of electronic order sets, with two surgeons who had not completed the required training session before the system went "live." The failure to document the catheter discontinuation order under these circumstances was considered to be special cause process variation, one of extreme impact but related to a clearly identified single source. If the team had modified the overall documentation process solely on the basis of the special cause factor, the underlying problem most likely would not have been improved for the long term.

"All One Team"

Effective team functioning is the third QI cornerstone, which embodies the principles of believing in people; treating everyone in the workplace with dignity, trust, and respect; and working toward win-win situations for all customers, employees, shareholders, suppliers, and perhaps even the broader community as a whole. For people to work this way, they must believe it is in their best interest to cooperate; they need to be more concerned with how the system as a whole operates rather than optimizing their own contributing area. In other words, all team members must rely more on cooperation and less on competition.

Example

Suzanne's example is one that demonstrates the following three principles of QI:
- *Quality:* Suzanne began to consider the patient as the one who would define the quality of her hospital stay. The nurse recognized that the perceived quality of the entire hospital stay could suffer if the prevention of complications could not be improved.
- *Scientific approach:* Suzanne was supported organizationally by her manager, who provided the opportunity for Suzanne to collaborate with other key members of the health care team to better comprehend the current status of catheter-associated UTIs through analyzing data and examining variations in the process. This group's work led to a clearer understanding of the interrelationship of the processes across multiple health care professionals, which together affected the overall timeliness of urinary catheter discontinuation and enabled the group to make the necessary improvements to achieve the desired result.

- "*All one team*": Managers in Suzanne's hospital had faith in the people who were working on the catheter-associated UTI team. They were recognized as the people who had the best understanding of how the postoperative care processes were happening and where the system was breaking down.

ADVANCING QUALITY THROUGH REGULATION AND ACCREDITATION

Today, almost all health care regulatory and voluntary accrediting agencies require QI in some form. The Centers for Medicare and Medicaid Services (CMS), which administers the U.S. Medicare program, has "conditions of participation" for its quality foundation, and most state licensing authorities also have required QI standards. The Joint Commission (TJC), an organization that offers voluntary accreditation for health care settings, has a strong focus on quality standards, as discussed in the following sections.

The Joint Commission

The Joint Commission was one of the first accreditation agencies to embrace QI principles as an accreditation requirement in hospital-based settings. TJC accredits and certifies more than 21,000 health care organizations and programs in the United States, including hospitals and health care organizations that provide ambulatory and office-based surgery, behavioral health, home health care, laboratory and nursing care center services. Health care organizations voluntarily seek TJC accreditation to demonstrate that they have achieved a "gold seal of approval" by following the quality and safety standards established by TJC (TJC, 2017b). TJC standards address the organization's level of performance in key functional areas, such as patient safety, patient rights, patient treatment, and infection control. The TJC accreditation system not only focuses on an organization's ability to provide safe high-quality care but also requires evidence of actual performance and continued improvement. Health care organizations that are accredited by TJC receive "deemed status" to automatically meet foundational approval from CMS.

Core Measures: National Hospital Quality Measures

In 1997, TJC introduced ORYX, a performance measurement and improvement initiative, as part of the accreditation process. The ORYX measurements were intended to support organizations in their quality improvement efforts as well as supplement their accreditation process. In 2002, as part of the ORYX initiative, accredited hospitals began collecting data on standardized "core" performance measures, and by 2004, TJC and CMS were working together to align current and future measures common to both organizations. These standardized measures are now referred to as National Hospital Inpatient Quality Measures and can be found on TJC's website (https://www.jointcommission.org/specifications_manual_for_national_hospital_inpatient_quality_measures.aspx). The performance data for hospitals across the country are now publicly reported on TJC's website Quality Check (http://www.qualitycheck.org) and through the CMS Hospital Compare website (http://www.medicare.gov/hospitalcompare/).

The National Hospital Inpatient Quality Measures now have an added level of significance beyond the public reporting aspect. These measures, in concert with patient feedback and other select clinical outcome measures, are being used increasingly in programs designed to "pay for performance" in moving health care payments away from simply paying for the provision of services to paying on the basis of the quality and outcomes associated with those services.

As part of the Patient Protection and Affordable Care Act of 2010, CMS was authorized to begin its Value-Based Purchasing program, whereby hospital inpatient Medicare payments are reduced annually (from 1% in the first program fiscal year of 2013 up to a maximum of 2% by fiscal year 2017 and beyond). Hospitals may earn back the reduced payments or even exceed the original payment amount on the basis of their performance results. Other commercial insurance carriers and state agencies are beginning to deploy similar strategies in their payment agreements. For more information on Value-Based Purchasing, including quality initiatives for other settings such as home health and nursing homes, visit the Innovation Center section of the CMS website (https://innovation.cms.gov/).

It is especially important for nurses to be knowledgeable about the National Hospital Inpatient Quality Measures and Value-Based Purchasing program because they are in the unique position of supporting the overall management of patient care, working collaboratively with other health care professionals to initiate changes, and monitoring ongoing effectiveness of the care and follow-up provided. For more information, nurses are encouraged to visit the Performance Measurement section of the TJC website (https://www.jointcommission.org/performance_measurement.aspx).

CLINICAL INDICATORS AND PROCESS IMPROVEMENT TOOLS AND SKILLS

The basic foundation of the monitoring and evaluation process required by QI principles is in the use of clinical indicators, measurable items that reflect the quality of care. Just like the National Hospital Inpatient Quality Measures previously referenced, clinical indicators are aspects of clinical care that can be measured to show the extent to which care is or is not being implemented as it should be. Indicators focus on clinical actions or outcomes of clinical care; indicators should not focus on procedures that support clinical care. For example, replacing the intravenous (IV) solutions on the IV supply cart as they are used is a procedure that supports clinical care. Administering the correct IV solution at the correct rate as prescribed is appropriate clinical care. Both items are measurable, but only the latter is truly a clinical indicator. Indicators are meant not to define quality but, rather, to point the way to assessment of areas in which quality issues may be present.

How do process improvement skills and tools fit with clinical indicators? Clinical indicators help identify the goals of QI, whereas process improvement skills and tools support the quantitative understanding of key work processes. Several different methods are used by health care facilities for QI and process improvement, including Lean methodology, Lean Six Sigma, and failure mode and effects analysis (FMEA). The tools described within this section (e.g., flowcharts, Pareto charts) are all used in each of these various methods of QI. Addressing these specific improvement strategies is not within the scope of this chapter, but it is important to note that all improvement models generally have the following activities in common:

- Analyzing and clearly understanding the process
- Selecting key aspects of the process to improve
- Establishing "trial" targets to guide improvement measures
- Collecting and plotting data
- Interpreting results
- Implementing improvement actions and evaluating effectiveness

Various tools, such as flowcharts, Pareto charts, cause-and-effect diagrams, and run charts, may be used to accomplish each of these six steps. Through use of these tools, results can be analyzed with interpretations subsequently guiding appropriate improvement actions. Once improvements are initiated, ongoing monitoring is initiated to evaluate the effectiveness of the changes implemented. It will become increasingly necessary for professional nurses to understand improvement models and develop the ability to apply these tools.

Flowchart

The analysis of a work process is usually initiated through construction of some sort of flowchart or flow diagram. These are indispensable tools in mapping out what actually occurs during the process versus what is intended. There are several different types of flowcharts, each of which is valuable in its own way. A top-down flowchart simply lists the main steps and substeps of a process in a linear fashion (Fig. 22.1). A deployment flowchart maps out the steps of a process under headings that designate the people or departments carrying out each step. This type is especially helpful to deal with processes that involve multiple areas or caregivers and when there is a need for common understanding of what the process is doing as a whole

Fig. 22.1 Top-Down Flowchart of Process for Administering Intravenous Solutions.

(Fig. 22.2). As illustrated in Figures 22.1 and 22.2, top-down and deployment flowcharts can be used to view the process of administering the correct IV solution at the correct rate.

Pareto Chart

For selecting key aspects on which to focus within the process, a Pareto chart may be an appropriate tool. Collecting data on presumed or known problems in a given process can achieve areas of focus or concentration. This tool itself is a type of bar graph, with the height of bars reflecting the frequency with which events occur or the effect events have on a process problem. The bars are arranged in descending order so that the most commonly occurring problems are readily visible. Figure 22.3 is based on the Pareto principle, which proposes that 80% of process or system problems are generated from only 20% of the possible causal factors. Therefore, focusing on the significant few causes can achieve a much broader effect on improvement efforts.

Fig. 22.2 Deployment Flowchart of Process for Administering Intravenous Solutions.

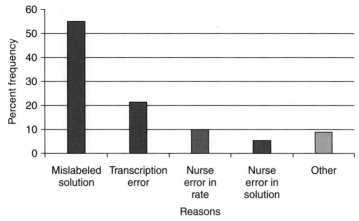

Fig. 22.3 Pareto Chart of Reasons for Incorrect Intravenous Solution Administration.

Cause-and-Effect Diagram

The **cause-and-effect diagram** is another worthy tool that can help determine potential sources of a problem. Such a diagram is a list of potential causes arranged by categories to show their potential effect on a problem. The categories are usually broad, with subsequent levels of detail to illustrate what "might cause" the effect in question. This diagram is sometimes referred to as a "fishbone diagram" because it resembles a fish skeleton when complete (Fig. 22.4). Cause-and-effect diagrams are helpful when the major problem areas have been localized through the use of the Pareto chart.

Run Chart

Measuring data over time to evaluate patterns in process variation typically is suited for tools such as the run chart and the control chart. Run charts, also known as time plots, are graphs of data points as they occur over time (Fig. 22.5). Valuable information can be obtained regarding process variation through study of the trends in the run chart. A control chart is a slightly more sophisticated tool to help distinguish between common cause and special cause variations. A control chart is basically a run chart with statistical control limits added.

UNDERSTANDING, IMPROVING, AND STANDARDIZING CARE PROCESSES

Standardized processes, otherwise referred to as "best known methods" or "best practices," when effectively managed, have been shown to be the foundation for

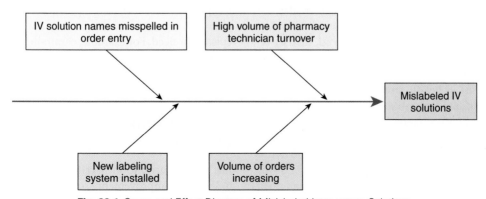

Fig. 22.4 Cause-and-Effect Diagram of Mislabeled Intravenous Solutions.

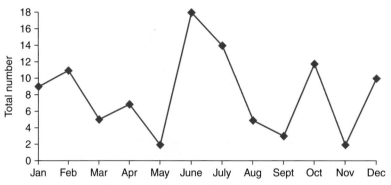

Fig. 22.5 Run Chart of Number of Mislabeled Intravenous Solutions.

improvements in all areas of business today, but especially in the clinical care setting. There is a typical resistance to standardizing practices, especially when they involve providing patient care, but the realistic effect of care without standardization must be considered in the following context as described by Joiner (1994):

- Most employees receive little training on how to do their jobs. Instead the majority are left to learn by watching a more experienced employee.
- Most employees have developed their own unique versions of any general procedures they witnessed or were taught. They think, "My way is the best way."
- Changes to procedures happen haphazardly; individuals constantly change details to counteract problems that arise or in hopes of discovering a better method. Tampering is rampant.

Each of the quality improvement cornerstones could easily be applied to caregiver situations. At first glance, it would be assumed that all care practices are based on scientific evidence and research, and although many are, others exist simply because that was how the practitioner originally was educated. Those practices that are research based, even though they represent best known methods, may still not be widely practiced, thereby resulting in lack of standardization.

During the past few years, a number of methods have been used in health care settings for the purpose of supporting standardization of care processes. Clinical guidelines, critical pathways, and clinical protocols or algorithms are standardization methods that are more prevalent and familiar. Although these terms sometimes are used interchangeably, the following is offered as a context in which to understand their potential differences.

Clinical Pathways or Critical Pathways

Clinical pathway or *critical pathway* typically defines the optimal sequencing and timing of interventions by physicians, nurses, and other interprofessional team members when providing care for a patient with a particular diagnosis or procedure, such as a patient who is hospitalized for a coronary artery bypass graft. These pathways are usually developed through collaborative efforts of the interprofessional team, which includes physicians, nurses, pharmacists, and others, to improve the quality and value of the patient care provided. Among the most obvious benefits of using clinical pathways are (1) reduction in variation of the care provided, (2) facilitation and achievement of expected clinical outcomes, (3) reduction in care delays and lengths of stay in the inpatient setting, and (4) improvements in cost-effectiveness of the care delivered while maintaining or increasing patient and family satisfaction.

Clinical Protocols or Algorithms

Clinical protocols or algorithms are different from clinical pathways because they represent more of a decision path that a practitioner might take during a particular episode or need. For example, common algorithms exist for treatment of hypertension, provision of both basic and advanced life support, and general diagnostic screening (Fig. 22.6).

BREAKTHROUGH THINKING TO IMPROVE QUALITY

Just as standardization is critical to the foundation of health care improvement, so is the notion of breakthrough thinking and swift application of best known

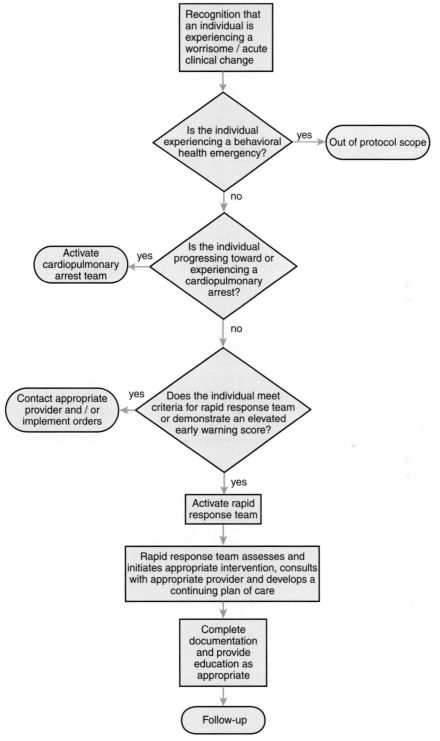

Fig. 22.6 Clinical Algorithm—Health Care Protocol: Rapid Response Team.

methods for practice. The premise behind breakthrough thinking and its resulting action is threefold: (1) substantial knowledge exists about how to achieve better performance than currently prevails; (2) strong examples already exist of organizations that have applied that knowledge and broken through to substantial improvements; and (3) the stakes are high and relevant to the most crucial strategic needs of health care (Berwick, 1997).

The Institute for Healthcare Improvement (IHI), a voluntary organization formed to assist leaders in all health care settings actively involved in improving quality, recommends a QI model developed by Langley and colleagues (2009) and is composed of two parts. Part one asks three fundamental questions:

1. What are we trying to accomplish?
2. How will we know that a change is an improvement?
3. What changes can we make that will result in improvement?

Part two uses a sequence of steps, starting with developing an action plan based on the three questions and going on to taking actions to test the plan, making refinements as needed, and implementing the resulting changes in real work settings. This is known as a plan–do–check–act (PDCA) cycle (Fig. 22.7). For more in-depth information, visit the IHI website (http://www.ihi.org).

PATIENT SAFETY

Nowhere is the need for QI more evident than in the area of health care errors. As discussed previously, the IOM report *To Err Is Human: Building a Safer Health System* (2000) placed the issue of medical mistakes and patient safety on the pages of many national newspapers, on the agendas of health care governing boards, and at the forefront of federal government legislation. In response to the focus on patient safety and the need for data to better understand the priority concerns, several national initiatives were implemented and are discussed in the following sections.

Institute for Safe Medication Practices

An outcome of the patient safety and QI movement was establishment of the Institute for Safe Medication Practices (ISMP), a nonprofit organization that is now well known as an education resource for the prevention of medication errors. The ISMP provides independent,

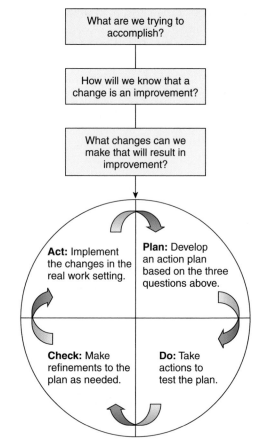

Fig. 22.7 Institute for Healthcare Improvement (IHI) Quality Improvement Model.

multidisciplinary, expert review of errors reported through the ISMP Medication Errors Reporting Program (MERP). Through MERP, health care professionals across the nation voluntarily and confidentially report medication errors and hazardous conditions that could lead to errors. The reporting process is simple and easily accessible by clinicians. All resulting information and error-prevention strategies are shared with the U.S. Food and Drug Administration (FDA).

The ISMP has also developed *Medication Safety Self-Assessments* to allow nurses and other health care professionals to assess the medication safety practices in their work setting. These tools contain items that address the use of medications in the clinical setting, use of high-alert medications, and system improvements and safeguards that the ISMP has recommended in response to analysis of medication errors (ISMP, 2017).

The assessments are publicly available on the ISMP website (https://www.ismp.org/self-assessments).

Role of Regulatory and Accrediting Agencies in Promoting Patient Safety

The leaders of regulatory agencies (e.g., CMS) and accrediting agencies (e.g., TJC) have developed standards and programs to promote patient safety. Three such programs are discussed in the following sections.

Sentinel Event Standard. As one response to the increasing emphasis on patient safety, TJC established its sentinel event standard in 2000. This standard, which continues today, requires organizations to carry out designated steps to fully understand the factors and systems associated with adverse patient events. The steps revolve around a "root cause analysis (RCA)," which is a direct application of the quality improvement principles and methods defined earlier in this chapter. The intention behind the root cause analysis is to understand the systems at fault within the organization so that improvements can be determined and implemented to prevent any future occurrences. TJC allows organizations some latitude in determining the policy for disclosure of these events to the commission.

National Patient Safety Goals. The purpose of TJC's national patient safety goals is to help accredited organizations address specific areas of concern in regard to patient safety. These goals are based on ongoing analyses of reported sentinel events and the identified root causes of these events. An annual review of these goals generally results in modification of existing goals and the creation of new ones, as evidenced in the published list for 2018, which modified requirements for hospitals, critical access hospitals, and nursing care centers in the health care–associated infections category (Box 22.1).

BOX 22.1 2018 Hospital National Patient Safety Goals

1. Improve the accuracy of patient identification.
   - Use at least two patient identifiers when providing care, treatment, and services.
   - Eliminate transfusion errors related to patient mis-identification.
2. Improve the effectiveness of communication among caregivers.
   - Report critical results of tests and diagnostic procedures on a timely basis.
3. Improve the safety of using medications.
   - Label all medications, medication containers, and other solutions on and off the sterile field in perioperative and other procedural settings.
   - Reduce the likelihood of patient harm associated with the use of anticoagulant therapy.
   - Maintain and communicate accurate patient medication information.
4. Reduce the harm associated with clinical alarm systems.
   - Improve the safety of clinical alarm systems.
5. Reduce the risk of health care–associated infections.
   - Comply with either the current Centers for Disease Control and Prevention (CDC) hand hygiene guidelines or the current World Health Organization (WHO) hand hygiene guidelines.
   - Implement evidence-based practices to prevent health care–associated infections due to multidrug-resistant organisms in acute care hospitals/critical access hospitals.
   - Implement evidence-based practices to prevent central line–associated bloodstream infections.
   - Implement evidence-based practices for preventing surgical site infections.
   - Implement evidence-based practices to prevent indwelling catheter–associated urinary tract infections.
6. The hospital identifies safety risks inherent in its patient population.
   - Identify patients at risk for suicide.
7. Universal protocol is used for preventing wrong site, wrong procedure, and wrong person surgery.
   - Conduct a preprocedure verification process.
   - Mark the procedure site.
   - Procedure time-out is performed before the procedure.

Adapted from The Joint Commission. (2017). *National patient safety goals effective January 2017.* Retrieved from https://www.jointcommission.org/assets/1/6/NPSG_Chapter_HAP_Jan2017.pdf; and The Joint Commission. (2017). *Changes for national patient safety goal 7 on health care–associated infections.* Retrieved from https://www.jointcommission.org/assets/1/6/Changes_NPSG_7_hai.pdf. Reprinted with permission.

Never Events. In 2006, CMS began to investigate ways that Medicare could help decrease or eliminate the occurrence of never events—serious and costly errors in health care delivery that should never happen. Examples of such events include wrong site surgery and mismatched blood transfusions, which can cause serious patient injury or death and can result in increased costs to Medicare. CMS worked with the National Quality Forum (NQF) to identify hospital-acquired conditions determined to be reasonably preventable and for which the additional cost of hospitalization for treating these conditions should not be paid. Box 22.2 presents the most current list of hospital-acquired conditions for which Medicare will no longer make additional payments for treatment.

Beginning in the CMS fiscal year 2015 and still in place today, reimbursement penalties are applied to hospitals performing in the bottom quartile nationally for a selected subset of the hospital-acquired conditions. The penalty consists of a 1% deduction of an organization's

---

BOX 22.2 Never Events: The Centers for Medicare and Medicaid Services Listing of Hospital-Acquired Conditions for 2018

- Foreign object retained after surgery
- Air embolism
- Blood incompatibility
- Stage III and IV pressure ulcers
- Falls and trauma
- Catheter-associated urinary tract infection
- Vascular catheter–associated infection
- Surgical site infection—mediastinitis after coronary artery bypass graft
- Manifestations of poor glycemic control
  - Deep vein thrombosis/pulmonary embolism with total knee or hip replacement
- Surgical site infection—bariatric surgery
- Surgical site infection following certain orthopedic procedures of spine, shoulder, and elbow
- Surgical site infection following cardiac implantable electronic device procedures
- Iatrogenic pneumothorax with venous catheterization

From the Centers for Medicare and Medicaid Services. (2018). *Hospital-acquired conditions.* Retrieved from https://www.cms.gov/Medicare/Medicare-Fee-for-Service-Payment/HospitalAcqCond/Downloads/FY-2018-Hospital-Acquired-Conditions-List.zip.

---

baseline annual Diagnosis-Related Group (DRG) Medicare reimbursement. Like Value-Based Purchasing, this program is a result of the Patient Protection and Affordability Act of 2010.

THE PROFESSIONAL NURSE AND PATIENT SAFETY

For nurses, the challenge starts with making patient safety improvement and error reduction not just an organizational priority but a personal one as well. This means adopting a state of mind that recognizes the complexity and high-risk nature of modern health care, implementing standardized best practices, and working to eliminate never events. Two significant nursing functions that most closely affect patient safety, quality of care, and resulting outcomes are:

1. Monitoring for early recognition of adverse events, complications, and errors.
2. Initiating deployment of appropriate care providers for timely intervention, response, and rescue of patients in these situations.

A critical factor in supporting a nurse's ability to carry out these two functions is nurse staffing. Although defining the appropriate level of staffing is a matter of debate, there is widespread recognition that a strong linkage exists between patient outcomes and nurse staffing (Martsolf et al, 2014; McHugh and Ma, 2013; Smeds Alenius et al, 2014; Tubbs-Cooley et al, 2013). Chapter 13 presents a thorough discussion of strategies nurses can use to promote quality care and a safe work environment.

Nursing Quality Indicators

The governing body of the American Nurses Association (ANA) established the National Database of Nursing Quality Indicators (NDNQI) in 1998 as part of the ANA's safety and quality initiative. This national database program collects information on designated indicators that strongly affect patient clinical outcomes for two major purposes: (1) to provide comparative data to health care organizations to support QI activities and (2) to develop national data to better understand the link between nurse staffing and patient outcomes (Box 22.3). The NDNQI is unique in that it is the only national nursing quality measurement program that allows comparison measures of nursing quality among national, regional, and state hospitals of similar type

BOX 22.3   Nursing-Sensitive Quality Indicators

Clinical Indicators

Structure
- Nurse Turnover
- Patient Volume and Flow
  - Admissions, Discharges, and Transfers
  - Emergency Department Throughput
- RN Education/SpecialtyCertification
- Staffing and Skill Mix*

Process
- Care Coordination
- Device Utilization
- Patient Falls*
- Pressure Injuries
- Pediatric Pain Assessment/Intervention/Reassessment (AIR) Cycle
- Restraints

Outcome
- Assaults by Psychiatric Patients
- Assaults on Nursing Personnel

- Catheter-Associated Urinary Tract Infections (CAUTI)
- Central Line Catheter Associated Blood Stream Infections (CLABSI)
- Hospital Readmissions
- Multidrug-Resistant Organisms (MDRO)
  - *C. difficile* Infections
  - MRSA Infections
- Patient Falls*
- Pediatric Peripheral Intravenous Infiltrations
- Pressure Injuries
- Ventilator-Associated Events (VAE)
- Ventilator-Associated Pneumonia (VAP)

RN Survey Options

Structure, Process, and Outcome
- RN Survey with Job Satisfaction Scales
- RN Survey with Practice Environment Scale (PES)*

*Includes National Quality Forum-endorsed measures.
RN, Registered nurse.
Adapted from Cuddigan, J. (2016). *NDNQI®: Getting the numbers—pressure injuries across the US.* Retrieved from http://www.npuap.org/wp-content/uploads/2017/03/Cuddigan-NDNQI-Staging-FINAL.pdf.

and size, from the unit level perspective. As of 2017, 2000 hospitals have joined the database, and quarterly reports are provided to these organizations for analysis of their own care processes and support systems as related to nurse staffing (Press Ganey, 2017). In 2014 the NDNQI database was acquired by Press Ganey, a national provider of patient satisfaction surveys and other strategic resources for health care organizations.

Interprofessional Teamwork

Equally critical in its effect on patient safety is the work environment that supports the interdependence and effective communication among nurses and other health care professionals. Most nurses and other clinical staff assume they already work in teams; however, teamwork concepts are infrequently taught in health professional educational programs. Patient care depends on effective interprofessional communication to support the coordination of activities that promote efficiency and safety. One strategy to improve interprofessional teamwork is TeamSTEPPS (Team Strategies and Tools to Enhance Performance and Patient Safety). TeamSTEPPS was developed

by the AHRQ and the U.S. Department of Defense as an evidence-based teamwork system aimed at optimizing patient outcomes by improving communication and teamwork skills among health care professionals. Comprehensive information about TeamSTEPPS, including readiness assessments and training materials, is available on its website (http://teamstepps.ahrq.gov*)*.

QSEN (QUALITY AND SAFETY EDUCATION IN NURSING) COMPETENCIES

This chapter has examined the vital need to transform today's health care systems to improve quality and safety for patients. Nurses are emerging as leaders in this transformation and, as such, need to incorporate into their nursing practice the six competencies recommended by the IOM (2003) as essential for all health professionals:
- Patient-centered care
- Teamwork and collaboration
- Evidence-based practice
- Quality improvement

- Safety
- Informatics

To support nursing education around these six competencies, the national Quality and Safety Education for Nurses (QSEN) project was created through support from the Robert Wood Johnson Foundation (Cronenwett et al, 2009). In support of the importance of these six competencies to nursing practice, they have been incorporated into nursing education standards and the nurse licensure examination (American Association of Colleges of Nursing, 2008; Smith et al, 2007) so that all nurses will be held accountable for being competent in these six areas.

Although these six competencies may seem familiar to nurses, it is important to understand them as intended by the IOM so that all disciplines (e.g., nursing, medicine, pharmacy) have the same frame of reference for incorporating the competencies into practice. Table 22.1 presents

TABLE 22.1	QSEN (Quality and Safety Education for Nurses) Competencies			
Competency	**Definition**	**Knowledge**	**Skills**	**Attitudes**
Patient-Centered Care	Recognize the patient or designee as the source of control and full partner in providing compassionate and coordinated care based on respect for patient's preferences, values, and needs	Integrate understanding of multiple dimensions of patient-centered care	Elicit patient values, preferences, and expressed needs as part of clinical interview	Value seeing health care situations "through patients' eyes"
		Describe how diverse cultural, ethnic, and social backgrounds function as sources of patient, family, and community values	Communicate patient values, preferences, and expressed needs to other members of health care team	Respect and encourage individual expression of patient values, preferences, and needs
Teamwork and Collaboration	Function effectively within nursing and interprofessional teams, fostering open communication, mutual respect, and shared decision making to achieve quality patient care	Describe own strengths, limitations, and values in functioning as a team member	Demonstrate awareness of own strengths and limitations as a team member	Acknowledge own potential to contribute to effective team functioning
		Describe examples of the impact of team functioning on safety and quality of care	Follow communication practices that minimize risks associated with handoffs among providers and across transitions in care	Appreciate the risks associated with handoffs among providers and across transitions in care
Evidence-Based Practice (EBP)	Integrate best current evidence with clinical expertise and patient/family preferences and values for delivery of optimal health care	Demonstrate knowledge of basic scientific methods and processes	Participate effectively in appropriate data collection and other research activities	Appreciate strengths and weaknesses of scientific bases for practice

TABLE 22.1	QSEN (Quality and Safety Education for Nurses) Competencies—cont'd			
Competency	**Definition**	**Knowledge**	**Skills**	**Attitudes**
		Discriminate between valid and invalid reasons for modifying evidence-based clinical practice on the basis of clinical expertise or patient/family preferences	Consult with clinical experts before deciding to deviate from evidence-based protocols	Acknowledge own limitations in knowledge and clinical expertise before determining when to deviate from evidence-based best practices
Quality Improvement	Use data to monitor the outcomes of care processes, and use improvement methods to design and test changes to continually improve the quality and safety of health care systems	Describe strategies for learning about the outcomes of care in the setting in which one is engaged in clinical practice	Seek information about outcomes of care for populations served in care setting	Appreciate that continual quality improvement is an essential part of the daily work of all health professionals
		Describe approaches for changing processes of care	Design a small test of change in daily work	Appreciate the value of what individuals and teams can do to improve care
Safety	Minimize risk of harm to patients and providers through system effectiveness and individual performance	Examine human factors and other basic safety design principles as well as commonly used unsafe practices	Demonstrate effective use of technology and standardized practices that support safety and quality	Value the contributions of standardization/reliability to safety
		Discuss potential and actual effect of national patient resources, initiatives, and regulations	Use national patient safety resources for own professional development and to focus attention on safety in care settings	Value relationship between national safety campaigns and implementation in local practices and practice settings
		Knowledge	Skills	Attitudes
Informatics	Use information and technology to communicate, manage knowledge, mitigate error, and support decision making	Identify essential information that must be available in a common database to support patient care	Navigate the electronic health record	Value technologies that support clinical decision making, error prevention, and care coordination
		Describe examples of how technology and information management are related to the quality and safety of patient care	Respond appropriately to clinical decision-making supports and alerts	Value nurses' involvement in design, selection, implementation, and evaluation of information technologies to support patient care

Abbreviated from Cronenwett, L., Sherwood, G., & Gelmon, S. B. (2007). Quality and safety education for nurses. *Nurs Outlook,* *55*(3), 122-131.

each competency with its definition and a sample of knowledge, skills, and attitudes related to it. The QSEN website (http://www.qsen.org) is a good resource offering extensive information about each competency, including annotated bibliographies, peer-reviewed teaching strategies, and instructional videos. Readers are encouraged to visit the QSEN website to learn more about these competencies, which are essential to today's nursing practice.

ROLE OF PROFESSIONAL NURSES IN QUALITY IMPROVEMENT

There are lessons for all nurses from one of the original patient safety and quality improvement mentors, Florence

Nightingale. Nightingale used data to support her efforts to reduce the incidence and spread of infections in the patient wards she was accountable for during the Crimean War. What resulted from her work was a broader shift in the culture of health care at that time. What can result from the current emphasis on quality and patient safety is a new cultural shift in health care, with "building health care systems that do no harm" increasingly being the shared value and goal of all those involved in health care delivery. Nurses are in the perfect position to lead this cultural change. Quality improvement should be considered not a separate function within the role of care provider but, rather, an ongoing part of the professional role for all health care professionals.

SUMMARY

For today's graduating nurses, the challenge is to find whatever means are available to refine the knowledge and skills fundamentally necessary to enter a partnership with all other interprofessional team members in the ongoing improvement of health care. Just as essential to professional nursing practice as knowing, for instance, the symptoms of diabetic ketoacidosis or how to give an injection, are understanding the basic principles of QI, process

improvement, and variation; using clinical indicators, process improvement tools, and standardized care processes; and addressing patient safety in every aspect of care. Every nurse should enter practice accepting accountability for the quality of care provided by the health care organization and taking a leadership role to implement improvements to achieve health care that is safe, timely, effective, efficient, equitable, and patient centered.

REFERENCES

Agency for Healthcare Research and Quality. (2014, May). *National healthcare quality report, 2013.* Publication No. 14-0005. AHRQ. Retrieved from https://archive.ahrq.gov/research/findings/nhqrdr/nhqr13/index.html.

Agency for Healthcare Research and Quality. (2017, July). *National healthcare quality and disparities report, 2016.* Publication No. 17-0001-1-EF. AHRQ. Retrieved from http://www.ahrq.gov/research/findings/nhqrdr/index.html.

American Association of Colleges of Nursing. (2008). *The essentials of baccalaureate education for professional nursing practice.* Washington, DC: American Association of Colleges of Nursing.

Berwick, D. (1997). The breakthrough series. *Quality Connection, 6*(2), 11.

Cronenwett, L., Sherwood, G., & Gelmon, S. B. (2009). Improving quality and safety education: the QSEN learning collaborative. *Nursing Outlook, 57*(6), 304–312.

Institute of Medicine, Kohn, L. T., Corrigan, J. M., & Donaldson, M. S. (Eds.), (2000). *To err is human: Building a safer health system.* Washington, DC: National Academies Press.

Institute of Medicine. (2001). *Crossing the quality chasm: a new health system for the 21st century.* Washington, DC: National Academy Press.

Institute of Medicine, Greiner, A. C., & Knebel, E. (Eds.), (2003). *Health professions education: A bridge to quality.* Washington, DC: National Academies Press.

Institute of Medicine. (2007). *Preventing medication errors: Quality chasm series.* Retrieved from https://www.nap.edu/read/11623/chapter/1.

Institute for Safe Medication Practices. (2017). *ISMP self assessments.* Retrieved from http://www.ismp.org/selfassessments.

James, J. T. (2013). A new, evidence-based estimate of patient harms associated with hospital care. *Journal of Patient Safety, 9*(3), 122–128.

Joiner, B. L. (1994). *Fourth generation management.* New York: McGraw-Hill.

Langley, G. J., Nolan, K. M., Nolan, T. W., Moen, R. D., Norman, C. L., & Provost, L. P. (2009). *The Improvement Guide: A Practical Approach to Enhancing Organizational Performance* (2nd ed.). San Francisco: Jossey-Bass.

Martsolf, G. R., Auerbach, D., Benevent, R., Stocks, C., Jiang, H. J., Pearson, M. L., et al. (2014). Examining the value of inpatient nurse staffing: An assessment of quality and patient care costs. *Medical Care, 52*(11), 982–988.

McHugh, M. D., & Ma, C. (2013). Hospital nursing and 30 day readmissions among Medicare patients with heart failure, acute myocardial infarction and pneumonia. *Medical Care, 51*(1), 52–59.

Press Ganey. (2017). *Nursing quality (NDNQI).* Retrieved from http://www.pressganey.com/solutions/clinical-quality/nursing-quality.

Smeds Alenius, L., Tishelman, C., Runesdotter, S., & Lindqvist, R. (2014). Staffing and resource adequacy strongly related to RNs' assessment of patient safety: a national study of RNs working in acute-care hospitals in Sweden. *BMJ Quality & Safety, 23*, 242–249.

Smith, E. L., Cronenwett, L., & Sherwood, G. (2007). Current assessments of quality and safety education in nursing. *Nursing Outlook, 55*(3), 132–137.

The Joint Commission. (2017a). *Sentinel events.* (website). https://www.jointcommission.org/sentinel_event_policy_and_procedures/.

The Joint Commission. (2017b). *About the Joint Commission.* Retrieved from https://www.jointcommission.org/about_us/about_the_joint_commission_main.aspx.

Tubbs-Cooley, H. L., Cimiotti, J. P., Silber, J. H., Sloane, D. M., & Aiken, L. H. (2013). An observational study of nurse staffing ratios and hospital readmission among children admitted for common conditions. *BMJ Quality and Safety, 22*(9), 735–742.

23

Health Policy and Politics: Get Involved!

Barbara Cherry, DNSc, MBA, RN, NEA-BC,
Carole R. Myers, PhD, RN

Nurses must be powerful, informed advocates for health policy that improves health and health care!

(e) Additional resources are available online at: *http://evolve.elsevier.com/Cherry/*

LEARNING OUTCOMES

After studying this chapter, the reader will be able to:

1. Differentiate between policy and politics.
2. Discuss roles of the legislative, administrative, and judicial branches of government.
3. Differentiate among federal, state, and local governments and their roles in governing and influencing health care and nursing.
4. Identify three policy issues of significant consequence to nurses and nursing.

5. Demonstrate knowledge needed to be a responsible and informed, politically active nurse.
6. Use diverse technologic resources to obtain information about current health policy developments and political issues.

KEY TERMS

Constituent A citizen who has the opportunity to vote for candidates in elections for representation at the local, state, and federal levels.

Constituent/State Nurses Association (C/SNA) The professional organizational unit member of the American Nurses Association that represents all professional nurses within a state or territory or other defined organizational entity or boundary—also known as the state nurses association (SNA).

Grassroots lobbying Personal advocacy by individual constituents—everyday citizens—in support of a problem/position/option related to a policy issue.

Health policy A set course of action(s) undertaken by governments or health care organizations in order to achieve a particular health outcome. Private health policy is made by health care organizations, such as hospitals, whereas public health policy refers to local, state, and federal legislation, regulations, and court rulings that govern health care within a certain arena.

Lobbying Acting to persuade or educate policymakers to respond positively to a particular position on an issue or to follow a particular course of legislative, regulatory, or funding activity.

Platform The statement of principles and policies of a political party, candidate, or elected official.

Policymaker A local, state, or federally elected or appointed official who can propose and directly affect legislation, regulations, or programs that can become actualized.

Regulations Rules used to implement legislation and translate concepts into actions that can be put into practice.

Stakeholders Individuals, groups, or organizations who have a vested interest in and may be affected by policy decisions and actions being taken, and thus may attempt to influence those decisions and actions.

PROFESSIONAL/ETHICAL ISSUE

Tashauna Banks works in a very busy outpatient surgical center where the nurses often stay past the end of their shifts to care for patients who are not yet stable enough to go home. Tashauna and other nurses in the center typically work more than 50 hours per week. Although the pay is very good, Tashauna is often so fatigued, especially at the end of the week, that she is concerned about making mistakes that might harm her patients. Tashauna also knows that two of her colleagues work as agency nurses on their days off from the surgical center, which means they may be working up to 65 to 70 hours per week. Tashauna has begun to notice that nurse fatigue is a problem in their surgery center, negatively affecting the nurses' motivation and energy levels. She also notices lapses in attention to detail and what sometimes seem to be slow reactions to urgent situations. She becomes very concerned as she realizes that fatigue could have extremely serious legal ramifications if a medical error caused by fatigue were to lead to patient harm.

When visiting with some of her nurse friends who work at the local medical center, Tashauna learns that nurse fatigue is a concern there as well. Tashauna and her nurse friends discuss their responsibility to make good decisions when agreeing to work overtime and using the *Code of Ethics for Nurses* as a guide. After the discussion with her friends, Tashauna is motivated to take action to address the problem of nurse fatigue in her own work setting as well as at a broader level through the state nurses association. She understands that together, nurses can have a powerful voice to effect change both in the work setting and at state and national policy levels.

- What resources are available for Tashauna and her colleagues to learn more about nurse fatigue?
- How can the *Code of Ethics for Nurses* guide nurses to make balanced decisions about their work hours?
- What responsibility do the managers in health care organizations have to implement policies to address nurse fatigue and keep nurses and patients safe?
- Discuss steps Tashauna can take to begin to address the problem of nurse fatigue as a policy issue in her own work setting and through the state nurses association.

VIGNETTE

Juan Hernandez is one of only four registered nurses (RNs) now staffing the 7 AM to 7 PM shift in a 12-bed medical intensive care unit (MICU) as two RN colleagues have just transferred to positions in the hospital's rapidly growing case management service. The chief nursing officer (CNO) and MICU nurse manager are actively recruiting permanent RNs for the vacant positions but have not been successful as yet. Temporary service RNs and nursing assistive personnel are filling in within the staffing mix. Juan is aware that all posted openings for RNs throughout his hospital system now include "BSN (Bachelor of Science in Nursing) preferred" as a descriptor following the hospital's recently announced plans for achieving Magnet Hospital status.

When Juan begins to inquire about the issues in hiring BSN-prepared nurses, he is both relieved and alarmed by what he hears. First, the hospital administrators clearly support his position that adequate numbers of permanently employed, well-educated RNs are essential to provide high-quality, safe patient care. The hospital's rapidly evolving care models and driving force to succeed on the Magnet journey require giving a preference to nurses with a BSN or higher degree. However, an underlying complicating issue for health care organizations in Juan's state and region is that the numbers of nurses with the needed education and credentials simply are not adequate to meet the demand, and hiring is taking much longer than in the past, further complicating issues of safety, quality, and continuity of care in Juan's MICU.

Juan calls his state nurses association (SNA) to discuss his concerns and to learn more about the nursing workforce trends. Through that call, he discovers that other nurses and hospitals across the United States are facing many of the same dilemmas. Meeting nurses' current professional responsibility to provide and advocate for safe care for patients is colliding with the larger national and employer issues of securing a higher number of better educated, more broadly skilled nurses to meet the rapidly evolving expectations in complex care systems. Therefore, Juan makes a commitment to engage in discussions about policy and political strategies that are needed now to promote and protect models of care that will facilitate professional nursing practice; promote development of a highly educated nursing workforce to meet his state's and region's needs; and ensure his ability to grow in his own professional career.

Questions to Consider While Reading This Chapter:

1. What types of local, state, and federal health policies affect Juan's nursing practice?
2. What are the major steps in health policy development that Juan must understand in order to engage in policy improvements for the nursing workforce and his own professional career?
3. How can Juan relate his knowledge of the nursing process to an effective plan for policy development related to improving the nursing workforce and his own professional career?
4. What types of grassroots political strategies can Juan use to ensure that policymakers hear his interests and concerns about quality, safe patient care, and the supply of professional nurses?

CHAPTER OVERVIEW

Perhaps at no other time in the history of the nursing profession has there been such an imperative for strong, involved, informed nursing leadership. The challenges currently faced by the U.S. health care system—ongoing and serious patient safety issues; a shortage of appropriately educated and geographically dispersed nursing and other essential health professionals; complex, high-tech work environments; a fragmented delivery system; an aging population; the drive for improved population health; and dramatic health care system changes to provide higher quality care at lower costs—affect the health and well-being of patients, families, and communities across the country. Nurses can no longer simply move forward and participate in the delivery of patient care without also addressing these larger issues that have a direct impact on the whole of the health care system. Frequently, these critical issues can be understood, addressed, and resolved only through the policy process. Without a doubt, legislation, regulation, and health policy directly affect how health care is delivered and how the health care system responds to the very real challenges and opportunities it faces. *Nurses must get involved now* in the policy process and provide strong leadership among the health care professions to ensure evolution to an efficient, effective health care system that promotes and protects the health and well-being of each person in our society.

This chapter explores the effect of governmental roles, structures, and actions on health care policy and demonstrates how nurses' participation in the policy process can shape the U.S. health care system. Local, state, and federal legislative concerns, including the involvement of professional nursing organizations in policy and politics, are discussed. Nurses' very important role in the policy process and involvement in political advocacy and campaigns is described. This chapter provides the reader with a basic understanding of policy development and political processes, tools to gain political savvy, and methods for getting politically involved.

NURSES' INVOLVEMENT IN HEALTH POLICY AND POLITICAL ACTION

Nurses' involvement in policy and politics has become considerably more important in recent years for the following reasons:

- State and federal governments play an increasingly important role in health care by putting in place new rules and regulations, which are obligating health care organizations and providers to adjust to totally new payment models based on quality, care coordination, and population health.
- Nursing practice is directly affected by health policy development, which is, in turn, affected by the political action of citizens—nurses and many others.
- National attention on nurses and nursing has intensified—our numbers, education, scope of practice, and overall value to the health care system.

Decisions affecting the health care system, patient care, and the nursing profession will be made with or without the input of nurses. As the reader will see from health policy examples provided throughout this chapter, patient care and nursing practice are highly political endeavors, with health policy determining the types of care systems in place and how that care is paid for. Thus, it is absolutely essential that nurses become actively engaged in the policy process and use effective political action to successfully achieve the development of health policies that are reflective of nursing's perspective on the preferred future for the profession and for the health of people in the United States.

WHAT IS HEALTH POLICY?

Health policy is a set course of action(s) undertaken by governments or health care organizations to obtain a desired outcome. Private health policy is made by health care organizations, such as hospitals, and includes those policies instituted to govern innumerable employer/ employee practices and processes in the delivery of the health care services provided within the organization. A hospital's specific plan to report errors in patient care is an example of private health policy. *Public health policy* refers to local, state, and federal legislation, regulations, and resource allocation related to health, health care service delivery, coverage, workforce, and reimbursement. The mandatory requirement for licensure to practice professional nursing is an example of public health policy. There is a close link between private policy and public policy, in that the policies of health care organizations must conform to (and are actually frequently developed and implemented to comply with) a public policy. Although it is vital that the RN be an informed participant in policy development at his or her employing health care organization, this chapter focuses on the development of public or governmental health policy, which will be referred to simply as *health policy*.

Health Policy at the Local, State, and Federal Levels

Health policies may be developed and implemented at the local, state, or federal level, and they apply to all residents within the jurisdiction of the respective governmental authority. Local health policy applies only to those people who are residents of the local community, whereas health policy enacted at the federal level applies to all residents of the United States.

Local Health Policy. At the local level, many cities or counties offer a variety of health care services to meet the needs of their residents. For example, as part of a city's health policy, free or reduced-rate immunizations may be offered to all children in the community. Allocating funds to employ RNs as school nurses in public schools is another example of local health policy. A more comprehensive (and thus perhaps more controversial) policy is a community's requirement for tobacco-free public areas such as restaurants and office buildings. Local health policy varies considerably across the United States, with some communities funding an extensive variety of health programs and others offering very limited health services or none at all. However, even the smallest communities are involved to some extent in health policy through partnerships with their state governments to provide public health programs such as safe drinking water, enforcement for seat belt and child restraint laws, and emergency medical systems.

State Health Policy. Health policy at the state level has a powerful influence on the health and safety of each state's residents. In addition to its lead role in governing nursing and other health professions' scope, practice, and performance through the state's professional practice acts, each state also has innumerable health policies that may not be visible. These policies include maintaining a safe meat supply through livestock inspections; ensuring safe food storage, preparation, and serving in restaurants; monitoring infectious disease outbreaks; and ensuring that health care facilities provide safe, quality care through regulatory compliance. Only when these activities fall short of preventing problems—as in cases of *Escherichia coli* (*E. coli*) outbreaks—do most residents of the state realize the critical nature of these health policies.

State health policy also involves paying for some individual health care services. The Medicaid program, which is funded through a blend of state and federal funds, is a health insurance program for health care services for eligible people at (or below) a specific income level and other designated categories (as defined by a combination of federal and individual state standards). Most states also have a state Children's Health Insurance Program (CHIP) that provides health insurance coverage to uninsured children who do not qualify for the state Medicaid program. The CHIP is funded through a partnership between federal and state governments. State and federal governments are also the prime sources of funding for public mental health and substance abuse services, long-term care services for older adults and disabled persons, and health care services for prisoners.

A key piece of the Patient Protection and Affordable Care Act of 2010 (PPACA) was the provision for states to implement State Health Insurance Exchanges (SHIEs). An SHIE is a set of state-regulated and standardized health care plans from which individuals may purchase health insurance eligible for federal subsidies; such plans offer affordable and credible coverage that meet national standards for covered services with individual state benchmarks.

Federal Health Policy. State government and state health policies have an enormous effect on people's health and safety. Likewise, the federal government plays a vitally important leadership role in the health of Americans, including passage of the PPACA by the 111th Congress. The federal government's role in health care includes significant funding for health and disease prevention and research; supplemental funding for education for health professionals, such as nurses and physicians; and paying for individual health care services through Medicare, Medicaid, CHIP, Veterans Health Administration, and Indian Health Services.

Federal health policies have played and continue to play a pivotal role in shaping nursing practice. The first federal policy to provide funding for nursing services was the Sheppard-Towner Act of 1921. This act, passed by Congress despite objections from the American Medical Association (AMA), provided states with matching funds to establish prenatal and child health centers staffed by public health nurses. The goal of the act was to reduce maternal and infant mortality rates by teaching women about personal hygiene and infant care. Eventually, this highly successful program was discontinued when the AMA successfully persuaded Congress that physicians should perform these health activities (Starr, 1982), but these services were later reinstated (and continue today) within Title V of the Social Security Act of 1935.

Another example of federal legislation that has significantly influenced the context of nursing practice over the past seven decades was the Hill-Burton Act of 1950. This act provided funding to local communities that resulted in a boom in the construction of hospitals across the country. As the number of hospitals increased rapidly, so did the need for nurses to staff them. Thus, the professional nurse's historic role has shifted from community and public health settings to be predominantly hospital/acute care settings over the last six decades. Other key federal legislation has affected nursing practice through expanding Medicare and Medicaid reimbursement directly to advanced practice nurses and implementing policies and programs to enlarge the supply of nurses through enhancing access to nursing education at all levels of nursing, from BSN to Doctor of Nursing Practice (DNP) and Doctor of Philosophy (PhD). Table 23.1 provides some historic examples of how health policy enacted at the federal level has affected nursing practice and health care. Current policy issues affecting nursing practice and health care are addressed later in this chapter.

TABLE 23.1 Examples of Health Policies that Have Influenced Professional Nursing Practice

Legislation	Influence on Professional Nursing Practice
Nurse practice acts and registration of nurses were established (1910).	Established scope of practice and minimal educational requirements for nurses; implemented by most states.
Sheppard-Towner Act (1921) funded prenatal and child health centers staffed by public health nurses.	First federal policy to provide funding for nursing services.
Hill-Burton Act (1950), also known as the Hospital Survey and Construction Act, provided federal funding for hospital construction.	Caused a boom in hospital construction, shifting nurses' primary employment setting from public health to hospitals.
Nurse Training Act (1964), Public Law 88-581 (78 Stat. 908), provided enhanced funding for collegiate nursing programs.	Expanded university education for nurses, and laid the groundwork for the development of advanced practice nurses (APRNs).
Medicare program (1965) provided funding for health care services for older adults and the disabled.	Led to an increased number of hospitalized older adults and a greater need for nurses in acute care settings.
Renal Disease Program (1972) provided funding for dialysis treatments and renal transplantation for patients with kidney failure.	Led to the development of a new area of nursing practice that is now a recognized specialty—nephrology nursing.
Diagnosis-related groups (DRGs) (1983) changed Medicare reimbursement to hospitals from a fee-for-service method to a fixed-fee method.	Forced hospitals to reduce patients' lengths of stay, cut costs, and initially reduced staff, including nurses; led to the development of new nursing roles—nursing case management and utilization review.

TABLE 23.1   Examples of Health Policies that Have Influenced Professional Nursing Practice—cont'd

Legislation	Influence on Professional Nursing Practice
Balanced Budget Amendment (1997), Title 42 Sect 4511 CFR 410.75 and 410.76, provided for direct reimbursement of nurse practitioners (NPs) and clinical nurse specialists, regardless of geographic location, following state nurse practice act requirements for scope and practice.	Expanded the practice opportunities for APRNs, and further increased the importance of political action at the state level to remove barriers to APRN practice, such as medical supervision and other unwarranted limitations on scope and independence.
Medicare Modernization Act (Medicare Part D) (2003), PL 108-173 117 Stat 2066, added a prescription drug benefit for Medicare enrollees.	Provided needed access to medications for Medicare enrollees, and called attention to cost-and-effectiveness outcome from policymakers, requiring nurses to stay alert to proposed legislation and to advocate for appropriate benefits for the nation's older adults.
Mental Health Parity and Addictions Equity Act (MHPAEA) (2008), PL 110-343 Sect 511, removed discrimination in insurance coverage and benefits for mental illnesses and substance abuse disorders.	Greatly increased access to a continuum of mental health/substance abuse services, and put pressure on development of a nursing workforce with sufficient numbers and knowledge to address these illnesses as integrated with other chronic illnesses and as specialty services.
Patient Protection and Affordable Care Act (2010), Public Law 111-148.	Comprehensive health care reform legislation providing a health insurance program requiring U.S. citizens and legal residents to secure quality health insurance at reasonable rates with income-based subsidies while also providing for provisions to improve the quality of health care and reduce costs.

HOW IS HEALTH POLICY DEVELOPED?

The development of health policy at the state or federal level is a complex, dynamic process that occurs in the following three ways (Chaffee et al, 2015):

- Enactment of legislation and the accompanying rules and regulations that carry the weight of law
- Administrative decisions/directives made by various governmental agencies of the executive branch
- Judicial decisions that interpret statutes and regulations, and that settle legal disputes/conflicts within society

Numerous players (individuals and groups) are involved in developing health policy, including: elected officials and their staffs; officials/staffs of executive branch governmental agencies; individual experts in a health-related area; citizens who may be affected by a health problem; stakeholders, such as corporate representatives, who may be affected by a health problem or policy; and representatives from special interest groups who have a particular focused interest in one or more

policy options. As a special interest group representing the interests of 3.1 million professional nurses throughout the United States, the American Nurses Association (ANA) carries a strong voice and high visibility in influencing health policy and nursing practice. At the state level, the Constituent/State Nurses Associations (C/SNAs) of the ANA are the policy voices of the nursing profession with state governors and legislatures.

The development of health policy involves all three branches of government: executive, legislative, and judicial. A basic knowledge of the functions of the three branches of government is necessary to understand health policy development. Table 23.2 presents a brief review of the three branches of the federal government and their differing roles in health policy. Although most state governments parallel the structure and functions of the federal government, there are differences among states. Each nurse is encouraged to learn about the governmental structure of his or her state. In addition to understanding the branches of government, nurses also need to understand the influence of legislation and

TABLE 23.2	The Three Branches of the Federal Government		
	Executive	**Legislative**	**Judicial**
Composition	Office of the President and 15 executive departments (State, Treasury, Defense, Agriculture, Energy, Housing and Urban Development, Justice, Commerce, Education, Health and Human Services, Interior, Labor, Transportation, Veterans Affairs, and Homeland Security)	Senate and House of Representatives, known collectively as Congress, with 535 elected members	U.S. Supreme Court, federal district courts, and U.S. circuit courts of appeals
Role in health policy	Recommends legislation and promotes major policy initiatives Implements laws and manages programs after they have been passed by Congress through regulation, oversight, and presidential funding priorities Writes regulations that interpret statutes (laws) Has the power to veto legislation passed by Congress	Possesses the sole federal power to enact legislation and to tax citizens and allocate federal spending Able to originate and promote major policy initiatives Has the power to override a presidential veto	Judicial interpretations of the Constitution or various laws may have a policy effect Resolves questions regarding agency regulations that may affect policy
Restrictions to power	Unable to enact a law without the approval of Congress (legislative branch)	U.S. Supreme Court may invalidate legislation as unconstitutional	Unable to recommend or promote legislative initiatives

regulation on health policy as discussed in the following sections.

Legislation and Health Policy Development. The *development of health policy* refers to the steps through which a health issue moves from being a societal problem to becoming an actual health program that can be funded, implemented, and evaluated. The legislative process is fundamental to the movement from a public problem to a public solution: a public plan, program, or service. Although there are many problems related to health care and nursing practice, problems that attain policy solution status are those that are brought to the attention of a policymaker who is willing to take definitive action through legislative, regulatory, or funding processes.

Generally, interested individuals or citizens' groups approach policymakers either to present a problem to be solved or to suggest a policy option to a health problem that they have identified. However, policymakers may also become aware of problems through their personal experiences or that of their constituents and may take on development of policy solutions independently. At the federal level, only members of

Congress can introduce legislation. The congressional member who introduces a specific piece of legislation becomes the prime sponsor of that legislation. Legislation is introduced by a member of Congress after careful analysis of the problem, which likely includes the following:
• Public perception of the problem
• Definition of the problem
• Societal consequences of action or inaction and the number of people affected by the problem and/or the options for resolution
• Levels of support and opposition from other members of Congress, special interest groups, business leaders, and the general public, especially the member's constituents

After the problem is thoroughly analyzed and a decision is made to move forward with a policy solution, the sponsoring congressperson drafts the legislation, and congressional staff translates the option into legal, technical, and constitutional language that the congressperson then introduces through the appropriate process. Only then does the health problem addressed by a policy option/solution become a bill—a proposed legislative policy solution. Visit http://www.votesmart.

org/education/how-a-bill-becomes-law to review all the necessary steps in how a bill becomes law.

Although the legislative process to enact a new law appears to be simple and straightforward, it is actually very complex and convoluted, with only a fraction of introduced legislation actually making it through the final process to become law. In the 114th U.S. Congress (2015 to 2016), 2062 bills were introduced, but only 322 of those actually became public law (Congressional Record, 2017). In other words, only 15.6% of bills introduced in the 114th Congress actually became public law!

Once a bill becomes a law (a public policy), implementation falls to the jurisdiction of one of the departments under the executive branch of government. (See Table 23.2.) At the federal level, most health-related policies fall under the jurisdiction of the U.S. Department of Health and Human Services (DHHS) and its related agencies. The agency that will administer the law develops the regulations to implement the law. Implementation of new legislation can often be very different from what was originally intended when Congress debated and passed the bill. It is extremely important that supporters of any new law take steps to ensure that its advocates and the legislative policymakers implement the law as intended. This important caution leads us to the discussion about regulation and health policy.

HEALTH POLICY THROUGH REGULATION

The regulatory arena is an important but often overlooked area of policy that significantly affects nursing practice. An understanding of regulatory authority and processes provides nurses with the knowledge necessary to become involved and more successfully influence the future of nursing. Regulations refer to written sets of rules issued by an executive branch agency that has responsibility for administering a law. Because regulations carry the force of the law, they directly shape the implementation of health policy. Thus, it is very important that regulations reflect the intent of the law as enacted by the legislative body. Once the proposed regulations are developed, they must be published and open to public comment for a specified time before being adopted as final rules. As regulations are being developed by the government agency, public hearings are held to allow interested individuals and groups to comment on the draft content of the regulations and to suggest amendments or substitutions. At this stage in the development of a health care law, nurses can and must play an influential role in shaping the final regulations by writing to the regulatory agency or speaking at public hearings. Informed comments are critical for the development of administrative law. Each comment received must be considered and responded to before final regulations are issued. The time between the interim rules and final rules is critical for assessing the effect of the proposed rules and requires concerted nursing vigilance and action to react to the proposed rules either positively or negatively. Final published regulations carry the force of the law and will dictate how the law is actually implemented.

At the federal level, the proposed (or interim) regulations are published in the *Federal Register*. The *Federal Register* (located online at https://www.federalregister.gov) is the best source of information about proposed new rules as well as proposed changes to existing rules for federal programs. It is published each day and contains complete directions about where to send comments in addition to the deadlines for the public comment period. Most states have a parallel publication (e.g., *Texas Register*) with information about proposed rules and regulations at the state level for state legislation. It cannot be overemphasized that supporters of any new law must be vigilant and involved in the development of rules and regulations long after the legislation has passed and been adopted as law to ensure its implementation as planned and supported.

A great deal of thoughtful, focused effort goes into the development of health policy—from the time a public health problem is identified; through when a legislative solution is conceived; a bill is passed; and a health policy is actually implemented through regulation and funding. By understanding and becoming involved in these processes, nurses can protect and influence nursing practice and create and shape positive change throughout the health care system.

HEALTH POLICY AND POLITICS: A KEY CONNECTION

Many people may view politics as somewhat "shady" activities that occur in and around federal, state, and local governments to influence the outcomes of candidate elections and/or the passage of legislation. Chaffee and colleagues (2015) have defined politics as "the process of influencing the allocation of scarce resources." Politics can also be defined as the process used to influence decisions and exert control over policy, circumstances, and events. As the reader will see, "influence" is the common denominator in any definition of politics. Political influence can be achieved through many methods, including:

- Campaign activity and contributions
- Knowledge
- Relationships
- Information/data
- Talent
- Perceived control over large groups of votes

Florence Nightingale was the consummate political nurse. She understood how to use data and expert knowledge to influence the British Parliament to allocate funds to reform British military hospitals and substantially improved the health conditions for the troops through changes in sanitary practices (Nightingale, 1859).

Politics is a necessary part of the policy process. Multiple interest groups (such as government officials, special interest groups, and corporate leaders) are all competing to achieve their potentially different policy goals/ outcomes. The process becomes even more interesting when the varied and increasingly polarized agendas of the Democratic, Republican, and emerging independent parties are added to the mix. Groups and individuals who have a stake in the fate of a piece of legislation or the election of a candidate use political strategies to obtain their desired outcome(s). Thus, it is through *effective* political action that nurses can positively influence legislative and regulatory decisions and the development of health policies that will affect nursing practice and the health of Americans in a positive way. Following is a discussion of how nurses can get involved in the political process and use effective political strategies to influence health policy.

Health Policy and the Nursing Process

The first step for nurses to get involved in health policy development and politics is to learn to recognize nursing and health care issues that are amenable to and/or require policy action. During nursing school, students learn the nursing process as the foundation for professional nursing practice. Once nursing students graduate, they appreciate the nursing process as the basis for making sound clinical judgments. As nurses commit to being more policy focused and politically active, they will find that applying the nursing process is a natural and comfortable approach to identifying and taking on broader professional and health care issues. Just remember the following steps:

1. *Assessment:* Collecting information and understanding the information about the issue of concern are important first steps for approaching policy issues.
2. *Analysis and diagnosis:* Analyzing the information and identifying the fundamental issue or underlying problem that needs to be addressed follow.
3. *Planning:* Developing options for an effective policy plan involves input from many sources and perspectives.
4. *Implementation:* Implementing a policy requires political action and a set of strategies and strategic interventions.
5. *Evaluation:* Assessing evidence that determines the success (or not? and the why or why not?) of the intervention is the last step.

Nurses' ability and inclination to observe, use data, analyze it from a variety of perspectives and then make a plan prior to taking action make them "naturals" for policy activity and involvement. Policy work is challenging, important, and, in so many instances, fun and exciting and should become a part of the professional nurse's skill set.

GRASSROOTS POLITICAL STRATEGIES

Grassroots lobbying, or political strategies are actions taken at the local level to influence policymakers. Nurses as political constituents have a right (and a responsibility!) to petition, lobby, or persuade policymakers to ensure that their interests and concerns are heard. Such advocacy actions (frequently referred to as *lobbying*) offer individuals and groups who are stakeholders in a particular issue an opportunity to be heard. The lobbying process also provides policymakers with needed information from health experts upon which to base their decisions. Following are various methods through which nurses can be effective grassroots participants/players:

- Registering to vote and voting in *all* elections
- Joining professional nursing organizations with policy advocacy agendas
- Working on political candidates' campaigns
- Meeting with policymakers or their staff members

- Attending and speaking up at "meet-the-candidates" town hall meetings
- Communicating with policymakers by e-mail, fax, and telephone

Register to Vote and Vote in All Elections

Voting is a must for *every* nurse. However, voting is not enough. *Informed voting* is necessary to enhance nurses' political power to ultimately improve the health of patients and the care that they receive. Becoming informed involves reading legislative newsletters and finding out about policymakers' backgrounds, voting records, and current party and candidate platforms. Discussing your findings on these issues with nurse colleagues and others in the community enhances everyone's understanding of candidates and their positions and facilitates informed voting. Nurses must participate in identifying and electing "nurse-friendly" candidates and then must become candidates and policymakers themselves.

Join a Professional Nursing Organization

Another must for the professional nurse seeking to make a policy difference is to join a professional nursing organization. The value of the ANA, its C/SNAs, and its organizational affiliates, is that, *together,* the nursing profession is much more powerful than any individual RN speaking alone. Within a professional collective, nurses know more, have more resources, and are able to pool their strengths and direct resources toward "winning" the health policy competition and thus ensuring a more "nurse-friendly" public policy.

The ANA is the foremost recognized professional nursing organization for federal health and nursing public policy. The ANA speaks for all professional nurses, regardless of specialty. All nurses should consider ANA membership as one of their fundamental professional investments. The nurse who chooses to also be a member in a specialty organization that represents his or her focus arena of nursing practice has the additional advantage of receiving clinical and health policy information related to that specialty.

Because professional nursing organizations monitor public policy and offer avenues for their members to learn about health policy, they serve as invaluable resources for reliable information related to policy issues and policymakers. Joining a professional nursing organization that has a political action committee (PAC) can help nurses develop the necessary skills to understand and participate in political issues and elections and can give nurses increased access to policymakers.

A PAC is an arm of a corporation, association, or union formed to provide support and resources either to work toward the election or reelection of policymakers who support the organization's overall goals or to persuade a policymaker to support a certain policy. Not all professional nursing organizations have PACs, but those that do so may choose to endorse a specific candidate for office. Endorsement simply means that, in a particular political race, the nursing organization selects a particular candidate to support because of that candidate's platform or record supporting specific issues or policy goals. Although endorsement does not mean that everyone in the organization *must* vote for the selected person, it does mean that the organization has carefully screened the candidate, and the nurse can be reasonably sure that, if elected, the candidate will support the organization's preferred outcomes and interests. Nursing organizations are looking for health-friendly and nurse-friendly candidates who will champion laws and programs to improve health and nursing.

Work in Political Candidates' Campaigns

Most political candidates are not health professionals and do not fully understand health-related issues. By becoming involved in political campaigns, nurses can (and should) educate and inform candidates about health care issues. Other activities that the nurse may undertake on behalf of the candidates include assisting in writing health care position statements; working in campaign offices; attending local debates; displaying the candidates' political buttons, signs, and stickers; and participating in fundraising events. Nurse supporters may also write letters/e-mails to and/or call other nurses in the region to tell them about their support of the candidate and to ask for their vote. Having nurse-friendly candidates win and become nurse-friendly policymaking officials is critical to achieving nursing's policy agenda.

Visit with Policymakers and their Staff Members

Personal visits to policymakers and their staff members can be one of the most effective methods of advocacy for or against a health care policy. Nothing is more effective in communicating nursing's position on an issue than face-to-face contact between a group of well-informed nurses and a policymaker and his or her staff. Face-to-face meetings provide a great opportunity for nurses to educate policymakers about health care issues while enhancing the image of the nurse as an informed, trustworthy constituent. Policymakers are very interested in information that will increase their knowledge about health care and help them develop options for future health care policy. For more information, the ANA website offers *Tips and Tricks for Visiting your Senator's Office* under the "Policy and Advocacy" link (https://www.nursingworld.org).

Participate in "Meet-the-Candidates" Town Hall Meetings

A strategy that nursing associations can use to determine which candidate(s) to endorse is to invite all candidates running for a particular office to a town hall meeting to discuss their positions and platforms directly with nurses. Town hall gatherings with nurses allow the candidates to talk about their platform to a group of interested likely voters and afford nurses an opportunity to voice their experiences, opinions, and concerns about health care issues and assess the candidates' views. Box 23.1 provides the correct titles to use when addressing state elected officials.

Hosting a meet-the-candidates town hall meeting can be an exciting activity for student nurses and faculty. Just as in preparing for a personal visit to a policymaker, nursing students should also prepare carefully to host a town hall meeting:

1. Before the town hall meeting, become familiar with each candidate's background, including his or her voting record on health policy issues, party affiliation, major contributors, personal occupation,

family information, and hobbies. This information can provide insight into the candidate's positions on issues.

2. Identify current issues that would be relevant for discussion with the candidates. Collect and review information related to the issues and then prioritize the issues. Time may not be sufficient to discuss all of the issues of interest.

3. Prepare to give concise examples of how the issue affects the individual, community, health care consumers, and other members of the nursing profession. Be prepared to debate the pros and cons of health positions that may arise.

4. Plan the agenda for the meeting to allow ample time for discussion.

5. After introductions are made, listen carefully as each candidate presents his or her campaign platform, and then be prepared to clearly and concisely discuss the issues with relevant examples. Real-world stories put a human face on health policy issues.

6. At the conclusion of the meeting, provide the candidate with contact information (names, addresses, telephone numbers, and e-mail addresses) for key members of your group.

Communicate with Policymakers through E-mail, Fax, and Telephone

Contacting policymakers through letters, e-mail, fax, and telephone can be effective if properly planned and implemented. The timing of the communication is important; it should be made early, before policymakers publicly commit to a certain policy option. It is easier to persuade an undecided policymaker than to get him or her to switch positions. A second very effective step is to send a follow-up communication immediately before the vote on a particular bill is scheduled. Information about voting schedules can be obtained online in most states and certainly from your SNA.

Because of the security slowdowns that may affect delivery, U.S. mail to Congress and the White House may be subject to delay, making letters a less effective means of communicating with federal policymakers. Using e-mail or sending a fax is really the best way to make sure your voice will be heard in a timely way to make a difference. Suggestions for communicating effectively with policymakers include:

1. *Be brief.* Short, direct e-mail and faxes are the most effective.

BOX 23.1   How to Address the Governor, Lieutenant Governor, Legislators, or Staff

Governor: Governor (last name)
Lieutenant Governor: Lt. Governor (last name)
Speaker of the House: Mr. Speaker or Madam Speaker
Senator: Senator (last name)
Representative: Representative (last name) or Mr. or
  Ms. (last name)
Staff: Mr. or Ms. (last name)

2. *Be specific.* Deal with just one subject or issue in the communication; state your topic clearly in the first sentence. The subject of an e-mail message should contain the number of the bill to which you are referring in the message. For example, "In Opposition to Senate Bill 123." The message itself should be just a few short lines to relay a clear and strong message related to the issue. Brief examples of how the issue/policy affects people in the policymaker's district are often most persuasive.

3. *Be personal.* Communication is most effective when it reflects your personal experiences and presents your views in your own words; mass-produced letters, e-mails, and faxes do not carry as much weight as a communication that you have written/modified in your own words.

4. *Provide your name and address.* Policymakers pay most attention to communications that come from their constituents—the very people who may be voting for or against them in their next election. So it is important to let them know whether you are from their district. Include contact information so that the elected official may respond to your concerns.

5. *Be persistent.* Communicate often, especially if the policymaker is undecided on an issue.

Telephone calls are usually taken by a staff member; ask to speak to the staff person assigned to the bill or issue for which the call is being made. After introducing yourself, give a brief and simple message, such as "Please tell Senator or Representative [name] that I support/oppose [bill number]." You may briefly state your reasons for supporting or opposing the bill and ask for the policymaker's position on the bill. Conclude the call by leaving your name, telephone number, and address; if appropriate ask for a written response to your telephone call.

Rosters of state legislators can be found online in most states. The roster contains contact information for each policymaker and usually includes information about his or her committee memberships. Contact information for members of the U.S. House of Representatives is available online (https://www.house.gov). This site shows committee memberships and has links to individual representatives' websites. Similar information for U.S. senators is also available online (https://www.senate.gov).

THE AMERICAN NURSES ASSOCIATION

The ANA is the professional nursing organization representing the nation's entire RN population—approximately 3.6 million RNs. The ANA is composed of 51 **Constituent/State Nurses Association (C/SNA)** plus other direct membership categories that represent state and U.S territory nursing associations and includes key corporate affiliated entities such as the American Nurses Credentialing Center (ANCC), the American Nurses Foundation (ANF), the American Academy of Nursing (AAN), and more than 35 specialty organizations, such as the American Psychiatric Nurses Association and the American Association of Critical-Care Nurses. A complete list of ANA-affiliated organizations and links to their websites can be found on the ANA website.

Through legislative, regulatory, and political activities, the ANA has taken firm and visible positions on a huge variety of health policy issues of great importance to the nation and to the profession. A few of these are passage of Medicare and Medicaid bills and then significant reforms of these programs over time, including APRNs' direct reimbursement in the plans; patients' rights; the importance of safe workplaces and safe health devices and practices, such as safe needles, safe patient handling, and whistle-blower protection for health care workers; adequate reimbursement for health care services; access to health care; and, most recently, comprehensive health care reform. Most important, it is the ANA members—the state nurses associations—that carry forward on the policy and political activities for health policy and nursing practice, roles, and reimbursement within a given state. A tremendous amount of health policy development and implementation occurs within state boundaries, and in order for the nursing profession's voice to be heard, SNA membership and participation are a must, because very few of the specialty nursing organizations have an individual state presence for policy and political activity. Students are encouraged to spend time browsing the ANA website at to learn more about this nursing organization so important to us all.

Students are also encouraged to visit ANA's Action Center and sign up to receive legislative updates and action alerts important to nurses and health care (www.rnaction.org). Through action alerts, members are informed about when e-mails, telephone calls, and faxes will have the most effect. Being connected through the ANA Action Center website makes the political process less intimidating by keeping nurses informed of political issues and providing strategies for making their opinions known.

CURRENT HEALTH POLICY ISSUES

Policy issues come and go as societal, health care, and public needs, demands, and priorities ebb and flow. However, several policy topics bear watching over the next decade: (1) health care reform through the PPACA along with Medicare's drive for value through innovative payment models that reward safety, quality, and care coordination; (2) building a culture of health throughout the nation; and (3) enhancing/shaping the nursing workforce and nursing leadership. The critical importance of these topics will keep them on the policy agenda for many years to come.

Health Care Reform and Innovative Payment Models

Health care reform is the general term used to refer to health policy initiatives to effect significant changes in how health is promoted and health care is accessed, delivered, and paid for in the United States. The U.S. health enterprise has historically yielded poorer outcomes with significantly higher costs than that of any other industrialized nation in the world (Davis et al, 2014). Many Americans, consumer groups, and health care organizations such as the ANA, as well as vocal individuals including many professional nurses, have long supported bold and comprehensive health care reforms to address critical issues facing our nation and its citizens. These issues include high health care costs that are not sustainable, barriers in access to care, health care disparities, concerns about quality and safety, and a system that is focused on illness care rather than one that promotes health and wellness.

Comprehensive health care reform became a reality when the PPACA was passed in 2010 with a complex, multiyear implementation plan to address some of the issues plaguing our nation's health care system. One major component of the PPACA was to provide funding for a health insurance program, allowing U.S. citizens and legal residents to secure quality health insurance at reasonable rates. The ability to obtain/maintain affordable, credible health insurance coverage was perhaps the most significant inequity of the prior system. In 2013, prior to implementation of health insurance through the PPACA, 13.4% of the population, or 42.0 million people, were without health insurance for the entire calendar year (U.S. Census Bureau, 2014). In 2016, that

percentage was down to 8.8%, or 28.1 million people without health insurance (U.S. Census Bureau, 2017). Obviously, the plan for expanding affordable health insurance provided through the PPACA has been successful. See Chapter 7 for a full discussion about the lack of health insurance and its tremendous negative effect on an individual's overall health status.

The second major component of the PPACA was to improve the quality of health care and reduce costs by requiring the Centers for Medicare and Medicaid Services (CMS) to implement specific changes to how hospitals are paid, as follows:

- Medicare payments to some hospitals are reduced or eliminated for treating hospital-acquired conditions, such as falls, decubitus ulcers, and infections.
- The Hospital Value-Based Purchasing Program was established, in which hospitals are paid based on their performance on quality measures including patient satisfaction.
- Medicare payments to hospitals are reduced for preventable hospital readmissions.

As the reader can see, nurses are critically important to influence these components of Medicare payments by preventing hospital-acquired conditions, promoting patient satisfaction and other quality measures, and reducing preventable hospital readmissions through appropriate discharge planning and care transitions.

To continue to promote population health, quality care, and reduced costs, Congress also authorized CMS to establish the Center for Medicare & Medicaid Innovation, which allows for creation and testing of new care delivery models designed to improve care quality, reduce costs, support patient-centered practices, and keep people healthier (CMS, 2017). Such new models include Accountable Care Organizations, Medical Home Models, and episode-based payment initiatives. Students are encouraged to visit the CMS Innovation Center to learn more about these new models of care delivery, which will all require active, engaged nursing practice to be successful (https://www.cms.gov).

It is vitally important that nurses pay particular attention to evolving developments about the PPACA and other national and state health care reforms. The ANA/SNAs provide the professional venue for nurses to stay current—and become involved—as health care reform moves forward. Comprehensive health system change will not be smooth or seamless or without continuing controversy, but it is critical. Through informed participation in health care reform initiatives, nurses can advocate for their profession and the safety, quality, value, and availability of health and nursing care for all Americans.

A Culture of Health

In 2014 the Robert Wood Johnson Foundation (RWJF) launched a new initiative, Culture of Health. A Culture of Health recognizes health as inextricably linked to all aspects of a person's and community's life, inclusive of where people live, work, and play and the choices they make. Collaboration among community stakeholders and sectors, including business, government, and organizational sectors, engagement with patients and community members, and supportive policies are essential to create environments that support healthy choices. A Culture of Health celebrates diversity and aims to achieve health equity across diverse individuals, communities, and populations. At the center of the

grand vision of a Culture of Health is the certainty that "everyone deserves to live the healthiest life possible" and that "we must [as a nation] ensure all people have equal opportunity to make healthy choices" (RWJF, 2014).

The Culture of Health initiative transcends the idea that health is equated with health care. Health care is necessary for health but alone it is not sufficient. The evidence-based County Health Rankings Model (Figure 23.1) depicts health outcomes as a composite of several health factors and determines the contribution of each factor to overall health. Clinical care (health care) accounts for 20% of overall health outcomes, social and economic factors for 40%, health behaviors for 30%, and physical environment for 10%. Improvements in these factors can improve individual health outcomes and make communities healthier (County Health Rankings, 2016). Part of the call to action to nurture a Culture of

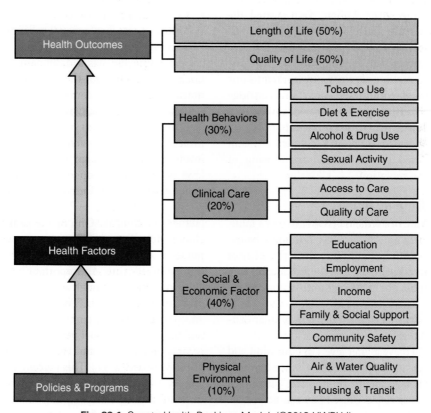

Fig. 23.1 County Health Rankings Model. (@2016 UWPH.I)

Health is the recognition that the U.S. health care system must change in fundamental ways to be more community-oriented and patient- and population-centered, all of which represent a major transition.

Nurses are uniquely qualified to be leaders in developing a Culture of Health. Nurses' holistic perspective of health is congruent with a focus on social factors that influence health outcomes (these are sometimes called "social determinants of health"). The nursing profession has a rich historical legacy of working with diverse and often disadvantaged populations. Nurses have long understood how environmental and other social factors can enable or constrain choices available to people and have worked to improve circumstances that have an impact on health and empower people to take better care of themselves. Examples of nurse leaders known for addressing social determinants of health include Florence Nightingale, Lilian Wald, Clara Barton, and Mary Breckenridge. Florence Nightingale is remembered for her attention to improving the environment to promote healing among wounded soldiers of the Crimean War in the 1850s. Lillian Wald started the Visiting Nurses Service in 1893 to serve poor immigrants in New York City. Wald was also the founder of the Henry Street Settlement, which provided community-based nursing services and worked to improve neighborhood conditions. Mary Breckenridge established the Frontier Nursing Service in eastern Kentucky in 1920, which provided services to the rural, poor, and isolated communities and included a system of community-based clinics, central monitoring of patients, and home visitation.

The Future of Nursing Report

In 2010, the Institute of Medicine (IOM) issued a landmark report, *The Future of Nursing: Leading Change, Advancing Health,* calling attention to the essentiality of nursing in the success of reforming the U.S. health care system. In this report, the IOM had four major recommendations:

- Nurses should practice to the full extent of their education and training.
- Nurses should achieve higher levels of education and training through an improved education system that promotes seamless academic progression with a goal that 80% of nurses in the United States hold at least a bachelor's degree by 2020.

- Nurses should be full partners, with physicians and other health care professionals, in redesigning health care in the United States.
- Effective workforce planning and policy making require better data collection and information infrastructure.

Although the *Future of Nursing* report was released almost a decade ago, extensive work continues to ensure that its recommendations become reality. Implementation of the recommendations and tracking of progress occur through a national initiative entitled the Future of Nursing Campaign for Action. As part of the Campaign for Action, coalitions at the state and local levels are driving action and policy change to transform nursing and health care. Specific issues being actively addressed by the Campaign for Action are as follows (Future of Nursing Campaign for Action, 2017):

- Improving access to care
- Transforming nursing education
- Promoting nursing leadership
- Increasing diversity in nursing
- Collecting workforce data
- Fostering interprofessional collaboration
- Building healthier communities

The Campaign has a dashboard available online to track progress through the years in each of these areas noted. Students are encouraged to visit the Campaign for Action website (https://www.campaignforaction.org) to learn much more about how this initiative is advancing professional nursing practice and health care. Becoming involved in the Campaign for Action at your local or state level is an excellent opportunity to affect health care policy and drive transformation in your own area.

Nurses on Boards. One of the recommendations included in the *Future of Nursing* report (IOM, 2010) is for nurses to be equal partners with other leaders in redesigning health care. An important way for nurses to be equal partners is through serving as members of health care governing boards. The majority of U.S. hospitals and health systems do not have nurse board members, and the overall national percentage of nurses on boards is only 5% (American Hospital Association [AHA], 2014; Reinhard, 2017). This percentage needs to change! Nurses have a unique perspective and skill set that will facilitate diversification of boards and help boards address priority issues facing health care organizations in today's challenging environment (Hachten & Mershon, 2017; Reinhard, 2017).

Nurses can help boards address critical problems, including medical errors and issues related to patient safety, quality of care, and changing models of reimbursement. Nurses' proximity to patients, understanding of the patient experience, and quality improvement and caregiving expertise are value-added knowledge and skills that are needed as health care organizations adapt to the greater diversity of patients served and demands to increase value by reducing unnecessary costs while concomitantly improving outcomes and patient engagement and satisfaction.

Serving on a board requires professional preparation. Nurses must actively seek board positions. Early career nurses are encouraged to seek opportunities to serve on various community and professional boards.

Examples of these types of boards include: county and district boards of health, boards of nonprofit organizations that serve the community and special populations, and the boards of state and district nursing associations and specialty nursing associations.

There are many resources available for nurses to learn more about serving on boards. Sigma Theta Tau, the international honor society for nursing, published a book on charting a course for becoming a board member (Curran, 2016) and also offers board member (or trustee) training, as do many of the Campaign for Action state coalitions. One initiative that aims to accelerate nurses serving on boards to catalyze changes needed to improve outcomes and promote equity is the Nurses on Boards Coalition (https://www.nursesonboardscoalition.org). Students are encouraged to visit this website to learn more about serving on boards.

▌ SUMMARY

Nurses must be powerful advocates for health care for all and for their profession. By understanding the policy and political processes presented in this chapter, nurses can make significant contributions to the development of health policies that promote a healthier society. A basic professional responsibility is to be involved in professional nursing organizations and to be politically active in supporting meaningful health policies. Just as the first politically active nurse, Florence Nightingale, used expert knowledge to shape health policy to make a difference, so can *we make a difference* in the lives of people we care for, in our own lives, and in the future of our profession.

REFERENCES

American Hospital Association Center for Health Care Governance. (2014). *2014 National healthcare governance survey report* (p. 12). Retrieved from http://www.kha-net.org/trustees/resources/2014-national-health-care-governance-survey-report_124088.aspx.

Centers for Medicare and Medicaid Services. (2017). *About the CMS Innovation Center*. Retrieved from https://innovation.cms.gov/About/index.html.

Chaffee, M. W., Mason, D. J., & Leavitt, J. K. (2015). A framework for action in policy and politics. In D. J. Mason, J. K. Leavitt, & M. W. Chaffee (Eds.), *Policy and politics in nursing and health care* (7th ed.). Philadelphia: Saunders.

Congressional Record. (2017). *Bill summary & status for the 114th Congress*. Retrieved from https://www.congress.gov/search?searchResultViewType=expanded&q=%7B%22source%22%3A%5B%22legislation%22%5D%2C%22search%22%3A%22summary+114th+congress+%22%2C%22congress%22%3A%22114%22%7D.

County Health Rankings. (2016). *County Health Rankings Model*. Retrieved from http://www.countyhealthrankings.org/county-health-rankings-model.

Curran, C. (2016). *Nurse on board. Planning your path to the boardroom*. Indianapolis: Sigma Theta Tau International.

Davis, K., Stremikis, K., Schoen, C., & Squires, D. (2014). *Mirror, mirror on the wall, 2014 update: How the U.S. health care system compares internationally*. Retrieved from http://www.commonwealthfund.org/publications/fund-reports/2014/jun/mirror-mirror.

Future of Nursing Campaign for Action. (2017). *Campaign for Action*. Retrieved from https://campaignforaction.org.

Hachten, R., & Mershon, K. (2017). Hospital impact: In uncertain times healthcare boards have even more reason to embrace nurse leaders. *FierceHealthcare*. Retrieved from https://www.fiercehealthcare.com/hospitals/hospital-impact-uncertain-times-healthcare-boards-have-even-more-reason-to-embrace-nurse?utm_medium=nl&utm_source=

internal&mrkid=4586458&mkt_tok=eyJpIjoi-
WkRBek1qQXlPVEZpTlRRnMSIsInQiOiJHdG-
drUXlvc2hkS3BlYmRCQkpQN1A3.

Institute of Medicine. (2010). *The future of nursing: Leading change, advancing health*. Washington, DC: National Academies Press.

Nightingale, F. (1859). *Notes on hospital*. West Strand, London: John W. Parker and Sons.

Reinhard, S. (2017). Getting nurses on boards. *Trustee*. Retrieved from https://www.trusteemag.com/articles/1212-getting-nurses-on-the-hospital-board.

Robert Wood Johnson Foundation. (2014). *2014 President's Message*. Retrieved from https://www.rwjf.org/en/library/annual-reports/presidents-message-2014.html.

Starr, P. (1982). *The social transformation of American medicine: The rise of a sovereign profession and the making of a vast industry*. New York: Basic Books.

U.S. Census Bureau. (2014). *Health insurance coverage in the United States: 2013*. Retrieved from http://www.census.gov/library/publications/2014/demo/p60-250.html.

U.S. Census Bureau. (2017). *Health insurance coverage in the United States: 2016*. Retrieved from https://www.census.gov/library/publications/2017/demo/p60-260.html.

24

Moving from student to professional can be frightening; plan your strategies.

Making the Transition from Student to Professional Nurse

Tommie L. Norris, DNS, RN

ⓔ Additional resources are available online at: *http://evolve.elsevier.com/Cherry/*

LEARNING OUTCOMES

After studying this chapter, the reader will be able to:

1. Compare and contrast the phases of **reality shock** with the phases of **transition shock**.
2. Differentiate between the **novice nurse** and the expert professional nurse.
3. Design strategies to ease the **transition** from novice nurse to professional nurse.
4. Differentiate between **compassion fatigue** and burnout.
5. Make the transition from novice nurse to professional nurse.

KEY TERMS

Biculturalism The merging of school values with those of the workplace.

Compassion fatigue The gradual decline of compassion over time as caregivers are exposed to events that have traumatized their patients.

Horizontal violence (also known as lateral violence) The covert or overt directing of dissatisfaction toward peers, themselves, or those less powerful (Falletta, 2017). Eye-rolling, badgering, belittling, and withholding information are examples.

Intuition Extracting clues from one's subconscious so decisions are based on a holistic view of the patient and surroundings.

Mentoring A mutually interactive method of learning in which a knowledgeable nurse inspires and encourages a novice nurse.

Novice nurse A nurse who is entering the professional workplace for the first time; usually applies from the point of graduation until competencies required by the profession are achieved.

Preceptor An experienced professional nurse who serves as a mentor and assists with socialization of the novice nurse.

Reality shock Occurs when a person prepares for a profession, enters the profession, and then finds that he or she is not prepared.

Role model A person who serves as an example of what constitutes a competent professional nurse.

Socialization The nurturing, acceptance, and integration of a person into the profession of nursing; the identification of a person with the profession of nursing.

409

Transition Moving from one role, setting, or level of competency in nursing to another; change.

Transition shock The abrupt shock that can occur with moving from student to professional nurse; associated with doubt, confusion, disorientation, and loss (Duchscher, 2009).

Trust Confidence that one's peers in the workplace have good intentions toward one.

Workplace violence Sexual harassment and abusive acts from patients or coworkers that can be physical, verbal, and emotional and can lead to a hostile work environment. It has been suggested that identifying workplace violence is difficult owing to its subjectivity (how it is seen by the recipient).

PROFESSIONAL/ETHICAL ISSUE

Lauren, a new nurse, who has just graduated with her bachelor of science in nursing (BSN), is interviewing with the nurse manager. She comes with questions and asks, "Can you tell me about the culture of your unit?" The nurse manager describes the culture as "accepting, diverse, and dynamic." Laura decides to accept this position.

Lauren is excited to have such a culture to begin her nursing career. She attends new employee orientation for 3 days and looks forward to beginning her career on her first nursing unit. She arrives 30 minutes early and enters the nursing lounge. She scans the lockers to determine whether one is available. She notices several of the night shift nurses watching, so she asks, "Do we have assigned lockers or should I just chose one that is empty?"

One nurse rolls her eyes and mumbles, "New BSN nurses think they deserve what we have worked for."

Lauren hopes she didn't understand her correctly and waits for her preceptor to arrive. She shares with the preceptor her concern with choosing a locker and what she thought she heard from the night nurse.

Lauren's preceptor replies, "Never mind her. She is always like that. She doesn't like anyone, especially new nurses with a BSN."

Lauren takes report the following day from the night nurse and is told that the "patient is monitoring her own blood sugar" and that the nurse did not report lab values ordered at midnight. Lauren is surprised when she finds the results from the lab posted from the previous night showing that the patient's blood glucose was actually 400 mg/dL.

When she reports this second experience to her preceptor, she is told, "Sometimes the night nurse forgets to check lab results." Lauren feels anxiety and wonders whether she can ever work under these conditions.

1. Was Lauren being targeted for horizontal violence?
2. Was information being purposefully withheld?
3. What are the signs of horizontal violence?
4. Should Lauren report the night nurse to the nurse manager?

VIGNETTE

Every nurse has experienced the transition from student to professional nurse. Why can't we learn from our experiences and help our future nurses have a positive first impression of nursing? The cost alone of the revolving door for new nurses should be enough for organizations to reconsider not only how novice nurses are orienting to the facility but also what proactive measures are in place to ensure that experienced nurses stay rather than leave due to violence or burnout.

Questions to Consider While Reading this Chapter:

1. What could educators incorporate into the curriculum to decrease the "reality shock" of transition from student to professional nurse?
2. What could employers of novice nurses do during the orientation phase to help nurses learn the ropes of their organization, which may differ somewhat from the learning environment?
3. What strategies should novice nurses use to gain self-esteem and prove themselves capable of having the required skills while still needing help with specific tasks and skills that come with experience?
4. Should professional nurses form official teams to look at the role of mentoring as one means of transitioning novice nurses into the profession?

5. What could orientation for new employees include to help novice nurses be proactive in preventing or reacting to violence at work?

CHAPTER OVERVIEW

According to *The Merriam-Webster Dictionary* (2018), *transition* is defined as "change" or the "passage from one state, stage, subject, or place to another" (https://www.merriam-webster.com/dictionary/transition). As nurses prepare to enter the profession and make the transition from student to registered nurse (RN), they move not only from one role to another, but also from the school or university setting to the workplace. Transition is a complicated process during which many changes may be happening at once. The novice nurse tries to juggle all these changes while continuing a life outside of nursing (e.g., as mother, father, husband, wife, daughter, son, active church leader, or community volunteer).

To help students gain an understanding of the issues involved in the transition from the student role to that of the professional nurse, this chapter discusses the various stages of reality shock. Strategies that may alleviate this shock and ease the transition are also suggested.

REAL-LIFE SCENARIO

The first impression the novice nurse has of his or her chosen profession is valuable and sets the stage for entry into nursing. This first impression occurs during the transition phase from student to professional. Consider Case Study 24.1.

CASE STUDY 24.1

Rachel Stevens had wanted to be a nurse for as long as she could remember. As a child, she donned a pretend laboratory jacket and set to work providing care to teddy bears and dolls. She softly spoke to her pretend patients, explaining that she was a nurse and would make everything better. After graduation from high school, Rachel entered nursing school and visualized her dream coming true. She was a high achiever and received comments from her instructors such as "shows evidence of applying the nursing process to the clinical environment," "psychomotor skills improving," and "becoming more autonomous." Her patients complimented her nursing abilities and caring attitude. Finally, Rachel graduated from nursing school, passed the national licensure examination, and accepted her first position as an RN. She proudly entered the hospital and felt confident that she would be a caring nurse and would help patients achieve their highest level of health.

The hospital provided a 2-month orientation period. The first week consisted of classes to explain benefits, safety education, Standard Precaution protocols, and computer skills. Rachel loved her new job. The next step in her employment was orientation to the medical-surgical unit where she would be working.

The nurse manager welcomed her to the unit and introduced her to the staff. Because all the seasoned nurses wanted to transfer to the day shift, Rachel was hired to work the evening shift, which had a higher nurse-patient ratio than the day shift. Rachel proudly sat through the shift report, jotting down reminders that were stressed by the previous shift, such as "The patient in room 200 needs a blood glucose sample drawn at 6 PM," and "The patient in room 215 is to receive a unit of blood." Rachel's assignment consisted of six patients. The charge nurse encouraged Rachel to ask if she had any questions. The nursing assistants hurried to complete their tasks.

Rachel reread her assignment and entered the first room, saying, "Hello, my name is Rachel Stevens, and I'll be your nurse tonight." She assessed each of her patients and reviewed their medication sheets. No medications were due until 6 PM, so she began researching those medications with which she was not familiar. At 5:30 PM, the charge nurse informed Rachel that the only other nurse on the floor would be going for dinner and that Rachel should respond to that nurse's patients during her absence. Rachel was a little nervous about the responsibility but positively acknowledged the assignment.

Moments later, Rachel was paged to respond to a newly admitted patient who was assigned to the nurse on break. As soon as Rachel entered the room, the patient complained of nausea and began vomiting. Rachel assessed and comforted the patient and reviewed the medication record for orders related to antiemetics. The physician had not ordered medication for nausea, so Rachel quickly telephoned his office to report the patient's condition. She received an order to insert a nasogastric tube and place to suction. Rachel was anxious; she had inserted only one such tube, and that with her instructor's

Continued

CASE STUDY 24.1—cont'd

assistance. She gathered supplies and reentered the patient's room. She measured for correct placement and was just positioning the patient when she received a page that the blood had arrived for the other patient, and that the laboratory assistant could not obtain a blood culture specimen ordered on yet another of Rachel's patients.

After numerous unsuccessful attempts to insert the nasogastric tube, Rachel became more anxious and requested assistance from the charge nurse. The charge nurse replied, "I'm admitting a new patient and can't help you. Don't you know how to insert the nasogastric tube?" Rachel explained that she had made numerous attempts, and the patient was continuing to vomit.

Rachel returned to the patient's room and attempted again to insert the tube. The nurse originally assigned to the patient returned to the floor; however, neither the secretary nor the charge nurse informed the returning RN

of the new admission with orders. Not knowing this, Rachel proceeded to care for her other patients. Finally, Rachel again requested help, and the charge nurse inserted the tube to the relief of Rachel and the patient.

Now the medications were late, she had forgotten to check the patient's blood sugar, and she had not completed the charts. "Where are my notes?" she asked herself. Oh, well, she would just have to remember.

Finally, at 10 PM, 1 hour before the shift ended, Rachel sat down to chart. She took out scrap paper and began writing her notes, but what time had she started the blood? She became more and more anxious. The clock continued to advance to 11 PM, and Rachel was still charting.

"You need to give the shift report to the oncoming shift," said the charge nurse. Rachel complied and 15 minutes later returned to her charting. At 1 AM, Rachel left the unit feeling depressed and incompetent.

IMPACT OF SHOCK IN NOVICE NURSES

Novice nurses describe feelings of being overwhelmed and isolated. Taking critical thinking from a hypothetical situation to real life is the most difficult part of the first year (Johnson, 2016). When the expert student moves into the novice nurse role, uncertainty takes over, and the support of classmates and the nursing instructors is gone. This time marks the end of one era as a student and the beginning of a new era in a nursing career.

The phases of transition into practice were first recognized by Kramer in the 1960s, and more recently, Duchscher (2009) coined the term "transition shock" to reflect that transition in today's dynamic environment. Kramer (1974) describes *reality shock* as the result of inconsistencies between the academic world and the world of work. Reality shock was believed to occur in novice nurses when they became aware of the inconsistency between the actual world of nursing and that of nursing school. The excitement of passing the licensure examination quickly fades in the struggle to move from the student to the staff nurse role. Both reality shock (Kramer, 1974) and transition shock (Duchscher, 2009) lead to stress, threatening the well-being of new nurses and resulting in anxiety, phobias, depression, change in mood and behavior, and physical illness (Sullivan and

Decker, 2018). Stress also contributes to nurse turnover (Choi and Lee, 2017).

The National Council of State Boards of Nursing (NCSBN) (2018) states that 25% of new nurses leave their positions within the first year, a fact that has a substantial impact on employers. Care of sicker patients and increased stress levels have led new nurses to report more practice errors and negative safety practices. New nurse turnover in the United States is estimated to cost between $1.4 and $2.9 billion per year (Shatto and Lutz, 2017). Age less than 30 years, obtainment of a bachelor's degree, hospital bed size less than 199, Magnet hospital status, and transition to practice programs (TTPs) have been found to reduce turnover rates for new nurses (Silvestre et al, 2017). An Institute of Medicine (IOM) report recognized the need to assist novice nurses in their transition to practice (2011). The four phases of reality shock, *honeymoon, shock or rejection, recovery,* and *resolution,* first described by Kramer in 1974, continue to be recognized in novice nurses today. This theory still holds for those transitioning to practice 42 years later (Guinan, 2016; Zerwekh and Garneau, 2018).

This chapter offers a brief tour of Kramer's reality shock theory to give a historical perspective on the "shock" phenomenon. Then it explores "transition shock" to help the reader understand the causes and how to be proactive to prevent it from happening or at least to reduce its effects.

REALITY SHOCK

Kramer describes the four phases of reality shock, from the honeymoon phase to the shock phase through recovery to the resolution phase, when the novice transitions into the role of "nurse."

Honeymoon Phase

During the honeymoon phase, everything is just as the new graduate imagined. The new nurse is in orientation with former school friends or other new graduates who often have similarities. Many novice nurses in this phase are heard making the following comments: "Just think; now I'll get paid for making all those beds" and "I'm so glad I chose nursing; I will be a part of changing the future of health care." When asked, novice nurses today admit to calculating budgets on the basis of their anticipated salary.

Shock (Rejection) Phase

Then orientation is over, and the novice nurse begins work on his or her assigned unit. This nurse receives daily assignments. "But wait. I've only observed other nurses hanging blood. Where is my instructor?" Now the shock or rejection phase comes into play. The nurse comes into contact with conflicting viewpoints and different ways of performing skills, but lacks the security of having an expert available to explain uncertain or gray areas. Novice nurses discover flaws in the system and communication breaks down (Guinan, 2016). Duchscher (2012) described transition similarly as an obstacle course. Kramer (1974) suggests that during this phase, novice nurses ask themselves two important questions:

1. What must I do to become the kind of nurse I want to be?
2. What must I do so that my nursing contributes to humankind and society?

Kramer described several approaches novice nurses take to deal with reality shock.

Natives. Many nurses choose to "go native" (Kramer, 1974). That is, they decide they cannot fight the experienced nurses or the administration, so they adopt the ways of least resistance. These nurses may mimic other nurses on the unit and take shortcuts, such as administering medications without knowing their actions and side effects and the associated nursing responsibilities. Unfortunately, the NCSBN (2018) identified this shortcut as a current issue leading to errors.

Runaways. Others choose to "run away." They find the real world too difficult. These new nurses may choose another occupation or may return to graduate school to prepare for a career in nursing education to teach others their "values in nursing." The NCSBN (2018) reported that novice nurses continue to leave the workplace; however, residency programs have provided resources to reduce nurse turnover.

Rutters. Some adopt the attitude that "I'll just do what I have to do to get by," or "I'm just working until I can buy some new furniture." These nurses are called *rutters*. They consider nursing just a job. A focus on professionalism and involvement in professional organizations may prevent this behavior. Have you witnessed a "rutter" on any of the nursing units where you have had clinical experiences?

Burned Out. Some nurses bottle up conflict until they become burned out. Kramer (1974) describes the appearance of these nurses as having the look of being chronically constipated. In this situation, patients may feel compelled to nurse their nurse. One third of all nurses in the U.S. experience "high burnout," resulting in stress, emotional indifference, and persistent fatigue; burnout can lead to poor decision making, an increase in hospital-acquired infections, and poor patient relationships (DeKeyrel, 2017). With a focus on working as a team and not accepting horizontal violence, nurses have support to prevent or at least reduce burnout. Heavy workload assignments and complex patient situations continue to contribute to burnout. The Mayo Clinic, which is committed to recognizing and dealing effectively with nurse burnout, has developed the Well-Being Index to enable organizations to evaluate distress among their nurses and prevent burnout (https://www.mededwebs.com/nurse-wbi/nurse-burnout-assessment-tool).

Compassion Fatigue. Not to be confused with burnout, which evolves over time, compassion fatigue has a swift onset (The American Institute of Stress, 1979-2017).

Even Mother Teresa recognized compassion fatigue, recommending that her nuns take off an entire year every 4 to 5 years to recover from the care they provided. Burnout and compassion fatigue do share some of the same symptoms, such as emotional, mental, and physical exhaustion and lack of meaning from work. Loss of hope and self-worth and effects on well-being are common in compassion fatigue. The single greatest risk for compassion fatigue is sacrificing one's own self-care (Sheppard, 2016). The American Institute of Stress offers the ABCs of prevention: Awareness, Balance, and Connections. The compassion fatigue process is depicted in Figure 24.1.

Loners. The nurses who react to reality shock by becoming loners create their own reality. They adopt the attitude "Just do the job and keep quiet." These nurses may prefer night shifts, during which they often are "left alone." Have you observed a loner on any nursing units?

New Nurse on the Block. Some nurses change jobs frequently. They go from the hospital setting to community health to the physician's office. They are always the new nurse on the block in their settings and therefore adopt the attitude "Teach me what you want; I'm new here." During orientation you may meet some individuals who report being new but who have just completed a short stay at another health care facility.

Change Agents. Nurses who are called change agents care enough to work within the system to elicit change. They frequently visit the nurse manager or head nurse to suggest change or a better way. They keep the welfare of the patient at the forefront. Leaders, whether in formal or informal positions, are often adept at leading and/or supporting change. See whether you can identify the change agents on the units where you have had clinical experiences as a student or novice nurse.

Recovery Phase

Usually the first sign that a nurse has entered the recovery phase is the return of his or her sense of humor or desire to succeed. The novice nurse begins to understand the new culture to a certain degree, so feels less tension and anxiety, and healing begins. The nurse in this phase may comment, "I'll hang that blood, and I'll bet I can infuse it before 8 hours this time."

Resolution Phase

The resolution phase is the result of the shock phase combined with the novice nurse's ability to adjust to the new environment. If the nurse is able to positively work through the rejection phase, he or she grows more fully as a person and a professional nurse during the resolution phase. Work expectations are more easily met, and the nurse will have developed the ability to elicit change.

Individual Experiences of Reality Shock

Most novice nurses experience each phase of reality shock (honeymoon, shock or rejection, recovery, and resolution); however, the degree of shock is individualized. For example, the new graduates who complete their clinical rotation during school in the same institution as

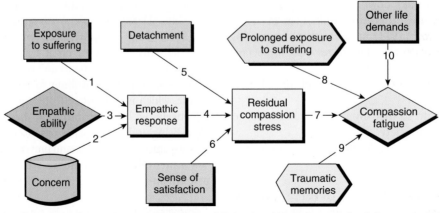

Fig. 24.1 Compassion Fatigue Process. (From Figley, C.R. [updated 2014]. Compassion fatigue: an introduction [website]. Retrieved from http://www.giftfromwithin.org/html/What-is-Compassion-Fatigue-Dr-Charles-Figley.html. Accessed January 20, 2018.)

they choose to begin their career may suffer reality shock to a much lesser extent because they are already familiar with the environment, staff, and overall personality of the nursing unit. The staff in the institution where novice nurses were educated may continue to see them as only "student nurses," however, an attitude that simply presents another barrier for novice nurses to overcome. Many students choose another institution for various reasons, such as better hours, better pay, and less travel time to work.

Zerwekh and Garneau (2018) suggest that nurses complete a reality shock inventory to make them more aware of how they feel about themselves and the situation at present. The higher the score, the better the nurse's attitude. It might be helpful to take the test at different times throughout one's career or when one is trying to decide whether a career change would be advantageous (Box 24.1).

TRANSITION SHOCK

As previously mentioned, Duchscher (2009, 2012) built on Kramer's theory of reality shock in recognizing the following fundamental elements of transition of new nurses to the professional role:

- *Stability* is described as being "steady" or what is unlikely to change for you as a new nurse. Asking the following interview questions can help you judge the likelihood of stability on the unit: (1) How many nurses have left in the past year? (2) What are the staffing levels? (3) What are the acuity and average length of stay for patients? (4) Are any socialization activities planned? (5) Do people like working here? and (6) What does a routine day look like on this unit?
- *Predictability* is knowing with some certainty the types of patients you will encounter, who is staffing the unit, and what your work schedule will be.

BOX 24.1 Reality Shock Inventory

Respond to the following statements with the appropriate number.

1—strongly agree
2—agree
3—slightly agree
4—slightly disagree
5—disagree
6—strongly disagree

1. _____ I think often about what I really want from life.
2. _____ Nursing school and/or my work has brought stresses for which I was unprepared.
3. _____ I would like the opportunity to start anew, knowing what I know now.
4. _____ I drink more than I should.
5. _____ I often feel that I still belong in the place where I grew up.
6. _____ Much of the time my mind is not as clear as it used to be.
7. _____ I am experiencing what would be called a crisis in my personal or work setting.
8. _____ I cannot see myself as a nurse.
9. _____ I must remain loyal to commitments, even if they have not proven as rewarding as I had expected.
10. _____ I wish I were different in many ways.

11. _____ The way I present myself to the world is not the way I really am.
12. _____ I often feel agitated or restless.
13. _____ I have become more aware of my inadequacies and faults.
14. _____ I often think about students or friends who have dropped out of school or work.
15. _____ I am still finding new challenges and interest in my work.
16. _____ My own personal future seems promising.
17. _____ There is no sense of regret concerning my major life decision of becoming a nurse.
18. _____ My views on nursing are as positive as they ever were.
19. _____ I have a strong sense of my own worth.
20. _____ My sex life is as satisfactory as it has ever been.

Scoring

To compute your score, reverse the number you assigned to statements 1, 3, 9, 10, 11, and 19. For example, if you responded to a statement with a 1, your score for that statement would be a 6. Likewise, 2 would become a 5; 3 would become a 4; 4 would become a 3; 5 would become a 2; and 6 would become a 1. Total the numbers. The higher your score, the better your attitude. The range is 20 to 120.

From Zerwekh, J., & Garneau, A. Z (2018). *Nursing today: transition and trends* (9th ed)., St. Louis: Elsevier.

- *Familiarity* is developing routines and becoming familiar with the staff and layout of the unit.
- *Consistency* can be described as "sameness"—whether you can expect similar types of patients and staff.

Duchscher stressed that it takes 6 months to find your "sea legs" as a novice nurse.

To help novice nurses deal with transition shock, Duchscher provides "need to know," "need to think about," and "need to do" approaches. The "need to know" concepts are the need to understand that although you are educationally prepared it is not possible to be a polished practitioner right away. Transition shock is intellectual, cultural, social, physical, emotional, and spiritual. The "need to think about" questions to ask yourself include "What is the SAFEST place for me to work that will allow me the environment needed for transition?" "Need to do" comprises understanding transition shock. You must know your capabilities and boundaries and you must learn to say "no" if you do not feel comfortable with an assignment. Consider how you deal with stress, let your friends, family, and significant other know you will be under stress as you transition, and recognize how you deal with stress. Get plenty of sleep, make wise healthy decisions, and use positive coping strategies. The stages of transition according to Duchscher—doing, being, and knowing—are shown in Figure 24.2.

CAUSES OF SHOCK IN NOVICE NURSES

Many nurses are familiar with the term culture shock. Culture shock occurs when people are immersed into a culture different from their own with norms that are unfamiliar and uncomfortable. Kramer described reality shock as exactly that. Duchscher (2012) described the transition phase as "back pedaling" as the novice nurse focuses more on doing than knowing. Entry into practice in acute care areas, where patients have high acuity but with fewer care resources, is one contributing factor. Because health care delivery still focuses on illness or disease models rather than primary health care, there is a gap between nursing education and nursing practice. When this disparity is paired with lack of experience in delegation and working with teams, the novice nurse may feel unprepared for such a demanding role. Patient-centered nursing is prioritized in nursing school, whereas in the workforce the priority is often the management of tasks and time lines. This disconnect may lead the novice nurse to feelings of failure because of the inability to provide holistic care. First, one should consider how students were taught to think in nursing school. When they prepared a care plan that took hours to complete, how were they to view the patient? The Quality and Safety Education for Nurses (QSEN) competency for patient-centered care is based on the premise of diversity and individual values of the patient, also requiring a more holistic view.

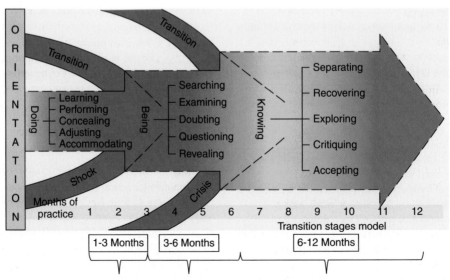

Fig. 24.2 New Grad Transition Stages. (From Duchscher, J. B. [2012]. *From surviving to thriving: navigating the first year of professional practice.* Saskatoon, Saskatchewan: Saskatoon Fastprint.)

BOX 24.2 Whole-Task and Partial-Task Checklists

Whole-Task Checklist		Partial-Task Checklist	
(Completed By Same Nurse)		(Completed by Different Members of the Health Care Team)	
Initials	*Task*	*Initials*	*Task*
TN	✓ Nursing history	SJ	✓ Nursing history
TN	✓ Nursing assessment	TN	✓ Nursing assessment
TN	✓ Patient education	BC	✓ Patient education
TN	✓ Medication teaching	CS	✓ Medication teaching
TN	✓ Bed made	CS	✓ Bed made
TN	✓ Intake and output recorded	SJ	✓ Intake and output recorded
TN	✓ Dressing changed	SJ	✓ Dressing changed
TN	✓ IV fluids hung	CS	✓ IV fluids hung
TN	✓ Patient turned	BC	✓ Patient turned

However, in the workforce, nurses may function with a partial-person or functional approach, in which different members of the health care team divide the patient care into parts. This care delivery approach, in which care is divided into tasks, is associated with higher nurse turnover (Choi and Lee, 2017).

Partial-Task versus Whole-Task System

The *partial-task system* of health care, in which different members of the health care team divide the patient care into parts, requires only partial knowledge (Kramer, 1974). For instance, one nurse may be assigned to administer all medications, whereas another may be assigned to dressing changes. The nursing assistant aids with personal hygiene and grooming, the physical therapist provides range-of-motion exercises, and the respiratory therapist teaches pulmonary hygiene techniques. There are many other nursing care delivery models in which the role of the RN varies considerably. The partial-task system just described is also congruent with the model known as "functional nursing," which places a high emphasis on completion of tasks. It is an efficient method for working with large numbers of patients, but the nurse cannot provide holistic care within such a system (Sullivan and Decker, 2018). With functional nursing and the partial-task system, the nurse is seen as only part of the care picture, but the RN is the central organizer who is responsible for follow-through on all care given by other members. This type of system is popular because fewer professional staff members are required, and it is frequently used on the evening and night shifts, when staffing is

considerably lower. This type of system also encourages loyalty to the organization because it forces the nurse to focus on task completion and productivity. The nurse ensures that all tasks are carried out but is not the sole provider of care. A simple checkmark is often the only quality assessment, with initials being placed next to completed tasks (Box 24.2).

Most novice nurses are more comfortable with the *whole-task system* because it is more consistent with what they were taught in school. The whole-task system requires complete knowledge and encourages loyalty to the profession. The nurse provides total patient care, incorporating physical, emotional, spiritual, and cultural components. The model of nursing care consistent with the whole-task system is primary nursing, in which the nurse is responsible for all the needs of the patient (Sullivan and Decker, 2018). This model provides greater satisfaction for the patient and the nurse. However, because of the need to use an increasing number of lower-salaried employees and the shortage of RNs, few institutions continue to use this model.

Evaluation Methods

Another inconsistency between school and work environments is the means of evaluation (Kramer, 1974). The school environment evaluates care from the "correct step" aspect, whereas the evaluation phase in the work environment is based on whether components of care were completed according to established policies and procedures. Were all the steps carried out in a logical, correct, and efficient way? This approach is exemplified in Case Study 24.2.

CASE STUDY 24.2

A graduate nurse was involved in a resuscitation effort. After the incident, she exclaimed, "I remembered to keep the time recorded and even had all the needed equipment on hand. I did everything right." But what about the patient? This nurse may have enacted all the steps correctly but may not have completed the components of care according to policies and procedures.

Think back to your first days in the nursing skills course. Can you remember the hours of practice you spent in learning the six "rights" of medication administration and technique of parenteral medication administration? Remember the stress you felt when the instructor observed you drawing up and administering your first intravenous (IV) push medication? How much error did the instructor allow? Probably not much. This is not to say that you should become lax in your tolerance for error. For example, it is never acceptable to have errors in the six "rights" of medication administration. You must and will develop your own system and quality check for performing nursing care. Nursing texts often list supplies followed by a flow diagram for procedures in which each step is listed. For instance, in the resuscitation scenario in Cast Study 24.2, even basic and advanced life support courses focus on algorithms that direct the care of the patient step by step. Always remember that patient safety comes first.

The transition from student to professional nurse is difficult, and changes in the health care environment have only added to the strain. Socialization and caring relationship with colleagues are key to a nurse's ability to transition, and preceptors are believed to assist novices by working together with them to close the gap between education and practice (Lalonde and Hall, 2016). Often new nurses are greeted with open hostility rather than being welcomed. Rather than being mentored they are assigned the most complex patient to "see what they are made of" (Hospital News, 2017). According to Johnson (2016), new nurses' willingness to stay in the nursing profession is either negatively or positively influenced by how they are treated. Nursing administrators may not support the novices' need to learn and may expect them to perform at the same level as experienced nurses. Unfortunately, the novice nurse may become bewildered and discouraged.

FROM NOVICE TO EXPERT

Benner (1984) described the following five stages through which novice nurses proceed to become clinically competent:

- *Stage 1:* The nurse has few experiences with clinical expectations, and skills are learned by rote; this stage usually occurs while the nurse is completing nursing educational requirements.
- *Stage 2:* Exemplifies the situation of advanced beginners, who are able to perform adequately and make some judgment calls on the basis of experience; most novice nurses enter the workforce during this stage.
- *Stage 3:* Describes competent nurses who are able to foresee long-range goals and are mastering skills.
- *Stage 4:* Proficient nurses who view whole situations rather than parts and are able to develop a solution are in stage 4.
- *Stage 5:* Describes expert nurses for whom intuition and decision-making are instantaneous.

Stressors common during transition include incivility, with workload being the highest stressor (Halpin et al, 2017).

SPECIAL NEEDS OF NOVICE NURSES

The following skills have been identified as needing further refinement in novice nurses. However, it is important to remember that a novice nurse's "need for support" does not end with orientation.

- Interpersonal skills and communication skills (Chanya and Pataraporn, 2017; University Alliance, 2014; Zerwekh and Garneau, 2018)
- Clinical skills/judgment/problem solving (Chanya and Pataraporn, 2017; Zerwekh and Garneau, 2018)
- Organizational skills (Chanya and Pataraporn, 2017; Zerwekh and Garneau, 2018)
- Delegation skills (Huber, 2013; Zerwekh and Garneau 2018)
- Priority-setting skills (Huber, 2017; Zerwekh and Garneau, 2018)
- Assertiveness skills
- Dealing with horizontal violence (Germann and Moore, 2017)
- Intuition

Discussion of each of these areas follows.

Interpersonal Skills

Most physicians, administrators, and nurse managers expect the novice nurse to immediately develop interpersonal skills that they take for granted. These feelings probably are rooted in the past, when nurses in training spent most of their time on units caring for patients and received little theoretic information or content in the classroom setting. They had time to get to know the members of the health care team and felt comfortable interacting with them. It is difficult for many people, including novice nurses, to be comfortable with interpersonal skills at work when they feel incompetent and inadequate as members of the interprofessional health care team. They are often uncomfortable making rounds, clarifying orders, and participating in interprofessional team conferences. However, effective communication is critical. Development of communication and interpersonal skills is a key success factor for new nurses (Blevins, 2016). These skills are especially important for nurses, who must be able to communicate with other members of the health care team, patients, and coworkers in a fast-paced environment (University Alliance, 2014). For example, consider the following scenario:

A novice nurse receives the following order from the patient's physician: "Give Tylenol as needed for pain."

The unit secretary transcribes the order and hands the chart to the new nurse, stating, "You will need to clarify this order: I can't take the new order."

Feelings of fear and uncertainty invade the novice nurse as he or she practices what to say to the physician. This fear and sense of insecurity can make the novice nurse avoid future contact with the physician, thus compromising patient safety. The nurse must, however, find some way to communicate, and may consider the following: "Can you clarify the Tylenol order on your patient?" or, possibly, "How much Tylenol did you want your patient to have?" or maybe even "Hey stupid, can't you write your orders using the six 'rights'?"

Perhaps the nervous nurse speaks as follows: "Dr. Jones, this is the student nurse. I mean the nurse taking care of your patient. I don't understand your order. I mean can you clarify how much Tylenol you want me to take? I mean how much Tylenol do you want the patient to have?" Then the inexperienced nurse hangs up, feeling ineffective, and the physician questions the nursing care the patient is being given.

Before asking a physician to clarify an order, it is a good idea for the novice nurse to practice what to say and even write it down so as not to forget. Then, when face to face with the person, he or she can state the facts simply and allow the physician time to consider the correct answer. A smile during the exchange in conversation might provide the receiver with a little more patience.

Gaps in communication may also occur between the novice nurse and the experienced staff because staff are so familiar with the routines that they may leave out information, unintentionally making the novice unable to complete the task.

Novice nurses need to develop interpersonal communication skills by building self-confidence (Pfaff et al, 2014). Reflecting back over transitions in her career, Donnelly (2017) suggests, "Carefully launder angry letters, memos, or e-mails before sending them. Sometimes a message needs 2, even 5 rinses, and occasionally a bit of fabric softener before sending. The 5-rinse message is an exercise in perspective building and in getting at the heart of the matter. Focus on data, facts, and constructive action when having difficulties at work."

Clinical Skills

Novice nurses report being caught unaware of the complexity of problem solving in the clinical environment or "thinking like a nurse." Students are taught skills in terms of objective attributes without situational experience. For example, the instructor asks the student to listen to heart sounds; as a student you simply follow the pattern of assessment (Zerwekh and Garneau, 2018). A 2017 study found that only 10.7% of new nurses felt comfortable performing clinical skills (Chanya and Pataraporn, 2017). Practice increases the effectiveness, efficiency, and correctness of performing skills. However, until the novice nurse has actual experience, there are actions he or she can take. For example, it is wise to be familiar with the procedure manual on the unit. Also, during the orientation phase the novice nurse should ask for a mentor to observe or assist with procedures for which he or she has a lower comfort level or a lesser degree of experience, to role-model excellent communication skills, and to answer the mentee's questions. It is important to remember that "practice does make perfect" or at least competent. Every new nurse needs a mentor for support and professional relationships (Zerwekh and Garneau, 2018).

Remember, no one was born with a Foley catheter in one hand and the set of directions engraved in memory.

Organizational Skills

The novice nurse may lack organizational skills. This lack of proficiency may be exaggerated by feelings of being "overwhelmed" by the new environment. Typically, student nurses are responsible for a limited number of patients, and although they must answer for their care, they typically are not responsible for as many patients as they will be assigned as new nurses. Someone is usually with students to offer suggestions on how to organize their time. The instructor might question, "Now, what do you plan to do, and what supplies will you need to accomplish the task?" New nurses might consider asking these same questions of themselves. If unsure, the procedure book lists not only the steps to follow but also the supplies that will be needed. List specific time-limited tasks. Avoid scheduling time so tightly that a slight delay causes chaos. Planning and prioritization skills are seen as areas of concern of newly graduated nurses (Huber, 2017). Chapter 25 offers valuable tips on getting organized, setting priorities, and managing time.

Delegation Skills

Most students have limited exposure to delegation. Uncertainty about or feeling uncomfortable with delegation may be a result of the characteristics of the personnel to whom one is delegating. Consider the licensed practical nurse, the nursing assistant, and other unlicensed staff. Often these personnel are older and more experienced; therefore, the new nurse might feel intimidated when delegating to them. Novice nurses should familiarize themselves with policies concerning which tasks can be performed by which category or level of health care provider. The question "Who can perform this task other than myself?" should be considered. Teamwork not only can increase job satisfaction; it has been found to improve patient outcomes. As you learn to delegate within the team, you develop leadership skills and provide more cost-effective quality care (Hansten, 2018). Delegation relies on **trust** and leadership skills, both of which may be deficient in the novice nurse. Chapter 19 presents a comprehensive overview of delegation.

There are also times when the novice nurse should decline to accept a delegated responsibility because he or she may not be competent to perform the task even though it is within his or her scope of practice. Remember that patient safety is always the priority. Show your willingness to learn, and ask someone to demonstrate the task by simply stating, "I would appreciate you demonstrating the procedure and allowing me to observe, and when the next opportunity arises I would like for you to observe me completing the procedure."

Priority-Setting Skills

Priority setting is a skill that all nursing students must demonstrate. The difference between nursing school and the workplace is that serious consequences occur if prioritizing is not done effectively in the workplace. Sullivan and Decker (2018) suggest considering the following when determining priorities:
- What you must do
- What you should do if possible
- What you could do if you have time to spare

Many novice nurses need help in organizational skills. Novice nurses may derive more satisfaction from performing technical skills, such as starting an intravenous IV drip, than from cognitive skills, such as developing a plan of care. Once they are comfortable with basic skills, they move on to critical thinking skills. How many people make to-do lists? Many make grocery lists, lists of bills to be paid, or lists of important dates. The same should be done for work—tasks are crossed off as they are completed. At the end of the day, consider what time was spent in unproductive ways, what caused interruptions, and what could have been done to save time. The same list may cue the novice nurse to a "forgotten" task or intervention. Sullivan and Decker (2018) also suggest determining the importance and urgency of the problem.

Assertiveness Skills

When novice nurses are placed in a situation that could possibly jeopardize patient safety and cause distress, it is critical they use assertiveness skills to negotiate the expected orientation time allowing them to effectively care for their patients. Assertive communication allows the novice nurse to say "no" in a respectful way without feeling guilty. Demonstrating appropriate assertive communication skills can promote emotional well-being and mental resilience (Queensland Nurse, 2016). Students are often naive when they are told by recruiters, "Come work for us; we offer a 6-month orientation, and you can ask for an extension if you feel uncomfortable. You will not be placed in charge, and only after a full year's experience will you be allowed to independently care for patients requiring advanced technology, such as ventricular assist devices." Students may be misled into feeling that they are "advanced" in their learning and moving ahead of all the others if they agree to shorten their orientation or if, after only 6 months, they take on the responsibility of caring for patients with special equipment.

However, after 6 months, even though novice nurses are becoming more competent and confident, they lack the experience to make instantaneous decisions based on intuition. Unfortunately, novice nurses are often employed on the night shift working with nurses with the same or less experience. As newer novice nurses (those who graduated the following semester) are hired, the more experienced novice nurses may even be expected to serve as preceptors. Nursing faculty should invite recent graduates to speak to classes concerning expectations after employment. Faculty should also inform students that they will move through many stages during the next year, and that they should take full advantage of this learning opportunity.

VIOLENCE AT WORK

When you think of dangerous occupations, law enforcement and military careers may come to mind. However, nursing is one of the most dangerous professions in America. Nursing can actually be more dangerous than a career in law enforcement. More than 75% of nurses in one study said they had been abused by patients or visitors trying to get to patients or family members (Dvorak, 2017). According to the Occupational Safety and Health Administration (OSHA) almost 2 million American workers have been victims of workplace violence each year (OSHA, n.d.) but there are most likely many more because most events go unreported. Currently there is no federal requirement for workplace violence protection; however, following several highly publicized situations of violence on nurses, the American Nurses Association (ANA) developed a zero-tolerance policy on workplace violence. Workplace violence is prevalent in all settings (ANA, 2018). Student nurses are also leading recipients of vertical or nurse-to-student violence (Falletta, 2017; Sanner-Stiehr and Ward-Smith, 2017), a situation that perpetuates the cycle of lateral violence that continues in nursing. The ANA's continuing education module *Navigating the Work Environment: Embracing a Zero Tolerance for Bullying* is a resource for any nurse who has experienced or wants to be prepared for horizontal violence. Box 24.3 shows four types of workplace violence identified by Wild Iris Medical Education (2014).

Sanner-Stiehr and Ward-Smith (2017) describe horizontal violence and bullying as being prevalent in the

BOX 24.3	**Types of Workplace Violence**
Type 1. Violence by a stranger with criminal intent	These violent acts are not committed by employees; rather criminals are strangers without relationship to organization or employees. Robbery most common motive.
Type 2. Violence by customer or client	Patients or customers become perpetrators of violent acts.
Type 3. Coworker (worker to worker)	Employee or prior or disgruntled employees threaten or commit violence against current employees and/or management. This is referred to as vertical or horizontal violence.
Type 4. Violence by someone in a personal relationship	Individuals who have a relationship with a current employee commit a violent act in the health care environment.

From Wild Iris Medical Education. (2014). *Workplace violence.* Retrieved from https://wildirismedicaleducation.com/courses/workplace-violence. Accessed January 16, 2018.

nursing profession. Horizontal violence includes such acts against coworkers as withholding patient information, exclusion, belittling, refusing to assist, badgering, displaying errors for others to observe, eye-rolling, and scapegoating. These researchers suggest that horizontal violence leads to increased stress and job dissatisfaction, which can result in missed work days. In 1996, The Joint Commission (TJC) issued a sentinel event alert in response to a growing number of crimes in health care settings (2018). The Sentinel Event Database contains reports of permanent harm, death, and temporary harm requiring intervention to sustain life and homicide (which are suspected to be much higher due to underreporting). According to the Occupational Safety and Health Administration (nd), a well-written and implemented prevention plan to reduce workplace violence is recommended and a record log of Work-Related Injuries and Illness (OSHA Form 300) must be maintained. Lateral violence has been described as an epidemic and must be confronted as if it were an infectious disease because it threatens the health of nurses. Because lateral violence can be obvious or covert, it is often difficult to diagnose and even more difficult to deal with (Germann and Moore, 2017). The ANA (2018) states that "the nursing profession will no longer tolerate violence of any kind from any source."

INTUITION

A nurse walks into a patient's room and senses something is wrong, and even though the data show nothing has changed, the patient confirms feeling anxious. The nurse stops to use all her senses to observe and assess the situation. She is using intuition. Swanton (2017) describes intuition as "that gut feeling." Intuition is not guessing but a nonconscious pattern of recognition and experience. Others believe intuition is much more than a gut feeling; rather it has a place beside research-based evidence and objective data (Melin-Johansson et al, 2017). Benner (1984) described intuition as the function of an expert nurse—implying that intuition develops over time as nurses move from novice to expert.

STRATEGIES TO EASE TRANSITION

When interviewing for their first positions, novice nurses should determine the philosophies of the agencies and how the various orientation programs assist new nurses to enter the profession. There are many opinions on the best way to accomplish a smooth transition, and each nurse should evaluate the orientation options available.

The NCSBN developed an evidence-based model for transitioning novice nurses to practice. The care of patients with complex health needs and a gap in practice readiness were the stimulus for the Transition to Practice Model the NCSBN developed. This model prescribed that a graduate will have the same preceptor for 6 months. In some settings, a team of preceptors is used for ongoing support for an additional 6 months. The QSEN competencies constitute the five modules used in this model: patient-centered care, teamwork and collaboration, evidence-based practice, quality improvement, safety, and informatics. Feedback and reflection are elicited from the novice nurses throughout the 6-month period.

One nurse recommended, after her transition from student to professional nurse, "Take in every experience that you can during orientation, take the sick patients while there is someone to hold your hand, ask many questions, and read everything that interests you" (Hilton, 2015).

Biculturalism

Biculturalism is the joining of two contradictory value systems—in this context, those of school values with those of the workplace. Biculturalism is designed to enhance a positive self-image and help novice nurses set realistic goals for practice. This strategy, if accepted in the workplace, allows the new nurse to introduce ideas or values brought from nursing school and integrate them into the work environment. Kramer (1974) recommends that the novice nurse appraise both sides of an issue, determine how his or her behavior will affect other members of the interprofessional health care team, and single out accessible objectives. Have you ever heard, "We have always done it this way and it works"? Duchscher (2012) acknowledges that tradition is not easily changed but suggests that you "catch more flies with honey than vinegar" (p. 45). Ask yourself, "What is the process for change?" and remember that the solution is not just yours but ours.

Role Models and Mentors

Mentoring and role modeling are often considered to be the same, but in fact they are different. Mentoring is a personal relationship with a more experienced person willing to guide a novice or inexperienced person. It is a voluntary, ongoing two-way partnership of at least 2 years, according to Smith-Trudeau (2014), who suggests that the entire nursing profession would benefit from mentoring through the retention of nurses.

A new nurse described mentoring as the best way to learn the intangible skills (Quinn-Szcesuil, 2015). The first year of nursing is "tough," but having a mentor to ask questions and talk to about concerns related to the new role can positively affect the new nurse's overall career trajectory. Mentoring has been shown to be a key strategy for increasing the diversity of the nursing workforce when novice faculty are mentored by culturally competent faculty—thus retaining more diverse students. Sullivan and Decker (2018) remark that choosing the correct mentor is one of the most important tasks for the novice nurse.

Mentors are experienced nurses who must be willing to commit to a relationship with novice nurses to help them recognize their weaknesses and strengths. Mentors help novice nurses set and reach realistic goals by reinforcing and recommending appropriate courses of action and providing emotional support. Mentors help novice nurses to develop confidence and organizational skills and to validate intuitive notions (Smith-Trudeau, 2014). The benefactor of mentoring is termed a *protégé*. Smith-Trudeau (2014) lists the characteristics of both the mentor and protégé (Box 24.4).

BOX 24.4 **Characteristics of Mentor and Protégé**

Mentor	Protégé
Empathic and nonjudgmental	Intelligent
Has advanced personal, social, and professional skills	Self-starter
	Curious
Ethical and has moral integrity	Hard worker
	Risk taker
Welcomes change	Has a sense of humor
Excellent at communication (both listening and feedback)	Open to new ideas
Has commitment to excellence in nursing practice	Has a vision both personally and professionally
Sensitive to others' needs	
Has a positive outlook	Embraces challenges
Uses situations to teach	
Is a living example of the values, ethics, and practices of the nursing profession	Possesses interpersonal and communication skills

Adapted from Smith-Trudeau, P. (2014). Will you be my nurse mentor? *Vermont Nurse Connection, 17,* 3.

Some mentoring programs are aimed specifically at pairing male students and male novice nurses with male mentors. One resource for this impetus is the Minority Nurse website (https://www.minoritynurse.com). Just as women face special challenges when entering a predominantly male profession, so do men entering the predominantly female profession of nursing. Programs aimed at improving the retention of male nursing students, such as the pilot MENtorship Program, have been judged to be valuable (Milligan and Gillespie, 2017).

Preceptorships

Another popular orientation program is the use of preceptors during the nursing student's final semester of nursing school through his or her entering the workforce. Preceptor programs have gained popularity as a means to socialize the novice nurse into the profession and to ease the tension of transition from student to nurse. Preceptor programs often are incorporated into the senior nursing student's final practicum, but they also may be used as part of the orientation program in the first work experience. Preceptors orient novice nurses to the specific nursing area, aid in socialization, and teach skills that are deemed necessary. Recently, it has been shown that preceptors can help new graduates

learn to problem solve, bridging the gap between theory and knowledge (Sullivan & Decker, 2018). Preceptor programs lower economic costs by reducing turnover of new graduates and helping novice nurses meet the expectations of their employers and peers.

Self-Mentoring

Ultimately no one is as responsible for the transition into the nursing profession as the novice nurses themselves. Mentors and preceptors can ease the transition, but novice nurses can also help by using self-mentoring when preceptors or mentors are not available. Novice nurses must be willing to learn appropriate resources, develop problem-solving skills, and ask questions. Novices should reflect back over times when they were self-reliant and believed in themselves. Box 24.5 offers some coping skills new nurses can use for the transition.

Residency Programs

Residency programs are one innovative way to ease the transition from academia to practice and may also be incentives for graduates selecting that first job. Residency programs often provide didactic or program activities as well as one-to-one preceptor experiences for an extended time, with 12 months being typical. Although residency programs differ, they all focus on retention and increased satisfaction of new nurses with

BOX 24.5 **Coping Skills for New Nurses**

1. **Remember it's not personal**—Patients and family members are stressed and see you as part of the hospital. It is important to protect yourself and report to your supervisor.
2. **Practice deep breathing exercises**—Deep breathing causes release of endorphins that reduce stress and improve your mood.
3. **Take breaks**—Even better, take your breaks in a quiet environment if you sense you are becoming stressed or overworked.
4. **Keep a personal notebook**—Express yourself and perhaps come up with solutions to some of the stressful situations you are facing.

Data from Delzio, S. (2016). 4 coping skills for new nurses: learn easy ways to cope with stress at your nurse job. Nurse Zone. Retrieved from https://www.americanmobile.com/nursezone/new-graduates/4-coping-skills-for-new-nurses/. Accessed January 28, 2018.

the added bonus of improved patient outcomes and safety. Not all residency programs are the same. It is important for the new graduate to invest the time to research what a particular residency program has to offer. The Vizient/American Association of Colleges of Nursing (AACN) Nurse Residency Program is a one-year residency with evidence-based curriculum requiring an academic partner. This partnership has maintained an average first-year retention rate of 95%, compared with the national average of only 75% (AACN, 2017).

Preprofessional and Professional Organizations

Students who join preprofessional organizations, such as the National Student Nurses Association (NSNA), gain leadership opportunities and meet not only other students from across the nation and internationally but also leaders in nursing they thought they would only read about. Students participating in the NSNA leadership university network learn how to run for office, problem solve, and disseminate ideas (NSNA, 2017). The NSNA Foundation provides scholarships and mentors future registered nurses into the profession. The NSNA publishes a magazine with information on job opportunities and legislative issues that affect nursing practice. Participation in preprofessional organizations develops leadership skills that are useful in professional organizations and for potential employers after graduation.

The ANA and some state specialty organizations offer reduced rates for new graduates and student nurses and continue with the previously mentioned benefits after graduation. In addition to lobbying efforts, benefits of involvement in the ANA include access to current information on standards of practice, certification, and networking opportunities.

Self-Confidence and Self-Esteem

Do you ever feel like an impostor, masquerading as a confident oncology nurse?

Deborah Christensen

The Clance Impostor Phenomenon Scale can be used to identify the presence of the impostor phenomenon in new graduates. Take a moment and rate yourself to determine whether you are an impostor (http://paulineroseclance.com/pdf/IPTestandscoring.pdf). One new nurse remembered thinking that, even though she was in uniform and looked competent, she should have a neon sign above her head signaling her "new nurse" status (Pascale Blakey and Jackson, 2016). A relationship woven with encouragement can inspire self-esteem and self-confidence. It is easy to become discouraged and disillusioned when reality does not quite match our dreams and fantasies. Self-esteem, or belief in oneself, comes as the novice nurse passes through the stages of reality shock and into a career in nursing:

Self-esteem = Self-confidence + Self-respect

Individuals with high self-esteem can problem-solve critically, tackle obstacles, take sensible risks, believe in themselves, and take care of themselves (Positive Way, 2017). Nurses with good self-esteem are effective and respond to themselves and others in healthy ways (Figure 24.3). They can accomplish more because they feel comfortable with themselves. Take the self-esteem questionnaire in Box 24.6; then visit the Create Positive Relationships website. If your score is low, visit the Positive Way website to learn how to stop your inner critic (http://positive-way.com/stopping%20your%20inner%20critic.htm).

So far, we have discussed ways that the employer and novice nurse can use to ease the transition period—implementing biculturalism, preceptorships, mentoring,

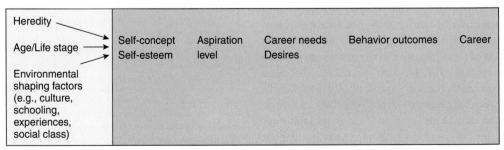

Fig. 24.3 Behavior Model. (From Schutz, C., Decker, P .J., and Sullivan, E. J. [1992]. *Effective management in nursing: an-experiential/skill building workbook.* Menlo Park, CA:, Addison-Wesley.)

BOX 24.6   Self-Esteem Questionnaire

Answer yes or no to the following questions:

_____ Do you have a hard time nurturing yourself?

_____ Have you ever turned down an invitation to a party or function because of the way you felt about yourself?

_____ Do you get your sense of self-worth from the approval of others?

_____ Are you supportive of others who berate you?

_____ When things go wrong in life, do you blame yourself?

_____ Do you react to disappointment by blaming others?

_____ Do you begin each day with a negative attitude?

_____ Do you feel undeserving?

_____ Do you ever feel like an impostor and that soon your deficiencies will be exposed?

_____ Do you have an inner critic who is disparaging or demeaning?

_____ Do you believe that being hard on yourself is the best motivation for change?

_____ Do your good points seem ordinary and your failings all important?

_____ Do you feel unattractive?

_____ Have you ever felt that your accomplishments are due to luck but that your failures are due to incompetence or inadequacy?

_____ Have you ever felt that, if you are not a total success, then you are a failure and that there is no middle ground and no points for effort?

_____ Do you feel unappreciated?

_____ Do you feel lonely?

_____ Do you struggle with feelings of inferiority?

_____ Do other people's opinions count more to you than your own?

_____ Do you criticize yourself often?

_____ Do others criticize you often?

_____ Do you hesitate to do things because of what others might think?

The more yes answers you have, the greater the opportunity exists for improving your self-esteem.

From The Positive Way. (1996-2014). *Self-Esteem Questionnaire.* Retrieved from http://www.positive-way.com/self-est1.htm. Accessed June 10, 2015.

---

and self-mentoring. However, each new nurse must begin by evaluating his or her own self-esteem. In addition, the novice nurse must realize his or her uniqueness and rely on instinct and past experiences when maturing and moving to a higher level of responsibility. The new nurse should remember to seek a role model or mentor for guidance through the transition. It is important to remember that it is difficult to be successful if one's personal and social lives are not kept in balance (e.g., in high school it was great to solve all the chemistry equations on an examination, but if "personal chemistry" was neglected, a void was felt that could plague future attempts at maturing).

Violence Prevention

Because new graduates are frequent victims of horizontal violence in their first year of practice, preceptors with zero tolerance for such activities are invaluable. It is also suggested that having nurses remember when they were a new nurse. Unit culture is impacted by high levels of fatigue creating a "toxic environment". Lateral violence was reported as both the cause and effect of this emotional and mental fatigue negatively impacting patient care and personal/professional lives (Wolf et al, 2017). Experienced RNs should consider the following to help

ease the transition of the novice nurse to the profession of nursing: The novice nurse should not be expected to enter the work environment and be as productive as experienced staff members. It is important for experienced nurses serving on agency committees to serve as advocates for novice nurses by reminding nurse managers and administrators that it is not possible for nursing students to learn everything necessary for professional practice during school. Also remind other members of the nursing unit about this fact. If a novice nurse develops initiative, autonomy, and a desire to become a team member, he or she will succeed. Newly graduated nurses are at high risk for lateral violence. Strategies that educators can use to prepare students prior to graduation to handle such situations include: identify and discuss occurrences of lateral violence when in clinical rotations; allow students to rehearse strategies when confronted with lateral violence; role-model professionalism; and develop a Code of Conduct that is consistently enforced (Sanner-Stiehr and Ward-Smith, 2017). Continuing nursing education is available to help new nurses identify and act to prevent lateral violence (Chu and Evans, 2016). Novice nurses entering the workforce will find the OSHA book *Guidelines for Preventing Workplace Violence for Health Care and Social Service Workers* helpful (https://www.osha.gov/Publications/osha3148.pdf). Novice nurses can also access the ANA website for continuing education resources on conflict competence for help with conflict management and should review the ANA position statement for recommended strategies to help eliminate lateral violence.

KEYS TO SURVIVAL DURING TRANSITION

Tingle (2000) offers four coping skills for new nurses to deal with stress at the first nursing job (Box 24.7). The College of Health Sciences at Jacksonville University suggests the following activities to cope with stress at work:

1. Breathe slowly, deeply, and easily to release endorphins.
2. Be organized—awaken earlier and leave for work earlier.
3. Stay hydrated and eat regularly.
4. Exercise to stay in good physical shape.
5. Develop a sleep schedule that allows uninterrupted sleep.
6. Use humor and laughter to reduce tension.

BOX 24.7 NURSES Transition Strategy

*N*ever fail to ask for help.
   If you do not ask, you may never receive help. The best way to get help is to ask.

*U*se available facility resources.
   Use other experienced staff, policy and procedure manuals, and staff development personnel.

*R*eenergize with professional associations.
   This helps to keep the novice nurse from losing sight of the profession in favor of the job.

*S*tay in contact with friends.
   Join the alumni association at your nursing school, and find out what your peers are doing.

*E*valuate your growth realistically.
   Develop short-term goals (e.g., open all charts by 9 AM), and then long-term goals (e.g., gain certification in your field).

*S*tay focused on your goals.
   Remember: Climbing the hill of professionalism is hard, but the pure "pride" becomes your armor.

From Tingle, C.A. (2000). Workplace advocacy as a transition tool. Retrieved from http://www.lsna.org/newpage12.htm. Accessed December 2007.

---

7. Avoid negative people and think positively.
8. Engage positive-thinking friends, family, and coworkers.
9. Take a break.

Hilton (2018) suggests taking time to consider these important issues before accepting your first nursing job: Ask about the first-year turnover rate (a rate higher than 20% is a concern); ask about clinical, social, and emotional support for new nurses; don't just tour the unit, stay for a few hours, and start on a specialty unit because it is more homogeneous; and consider accepting a "non-nursing" position in the organization prior to graduation to become familiar with the culture.

MEETING SPECIAL NEEDS OF THE NOVICE NURSE

It is important to review some common problems perceived by novice nurses and to offer suggestions to ease the transition period.

Organizational Skills

Lack of organization is common when the novice nurse's assignment becomes much heavier than that of a student nurse. The use of a report sheet can enable the novice nurse to note important information received during the shift report and from other members of the interprofessional health care team as the day progresses. The report sheet can also be used to document occurrences during the shift. Another suggestion for the novice nurse is to contact a former nursing instructor. Most students have developed a special rapport with one or two instructors. Novice nurses might telephone one of their former instructors to discuss the challenges they face during transition so that the instructor can help with problem solving. Hickerson (2017) suggests a checklist to mitigate stress and provide structure to the day. The checklist constitutes the following questions (p. 494):

- Why is the patient admitted?
- What new orders are entered?
- What are the patient's goals for the day? How can you reduce potential complications?
- What are the patient's recent vital signs, intake, and output?
- What does your patient and his or her environment look like? (Check identification band, IV fluids, and monitors.)

The basic report sheet (Box 24.8) also can be transformed into a unit-specific sheet. For instance, if the

---

BOX 24.8   **Basic Report Sheet for New Nurses**

Patient's Name _____
Room # _____
Diagnosis _____
Diet _____
Activity status _____
Lab ordered/time _____
IV fluids _____

Intake/Output
Urine _____ Stools _____
Other _____
IV primary _____
IV secondary _____
Other _____

Patient's Name _____
Room # _____
Diagnosis _____
Diet _____
Activity status _____
Lab ordered/time _____
IV fluids _____

Intake/Output
Urine _____ Stools _____
Other _____
IV primary _____
IV secondary _____
Other _____

Patient's Name _____
Room # _____
Diagnosis _____
Diet _____
Activity status _____
Lab ordered/time _____
IV fluids _____

Intake/Output
Urine _____ Stools _____
Other _____
IV primary _____
IV secondary _____
Other _____

Patient's Name _____
Room # _____
Diagnosis _____
Diet _____
Activity status _____
Lab ordered/time _____
IV fluids _____

Intake/Output
Urine _____ Stools _____
Other _____
IV primary _____
IV secondary _____
Other _____

---

novice nurse is on a telemetry floor, there might be a section for "rhythms." The orthopedic nurse could include "traction." This form also can be used to establish and set priorities. Once the care has been prioritized, the nurse can begin these critical interventions. However, it also may be possible to delegate tasks to ancillary staff if the tasks are within their scope of practice. This possibility requires the novice nurse to become familiar with the job descriptions of other nursing personnel, such as licensed professional nurses, nursing assistants, and unlicensed personnel, so delegation will be within their defined roles. Remember that the RN cannot do everything.

Clinical Skills

According to Benner's model (1984), the graduate nurse must be allowed to develop clinical skills on the basis of experiences. The novice nurse can develop competence with clinical skills during the orientation phase by asking

to observe an experienced nurse perform those skills with which the novice nurse is less familiar. The novice nurse also can provide the nurse manager and mentor with a list of his or her skills that need further practice. The unit's policy and procedure book is a valuable asset. It should describe in detail the steps to follow for performing a particular procedure. Spend time reviewing the manual before observing the procedure being performed, and then ask questions. Take into consideration that there is more than one correct way to perform a skill; remember, though, that it is not acceptable to take shortcuts that jeopardize the safety of the patient.

Interpersonal Skills

Developing interpersonal skills may be achieved by attending unit meetings, volunteering to serve on committees on the unit or within the agency, and taking an active interest in the nursing unit. These activities aid in the new nurse's socialization into the unit and profession. It is important for all nurses, regardless of their experience, to take part in professional organizations at the local, regional, state, or national level. Specialty organizations often provide valuable information and continuing education pertinent to the nurse's area of practice.

As the nurse becomes more confident in his or her nursing abilities and is less stressed by performing tasks, he or she can develop positive relationships with physicians and other members of the interprofessional team. Various methods that may be used to develop professional relationships should be emphasized during the orientation period. Nurses in staff development positions can be key players in assisting the novice nurse to develop professional communication skills. Making rounds with physicians and helping them with procedures open the door for communication. Asking pertinent and relevant questions ensures that the door remains open.

Delegation Skills

Another important skill that novice nurses need to learn is delegating. First, nurses should consider how others have delegated to them. Body language is important when delegating. Look at the person, be pleasant, and leave room for suggestions from the delegatee; however, do not allow the delegatee to resist or intimidate you so that you end up completing the task yourself. After communicating face to face, give a list of tasks in writing, or post it at the nurses' station; this leaves little room for misunderstanding. Be willing to change the assignment if there are changes in a patient's condition, new patients are admitted, or you realize that the time needed to perform a task was underestimated. If time allows, it is always good to help those to whom you have delegated tasks. For example, if a nurse passes by a door and the attendant is trying to turn a very large patient, the nurse should enter the room and ask, "How can I best help you turn the patient?" Always take time to give sincere positive reinforcement and say "Thank you."

Priority-Setting Skills

Now consider the best way to prioritize. How did you prioritize in nursing school? What worked then will probably work now with a few modifications. Remember: If it is not written down, it will probably be forgotten. Keep a notepad and pen in your pocket. Jot down reminders of things to be done, and place a number next to

each indicating its importance. For example, assume that you have already written the following list:

_____ Start the IV for Mr. B. in room 211
_____ Check the IV site for Mrs. C. in room 300
_____ Call the laboratory and check on blood sugar for Mrs. M. in room 215

Now you receive a call from the LPN that Mr. T.'s IV line is not dripping in room 212. Next the dietary worker calls to say that when she took the food tray to the patient in room 217, the patient vomited. Then the emergency light goes off in the bathroom of an older, confused patient. Now prioritize. What needs to be done first? First, answer the emergency light; do not even take time to write this one down. Now it is time to reprioritize. The new tasks have been added to the bottom of your previous list. Look over your new list (below). How would you prioritize these tasks?

_____ Start the IV for Mr. B. in room 211
_____ Check the IV site for Mrs. C. in room 300
_____ Call the laboratory and check the blood sugar for Mrs. M. in room 215
_____ Check Mr. T.'s IV line that is not dripping
_____ Assist the patient in room 217 who is vomiting

Now try out your delegating skills. Place a *D* next to any tasks that can be delegated in the list below.

_____ Start the IV for Mr. B. in room 211
_____ Check the IV site for Mrs. C. in room 300
_____ Call the laboratory and check on blood sugar for Mrs. M. in room 215
_____ Check Mr. T.'s IV in room 212 that is not dripping
_____ Assist the patient in room 217 who is vomiting

What had to be considered when you prioritized the tasks? First you needed to consider how much time was required for each task. It usually takes longer to start a new IV line than to check an existing IV site. It also requires less time to determine why an IV is not dripping. However, this fact is insignificant if the patient for whom the IV line must be started is in critical condition and needs the medication to reduce his or her blood pressure. Delegation may be needed. What tasks can other members perform? The unit secretary can call the laboratory to check on lab results, and a licensed practical nurse or nursing assistant can assist the patient who is vomiting, provided that you follow up very soon to assess the patient's condition. A nurse must know how to prioritize. Think through each situation. Change the priority as needed or as situations change throughout the shift.

Now that you know ways to develop organizational skills, refine clinical and interpersonal skills, delegate tasks, and set priorities, take time to remember other important areas of your life. Remember the people you may have neglected during school, and make it a priority to reestablish special relationships with friends, family, and loved ones.

SUMMARY

The period of transition from novice to competent practitioner is critical. New skills must be learned and refined, professional relationships established, and autonomy gained in nursing practice. Knowledge and skills must be refined over time. The transition from student to RN can be compared with that of butterflies as they emerge from their cocoons. It is unfair to judge them while still nymphs; therefore, the nursing profession must withhold scrutiny until novice nurses fly with their beautiful wings spread.

REFERENCES

American Association of Colleges of Nursing. *Vizient/AACN nurse residency program*. Retrieved from http://www.aacnnursing.org/Portals/42/AcademicNursing/NRP/Nurse-Residency-Program.pdf.

ANA (nd). Continuing Education. Retrieved from https://www.nursingworld.org/continuing-education/.

American Nurses Association. (2018). *Incivility, bullying, and workplace violence*. Retrieved from http://nursingworld.org/MainMenuCategories/WorkplaceSafety/Healthy-Nurse/bullyingworkplaceviolence.

American Nurses Association. (2018). *Zero tolerance*. Retrieved from http://www.theamericannurse.org/2015/11/01/zero-tolerance.

Asserting yourself in the workplace. (2016). *Queensland Nurse, 35*(5), 28–31.

Benner, P. (1984). *From novice to expert*. Menlo Park, CA: Addison-Wesley.

Blevins, S. H. (2016). Educators nurse residency programs: supporting nurse graduates. *Medsurg Nursing, 25*(5), 367–368.

Chanya, T., & Pataraporn, K. (2017). Experiences during the first year of practice among new graduate nurses. *Asian Journal of Nursing Education and Research, 7*(4), 461. doi:10.5958/2349-2996.2017.00090.8.

Choi, S. H., & Lee, H. (2017). Workplace violence against nurses in Korea and its impact on professional quality of life and turnover intention. *Journal of Nursing Management, 25*(7), 508–518. doi:10.1111/jonm.12488.

Christensen, D. (2014). Are you masquerading as a confident oncology nurse? *ONC Connect Blog*. Retrieved from http://connect.ons.org/ons-connect-blog/are-you-masquerading-as-a-confident-oncology-nurse.

Chu, R. Z., & Evans, M. M. (2016). Lateral violence in nursing. *Med-Surg Matters, 25*(6), 4–6.

DeKeyrel, A. (2017). How will nurse burnout affect the medical industry in 2017? *MedEd and Wellness Blog*. Retrieved from https://www.mededwebs.com/blog/how-will-nurse-burnout-affect-the-medical-industry-in-2017.

Delzio, S. (2016). 4 coping skills for new nurses: Learn easy ways to cope with stress at your nurse job. *Nurse Zone*. https://www.americanmobile.com/nursezone/new-graduates/4-coping-skills-for-new-nurses/.

Donnelly, G. F. (2017). Normative and Cataclysmic Career Transitions: A Nurse's Memoir . . . Gloria F. Donnelly. *Nursing Administration Quarterly, 41*(3), 223–232. doi:10.1097/NAQ.0000000000000232

Duchscher, J. E. (2009). Transition shock: the Initial stage of role adaptation for newly graduated registered nurses. *Journal of Advanced Nursing, 65*(5), 1103–1113.

Duchscher, J. E. B. (2012). *From surviving to thriving: Navigating the first year of professional nursing practice*. Saskatoon, Saskatchewan: Saskatoon Fastprint.

Dvorak, P. (2017). What's one of America's most dangerous jobs? Its not what you think. The Washington Post (February 11, 2017). Retrieved https://www.washingtonpost.com/local/whats-one-of-americas-most-dangerous-jobs-its-not-what-you-think/2017/09/11/71eae4d8-9715-11e7-87fc-c3f7ee4035c9_story.html?noredirect=on&utm_term=.c27692962d0b.

Falletta, E. (2017). Lateral violence in the workplace. *John Hopkins Nursing*. Retrieved from http://magazine.nursing.jhu.edu/2017/09/lateral-violence-workplace/.

Germann, S., & Moore, S. (2017). Lateral violence, a nursing epidemic? *Reflections On Nursing Leadership, 43*(1), 39–43.

Guinan, K. (2016). *Reality shock for nurses*. Retrieved from https://connected.unmc.edu/reality-shock-for-nurses.

Halpin, Y., Terry, L. M., & Curzio, J. (2017). A longitudinal, mixed methods investigation of newly qualified nurses' workplace stressors and stress experiences during transition. *Journal of Advanced Nursing, 73*(11), 2577–2586. doi:10.1111/jan.13344.

Hansten, R. I. (2018). Delegation in the clinical setting. In J. Zerwekh, & A. Garneau (Eds.), *Nursing today: Transition and trends* (9th ed.). St Louis: Elsevier.

Hickerson, K. A. (2017). Checklists for new graduates. *Journal of Continuing Education in Nursing, 48*(11), 494–495.

Hilton, L. (2018). *Six tips to survive your first year as a hospital RN.* Retrieved from http://allhealthcare.monster.com/benefits/articles/3846-six-tips-to-survive-your-first-year-as-a-hospital-rn.

Hilton, S. *How to Become a Nurse ©2006-2015: 1-6.* Retrieved from http://www.hackcollege.com/guides/how-to-become-a-nurse.

Hospital News. (2017). *A hidden truth: Hostility in healthcare.* Retrieved from http://hospitalnews.com/a-hidden-truth-hostility-in-healthcare/.

Huber, D. (2017). *Leadership and nursing care management* (6th ed.). Philadelphia: Saunders.

Institute of Medicine. (2011). *The Future of Nursing: Leading Change, Advancing Health.* Washington, DC: The National Academies Press.

Jacksonville University. (nd). How to reduce stress in your nursing job. Retrieved from https://www.jacksonvilleu.com/blog/nursing/how-to-reduce-stress-nursing/.

Johnson, N. (2016). Surviving your first year as a nurse. *Minority Nurse Winter/Spring*, 33–37.

Kramer, M. (1974). *Reality shock: Why nurses leave nursing.* St. Louis: Mosby.

Lalonde, M., & Hall, L. M. (2016). The socialization of new graduate nurses during a preceptorship programme: strategies for recruitment and support. *Journal of Clinical Nursing, 26*, 774–783. doi:10.1111/jocn.13563.

Melin-Johansson, C., Palmqvist, R., & Rönnberg, L. (2017). Clinical intuition in the nursing process and decision-making-A mixed-studies review. *Journal of Clinical Nursing, 26*(23/24), 3936–3949. doi:10.1111/jocn.13814.

Milligan, K. J., & Gillespie, G. L. (2017). Feasibility for the implementation of the MENtorship Program. *Journal Of Nursing Education and Practice, 7*(11), 84–91. doi:10.5430/jnep.v7n11p84.

National Council of State Boards of Nursing. (2018). *Transition to Practice.* Retrieved from http://www.ncsbn.org/transition-to-practice.htm.

National Student Nurses Association. (2017). *Leadership Conference.* Retrieved from http://www.nsna.org/meetings.html.

OSHA (nd). Guidelines for preventing workplace violence for healthcare and social service workers. Retrieved from https://www.osha.gov/Publications/osha3148.pdf

Pascale Blakey, E., & Jackson, D. (2016). Editorial: Reflections on being a new nurse: 10 insights after four weeks as a registered nurse. *Journal of Clinical Nursing, 25*(11/12), 1483–1485. doi:10.1111/jocn.13310.

Pfaff, K., Baxter, P., Jack, S., & Ploeg, J. (2014). An integrative review of the factors influencing new graduate nurse engagement in interprofessional collaboration. *Journal of Advanced Nursing, 70*(1), 4–20.

Positive Way. (2017). *Self-esteem questionnaire.* Retrieved from http://www.positive-way.com/self-est1.htm.

Quinn-Szcesuil, J. (2015). Skills for success what every new nurse needs. *Minority Nurse* (Fall): 10–15.

Sanner-Stiehr, E., & Ward-Smith, P. (2017). Lateral violence in nursing: implications and strategies for nurse educators. *Journal of Professional Nursing, 33*(2), 113–118.

Shatto, B., & Lutz, L. M. (2017). Transition from education to practice for new nursing graduates: a literature review. *Creative Nursing, 23*(4), 248–254. doi:10.1891/1078-4535.23.4.248.

Sheppard, K. (2016). Compassion fatigue: are you at risk? *American Nurse Today, 11*(1), 53–55.

Silvestre, J. H., Ulrich, B. T., Johnson, T., Spector, N., & Blegen, M. A. (2017). A multisite study on a new graduate registered nurse transition to practice program: return on investment. *Nursing Economics, 35*(3), 110–118.

Smith-Trudeau, P. (2014). Will you be my nurse mentor? *Vermont Nurse Connection, 17*(2), 3.

Sullivan, E. J., & Decker, P. J. (2018). *Effective leadership and management* (9th ed.). Menlo Park, CA: Pearson.

Swanton, C. (2017). Connecting person to person: the power of intuition in the holistic caring process. *Beginnings, 37*(5), 20–21.

The American Institute of Stress. (1979-2017). Transforming stress through awareness, education, and collaboration. Retrieved from https://www.stress.org/military/for-practitionersleaders/compassion-fatigue.

The Joint Commission (2018). Physical and verbal violence against health care workers. Sentinel Event Alert, (59). Retrieved from https://www.jointcommission.org/assets/1/18/SEA_59_Workplace_violence_4_13_18_FINAL.pdf.

University Alliance. (2014). *How to relieve stress in nursing.* Retrieved from http://www.jacksonvilleu.com/blog/nursing/how-to-reduce-stress-in-nursing/#. VDINbfldV8E.

Wild Iris Medical Education. (2014). *Workplace violence.* Retrieved from http://www.nursingceu.com/courses/455/index_nceu.html#top.

Wolf, L. A., Perhats, C., Delao, A. M., & Clark, P. R. (2017). Workplace aggression as cause and effect: emergency nurses' experiences of working fatigued. *International Emergency Nursing, 33*, 48–52.

Zerwekh, J., & Garneau, A. Z. (2018). Role transitions. In J. Zerwekh & A. Z. Garneau (Eds.), *Nursing today: Transition and trends* (9th ed.). St Louis: Elsevier.

25

Our lives revolve around time; use it as a way to ensure high performance, positive energy, and focus in all aspects of your life.

Managing Time: The Path to High Self-Performance

Genevieve J. Conlin, DNP, MEd, MS/MBA, RN, NEA-BC,
Patricia Reid Ponte, DNSc, RN, FAAN, NEA-BC

ⓔ Additional resources are available online at: *http://evolve.elsevier.com/Cherry/*

LEARNING OUTCOMES

After studying this chapter, the reader will be able to:

1. Understand the unique demands of complex health care environments in today's fast-paced world of high technology and communication transfer and its effects on personal time management.
2. Describe the relationship between personal performance and time management.
3. Articulate one's own time-management preferences and style.
4. Create an action plan to manage procrastination, distraction, and anxiety.
5. Describe how individual learning and communication styles interact with the ability to manage time effectively.
6. Adopt into daily practice a time-management strategy plan unique to one's own style to ensure high-level personal performance in work and home life.
7. Articulate the impact of personal time-related choices made by individuals on the risk to patients and the organization.

KEY TERMS

Energy management Ensuring that the right amount of effort matches the right task to optimize an outcome.

Goal A tangible, measurable, and attainable act in a specific time. It has broad-term results, experiences, or achievements toward which someone is willing to work.

Objective An identifiable, measurable act that implements one's goal and is typically short-term.

Prioritizing The act of deciding what should be done first and what activities should follow sequentially; establishing an ordered list or ranked items based on importance or urgency; method used to determine what actions need to be accomplished ahead of others; represents the execution of ranked items.

Procrastination The act of intentionally and/or habitually putting off doing something that should be done.

Technology management Application of information systems and equipment to enhance work and life activities to maximal benefit.

Time management The development of processes and tools that increase efficiency and productivity within the set standard of time.

PROFESSIONAL/ETHICAL ISSUE

Karen is a busy staff nurse working on a medical-surgical unit at the local community hospital. She has just returned to work from her vacation and is getting report for her patient assignment. While she was away, some significant updates were made to the clinical documentation system. Karen wasn't able to attend the training session to review the changes and is not familiar with the changes. Her manager had told her she needed to attend the training before she could return to practice. She hadn't been concerned, as she feels she has strong computer skills, and assumed she'd figure it out upon her return. "I mean, really, how hard can it be?" Karen had said. One of her colleagues offers to take a few minutes to show her some of the new workflows in the system, but Karen brushes her off, stating, "I don't have time to review this; I need to get my meds passed so I can go to the uniform sale in the café before it closes."

Karen soon discovers there are some big differences in how to document medications as well as some of the procedures. She quickly falls behind in her documentation and starts writing things on a piece of paper.

Karen has plans after work to meet friends for dinner. She's eager to finish her shift and get on with her evening. She has missed some important pieces of documentation, although she does give a thorough handoff to the next nurse at shift change report. The oncoming nurse asks about a patient's response to a pain medication given. Karen replies, "I need to remember to note that; I'll just deal with it next time I work. . . . Hopefully I'll remember everything I did!" She laughs it off as she leaves the unit at the end of her shift.

You are the nurse receiving report from Karen, and you realize her documentation is not complete. What do you do? What systems could have been put in place to ensure that Karen did not return to work before completing the new documentation system training? What could Karen have done when she realized the enormity of the gap in her knowledge and skills in using the new documentation system? What are the ethical considerations involved in this situation? Are they at the organizational as well as individual clinician levels?

VIGNETTE

Approximately 4 months ago, Susan Kenny transferred to a position as a staff registered nurse (RN) at an ambulatory cancer treatment center. Today Susan arrived at the chemotherapy infusion room 15 minutes before the start of her shift. She knew it was going to be a busy day, and given her lack of experience in this work setting, she thought she should get a head start on her assignment. She was heading toward the workstation when one of her colleagues stopped her to discuss a holiday party, and they both spoke fervently about how much fun it would be.

Ten minutes later, Susan resumed her trek to the workstation. Just as she arrived, the phone rang, and Susan answered it. A patient was seeking information about her appointment time. It took Susan quite a while to open up the computer screen, log in, and find the information, which she communicated to the patient. By now many of her colleagues were on site, already starting to work on their assignments. Susan looked at her assignment and realized that in addition to her other assigned patients, one of her patients would be receiving the first treatment of a new chemotherapy protocol. She knew that given the time necessary to work with the patient and family, triple-check orders with her physician and pharmacist colleagues, and administer the premedication and chemotherapy, all while monitoring this very ill patient, she would be very busy all day.

While she was reviewing the new chemotherapy protocol, one of Susan's primary patients came in unexpectedly with a fever and low blood pressure, needing hydration and platelets. The physician gave Susan orders to stabilize the patient and arrange for transfer to the inpatient unit. The hospital was full, so the transfer would take some time. Susan began to get very anxious about being able to complete all of her assigned duties while giving her patients the specialized care and attention they needed. Unfortunately, this anxious feeling was becoming a common occurrence in Susan's workday.

Meanwhile, Maura Callahan, a staff RN who had been working on the inpatient oncology floor for just less than a year, was passing out 10 AM medications when she received a call from Susan to take report before accepting the patient later in the day when a room became available. Maura was already behind in passing medications because of the new barcoding system now in use for medication administration. Despite the fact that this system would be safer and more efficient, using the new application took more time in the first few weeks. The training was great, but medication administration took longer. Maura asked the charge nurse whether she could take report for her, but the charge nurse said she was in the midst of transferring another patient to the medical intensive care unit.

Maura took the report from Susan and agreed to accept the patient at 1 PM, when another patient's discharge would be completed and the room cleaned. Maura wondered, "How will I ever get finished in time to pick up my daughter from daycare by 4 PM?" Her day was lining up like so many before, with her not being able to finish her work before the end of the shift. She would have to call her mother to help out again by picking up her daughter.

Both Susan and Maura were working frantically to ensure that patients' needs were met in a timely way, but it seemed impossible to both of them before they decided to call their respective managers and seek assistance.

Questions to Consider While Reading this Chapter:

1. When Susan arrived on duty, what are some strategies she could have used to be sure she made the most of her early arrival?
2. What factors should Susan and Maura consider when deciding how to prioritize their patient care assignment?
3. What strategies could Maura and Susan consider when deciding how to manage their learning needs and the need to be patient and family focused?
4. What are some strategies that Maura and Susan can use to ensure balance between their work and personal lives?

CHAPTER OVERVIEW

The previous scenarios are typical of what happens daily in the lives of busy professionals. Managing multiple priorities during a particular workday and integrating personal and work-related demands is the constant dilemma of so many men and women today. Additionally, performing well in both arenas is not only a goal of most working professionals but more importantly an obligation to ensure quality and safety in care delivery. To accomplish the important goals in life, it is necessary to understand your own preferred style of managing priorities, recognize your typical distractions, identify a personal performance approach, and consistently use strategies and tools to make the most of every minute. This chapter is designed to assist students and busy professionals in implementing self-management strategies to better use their time and energy to ensure a highly productive, focused life.

HEALTH CARE TODAY

Health care environments are fraught with incredible complexities: high-acuity patients, vigilant and knowledgeable family members, ever-growing information technology geared toward supporting staff in their work, often tight quarters in which to deliver high-tech and high-risk care, and little time to interact with patients on an interpersonal therapeutic level. Interprofessional practice models demand collaborative teamwork, when in reality disciplines often function in parallel work processes. The need to move patients quickly from one site of care to another on a constantly growing continuum that reaches into patients' homes is the norm in today's health care environment. Fast-paced clinics, high-tech ambulatory care practice settings, and quaternary care in high-intensity critical care units and operating rooms are typical. The nature of the intimate human element inherent in the delivery of health care makes it like no other work.

As health care continues to evolve with a focus on improving access and quality and reducing costs, efficiency has become a critical component of health care delivery. Managing time, organizing care, and maintaining personal health and a balance between work and home settings become much more demanding—and essential. Therefore, it becomes critical for each professional working in these dynamic settings to receive education and coaching in managing time, energy, balance, and focus to ensure high performance. Florence Nightingale's words resonate: "Knowing how you manage when you are there [at work] . . . impacts how your work should be done when you are not there" (1969).

PERSPECTIVES ON TIME

Each person has a specific perspective of time, which is based on his or her own experiences, values, education, socioeconomic factors, age, personality, culture, and genetic makeup. To understand one's own perspective on time and the resulting behaviors, it is necessary to create opportunities to think introspectively and examine personal preferences, traits, habits, and tendencies. This is the critical first step in achieving an individualized time-management strategy and plan.

In her book, *Time Management from the Inside Out*, Julie Morgenstern (2004) presents "10 psychological obstacles" that influence one's ability to create and sustain focused and productive work habits. As you review the following 10 obstacles, carefully consider how they might affect your ability to develop productive, energetic work habits.

1. *Unclear Goals and Priorities:* Within a particular work shift or within your life as a whole, if you lack clarity about purpose and expected outcomes, the ability to manage time to meet your desires becomes a futile task.

2. *Conquistador of Chaos:* If you are constantly overburdened with tasks, events, urgent requests, and last-minute cancellations, you are a better crisis manager than a manager of time.

3. *Fear of Downtime:* Some individuals fear the possibility of standing still too long. They feel guilty with time-outs or time off. Often this fear is a result of not wanting to address the larger issues in life. Staying too busy to think keeps long-term planning and personal introspection at bay.

4. *Need to be a Caretaker:* In professions such as nursing, the need to be a caretaker is a common devotion and can be very gratifying. However, when this need becomes unbalanced, it can cause you to feel resentful, unappreciated, and overwhelmed.

5. *Fear of Failure:* If you are unable to get to the things that are important to you and are unable to meet your personal goals, you may be afraid of failure. It can be very upsetting to go after your dreams and find out you cannot reach them. Sometimes it is easier to avoid making the effort. Take time to understand what your fears are and to openly address them.

6. *Fear of Success:* You may have been given a message somewhere in your life that you do not deserve to be a success. Therefore, it can be anxiety provoking to garner success and stand apart from others, who may distance themselves from you. Take time to think through whether or not this issue is playing out in your life.

7. *Fear of Disrupting the Status Quo:* Not pursuing your goals for fear of the reactions of those around you is very common. Your family, coworkers, or supervisors may be critical of what you want to pursue. Gradually approaching changes gives you and those around you time to acclimate.

8. *Fear of Completion:* If you are afraid of completing a project that is creative and fun because you are fearful that another similar project will not find its way to you or the project may no longer be important to you, take the time to understand why you are not completing a routine task or a major project that has been with you for some time.

9. *Need for Perfection:* If you are a perfectionist and feel that everything should be completed with the same level of excellence, you are not keeping things in perspective. If you demand extremely high standards for every single task you undertake, you simply will not get everything done.

10. *Fear of Losing Creativity:* Many creative people think that creating an organized time-management structure or approach to life will squelch their creative natures or tendencies. However, creating a framework to manage priorities will allow more freedom and time to enhance your creative juices.

Following are some of the benefits that will result if you take the time to uncover your own tendencies, fears, strengths, and weaknesses (Childre, 2008; Ponte and Koppel, 2008):

- Improved patient outcomes through implementation of a collaborative structure in the work environment
- Increased satisfaction with your work accomplishments as a result of applying something new in your setting
- Improved interpersonal relations because of your ability to be fully present and engaged to do your best work
- Better future direction because there is more attentiveness to proactively managing and engaging in the environment
- Improved personal health because of decreased anxiety and a restoration of emotional balance

It is more crucial than ever that you strive to understand what you value, recognize your purpose in life, and determine strategies to ensure that your focus and energy are geared toward your major goals in life. Whether you are trying to organize how to approach a particular workday or trying to balance your personal and work life, the strategies that you will learn and integrate into your daily activities now will play out the rest of your life. Managing energy to ensure high performance is the first step.

ENERGY MANAGEMENT

Sources of Energy

According to Loehr and Schwartz (2005), "Energy, not time, is the fundamental currency of high performance." Striving to be more efficient and more organized or to manage time and priorities better is all in the interest of becoming a better performer in either one's work or one's personal life. Loehr and Schwartz (2005) also state that only when we are fully engaged do we perform our best. Full engagement requires drawing on four separate but related sources of energy: (1) physical, (2) mental, (3) spiritual, and (4) emotional. Just as we build physical capacity through disciplined exercise and strengthening routines, we can also strengthen our emotional, spiritual, and mental capacities.

Consider Susan from our earlier vignette. Her decision to transfer to the chemotherapy infusion center, her third transfer in 18 months, came only after the sheer frustration of not being able to feel in control of her work life and home life. At work, Susan felt overwhelmed, underappreciated, and unprepared physically for the daily challenges of 12-hour shifts. She was exhausted every morning, and she fell into bed as soon as she got home. Her energy level was poor. She felt dissatisfied with her inability to spend more time with friends on weekends. Susan could not bear the thought of getting out of bed early another day, even if it was for something fun. Because of this, she gained weight over the past 6 months, and the only thing that seemed to make her happy was to visit her sister on Sunday afternoons for shopping and dinner. Getting to work the next day often proved difficult because her motivation was low and her energy level even lower. With this new job, Susan was attempting to get back on track. "It's going to be different this time," she said to herself. With a focus on physical, mental, spiritual, and emotional energy, Susan may really have a different—and much better—life and work experience!

Physical Energy. Key components of physical energy for a productive and highly energizing life include paying attention to a routine of eating properly, getting adequate sleep and exercise, taking appropriate breaks during long shifts, drinking plenty of water, and focusing on one activity while collecting thoughts about what to prioritize next. Once the physical capacity of your holistic self is working well, you can pay attention to your mental, spiritual, and emotional capacities.

Mental Energy. The mental energy that is most potent to ensure full engagement and high performance is that of realistic optimism. *Realistic optimism* is seeing the world as it is but always working toward an optimal solution or goal. *Mental energy* is the ability to maintain sustained concentration on a task and move flexibly between issues. Mental energy includes preparation, visualization, positive self-talk, effective time management, and creativity. Susan has begun to identify this mental energy in her desire to get back on track. She realizes that change is necessary. To move in this direction, Susan needs to spend some time to reflect on the following questions: (1) What are my major goals in life? and (2) What is my purpose?

Spiritual Energy. Often we do not take the time to reflect about what is important to us. Being in a quiet place helps us identify our vision of life—our purpose and direction in life. Having direction and purpose is the key factor in one's spiritual capacity.

Emotional Energy. Physical, mental, and spiritual energy provide fuel for building our emotional capacity. Managing emotions skillfully in the service of high positive energy and full engagement is called *emotional intelligence* (Goleman, 2006). Striving to increase one's emotional capacity—which includes improving one's self-confidence, self-control, self-regulation, social skills, interpersonal effectiveness, empathy, patience, openness, trust, and enjoyment—will result in a more positive, invigorating work experience and personal life.

Practicing Mindfulness

There is growing interest in and evidence of the positive impact of adopting a mindful attitude and incorporating mindfulness practices into one's personal and professional life. Mindfulness practices help you stay focused on the present and be attentive to what is happening in the moment so that distractions are held at bay while the mind continuously brings you back to the present moment. One mindfulness practice is to use focused breathing for 1 to 2 minutes to stay calm and reflect on the priority at hand, allowing yourself the opportunity to remember the importance of what is happening in the moment. This practice results in less rumination about the future or extraneous phenomena and allows you to be clear-minded, focused, and attentive to the situation at hand, whether it be the need to administer a medication, to calm an upset family member, or to document in the medical record.

Incorporating a mindful attitude and mindful practices into you way of life and way of being can result in a more balanced and effective focus to carry out activities of everyday life and nursing practice (Ponte and Koppel, 2015). Mindfulness practices can also have an impact on your greater well-being and perceived health. Mindfulness-based practices in addition to focused breathing include meditation, yoga, reflective journaling, and incorporating music, art, and nature into your daily life and into nursing practice.

Nurses who adopt a mindful attitude and practices are more apt to be better at time and energy management in all aspects of their work and personal lives.

TIME AND ENERGY DISTRACTIONS

We are all subject to distractions in our work and personal lives that may influence our propensity to procrastinate or not reach our goals. Nurses experience stress and distraction when they assume unplanned responsibilities while simultaneously conducting their planned work. This is referred to in the literature as "complexity compression" (Krichbaum et al, 2011). It is important to recognize and understand the distractions or complexities that inhibit our ability to complete tasks and to meet our objectives and goals in a planned way. Box 25.1 lists many common internal and external time and energy distractions that each of us may experience

BOX 25.1 Time and Energy Distractions	
External Distractions	**Internal Distractions**
Interruptions	Procrastination
Socializing or visitors	Inadequate planning
Meetings	Ineffective delegation
Excessive paperwork	Failure to set goals and
Understaffing	priorities
Lack of information	A cluttered desk or mind
Ineffective	Personal disorganization
communication	Inability to say no
Lack of feedback	Lack of self-discipline
Inadequate policies and	Responding to crises
procedures	Haste
Poor filing systems	Indecisiveness
Looking for misplaced	An "open-door" policy
files, and so on	Shifting priorities without
Personnel or coworkers	sound rationale
with problems	Leaving tasks unfinished
Lack of teamwork	Not setting time limits
Duplicating efforts	Daydreaming
Confusing lines of au-	Attempting too much at
thority, responsibility,	once
and communication	Over-involvement in routine
Bureaucratic red tape	detail
Junk mail	Making numerous errors
Waiting, meeting	Surfing the Internet
delays	Not listening

in a typical day. It is critical to be aware of the time distractions that affect us. The following section provides specific examples of how to strategically avoid these common time distractions.

TIME-MANAGEMENT STRATEGIES

It is easy to apply the perspectives-on-time concept to nurses because many nurses have type A personalities, meaning that they are oriented toward high achievement. As high achievers, nurses go above and beyond for their patients, colleagues, and families and are often attracted to activities that are challenging, difficult, and even risky. When high achievers mismanage themselves in relation to time, they experience frustration and stress. To assist nurses in improving their self-management and time management, various strategies are outlined in the following sections. Of important note is that *planning* is the most important step in time management.

Planning is the most important step in time management.

Planning, Organizing, and Implementing to Control the Use of Time

Planning, organizing, and implementing are the key actions a person can use to optimize the use of time. These three actions are sequential and build on each other for successful **time management**.

Planning for Control

Planning is the most important step in time management. Unfortunately, few people expend as much energy planning as they should. Some shy away from planning because they believe it is too time-consuming and never leads to closure. In reality, planning allows people to better use their time and can lead to completion of goals. For example, 1 minute of planning can transfer to at least 10 minutes of productivity, proving to be a great return on the investment of taking the time to review and plan for the day. If you arrive 10 to 15 minutes early for your scheduled shift and map out the day's priorities, your likelihood of executing those priorities is far greater than had you not taken the time to plan up front.

Having a priority-planning list as you work is useful in keeping you on track to accomplish tasks by the end of the shift or day. Those who plan well also tend to encounter fewer problems when Murphy's Law—*If anything can go wrong it will*—becomes a reality. Thus it is important to plan before beginning any task, project, or

day's activities. Planning involves (1) setting goals and establishing priorities, (2) scheduling activities, and (3) making to-do lists.

Setting Priorities. Prioritizing is about making choices about what to do and what not to do. To prioritize effectively, you need to be able to recognize what is important as well as to see the difference between urgent (must be done immediately) and important (must be done, but there may be flexibility as to when the task can be accomplished). A major component of planning is deciding what should be done first and what activities should follow sequentially. The factors that influence how to establish priorities include the following:

- Urgency of a situation
- Demands of others
- Closeness of deadlines
- Existing time frame
- Your level of familiarity with the task
- Ease of the task
- Amount of enjoyment involved
- Consequences involved
- Size of the task
- Congruence with personal goals

Unfortunately, not all of these factors carry the same weight in the consideration of the use of time. Several processes have been proposed to assist people in setting priorities, including the ABC approach, the Pareto principle, and the continuum approach.

The *ABC approach* is advocated by Lakein (1989) and Mancini (2003). In this approach, a person lists every task that needs to be done. An A is assigned to the high-value items, a B to the medium-value items, and a C to the low-value items. The A items should stand out from the others because of their worth to the person making the list. Also the A items are likely to require more energy and time, but they should be completed before any of the B or C items. As the A items are completed, you may find that the C items were of such low value that they did not need to be done at all. It is also possible that Monday's C item could become an A item on Friday, reflecting a change in values. Of course this is an arbitrary system that is based on a person's estimation of the value of activities within his or her own life. It allows for reflection and change while maintaining focus.

The *Pareto principle* is another process that is suggested for setting priorities. This principle is also referred to as the "80/20 rule," suggesting that 80% of the time expended produces 20% of the results, and 20% of the time expended produces 80% of the results (Koch, 2004). The essence is in determining the "vital few" activities that should be done and eliminating the "trivial many." This principle emphasizes selecting the most productive activities, eliminating trivia, and learning to say "no."

The continuum approach to setting priorities encourages a person to select priorities by categorizing or ranking items according to four continuums. As you read about the four continuums, think about Susan's assignment in the opening vignette and consider which of her tasks would have been high priorities according to this approach.

- *Intrinsic importance:* Very important and must be done; important and should be done; not so important and may not be necessary, but may be useful; or unimportant and can be eliminated entirely.
- *Urgency:* Very urgent and must be done now; urgent and should be done soon; not urgent and can wait; time is not a factor.
- *Delegation:* Must be done by me because I am the only one who can do it; can be delegated to A or B; can be dumped because task does not need to be done or delegated.
- *Visitations and conferences:* People I must see each day; people to see frequently but not daily; people to see regularly but not frequently; people to see only infrequently.

Obviously these continuums have varying usefulness, depending on the activity being scrutinized.

Overall it does not matter which method is used to establish priorities as long as priorities are established using a sound rationale. Fortunately, setting priorities becomes easier with practice. If Susan had established her priorities for the day, it is unlikely that talking about the holiday party or calling the inpatient unit to give a report on a patient that would not transfer for several hours would have taken precedence over reviewing the new chemotherapy regimen protocol she would be administering to a patient. Setting priorities would have allowed Susan to better use her time and decreased her anxiety about not managing her assignment appropriately.

Scheduling Activities. Scheduling activities is an important component of planning. It is one way to control Parkinson's Law, which states that work will expand to fill the time that is available. By scheduling activities, a person determines how much time is spent on a specific activity. Such time delineations tend to focus attention and activity so that the task gets completed more efficiently and effectively. A schedule of activities can be constructed using a variety of different methods, including hourly time schedules. Everyone has used an hourly schedule for appointments, classes, or leisure activities. In addition, nurses become adept at using hourly time schedules to administer medications appropriately. Unfortunately, most people, including nurses, do not use time schedules frequently or consistently enough.

The process of scheduling activities is an important part of planning to use your time more efficiently. However, scheduling needs to be done appropriately to ensure adherence. Remember to schedule activities so that they coincide with your internal "prime time," when you concentrate best, and your external "prime time," when you deal best with other people. As a general rule, 15 minutes of focused time and energy toward a project equates to 1 hour of productivity. Be sure to include some flexible time just for yourself.

Health care settings today have most aspects of the patient's health record in an electronic format. Technology continues to advance at a feverish pace and these systems are being enhanced with more logic to support a nurse's workflow and assist with prioritizing patient care activities by leveraging clinical decision support algorithms. For example, a nurse's patient assignment will have the medications coming due for administration highlighted.

Establishing a To-Do List. Writing something on paper often is the first step to accomplishing it. A to-do list tends to keep people on track and focused on specific activities. Thus the list should be reflective of your priorities and goals. To-do lists should be made and revised daily to be the most useful in managing your time. Sometimes they require revision more frequently, even hourly, when priorities shift for valid reasons. The list should be legible and easily accessible to review throughout the day. It is helpful to review the list at the end of the shift or day to assess how you achieved or did not achieve your goals. This is an opportunity to reflect on the distractions you experienced so that you can make note of what not to do when the next situation arises. The list will give you the opportunity to reevaluate your tasks to see what needs to be carried over to the next day. Different people find it useful to construct their lists on note cards, in day-planner calendars, on pocket calendars, in electronic recall devices, on computers, and myriad other ways. There is no right or wrong way to make a to-do list, but it should always be available to you.

Organizing for Control

Organizing yourself and your environment is an important component of time management. Such organization requires that you be able to deal effectively with the following:

- The stacked-desk syndrome
- The art of "no detourism"
- The art of "wastebasketry"
- E-mail and memo mania

The Stacked-Desk Syndrome. The stacked-desk syndrome is exactly what the label implies—a cluttered desk stacked with papers, books, and other things. The syndrome can also apply to the mind when it is cluttered with many thoughts and ideas. Both situations are distractions to accomplishing your goals and divert your attention sufficiently that you do not know where to begin. When you lose your concentration, you will again become distracted by the clutter. To deal effectively with this syndrome, you must clear both your work area and your mind. To effectively organize or clear a work area, you should:

- Remove everything from the work surface that does not directly relate to the project at hand; only things you need every day should be on your desk.
- Place the telephone out of sight, but within reach.
- Remove all personal items, such as calendars, clocks, and photographs, if they are distractors.
- Close the door to the work area when possible, but communicate to colleagues that you may be interrupted in the case of an emergency (Emmett, 2009).

For a nurse, desk management usually means eliminating clutter from a patient's room so that care can be delivered effectively and efficiently. Keep out in the open only things you need to use to carry out the task at hand. Another desk management strategy is to assign a work location at the nurses' station for each staff person working on a given shift so each has a dedicated space for computer access and other needs.

The Art of "No Detourism." To effectively organize, or clear the mind, you must practice the art of "no detourism." This requires complete concentration on one activity or task until—with no detours—it is completed. It mandates that only one activity at a time be undertaken and that it be completed before you move to a different task. This method also implies that the task should be completed correctly the first time so that you do not waste time redoing it. Inherent in the concept of "no detourism" is the fact that the tasks undertaken are directly related to personal goals and objectives; thus, completing them will result in internal satisfaction. Maura in the opening vignette may have benefited from practicing "no detourism." Perhaps she would not have become distracted by the telephone call from the infusion unit if she had been focused on passing the medications via the barcoding system.

The Art of "Wastebasketry." Perfecting the art of "wastebasketry" is mandatory for better use of time. The art of physical wastebasketry involves "circular filing" (in the trash can or with the delete key on the computer) of any documents, including e-mails and other paperwork, that has limited use or needs no response. The goal is to handle a paper (or e-mail) only once, then either act on it (do it), send it along to another appropriate person (delegate it), or throw it away (dump it). This art involves being sufficiently knowledgeable and skilled to ascertain which documents, e-mails, and paperwork are appropriate candidates for the "circular file" and then daring to follow through. Practicing this art daily also helps in managing the stacked-desk syndrome by reducing much of the clutter.

The art of mental wastebasketry also involves organizing your mind to deal with the established priorities. It requires using selective perception to attend only to those tasks at hand. It also assists in discarding useless information. Mental wastebasketry is a valuable skill to perfect in relation to achieving a better use of time.

E-Mail Mania. E-mail has become the primary method of communication for the majority of individuals in professional, health care, and academic settings. It is an expedient route to contact people, regardless of their location. It is also a useful way to conduct business with a group of people concurrently, when appropriate, because of the ability to share information with many parties at once. Keep in mind, however, that e-mail is a professional channel of communication, and messages should contain a greeting, a clear body of text, specific and clear requests for information, and an acceptable closing to the message. Messages should also be free of grammatical and typographic errors. Also keep in mind that a telephone call may be a sufficient and more efficient means of response and often is more appropriate.

Effective communication in health care is critical and it is important for a health care organization to recognize the diversity of its staff, noting that millennial nurses are steeped in technology. This technologic adeptness continues to evolve, and organizations are actively working to accommodate their staff by using multiple medias to communicate (Aurilio, 2017). Chapter 19 provides additional information about how to use e-mail effectively.

Implementing for Control

Implementing for control refers to carrying out activities that assist people in managing time use. Further exploring these activities in the following sections clarifies how they can be easily implemented in daily life.

Attacking the Priorities. It is important to attack your priorities early to gain control of your time. Delay in beginning tasks will only result in crises when deadlines or personal goals are not met. One of the most cited reasons for delaying this process is fear—a very real symptom of procrastination—usually fear of failure, although it could be a fear of something else. Regardless, it is important to analyze your fears to be able to identify the source and to determine whether the fear is valid or exaggerated so you can manage it to obtain the results you established (Emmett, 2009; Vestal, 2009). If the priority is a big project or large task, it can be successfully approached by examining how the project can be divided up into smaller, more manageable tasks.

Finding "Extra" Time. The concept of finding extra time seems paradoxical because in reality everyone has the same amount of time. The concept actually relates to how people choose to use their time. In some cases, a different use of time may result in additional time for accomplishing goals. A few ways to produce extra time are as follows:

- Use commuting time and coffee breaks to relax so that designated working hours are more productive.
- Institute working lunches periodically, such as twice a week.

Certainly there are other ways individuals might choose to alter their use of time. The key is knowing which activities can be altered without being detrimental to overall functioning. For example, perhaps giving up 30 minutes of television watching or reading each evening would work for some, but not if that is the only relaxation time that is available daily. Sacrificing downtime for more work may decrease overall productivity. It may be a case of working longer but not smarter, so less actually gets accomplished.

Avoiding Procrastination. Procrastination is a bad habit that ranks high on the list of time wasters. It has been referred to as an obstacle to success, "the cat burglar of time management," and a "hidden fear of conflict" (Mancini, 2003). It can wear many disguises, including fear, laziness, indifference, overwork, and forgetfulness. Procrastination is most frequently evident when a person is faced with an unpleasant task, a difficult task, or a difficult decision. Usually procrastination is easily recognizable because it involves doing low-priority rather than high-priority tasks, and it always welcomes interruptions. Procrastination is the art of "never doing today what can be put off until tomorrow." The result is less productivity, less internal satisfaction, and more stress.

The first step in avoiding procrastination is being able to recognize when it is occurring. The second step is being able to admit that what is occurring is procrastination. Once those two steps are accomplished, the work of overcoming procrastination can begin. Following are mechanisms for overcoming procrastination (Emmett, 2009):

- Identify the tasks that are being put off.
- Ask why the task is being avoided.
- Determine whether the task could or should be done by someone else.
- Identify consequences of the procrastination.
- Set priorities in relation to the task.
- Establish deadlines and adhere to them.
- Focus on one aspect at a time.
- Do not strive for perfection if 95% or 98% will be just as effective.

The last item is clearly one in which good clinical discernment must be exercised, because there are clearly instances in which providing nursing care that is anything less than 100% could cause harm. It also helps if you can eliminate those tasks that make up the procrastination. For example, if rearranging the desk, the furniture, or even the medication cart is part of how a person procrastinates, then eliminate that activity by changing the work location or environment. Most important, emphasize the benefits that are to be gained by completing the task and accomplishing the goals that will provide internal satisfaction.

Delegating Appropriately. Most simplistically, *delegation* is the art of giving other people tasks to be accomplished. In reality, however, there is nothing simple about delegation. It usually requires considerable time and energy to delegate, but the rewards are greater in the overall context of accomplishing goals. Following are some important benefits of delegation (Mancini, 2003):

- Extends the results that can be accomplished from what one person can do alone to what he or she can manage through others.
- Frees time for more important tasks.
- Assists in developing the initiative, skills, knowledge, and competence of others.
- Maintains the responsibility and decision level.
- Is often more cost-effective.

With these potential benefits, it would seem that everyone would want to use delegation. Unfortunately this is not the case. Many barriers, internal and external, can hinder the delegation process.

A brief exploration of those barriers may clarify why delegation is such a problem for some people. The internal barriers to delegating include: a personal preference for how tasks are accomplished, demanding that everyone know all the details, believing that no one else can complete the task as well, lack of experience in delegating, insecurity, fear of being disliked, lack of confidence in others, perfectionism resulting in over-control, lack of organizational skill, failure to delegate authority commensurate with the responsibility delegated, indecision, poor communication skills, and lack of commitment to the development of others.

The external barriers to delegating are inherent either in the situation or in the person to whom something is being delegated. External barriers within the situation may include stringent policies that mandate who can do what, low tolerance of mistakes, the criticality of the decisions, implementation of a management-by-crisis style, confusion regarding responsibilities and authority, and understaffing. External barriers to delegation that reside within the person to whom tasks are being delegated include lack of experience, lack of competence, avoidance of responsibility, overdependence on others, disorganization, procrastination, work overload, and immersion in trivia and clutter (Mancini, 2003).

When the barriers are identified and overcome, the delegation process can proceed. Implementing the following steps will facilitate appropriate delegation (also see Chapter 20 for a complete discussion of delegation in the clinical setting):

1. Identify exactly what is to be delegated and why.
2. Select the best person for the task; this may be the person most qualified or it may be the person whose development the delegator chooses to contribute to.
3. Communicate the assignment in detail, perhaps even including written instructions.
4. Involve the delegatee in establishing the objectives and deadlines for the task.
5. Have the delegatee repeat the details of the task.
6. Give the delegatee the authority for accomplishing the task.
7. Provide adequate resources and support as needed.
8. Follow-up regularly for progress reports.
9. Establish controls, and monitor the results.
10. Evaluate the process and progress of the delegatee.
11. Let the delegatee do the job.

It is not prudent to take shortcuts when delegating tasks because the results might be different from what was originally intended. Avoiding delegation shortcuts is an important consideration because the nurse who does the delegating also retains accountability for the task.

Delegation would have been useful to Susan in the opening vignette. It could have helped her meet her patient care goals and decrease her anxiety. Unfortunately Susan was overwhelmed, and she could not identify those things that needed to be done or direct someone else to do them. In addition, Susan had not established any priorities, so it was difficult for her to plan for appropriate delegation.

Controlling Interruptions. To focus on your priorities, it is important to establish uninterrupted blocks of time. Frequent causes of interruptions are telephone calls, meetings, and visitors, particularly the drop-in type. Learning how to control such interruptions helps you accomplish more in less time. One of the easiest ways to manage incoming calls is to not answer them during time that is scheduled for other activities. An answering machine, a voicemail service, or an assistant can take the message to be responded to later. "Later" should refer to the time that was preestablished for returning telephone calls. A good example of controlling interruptions in the opening vignette would have been for Susan to ask the unit secretary to help the patient requesting information about an appointment.

Most people schedule callbacks for times when their productivity level is lower or during their downtime. Also telephone calls can be controlled by the tone and verbiage used. If a person chooses to invite conversation and ensure a longer call, using a vague, open-ended greeting will accomplish that purpose. If a person chooses to focus the call specifically on its purpose, a specific, factual, informative greeting will enhance the productivity of the call and shorten its length. For example, "Hi, Bill, how are you? How are things going?" definitely invites the person to reply at length, whereas "Hi, Bill. I have two questions that I need for you to answer" tends to condense the telephone session. Also, being prepared for the conversation with all of the pertinent facts readily available helps focus the conversation and shorten the call.

Meetings can become a major time waster if they are poorly managed and nonproductive. The first step in controlling the interruption of a meeting is deciding whether to attend. Such a decision should be based on an evaluation of the potential productivity of the meeting. For example, ask such questions as Is the meeting absolutely necessary? Does the agenda contain items that you should be informed about? Is it necessary for you to contribute to the discussion? Will decisions be made that will affect you and your functioning? and Are you conducting the meeting? These questions should guide your decision (Mancini, 2003). Once a person is committed to attending a meeting, he or she is responsible for helping ensure that the meeting remains focused and productive. The person conducting the meeting not only shares these same responsibilities but also has a more direct role in affecting the outcome.

Visitors, particularly unplanned visitors, also create interruptions. One way to decrease the number of visitors is to seclude yourself during specific times by closing the door to others, physically and mentally. Managing visitors in today's health care environment can be difficult, given the fact that family members are able and welcome to accompany their ill members for extended periods and in a variety of settings. Educating family members can be a time-consuming task in a nurse's day. It is important to ensure that this time is factored into one's schedule because communicating with family members is an inevitable and important occurrence.

Learning the Art of Saying "No." "No" is such a small word, but it is sometimes more difficult to say than any 14-syllable word. The first step in learning the art of saying "no" is determining when to say it. The cost-benefit ratio of each opportunity must be evaluated in relation to the overall goals. If the activity will be a benefit overall, obviously it must be given careful consideration. If it will not be a significant benefit, you should decline gracefully but emphatically. There is no need to provide an elaborate qualifier to your "no" response; a clear, succinct reply is acceptable (Patterson et al, 2011). For example, when asked to review a clinical guideline, do not refuse on the basis of the fact that you are overworked and do not have a free minute for 3 weeks. The person requesting the review is likely to agree on the later time frame, in which case you will find yourself committed to doing something that has low benefit unless you create another excuse. Instead be polite and gracious in the refusal, but do not allow leeway so you are manipulated into saying "yes." Always consider the opportunity that "no" offers in terms of your overall goals.

Rewarding Yourself. All people function more productively when they are motivated. The sources of motivation vary from person to person. A person needs to identify his or her motivators and use them as rewards for accomplishing goals. It is important to identify long- and short-term rewards so that they can be implemented appropriately. Most people are familiar with rewarding themselves in exchange for doing something, and they do it frequently. For some it is a way of life. It usually amounts to bargaining with yourself to facilitate the completion of a task. For example, "If I finish reading these two work-related articles, then I can read my novel for 30 minutes," or "If I complete this paper, I will treat myself to ice cream." You should know which rewards work best and use them appropriately to accomplish long-term goals.

Using Technology. Many of today's technologic advances can be used to improve time management by improving technology management. Most health care settings have adopted more uses of technologic resources to better improve the use of time and enhance patient care. Most health care organizations use electronic health records (EHRs), which allows for multiple users to access a patient's record at the same time to document and to review information. There are also electronic order entry systems now in place, in which clinicians enter orders and activate orders that are then transmitted to the pharmacy to fill medication requests. Patient acuity rating systems are completed online and used by admitting departments to send patients to the appropriate units for care.

Just about every workplace has a professional office system that supports e-mail and scheduling activities. The scheduling features available can be very useful for staff in the planning phase of time management. Many people use smartphones to synchronize their personal and professional calendars. These devices also become valuable resources in the clinical setting if programmed with drug information and lab value databases, which allow a nurse to have a wealth of information at her or his fingertips without having to carry or look for resource manuals. However, when you are considering the many technologic devices available, keep in mind that the tools and devices should improve workflow and processes, not hinder them or create cumbersome ones (Brafman and Beckstrom, 2008). Also remember that taking time to learn to use new technology correctly will pay off in the long run by increasing your effective use of time. Once the strategies have been implemented, it is important to continue to use them to achieve your goals and gain internal satisfaction.

CONTINUING TO SUCCEED

Improving time management to enhance self-performance and accomplish goals is a lifelong process. The process becomes easier the longer you engage in it, but time management still requires continual attention and energy. Obviously, time management does not just happen—it requires a strong personal commitment. Lakein (1989) suggests that it is important to continue doing the following to succeed:
- When feeling overwhelmed, always stop and plan activities.
- Keep focused on priorities, and act accordingly.
- Avoid favorite forms of procrastination.
- Maintain a positive attitude about the established goals, or revise them so that they coincide with your value system.
- Do something for yourself every day.
- Continue to work on overcoming your fears.
- Resist doing the easy but unimportant tasks.

In addition, delete the words "if only" from your vocabulary. Regret is a luxury and a great time waster. You can spend significant time rehashing mistakes or determining how to make something perfect when it

was a one-time occurrence that is now over. Such time usually is not productive unless you will encounter similar situations in the future. It is more productive to admit mistakes, accept responsibility for them, identify how to prevent such mistakes in the future, and move on. The reader is encouraged to review the tips for continuing success in managing time presented in Box 25.2.

> **BOX 25.2 Tips for Successful Time Management**
>
> 1. Clarify objectives, put them in writing, and establish a priority list to work from.
> 2. Focus on objectives, not on activities.
> 3. Set at least one major objective for each day and achieve it.
> 4. Record a time log periodically to analyze how time is used and to document bad habits.
> 5. Analyze everything in terms of objectives.
> 6. Make a to-do list every day that includes daily objectives and priorities and time estimates to accomplish them.
> 7. Schedule time every day to ensure that the most important things are accomplished first.
> 8. Make sure the first hour of every workday is productive.
> 9. Set time limits for every task undertaken.
> 10. Take the time to do the task right the first time so that time will not be wasted doing it over.
> 11. Institute a quiet hour of uninterrupted time each day to work on the most important tasks.
> 12. Develop the habit of finishing whatever task is started.
> 13. Conquer procrastination and learn to do tasks now.
> 14. Make better time management a daily habit.
> 15. Never spend time on less important things when it could be spent on more important things.
> 16. Take time for yourself—time to relax, time to live, time to just be.
> 17. Develop a personal philosophy of time that is consistent with your values.
> 18. Know how you currently spend your time.
> 19. Identify your "prime productive time."
> 20. Do tomorrow's planning tonight.
> 21. Ask yourself often, "Why am I doing what I am doing right now?"
> 22. Handle each piece of paper only once.
> 23. Delegate whenever possible and delegate wisely.
> 24. Identify your high payoff items (80-20 principle).
>
> From Skillpath Seminars. (2011). *Managing multiple projects, objective and deadlines.* Mission, KS, Skillpath.

SUMMARY

This chapter has focused on how to better manage your energy to control one of our most precious and seemingly scarce resources—time. Time management is important to achieving any personal or professional goals, and it helps decrease frustration and anxiety in high achievers. Without time management, most professionals could never achieve their established goals, and for nurses many patient care activities would never be completed, perhaps resulting in poor patient outcomes. Susan's and Maura's experiences in the opening vignette are an example of what your life could be like in nursing unless you implement strategies for better self-management. Thus, it is important in your professional career to initiate habits related to time management that will continue throughout the years. Start asking yourself frequently throughout the day, "What is the best use of my time right now?" (Lakein, 1989). You may be surprised to learn that the answer does not coincide with your current activity. When that occurs, stop and implement the strategies for self-management to better control your time. You will become more productive and gain internal satisfaction as a result.

REFERENCES

Aurilio, L. A. (2017). Creating an inclusive culture for the next generation of nurses. *Nurse Leader, 15*(5), 315–318.

Brafman, O., & Beckstrom, R. A. (2008). *The starfish and the spider*. New York: Penguin Group.

Childre, D. (2008). *De-stress kit for the changing times*. Boulder Creek, CA: Institute of Hearthmath. Retrieved from https://www.heartmath.org/resources/downloads/de-stress-kit-for-the-changing-times.

Emmett, R. (2009). *Manage your time to reduce your stress: A handbook for the overworked, overscheduled, and overwhelmed*. New York: Walker and Company.

Goleman, D. (2006). *Emotional intelligence 10th anniversary edition: Why it can matter more than IQ*. New York: Bantam Books.

Krichbaum, K., Peden-McAlpine, C., Diemert, C., Koenig, P., Mueller, C., & Savik, S. (2011). Designing a measure of complexity compression in registered nurses. *Western Journal of Nursing Research, 33*, 7–25.

Koch, R. (2004). *Living the 80/20 way: Work less, worry less, succeed more, enjoy more*. Boston: Nicholas Brealey.

Lakein, A. (1989). *How to get control of your time and your life*. New York: Signet.

Loehr, J., & Schwartz, T. (2005). *The power of full engagement*. New York: Free Press.

Mancini, M. (2003). *Time management*. New York: McGraw-Hill.

Morgenstern, J. (2004). *Time management from the inside out*. New York: Henry Holt.

Nightingale, F. (1969). *Notes on nursing: What it is, and what it is not*. New York: Dover.

Patterson, K., Grenny, J., McMillan, R., & Switzler, A. (2011). *Crucial conversations: Tools for talking when stakes are high* (2nd ed.). New York: McGraw-Hill.

Ponte, P. R. (2008). Nurse executive: The four principles of management. In L. T. Adams & E. H. O'Neil (Eds.), *Nurse executive: The purpose, process, and personnel of management*. New York: Springer.

Ponte, P. R., & Koppel, P. (2015). Cultivating mindfulness to enhance nursing practice. *American Journal of Nursing, 115*(6), 48–55.

Senge, P. (2006). *The fifth discipline*. New York: Doubleday.

Skillpath Seminars. (2011). *Managing multiple projects, objective and deadlines*. Mission, KS: Skillpath.

Vestal, K. (2009). Procrastination: Frustrating or fatal? *Nurse Leader, 7*(2), 8–9.

26

The career path for nurses is long and wide.

Contemporary Nursing Roles and Career Opportunities

Susan R. Jacob, PhD, MSN, RN

ⓔ Additional resources are available online at: *http://evolve.elsevier.com/Cherry/*

LEARNING OUTCOMES

After studying this chapter, the reader will be able to:

1. Evaluate the effect of the current health care environment on the future role of nurses.
2. Analyze the influence of current demographic characteristics of registered nurses (RNs) in the United States on contemporary nursing roles.
3. Differentiate among various innovative nursing practice roles today.
4. Differentiate between the roles of advanced practice nurses and other RNs in various settings.

KEY TERMS

Advanced practice nursing Based on knowledge and skills acquired through basic nursing education, with licensure as a registered nurse RN and graduate education and experience that includes advanced nursing theory, physical assessment, psychosocial assessment, and treatment of illness. Includes nurse practitioners, certified nurse-midwives, certified registered nurse anesthetists, and clinical nurse specialists.

Interprofessional team Health care team composed of professionals from different disciplines, including chaplains, nurses, dietitians, pharmacists, physical therapists, physicians, respiratory therapists, social workers, and speech-language pathologists, who cooperate, collaborate, communicate, and integrate care to ensure that care is continuous and reliable.

Nursing roles (1) Traditional duties and responsibilities of the professional nurse, regardless of practice area or setting, such as the roles of care provider, educator, counselor, client advocate, change agent, leader and manager, researcher, and coordinator of the interprofessional health care team. (2) Duties and responsibilities of the professional nurse that are guided by specific professional standards of practice and usually carried out in a distinct practice area (e.g., flight nurse, forensic nurse, occupational nurse).

We thank Robert W. Koch, DNS, RN, for his contributions to this chapter in the first through the seventh editions.

PROFESSIONAL/ETHICAL ISSUE

Ashley Burton was excited to begin her new job in a small home care agency in a rural area some 30 miles from her city home. Although she had been a medical-surgical nurse for several years, she decided to try home care nursing after completing her population-focused community health course in her registered nurse to bachelor of science in nursing (RN-to-BSN) program. She was sure she could be a positive asset to the meet the growing needs of this rural community.

Ashley makes an initial evaluation home visit to see 78-year-old Mr. Horace Brown, who lives with his granddaughter, Megan, and her three preschool children. He is being monitored after hospital discharge for complications of congestive heart failure. His blood pressure is elevated, and Ashley assesses some edema in his lower extremities. She also notes that Mr. Brown's room is littered with newspapers and paper plates of half-eaten food. Ashley asks about his intake and finds out that he is not eating a low-sodium diet. Megan states that she tries to fix food that everyone can eat and struggles to keep the house clean while working a part-time job. She tells Ashley that she does not know how they would make it without Mr. Brown's social security check each month. Mr. Brown keeps the children while Megan works, but she admits he has spent more time in bed the last week.

Ashley considers how to address the fact that the money from Mr. Brown's check should be used for low-sodium foods. She also worries that the children are not being properly supervised by Mr. Brown when he is in bed and not well. The home situation is not optimal for Mr. Brown nor his grandchildren. Should Ashley chart what she sees or call her supervisor for advice? Should she discuss her concerns with Megan first? Is the situation one that should be reported to the Department of Human Services or maybe referred to the home care agency social worker? As a home care nurse, does she have the right or obligation to critique this home situation? This situation is so different from the hospital setting where she previously practiced!

VIGNETTE

When Eric Sanders graduated 15 years ago, he thought he would work in the hospital his entire career. However, with so many changes in the economic forces affecting health care and the resulting shift of clients outside acute care, more opportunities exist for him. Eric can take his skills and seek new ones to have a choice of practice roles and settings. Being an RN now gives him more options for practice than he ever thought possible.

Questions to Consider While Reading this Chapter:

1. What practice opportunities exist for graduate nurses?
2. How can a new nurse gain knowledge about the role of the faith community nurse, forensic nurse, or other unique nursing roles?
3. What special skills do nurses working in community settings need?

CHAPTER OVERVIEW

The health care system continues to change as social and economic factors create a state of constant evolution. Professional nurses respond by creating innovative alternatives to traditional nursing practice to meet these new challenges. As nurses proactively define solutions to today's health care challenges, multiple career opportunities emerge.

Since the 1950s, when medical innovations moved nursing from the community into hospitals, most nurses considered acute care hospitals the main practice setting available upon graduation. Few other career choices were available. Public health nursing was one of the exceptions, providing some variety in the nursing job market. As health care moves from inpatient treatment to outpatient and home care, and acute care shifts to health promotion and disease prevention, the U.S. culture seeks alternative options to meet the growing need for alternative care. This shift in health care settings creates a variety of choices for nurses exploring career opportunities.

Nurses today have more liberty to explore and create job opportunities. Nurses may continue to select the hospital acute care setting or may venture into less traditional nursing roles. Nurses must claim ownership of nontraditional roles as they emerge in the health care job market. As professionals, they should exercise their influence to develop and support new nursing roles.

This chapter presents an overview of some key opportunities available for RNs today in the United States. Included are demographics of today's nurses in addition to implications for the future. This chapter examines the traditional and less traditional options available and the current and future issues for roles in professional practice.

NURSING—MUCH THE SAME, BUT BIGGER AND BETTER

In the past, describing the role of the RN was simple because there were few opportunities for variation. Today, exploring job opportunities for RNs is more complicated because nurses can practice in literally hundreds of diverse settings with a broad variety of clients. Career opportunities for nurses are proliferating. Although nursing roles have expanded, the traditional functions of the nurse remain intact. Box 26.1 summarizes the roles nurses assume in any employment role or setting, discussed here.

Care Provider

The role of care provider is basic to the nursing profession. The nurse assesses client resources, strengths and weaknesses, coping behaviors, and the environment to optimize the problem-solving and self-care abilities of the client and family. The nurse plans therapeutic interventions in collaboration with the client, physician, and other health care providers. In addition, the nurse takes responsibility for coordination of care that involves other health care professionals or resources, providing continuity and helping the client deal effectively with the health care system. Caring is always central to nursing interventions and is an essential attribute of the expert nurse.

Educator and Counselor

Multiple factors increase the need for nurses to serve as educators. Today, the emphasis is on health promotion and health maintenance in addition to management of disease conditions. The role of nurse counselor has been elevated to new heights. Nurses encourage clients to look at alternatives, recognize their choices, and develop a sense of control in a rapidly changing health care environment.

Client Advocate

Professional nurses find that the role of client advocate is essential in various situations with a multitude of

---

BOX 26.1   **Professional Nursing Roles**
Care provider
Educator and counselor
Client advocate
Change agent
Leader and manager
Researcher
Coordinator of the interprofessional health care team

---

client populations. Promoting what is best for the client, ensuring that the client's needs are met, and protecting the client's rights remain important responsibilities of the professional nurse.

Change Agent

When nurses first adopted the role of "change agent," few individuals anticipated to what extent nurses would fulfill this role. However, nurses have expanded their role as change agents in many ways. The profession continues to identify client, patient safety, and health care delivery problems; assess individual and organizational motivation and capacity for change; determine alternative and explore possible outcomes of the alternatives; and assess cost-effective resources in infinite health- related situations.

Leader and Manager

The leadership role of the professional nurse is paramount in the health care system. Nursing leadership varies according to the level of application and includes the following:

- Improving the health status and potential of individuals or families
- Ensuring that safe, high-quality care is provided across all health care settings
- Increasing the effectiveness and level of satisfaction among professional colleagues providing care
- Managing multiple resources in a health care facility
- Elevating citizens' and legislators' attitudes toward and expectations of the nursing profession and the health care system

The management role of the nurse has become more important. Nursing management includes planning, giving direction to, and monitoring and evaluating nursing care of individuals, groups, families, and communities.

Researcher

During the past decades, nursing has taken its place among other disciplines in the production and use of research specific to its profession. Although the majority of researchers in nursing are prepared at the doctoral and postdoctoral levels, an increasing number of clinicians with master's degrees are participating in research as part of their advanced practice roles. Nurses prepared at the baccalaureate and associate degree levels are also participating in research. These nurses may be assisting with data collection, critiquing research findings, and using these findings in practice. More nursing interventions are based on nursing research than in the past.

Coordinator of the Interprofessional Health Care Team

The interprofessional team consists of collaborative practice relationships among several disciplines of health care professionals. These disciplines may include nursing, medicine, pharmacy, nutrition, social work, case management, and other allied health professionals, such as physical therapists, respiratory therapists, occupational therapists, and speech therapists. Chaplains or pastoral care representatives also serve a valuable role on the interprofessional health care team. These teams are found in all health care delivery settings and function most effectively when their focus revolves around the needs of the client.

Interprofessional teams are valuable because professional members bring in-depth and specialized knowledge and skills to the interaction process. In an age of rapidly expanding information, the roles of interprofessional team members complement one another. Through the formal and informal communication of ideas and opinions of team members, health care plans are determined. A plan of care developed by the interprofessional team is considered a valuable health management tool.

Interprofessional teams foster coordination between and among disciplines involved in providing client care. The collaborative process required by interprofessional health care transcends a single health profession to create comprehensive work outcomes. This team process can improve the quality of care, enhance client satisfaction, strengthen nursing satisfaction, and reduce hospital costs by decreasing patient length of hospital stay and increasing nurse retention.

Successful health care team models that use concepts related to interprofessional health care include pain management, nutritional support, skin care, rehabilitation, mental health, and hospice. Discharge planning, a major focus of health care delivery in the 1980s, involves developing a plan of treatment that ultimately results in the discharge of the client from the health care facility. This practice is built on the concept of interprofessional care, with each discipline involved in developing the discharge plan.

Client education is another area in which collaboration of disciplines is absolutely essential. Health care professionals must understand one another's contributions to client education and must ensure that the information clients and families receive is consistent and complete. This collaboration will produce the best possible health outcomes for clients and families.

Box 26.2 lists some common roles of interprofessional health care team members with the websites of

---

BOX 26.2 Interprofessional Health Care Team Members

Nurse (RN)

Often the coordinator of the team. RNs take licensure examinations after completing associate degree, diploma, or baccalaureate degree preparation through an accredited school of nursing. RNs are able to obtain specialty certification for advanced skills and/or advanced degrees. RNs use the nursing process in client care in any health care setting.
    American Nurses Association: https://www.nursingworld.org

Physician (MD or DO)

Often the leader of the team, the physician diagnoses and prescribes treatment interventions for clients. Medical doctors (MDs) or doctors of osteopathy (DOs) complete 4 years of medical school and board examinations. Physicians can complete postgraduate training, including internship, residency, and fellowship training in a specialty area. Physicians also complete state licensing examinations and function in all health care arenas.
    American Medical Association: https://www.ama-assn.org
    American Osteopathic Association: http://osteopathic.org

Pharmacist (RPh or PharmD)

Responsible for providing drug therapy for positive client outcomes; activities include drug information services, client and health care staff education, dispensing medications and monitoring clients, adverse drug reaction reporting, research, concurrent drug use evaluation, and consultative services in areas such as pain management and nutritional support. Pharmacists complete baccalaureate preparation, an internship period, and licensing board examinations. Pharmacists can complete additional specialized training, certifications, and/or advanced degrees. In some states, the PharmD, or doctor of pharmacy degree, is now the educational requirement for entering practice.
    American Pharmacists Association: http://www.pharmacist.com/

Physician Assistant (PA)

Works under the supervision of the MD or DO and performs assessments, procedures, or protocols approved by the physician. PAs complete a baccalaureate degree

BOX 26.2 Interprofessional Health Care Team Members—cont'd

with specialized PA training (usually 2 years) and state licensure.

American Academy of Physician Assistants: https://www.aapa.org

Dietitian (RD or LD)

Provides nutritional therapy and support to ensure that the nutritional needs of the client are met. Activities include involving both client and family in dietary assessment and teaching, identifying resources for food purchase and preparation, and determining areas of food-drug interactions. Dietitians complete a baccalaureate degree from an accredited nutrition or food service administration program, take national board examinations, and may also complete state licensure and advanced educational preparation.

Academy of Nutrition and Dietetics: https://www.eatright.org

Physical Therapist (PT)

Attends to the client's needs for movement. Activities include assessing physical strength and mobility needs and developing a plan of strengthening exercises for the client with movement dysfunction, maintaining range of motion and muscle tone, and identifying assistive devices that may be needed. A physical therapist may also be expert in the area of wound care. The minimum educational requirement to practice physical therapy is a post-baccalaureate degree from an accredited education program. While some programs offer a master's degree, a majority of programs offer the Doctor of Physical Therapy Degree.

American Physical Therapy Association: http://www.apta.org

Speech-Language Pathologist (SLP)

Assists clients who are communicatively impaired by intervening in speech, language, and/or swallowing disorders related to receptive language, expressive language, speech intelligibility, voice disorders, alaryngeal speech, or prosody and cognitive impairments; plays an important role in evaluation and treatment of swallowing disorders. Therapists obtain a master's degree from an accredited school, complete a 1-year fellowship, and pass a national certifying examination.

American Speech-Language-Hearing Association: https://www.asha.org

Occupational Therapist (OT)

Plans activities that assist and teach clients with physical disabilities to become independent in activities of daily living, such as dressing, grooming, bathing, and eating. Once self-care goals have been met, the OT can help the client perform daily responsibilities of caring for a home and/or returning to work. Educational requirements include completion of an occupational therapy program of study at the baccalaureate, graduate certification, or master's degree level. Graduates must complete a period of supervised clinical experience and state licensure examinations.

American Occupational Therapy Association: https://www.aota.org

Respiratory Therapist (RT)

Responsible for assessment and maintenance of the client's airway and the respiratory equipment and procedures used for diagnosis and therapy of respiratory disorders. Activities include client assessment, aerosolized medication administration, sputum sampling, arterial and mixed venous blood sampling, pulmonary function testing, cardiopulmonary stress testing, and sleep studies; may also be involved in conducting pulmonary rehabilitation programs. RTs complete a program of study and take a national certifying examination. If the program of study is completed in an associate or bachelor's degree program, the level of credentialing examination is different.

American Association for Respiratory Care: http://www.aarc.org

Social Worker

Uses skills to help clients, families, and communities address psychosocial needs. Activities include educating clients, families, and staff about community resources; planning for discharge; financial counseling and identification of financial resources; crisis intervention; referring to community resources; reporting of abuse and neglect; completing advanced directives; assisting with resolving ethical dilemmas; evaluating behavior and mental disorders; and conducting support groups. Social workers complete a minimum of baccalaureate preparation in the field and may pursue advanced degrees.

National Association of Social Workers: https://www.socialworkers.org/

Chaplain or Pastoral Representative

Attends to the spiritual and emotional needs of the client and family. Activities include providing pastoral counseling and support and sacramental ministry and liturgical celebrations. Pastoral representatives may not share the religion of the client or family members but they must be able to acknowledge the differences among religions and assist the person with spiritual needs. Basic education requirements vary according to the setting and religious affiliation.

Association for Clinical Pastoral Education, a multicultural, multifaith organization devoted to improving the quality of ministry and pastoral care offered by spiritual caregivers of all faiths: https://www.acpe.edu

their associated professional organizations. These team members are involved in client care to varying degrees, depending on client needs for the specific talents and knowledge of each team member. This list contains selected professional roles that contribute to the interprofessional health care team approach, but there may be more in a given team.

Case Study 26.1 provides an excellent example of the role of various members of the interprofessional health care team. Multiple professional caregivers provide health care within the limits of each provider's expertise. The joint efforts of all professionals provide the opportunity for a better overall outcome.

CASE STUDY 26.1

John was discussing a problem with a coworker over his cell phone as he approached the intersection. He did not notice the truck approaching on his left side, so he did not see the STOP sign. After evaluation in the emergency department, John was diagnosed as post–motor vehicle accident with multiple trauma, closed-head injury, several rib and leg fractures, lacerations, and internal injuries.

The physician ordered multiple diagnostic tests, laboratory tests, medications, and treatments. John's nurse monitored his physical status and carried out the orders written by the physician. The nurse organized the tests and procedures and managed his pain. The pharmacist reviewed and supplied the medications ordered and analyzed potential interaction effects of the multiple pharmaceutical agents. A respiratory therapist was consulted to perform breathing treatments to facilitate lung expansion and prevent respiratory complications. After surgical repair of his fractured leg, Physical Therapy was consulted to assess John's condition and his need for physical reconditioning. A plan of care was established to enhance his mobility. His long recuperation led to mild depression and spiritual distress. The nurse who assessed these symptoms made arrangements for the chaplain to visit John and discussed the possibility of pharmacotherapy for depression with the physician and pharmacist.

Throughout the period of John's care, all involved practitioners communicated their assessments and worked together to provide collaborative interventions for holistic care. In addition, all interprofessional team members collaborated in medical rounds and discharge planning meetings to plan and coordinate John's care.

NURSES TODAY: WHO ARE THEY, AND WHAT ARE THEY DOING?

The phrase "a typical nurse" became a misnomer as the profession entered the twenty-first century. Nursing roles are so diverse that no typical role or practice setting exists. Nursing is the nation's largest health care profession, with more than 3.1 million registered nurses nationwide. Of all licensed RNs, 2.6 million or 84.8% are employed in nursing (American Association of Colleges of Nursing [AACN], 2017), with the majority working in a hospital setting. Projections state that nursing jobs will grow faster than other occupations owing to the focus on preventive care, the prevalence of chronic disease, and increased demand for services by the aging baby boomer population. More specialties and diverse work options emerge as care shifts to outpatient settings for surgery, chemotherapy, and rehabilitation. The demand for RNs is projected to have an increase of 795,700 full-time employees (FTEs) between 2014 and 2030 (Health Resources and Services Administration [HRSA], 2017).

Nurses can specialize in basically four ways: work or treatment setting, disease category or condition, organ or body system, and population. Some nurses specialize in more than one. Examples of specialization in work or treatment settings include ambulatory care nurses, critical care nurses, trauma or emergency nurses, home care nurses, holistic care nurses, medical-surgical nurses, hospice nurses, perioperative nurses, transplant nurses, psychiatric nurses, and rehabilitation nurses. Examples of nurses who specialize in disease category or condition are oncology nurses, addictions nurses, ostomy and wound care nurses, developmental disabilities nurses, diabetes management nurses, human immunodeficiency virus–acquired immunodeficiency syndrome (HIV-AIDS) nurses, and genetics nurses. Organ or body systems can differentiate nurses, such as cardiovascular nurses, dermatology nurses, urology nurses, orthopedic nurses, nephrology nurses, gastroenterology nurses, gynecology nurses, ophthalmic nurses, and respiratory nurses. Nurses can be recognized from the population they serve, such as neonatology nurses, pediatric nurses, and gerontology nurses. Nurses such as clinical nurse specialists (CNSs), nurse anesthetists, nurse-midwives, and nurse practitioners (NPs) have more direct patient contact, whereas case management nurses, infection control nurses, forensic nurses, legal nurses, nurse educators, nurse administrators, and informatics nurse specialists have little or no contact with patients. Truly, these diverse opportunities are expanding in the world of health care.

Demographics for Registered Nurses

The National Council of State Boards of Nursing (NCSBN) 2015 survey estimated a national RN workforce of 3,895,600 FTEs by 2030. When asked to indicate highest level of education, 65% of respondents in the 2015 study responded that they had obtained a baccalaureate or higher degree, up from 61% in 2013. The study also found an increase in the percentage of respondents with a BSN as their initial nursing education, from 36% in 2013 to 39.0% in 2015. Additionally, almost 42% of RNs held either a BSN (39.0%) or graduate degree (3.0%) as their initial credential. Newly licensed RNs, those licensed from 2013 to 2015, were more likely to have obtained a BSN as their initial education (48.6%) than RNs licensed prior to 2000 (NCSBN, 2015).

Changes also are occurring in the educational preparation of RNs. The Institute of Medicine (IOM) nursing report *Future of Nursing: Leading Change, Advancing Health* recommended higher levels of education for nurses to prepare them for the more complex care needed by sicker patients coupled with higher and more sophisticated technologies. The IOM goals were to increase the proportion of nurses with baccalaureate degrees to 80% by 2020 and to double the number of nurses with doctorates. Indeed, for the first time ever, starting in 2012, the number of nurses graduating with a bachelor of science in nursing (BSN), including RN-to-BSN, surpassed the number earning an associate degree.

The number of RN-to-BSN program graduates increased 170% from 2010 to 2016. Enrollment in nursing-focused PhD programs and doctorate of nursing practice programs has also risen. Since 2010, the number of employed nurses with a doctoral degree has more than doubled. Approximately 30% of students at the baccalaureate, master's, doctoral, and doctor of nursing practice program levels represent minority populations. The number of men in nursing is also increasing as evidenced by 13.7% male graduates of prelicensure RN program graduates in 2015. In addition, significant progress toward the IOM goal of Nurses practicing to the full extent of their education and training. Has been made. Nurse practitioners are allowed to provide care to the full scope of their practice in 22 states and the District of Columbia.

Future of Nursing Campaign for Action (FNCA): Transforming. . . .

FNCA: Improving . . . . Hospital Opportunities

Despite enormous changes in health care, jobs in the hospital environment will be available for a long time. In the hospital, a nurse provides direct care for people who are ill and unable to care for themselves. Another function of the direct-care role is to help the client and family manage the illness event. Hospital positions can range from staff nurse to administrator and may entail any of the clinical specialties and most of the nursing roles identified in Table 26.1. Determining the area of clinical interest depends mainly on personal preferences.

Depending on the region of the United States, the new graduate's degree of choice in the clinical setting is highly variable. However, if the desired arena for work in hospital-based acute care is not available, it may be wise to accept an alternative position and to remain watchful for an opportunity to transfer when a position becomes available in an area of clinical preference. Such an approach is perceived as a willingness to be flexible and to learn. Accepting assignments in an open, cooperative spirit provides more opportunities for the novice nurse to learn about the organization and gain important experiences. Furthermore, working as a staff nurse offers diverse learning opportunities in addition to the immediate client-centered ones.

If the choice of the clinical setting has been based on experiences as a student, the new graduate needs to be prepared to have different perceptions in a new role. Experiences that are highly enjoyable on the limited-time basis of a student schedule may feel different when

TABLE 26.1 Trends in Health Care Delivery Systems	
From	**To**
Acute inpatient care	Lifespan care
Focus on the individual	Focus on aggregates or populations
Product of care orientation	Value of care orientation
Number of hospital admissions	Number of lives covered (capitation)
Managing organizations	Managing networks
Managing departments	Managing markets
Coordinating services	Documenting quality and outcomes

the new graduate functions in that role full time. It is good to have a mix of experiences and learning opportunities before making a definitive decision.

Misleading perceptions about functioning in various clinical arenas are not limited to new graduates. Often a person perceives or believes that one clinical area is the ideal choice, only to find that it is not what he or she wanted. Consider the following example:

Jane Patrick, RN, wanted to work with sick children. After a couple of years of experience as a staff nurse on an adult surgical wing, she obtained a position on the pediatric unit. Despite her eagerness for the position, however, Jane found it difficult to adjust to the unit. The distress of the children in the unit was painful to her, and she found herself depressed and unhappy. She began to dream about the children for whom she was caring and was increasingly unable to provide nursing intervention that entailed discomfort for the child. Jane was not in the right practice setting.

Nurses must stay attuned to their reactions and respond in a constructive manner to self-discovery. Internal transfers in large hospitals and health care organizations offer a continuum of care; the probability is high that the nurse will find a position that is deeply satisfying in another area.

In addition to clinical emphasis, nursing within hospitals offers almost endless opportunities for diversity. Staff-level positions in a hospital are available on many different units, and working different shifts on those units presents different work environments, approaches to work, and priorities for client care. Some examples follow.

Infection Control. The infection control nurse assesses the total incidence of infections within the hospital. Clients who suffer an infection while in the hospital are comprehensively reviewed to ensure prompt and accurate treatment and timely containment of the client's infection so that it is not passed to other clients or staff. The infection control nurse must also conduct a thorough analysis to determine the source of the infection and its onset. If the infection is determined to have been contracted during hospitalization, an investigation is initiated to assess the sequence of events leading up to the infection. An action plan is developed to prevent future occurrences. A position such as

infection control enables the nurse to have hospital-wide interactions and functioning. Knowledge of epidemiology and outstanding interpersonal skills foster full participation in the infection assessment process. Infection control nurses may work in community settings and hospitals.

Quality Management. Although the parameters of a position in quality management may vary from setting to setting, the basic premise is to ensure that outcomes in client care services are consistent with established standards. Benchmarking activities to establish such standards have been under way on a national level for the past few decades. Quality management nurses assess the compliance of the agency or institution with established standards and explore variations from these established standards. Chart reviews and ongoing interaction with the staff of the agency are integral components of a quality management position. Chapter 22 provides a more in-depth overview of the quality management process.

Specific Client Services. An almost endless list of specific client services can be found in hospitals, depending on the hospital's size and function within the community. Some nursing positions might be self-evident, such as the intravenous team, on which the nurse provides support and interventions with the insertion and maintenance of intravenous therapies. Other services might relate to ostomy care, counseling, support groups, or health education for a specialty area.

Coordinator Positions. Some hospitals have various coordinator positions, such as trauma nurse coordinator. The nurse in this position is responsible for the coordination and integration of the clinical and administrative requirements of the trauma victim. Consisting of equal parts of program and case management, the trauma nurse coordinator role involves overseeing the care of the client from the point of injury through acute care to rehabilitation and back home. Maintenance of a comprehensive database on the management of trauma victims is an important part of this position. Another example of a coordinator position for a highly specialized area is the organ donor coordinator, who procures organs and oversees the transplantation program. Coordinators require considerable experience in the specialties in which they practice.

Variations on Traditional Roles in Nursing

As clients shift from hospital to ambulatory and home care, the role of the community nurse has evolved beyond the traditional public health nurse concept. Although still based in the framework of the traditional public health nurse concept, community nurses today transfer their critical care skills from the acute care setting into the home, where clients recover from illness and surgery. Pharmacologic and technologic advances make the care of chronic and critically ill clients in their homes a cost-effective option. For example, therapies such as dobutamine administration and chemotherapy were once considered too risky for home administration. Today, adequate teaching of the client and family members and careful monitoring make these therapies a daily occurrence in clients' homes.

Clients can be monitored through home visits by RNs, expanded technology, radiographs, or telemetry at home. Uterine monitoring for high-risk obstetric clients is common; vital signs of the mother and baby are recorded and sent for review by nurses or doctors at a separate location by telephone modem. All of these changes increase the need for home health care nurses who are expert clinicians and client educators.

Hospice Nurse. As more clients with terminal illness choose to stop aggressive treatment, hospice nursing has flourished. About 4199 hospice programs exist in the United States. This estimate includes both primary locations and satellite offices. Hospices are located in all 50 states, the District of Columbia, Puerto Rico, Guam, and the U.S. Virgin Islands (NHPCO Facts and Figures, 2016).

Hospice and palliative care nurses treat the symptoms of clients with progressive terminal disease. These nurses work holistically with clients and families to maximize quality of life rather than focus on the quantity of life remaining. To learn more about the hospice concept, visit the NHPCO website (http://www.nhpco.org).

Informatics Nurse Specialist. As health care systems face the inevitable need for enhanced data management to enable decision making in diverse practice settings, another nursing role has emerged—the informatics nurse specialist. Nursing informatics (NI) focuses on management and processing of health care information. The American Nursing Information Association (ANIA) describes the specialty's charge as "integrating nursing science, computer science and information science to manage and communicate data, information, knowledge and wisdom in nursing and informatics practice." The organization claims the logo tagline "Where caring and technology meet" (ANIA, 2014).

The Joint Commission (TJC) recognized the increased need for information management in the clinical client care settings. The 1994 Joint Commission standards define information management as critical to organizational success. Nurses are well positioned to assume these roles because they best understand client care processes. The American Nurses Credentialing Center (ANCC) has developed a certification examination for nurses who demonstrate beginning levels of competency to become certified as informatics nurses. The American Nurses Association (ANA, 2008) *Scope and Standards of Nursing Informatics Practice* states: "Nursing informatics is a specialty that integrates nursing science, computer science, and information science to manage and communicate data, information, knowledge and wisdom in nursing practice. NI supports consumers, patients, nurses, and other providers in their decision making in all roles and settings. This support is accomplished through the use of information structures, information processes, and information technology." Emerging roles for informatics nurses include working as researchers, consultants, managers, educators, and product and web designers. More information is available on the ANA Informatics Association website (https://www.ania.org/).

Occupational Health Opportunities. Nursing within the framework of specific occupational groups (e.g., automobile factories, textile plants) has long been a career option for nurses. Within these settings, the nurse designs and implements a program of health promotion and disease prevention for employees and assists with immediate health needs as necessary. In this primary care milieu, the nurse assesses the need for programs about specific topics of importance to the health of the employees. Some examples of these are breast-screening programs for female employees and information on early identification of prostate cancer for male employees. Other programs might revolve around the management of developmental events such as empty nest syndrome, menopause, care for aging parents, and retirement.

In addition to services related to maintaining the health of employees, the occupational nurse is responsible for the assessment of the work environment to ensure the safety of the employees. Examples of significant environmental improvements in the health of U.S. workers are clean air programs, anti–smoking-on-the-job campaigns, and eliminating the use of asbestos in heating or insulation of buildings. All these activities pose special challenges to the occupational health nurse. The nurse in this setting develops procedures to be followed in the event of illness at work, including the management of health care emergencies.

Opportunities also exist in specific industries. For example, within the airline industry the nurse is responsible for airline safety through maintaining the health of employees. Protection of employees' health is a component of the role, as is the effect of the health of employees on the safety of the airline and its passengers. The nurse must be vigilant in the assessment of employee health problems that could affect overall airline safety. An obvious function is alcohol and drug screening. Protocols for the maintenance of employee health programs in the airline industry must be strictly followed and enforced as required by government regulation.

Nonetheless, the heart of this nursing position still lies with providing care to people, which sometimes can place the nurse in a difficult position. In the ongoing monitoring of the health of the employees, the nurse often is the first to spot a deviation from health that could affect the career and livelihood of an employee. Such an example is hypertension. If high blood pressure is developing in an employee, which will affect his or her employment status, that employee may encourage the nurse to "hear" the blood pressure in the qualifying range.

Occupational health and employment screening activities are entwined with urgent care and travel assistance for passengers. Although occasionally an emergency situation develops with a passenger or an employee, most of the client problems are neither emergency nor travel related. For example, international travel to some countries requires comprehensive precautions regarding immunizations and inoculations. Airport nurses were critical in screening passengers on

international flights during the severe acute respiratory syndrome (SARS) crisis in 2003 and the Ebola crisis in 2014. Also, passengers may forget prescribed medications, or medications may be lost in baggage. Short-term problems, such as fear of flying, are also managed by airport nurses.

Another form of transportation provides a career opportunity: cruise ship nurse. In general, when people think of taking a cruise, they do not plan on getting sick—nor do nurses usually consider career possibilities in the cruise ship industry. However, many cruise ships are as large as small cities. The role of the nurse in this setting is similar to that of the airline nurse with respect to the health of the employees and the safety of the passengers. The unique elements of the ship relate to special sanitation requirements, such as testing and culturing the water supply and managing the total health needs of the passengers. The nurse is responsible for instructing the staff on the basic elements of emergency care and transport. The nurse should be proficient in Basic Life Support (BLS) and Advanced Cardiac Life Support (ACLS). Primary patient care needs are similar to those found in an emergency department. Cruise ships also offer opportunities for nurse practitioners. Additional career information can be found on a website devoted to cruise ship employment (http://www.cruiseshipjob.com/medical.htm).

Quality Manager. Another role that is attractive to nurses is that of quality manager. This role reflects the need for health care providers to assess opportunities for process improvement, implement changes, measure outcomes, and then start the improvement process over again. Quality management nurses research and describe findings and look for opportunities to improve care. The result of quality assessment studies may produce critical pathways or algorithms defining care and expected client outcomes. Basic and advanced knowledge of quality management tools is essential for quality management nursing, although practice may vary from setting to setting. For instance, in the inpatient setting, the quality management nurse needs strong clinical skills, such as those that might be acquired in medical-surgical practice, intensive care units, or the operating room. Experience in home care would be an advantage for a quality management nurse employed in that setting. Interpersonal skills are important in all settings because to be successful in this role, the nurse must build relationships and rapport with people and groups across the organization. The role of quality manager is one that promotes improved care for health care recipients in a variety of settings. For more information, visit the quality management websites and see Chapter 22.

Case Manager. The role of case manager has had a rich tradition in community and public health nursing and now has gained more prominence in acute care. Case managers coordinate resources to achieve health care outcomes on the basis of quality, access, and cost. The complexity of case management practice is obvious in the era of chaotic systems caused by changes in the health care market, in which providers, services, and coverage details are constantly being modified. Case managers identify the best resources at the lowest cost to achieve the optimal health outcome for the client. Case managers are often nurses but can also be other professionals, such as medical social workers.

Flight Nurse. Flight nursing is a specialty for nurses who desire autonomous practice and the opportunity to use advanced clinical skills. Practice is diverse because clients are all ages and from all backgrounds with different health problems. Critical care experience, with certification in advanced cardiac life support, is necessary. Most programs prefer experienced nurses in critical care and/or emergency department nursing. The two types of flight practice available are military, such as in the Air Force Reserves or active duty, and civilian flight nursing. To learn more, visit the website titled "So, you wanna be a flight nurse?!" (http://seaox.com/wannabe.html). Nurses who enjoy a fast-paced diverse practice in an unstructured setting may find this role a good fit. For more information, call Flying Nurses International - R.N. Medical Escort Service" at 1-877-521-1333 or International: 1-808-521-1333 or visit their website (https://flyingnursesintl.net/) or visit their website (www.flyingnurse.com).

Telephone Triage Nurse (Telehealth Nurse). Another career option is that of telehealth nurse. Telehealth uses technology to provide health services through various telecommunication tools. With a shortage of nurses and the increase in the aging population with chronic diseases, telehealth can be a cost-effective way to reach more patients and monitor patient health in a timely way. The many opportunities to use telehealth are increasing with the expanding world of technology.

Telehealth nurses interact with clients through telephones, video devices, or computers to assess needs, intervene, and evaluate patient care. Telehealth nurses work in a variety of settings, including home telehealth care, by which patients who are homebound, have debilitating disease, or live in remote areas can be monitored. Patient education can be provided using telehealth with online videos, podcasts, MP3 files, and webcasts or webinars.

Telephone triage nurses utilize physician-approved protocols to guide clients to the most effective and cost-efficient level of care while educating and supporting clients to relieve anxiety. This position requires excellent communication and assessment skills, in addition to problem-solving and crisis management skills. Telephone triage is used in a variety of settings, including emergency departments, physician practices, crisis centers, and health maintenance organization (HMO) health plans (McGonigle and Mastrian, 2012).

Forensic Nurse. Forensic nursing may well be one of the fastest-growing nursing specialties in the twenty-first century, likely because of the epidemic increase in violence and resulting trauma in the United States. The ANA and International Association of Forensic Nurses 2009 report, *Forensic Nursing: Scope and Standards of Practice,* serves as a professional guide for nurses working in or entering this evolving specialty. Forensic nursing applies nursing science to public or legal proceedings in the scientific investigation and treatment of trauma and/or death of victims of violence, abuse, criminal activity, and traumatic accidents. The forensic nurse may provide direct services to individual clients and may consult with and/or be an expert witness for medical and law enforcement. To learn more about this exciting practice, visit the International Association of Forensic Nurses (IAFN) website (http://www.forensicnurses.org/). American Forensic Nurses, Inc., offers distance-learning programs through the Internet (http://www.amrn.com/).

School Nurse. Most registered professional nurses employed in school health are generalists prepared at the baccalaureate level who function as consultants or coordinators. The newer role for school nurses is school health manager or coordinator and includes functions such as policymaking, case management and program management activities, and health promotion and protection activities. The National Association of School

Nurses (NASN) defines the role as "a specialized practice of professional nursing that advances the well-being, academic success, and life-long achievement of students. To that end, school nurses facilitate positive student responses to normal development; promote health and safety; intervene with actual and potential health problems; provide case management services; and actively collaborate with others to build student and family capacity for adaptation, self-management, self-advocacy, and learning" (NASN, 2012).

Travel Nurse. For the person who wants to travel and still work as a nurse, travel nursing may be an answer. This role is expanding as the demand for nurses grows nationwide. Benefits and company programs vary, but many include travel reimbursement allowance for assignments in addition to free housing, free insurance, travel money, and free phone card use. Sign-on bonuses may also be offered. If these benefits are not important to the nurse, higher wages may be available. Some companies allow nurses' pets to travel with them. Assignments are usually for a minimum time, such as 12 weeks, but others may last as long as 1 year. For more information, visit the Healthcare Traveler website (http://health caretraveler.modernmedicine.com).

Faith Community Nurse. The role of faith community nurse (FCN), known previously as the parish nurse, is a recognized specialty in a growing professional practice. In 1998 the ANA, in collaboration with the Health Ministries Association (HMA), established the scope and standards of this professional practice. This role addresses holistic health promotion for oneself, others, and the community within the beliefs, values, and practices of various faiths, countries, and cultures. This professional practice focuses on the intentional care of the spirit as the client seeks wholeness in mind, body, and spirit (Westberg Institute, n.d.). In these contexts, health is seen as a sense of physical, psychological, social, and spiritual well-being. Health is further viewed as being in harmony with self, others, the environment, and God. "Nurses have long observed that when illness and brokenness occurs, health care consumers—whether individually or with their family and friends—may turn to their source of spiritual strength for reassurance, support, and healing" (ANA and HMA, 2012). "The primary focus of the FCN is the intentional care of the spirit, differentiating this specialty practice from the

general practice of the registered nurse" (ANA and HMA, 2012).

A faith community nurse is a registered professional nurse who is actively licensed in a given state and who serves as a member of the staff of a faith community. The FCN promotes health as wholeness of the faith community, its groups, families, and individual members through the practice of nursing as defined by that state's nurse practice act in the jurisdiction in which the FCN practices and the standards of practice set forth in the ANA/HMA *Scope and Standards of Practice: Faith Community Nursing* (2012).

The faith community nurse functions in either a paid or unpaid position as counselor, teacher, referral agent, volunteer coordinator, and integrator of spiritual care and health. Although not all communities have a hospital or clinic, most have a faith community, providing an exciting setting in which to teach disease prevention and health promotion.

The late Granger Westberg (1990), founder of this role in the mid-1980s, proposed that clergy can and already do more in the field of preventive medicine than traditional physicians. Westberg's efforts focused on getting the medical establishment to recognize faith communities as partners in keeping people well. He stated that churches, even though they may not realize it, are in the health business. In this role, faith community nurses participate in joint ministry with other staff members, helping to integrate faith and health for healing and wholeness. For more information on this practice, visit the website of Westberg Institute, a ministry of Church Health (https://westberginstitute.org).

Nursing Educator. Preparation for nursing educators occurs at the graduate and doctoral levels. Nursing educators should be competent in clinical practice either at the advanced generalist or specialist level. They should be prepared in the specialty area in which they teach and should match the needs of the institution that hires them. Nursing educators assume leadership in curriculum development, instruction, and evaluation. Knowledge of the learning process and classroom and clinical teaching methods that include engagement and "virtual teaching" is essential. Educators need to have a commitment to lifelong learning and to stay current in their practice. The role of faculty or nursing educator can be rewarding for those nurses who enjoy lifelong learning and mentoring. Individuals who assume these roles are usually expected to have not only teaching responsibilities but also evidence of scholarship and service to the community.

Other Unique Roles

Career opportunities described in this chapter should not be considered an exhaustive list of possibilities. Nurses now have selections for practice areas never before considered. Nurses should adopt an attitude of openness, an attitude of creativity, and a willingness to take a chance to explore these different possibilities. Nurses can allow their imaginations to take them to unknown settings or explore uncharted waters. To do so, they must develop confidence in their abilities and talents and must be willing to venture outside the norm. Many websites have been developed to portray nursing as an attractive career with endless opportunities.

There are those in the nursing profession who would limit the possibilities for the profession, claiming that many of the aforementioned alternatives are "not really nursing." However, this mindset severely diminishes the expansion of professional nursing in a changing health care environment. For nursing to thrive and the discipline to have success in the future, new roles need to be defined and refined.

One way to settle this dispute within the nursing profession is to evaluate new nursing roles through the definition established by the ANA in nursing's social policy statement (2010): "Nursing is the protection, promotion, and optimization of health and abilities, prevention of illness and injury, alleviation of suffering through the diagnosis and treatment of human response, and advocacy in the care of individuals, families, communities and populations."

Therefore, any evolving nursing role should be evaluated according to the ability of the new role to fit this accepted definition. Does the newly created role require assessment, diagnosis, planning, implementation, or evaluation of human responses? Does the newly created role require the knowledge and expertise of a professional nurse? By answering these questions, nurses can see that nursing is now more encompassing than "traditional" nursing.

ADVANCED PRACTICE NURSING

Much is written in the professional and lay literature about advanced practice nursing. Although new roles in advanced nursing may be forthcoming, the term *advanced practice nurse* (APN) includes nurse practitioners (NPs), certified nurse-midwives (CNMs), certified registered nurse anesthetists (CRNAs), and clinical nurse specialists (CNSs).

Each specialty of advanced practice nursing has unique differences, although they share key elements. All APNs make independent and collaborative health care decisions and engage in active practice as expert clinicians. APNs are educationally prepared through master's-level education to assume responsibility and accountability for the health promotion, assessment, diagnosis, and management of client problems, including the prescription of medication.

The Patient Protection and Affordable Care Act (PPACA) authorized a grant program that funds community-based Nurse-Managed Health Centers. These centers can be operated and managed by APNs who meet the qualifications of the law.

Nurse Practitioner

Nurse practitioners engage in advanced practice in a variety of specialty areas, such as family, adult, pediatric, geriatric, women's health, school health, occupational health, mental health, emergency, and acute care. Typically, NPs assess, diagnose, and manage medical and nursing problems. Health promotion and maintenance, in addition to disease prevention, are the emphases of their practice. Some NPs diagnose and manage acute and chronic diseases of their selected populations. NPs play a key role in the expansion of health care services under the PPACA. Almost half of the states in the United States allow NPs to practice without physician oversight. This means that NPs may set up individual practices. In most states, the NP collaborates with a physician at least weekly. The volume of people needing primary care under the PPACA means more opportunities for expanded practice by NPs (Nurse Practitioner Schools, 2013).

Job responsibilities of NPs include taking client histories; conducting physical examinations; ordering, performing, and interpreting results of diagnostic tests; and prescribing pharmacologic agents, treatments, and therapies for the management of client conditions. Frequently the NP serves as a primary care provider and consultant for individuals, families, or communities.

NPs have advanced education, with specific emphasis on pathophysiology and pharmacology. Certification is achieved via written examination after the completion of a master's-level program. Several professional organizations offer certification for NPs. For example, the National Certification Board of Pediatric Nurse Practitioners certifies pediatric NPs; adult NPs or family NPs may be certified by the American Academy of Nurse Practitioners. NPs achieve registration and licensure by state boards of nursing or other designated agencies. The state boards of nursing regulate NP practice and prescriptive authority, which can vary from state to state.

Clinical Nurse Specialist

A clinical nurse specialist is an APN who possesses clinical expertise in a defined area of nursing practice for a selected client population or clinical setting, such as oncology, pediatrics, geriatrics, psychiatric-mental health, adult health, acute-critical care, or community health. This practice specialty emphasizes the diagnosis and management of human responses to actual or potential health problems.

The CNS functions as an expert clinician, educator, consultant, researcher, and administrator. He or she monitors the care of clients and collaborates with physicians, nurses, and other members of the interprofessional health care team. The emphasis of this advanced nursing practice is to provide clinical support that improves client care and client outcomes.

CNSs are educated in graduate nursing programs. Their expertise is acquired from combining graduate study with clinical experience. The educational program for CNSs features an intense study of nursing theories and knowledge from other disciplines. Programs emphasize advanced scientific concepts, research methodologies, and supervised clinical practice.

CNSs practice within a systems model paradigm, which means that in performing their role CNSs evaluate each client in the context of his or her social environment. These APNs view clients as individuals who are part of a larger society entering a complex health care delivery system. This practice philosophy prompts the CNS to use a comprehensive approach to client care.

As consultants, CNSs are called on for expert clinical advice within and outside the clinical setting. Their consultation function frequently consists of problem solving with a client who may be a colleague, individual, family, group, agency, or community. Problems may be related to provider competence, equipment, facilities, or health care delivery systems.

CNSs contribute to research in their area of specialization, generating and refining research questions, interpreting research findings, applying them to clinical practice, and educating other nurses about them. As teachers, CNSs educate clients, families, and communities. The CNS functions as a role model or preceptor for nurse generalists and students in a variety of clinical settings (AACN, ; AACN, 2006).

Certified Registered Nurse Anesthetist

Established in the late 1800s, nurse anesthesia is recognized as the first clinical nursing specialty. Nurse anesthesia practice developed in response to requests from surgeons seeking a solution to the high morbidity and mortality attributed to anesthesia at that time. The most famous nurse anesthetist of the nineteenth century, Alice Magaw, called the "mother of anesthesia," worked at St. Mary's Hospital in Rochester, Minnesota. Magaw was instrumental in establishing a showcase of professional excellence in anesthesia and surgery. In 1909, the first formal educational programs preparing nurse anesthetists were established.

Since World War I, nurse anesthetists have been the principal anesthesia providers in combat areas of every war in which the United States has been engaged. Although nurse anesthesia educational programs existed before World War I, the war sharply increased the demand for nurse anesthetists and, consequently, the need for more educational programs.

Founded in 1931, the American Association of Nurse Anesthetists (AANA) is the professional association representing about 47,000 nurse anesthetists nationwide. The AANA promotes education, practice standards, and guidelines and affords consultation to private and governmental entities regarding nurse anesthetists and their practice.

The AANA developed and implemented a certification program in 1945 and instituted mandatory recertification in 1978. The association established a mechanism for accreditation of nurse anesthesia educational programs in 1952.

The educational preparation of CRNAs occurs at the graduate level or in association with traditional institutions of higher education, most commonly in schools of nursing or health sciences. The educational curriculum in the anesthesia specialty ranges from 24 to 36 months in an integrated program of academic and clinical study. The academic curriculum consists of a minimum of 30 credit hours of formalized graduate study in courses such as advanced anatomy, physiology, pathophysiology, advanced pharmacology, principles of anesthesia practice, and research methodology and statistical analysis. All programs require approximately 1000 hours of hands-on clinical experience. Students gain experience with clients of all ages who require medical, obstetric, dental, and pediatric interventions.

Admission requirements to a nurse anesthesia educational program include a bachelor of science degree in nursing, licensure as an RN, and a minimum of 1 year of acute care nursing experience. Nurse anesthetists are required to successfully complete a written examination for certification as CRNAs.

Recertification, which involves practice and continuing education requirements, must be performed every 2 years. CRNAs are qualified to make independent judgments relative to all aspects of anesthesia care on the basis of their education, licensure, and certification. CRNAs provide anesthesia and anesthesia-related care on request, assignment, or referral by a client's physician, most often to facilitate diagnostic, therapeutic, or surgical procedures. In other instances, CRNAs perform consultation or assistance for management of pain associated with obstetric labor and delivery, management of acute or chronic ventilatory problems, or management of acute or chronic pain through the performance of selected diagnostic or therapeutic blocks.

The laws of every state permit CRNAs to work directly with physicians or other authorized health care professionals, such as dentists, without being supervised by an anesthesiologist. TJC does not require anesthesiologist supervision of CRNAs, nor does Medicare. In some cases, a provider, payer, or medical staff bylaws may require anesthesiologist supervision. However, these decisions are not based on legal requirements (AANA, 2018).

Certified Nurse-Midwife

According to the American College of Nurse-Midwives (ACNM), certified nurse-midwives are primary care providers of women's health care, focusing particularly on pregnancy, childbirth, the postpartum period, care of the newborn, and the family planning and gynecologic needs of women (ACNM, 2018). This practice occurs within a health care system that provides consultation, collaborative management, or referral, as indicated by the health status of the client.

The CNM is educated in the two disciplines of nursing and midwifery and possesses evidence of certification according to the requirements of the ACNM. The CNM has successfully completed prescribed studies in midwifery, has met the requisite qualifications to be certified, and is legally qualified to practice in one or more of the 50 states.

The ACNM supports educational programs for CNMs at certificate and degree levels but opposes mandatory degree requirements for state licensure. The ACNM claims that mandatory degree requirements would limit women's access to maternity and gynecologic services. Several national reports specifically recommend placing greater reliance on CNMs to improve access to prenatal care for underserved populations. These reports also recommend that state laws be supportive of nurse-midwifery practice.

The entry-level nurse-midwife is a primary health care professional who independently provides care during pregnancy, birth, and the postpartum period to women and newborns within their communities. Therefore, the CNM is an individual who has successfully completed an ACNM-accredited educational program in nurse-midwifery and passed the national certification examination administered by the ACNM Certification Council. Midwifery care occurs within a variety of settings, including homes, birthing centers, clinics, and hospitals. The nurse-midwife works with each woman and her family to identify their unique physical, social, and emotional needs. Services provided by the CNM include education and health promotion. With additional education and experience, the nurse-midwife may provide well-woman gynecologic care, including family planning services. For situations in which the care required extends beyond the CNM's abilities, the midwife should have a mechanism for consultation and referral.

CNMs are an expanding group of professionals. Approximately 11,100 CNMs were active in the U.S. workforce in 2013. Trending forward to 2025, approximately 6,470 FTE CNMs will enter the workforce and 3,500 FTE CNMs will leave it. A net growth of 2,970 FTE CNMs will result in a projected national workforce of 14,070 FTE CNMs in 2025 (HRSA, 2016) (https://bhw.hrsa.gov/sites/default/files/bhw/health-workforce-analysis/research/projections/womens-health-report). Areas of practice include care to women from puberty through menopause, including gynecologic and wellness services, family planning and contraception care, preconception counseling, prenatal care, labor through childbirth and afterbirth care, and menopause counseling and care.

Nurse Administrator or Nurse Executive

Although not formally considered an APN, the nurse administrator or nurse executive has an important advanced role within nursing. It is vital that individuals be knowledgeable about the business of the health care system and the profession of nursing. Nursing administration unites the leadership perspective of professional nursing with the various aspects of business and health administration. The practice of nursing administration focuses on the administration of health care systems for the purpose of delivering services to groups of clients.

Individuals who assume a nurse executive role typically hold a master's degree. Master's-level and doctoral-level programs that offer degrees in nursing administration are available, although some nursing executives are educated in additional disciplines, such as business.

Nursing administration research focuses on organizational factors and management practices and their effect on nurses, health care delivery systems, and client outcomes. Nursing administration is concerned with establishing the costs of nursing care and examining relationships between nursing services and quality client care. Nurse executives view problems of nursing service delivery within a broader context of policy analysis and delivery of health care services.

Nursing administration is an integral part of any organization that provides health care. Nurse administrators lead and direct large groups of nurses and ancillary personnel. They manage large budgets and are responsible for provision of quality care at reasonable cost. They serve at all management levels in health care organizations and in the community.

WHAT ABOUT THE FUTURE?

The future of nursing is brighter than ever. Many new jobs will result from continuous change in the health care environment. Growth of the nursing profession will be prompted by technologic advances in client care, which allow an increased number of health problems to be detected early and managed quickly. A greater number of sophisticated health-related procedures are already performed not only in hospitals but also in a variety of settings such as clinics and physicians' offices. Health maintenance organizations, ambulatory surgical centers, and church health centers are only a few of the places where the public receives health care. Nursing can be a vital component of the alternative setting movement that is part of health care reform.

As the focus of health care shifts to disease prevention and lifestyle modification, the opportunities for nurses will follow. Nursing also can benefit from the increased emphasis on primary care, because prevention is the only true mechanism to reduce health care expenditures. Professional nursing services should be viewed as a cost-effective way to provide disease prevention and health promotion activities in multiple areas of the community, including industry, business, and commerce. Wellness and disease prevention, historically fundamental to the nursing profession, are becoming more meaningful and revitalized concepts within the larger health care system.

The need for the traditional role of the hospital nurse will always exist. In fact, with a shift to more community services, the intensity of hospital nursing care is likely to increase because only those in most need are treated there. Increases in client acuity will expand the need for professional nursing within the hospital setting. However, the most rapid growth for nursing employment is expected in outpatient facilities such as same-day surgery, rehabilitation, and chemotherapy infusion centers.

Nurses also will see job opportunities continue to develop in home health care. Many factors contribute to this phenomenon. The growing numbers of older persons with disabilities require nursing care to minimize their functional loss and optimize their quality of life. Another factor that promotes home care is the consumer's preference for care in his or her own home. Home care is a feasible option with recent technologic advances. Complex health care treatment that was once thought to be possible only in the hospital setting is now a reality in the home. Professional nurses who are able to perform complex procedures and comprehensive client assessments are invaluable to the home health care industry.

Financial pressures on hospitals to discharge clients as soon as possible are producing more admissions to nursing homes, skilled nursing facilities, and long-term rehabilitation units. In addition, because more individuals are living into their ninth and tenth decades, the number of people entering nursing homes or assisted-living facilities is increasing. The opportunity for nursing is tremendous in the long-term care arena because no other discipline can offer the multiple skills that nursing has to offer the aging population.

Despite this bright outlook, the nursing profession must heed the old cliché that "opportunity only knocks once." If nurses fail to seize their opportunities, other less qualified health care providers may attempt to move into this advantageous position. Nursing professionals must demonstrate their contributions to health care and publicly market their potential. Throughout history the nursing profession has requested a chance to prove its worth in producing cost-effective, quality health care—more than ever before, now is the time.

SUMMARY

This chapter has explored the various roles available to professional nurses today. Social and economic trends influencing the development of new nursing roles in innovative practice settings have been discussed. Nurses who are interested in developing new roles should be encouraged by the examples provided by nurses who first envisioned and created new roles. Traditional, nontraditional, and advanced practice nursing roles offer many exciting opportunities for professional growth and satisfaction. The diversity and challenge available to professional nurses today are unparalleled.

REFERENCES

American Association of Colleges of Nursing. (2006). *AACN statement of support for clinical nurse specialists.* Washington, DC. Retrieved from http://www.aacnnursing.org/News-Information/Position-Statements-White-Papers/CNS. Accessed January 17, 2018.

American Association of Colleges of Nursing. (2017). *AACN fact sheet.* Washington, DC. http://www.aacnnursing.org/News-Information/Fact-Sheets/Nursing-Fact-Sheet. Accessed January 16, 2018.

American Association of Nurse Anesthetists. *Certified registered nurse anesthetists' fact sheet.* Retrieved from https://www.aana.com/. Accessed January 17, 2018.

American College of Nurse Midwives. (2018). *Become a midwife.* Retrieved from http://www.midwife.org. Accessed January 17, 2018.

American Nurses Association. (2008). *Scope and standards of nursing informatics practice.* Washington, DC: American Nurses Publishing.

American Nurses Association. (2010). *Nursing's social policy statement.* Washington, DC: American Nurses Publishing.

American Nurses Association. (2010a). *Nursing: Scope and standards of practice* (2nd ed.). Washington, DC: American Nurses Association.

American Nurses Association & Health Ministries Association. (2012). *Scope and standards of practice: Faith community nursing* (2nd ed.). Silver Spring, MD: Nursesbooks.org.

American Nurses Association & The International Association of Forensic Nurses. (2009). *Forensic nursing: Scope and standards of practice.* Washington, DC: American Nurses Association.

American Nurses Informatics Association. (2018). *About Us.*

Future of Nursing Campaign for Action. (n.d.) *Transforming Nursing Education.* Retrieved from https://campaignforaction.org/issue/transforming-nursing-education/. Accessed January 17, 2018.

Future of Nursing Campaign for Action. (n.d.) *Increasing diversity in nursing.* Retrieved from https://campaignforaction.org/issue/increasing-diversity-in-nursing/. Accessed January 17, 2018.

Future of Nursing Campaign for Action. (n.d.) *Improving access to care.* Retrieved from https://campaignforaction.org/issue/improving-access-to-care/. Accessed January 17, 2018.

Health Resources and Services Administration, Bureau of Health Professions National Center for Health Workforce Analysis. *Nursing Workforce Projections by Ethnicity and Race 2014–2030.* Retrieved from https://bhw.hrsa.gov/sites/default/files/bhw/health-workforce-analysis/research/projections/hrsa-bhw-rn-lpn-factsheet-12-17.pdf. Accessed January 17, 2018.

IOM. (2011). *The Future of Nursing: Leading Change, Advancing Health.* Washington, DC: The National Academies Press. Retrieved from http://thefutureofnursing.org/sites/default/files/Front%20Matter%20%28R1-R26%29.pdf. Accessed Oct 1, 2014.

Lathrop, B., & Hodnicki, D. R. (2014, March 31). The Affordable Care Act: primary care and the doctor of nursing practice nurse. *OJIN: The Online Journal of Issues in Nursing, 19*(2), 7.

McGonigle, D., & Mastrian, K. (2012). *Nursing informatics and the foundation of knowledge* (2nd ed.). Burlington, MA: Jones and Bartlett. https://www.ania.org/about-us. Accessed September 7, 2015.

National Association of School Nurses. (2014). *Planning a career in school nursing*. Retrieved from http://www.nasn.org/RoleCareer/PlanningaCareerinSchoolNursing. Accessed October 1, 2014.

National Council of State Boards of Nursing. *The 2015 national nursing workforce survey*. Retrieved from https://www.ncsbn.org/workforce.htm. Accessed January 17, 2018.

NHPCO Facts and Figures. (2016). *Hospice Care in America*. NPHCO. Retrieved from http://www.nhpco.org/sites/default/files/public/Statistics_Research/2014_Facts_Figures.pdf. Accessed January 17, 2018.

Nurse Practitioner Schools and Degree Program Guide. (2013, February 27). *Nurse Practitioners and Their Role in the Affordable Care Act*. Retrieved from http://www.nursepractitionerschoolguides.org/nurse-practitioners-and-their-role-in-the-affordable-care-act/. Accessed October 1, 2014.

U.S. Department of Health and Human Services, Health Resources and Services Administration, Bureau of Health Workforce, National Center for Health Workforce Analysis. (2016). *National and Regional Projections of Supply and Demand for Women's Health Service Providers: 2013-2025*. Rockville, Maryland. https://bhw.hrsa.gov/sites/default/files/bhw/health-workforce-analysis/research/projections/womens-health-report.pdf.

Westberg, G. E. (1990). *The parish nurse: Providing a minister of health for your congregation*. Minneapolis, Minnesota: Augsburg Fortress Press.

Westberg Institute for Faith Community Nursing. (n.d.). *What is Faith Community Nursing*. Retrieved from https://westberginstitute.org/faith-community-nursing/. Accessed January 17, 2018.

27

Finding the right match can be exciting.

Job Search: Finding Your Match

Susan R. Jacob, PhD, MSN, RN

ⓔ Additional resources are available online at: *http://evolve.elsevier.com/Cherry/*

LEARNING OUTCOMES

After studying this chapter, the reader will be able to:

1. Use the interview process to evaluate potential employment opportunities.
2. Prepare an effective résumé and nursing portfolio.
3. Compare and contrast various professional nursing employment opportunities.
4. Summarize the employment process.

KEY TERMS

Orientation Activities that enhance adaptation to a new environment.
Portfolio A collection of evidence demonstrating acquisition of skills, knowledge, and achievements related to a professional career.

Professional objective Occupational position for which one aims.
Résumé Summary of a job applicant's previous work experience and education.

PROFESSIONAL/ETHICAL ISSUE

Alice and Renardo had just finished their senior seminar class, in which the nursing recruiters from the local hospital held a session on job interviewing. The recruiters told the class about potential job opportunities at their hospital and described their intensive 3-month orientation process for new graduates. The recruiters discussed the high cost of orienting one new nurse and told the class that it was well worth the investment to have the assurance that the new graduates would be skilled and

comfortable in their new positions. The recruiters added that once the hospital made an investment in a new nurse, they expected a commitment of at least 2 years.

Alice told Renardo she planned to apply at this hospital because it was likely there would be positions available, but she also planned to apply at the other local hospital closer to her home, where she really wanted to work, even though there were currently no openings for new graduates.

Renardo said, "I may hold out for the hospital I really want because I would hate to take a position and start orientation and then find out there were openings in the hospital that is my first choice."

Alice responded, "Not me! I will take the first position I am offered, because I can always quit if I get a better offer."

We thank Kathryn S. Skinner, MS, RN, CS, and Laura H. Day, MS, BSN, RN, for their contributions to this chapter in the 4th edition.

"Even if you have already started orientation?" asked Renardo.

"Yes sir," Alice said. "I need to do what is best for me and my family."

What are the professional and ethical issues involved in Alice's plans to take a job and quit if a better offer comes along? What are the implications for the hospital and for other new graduates if Alice quits a job at the hospital after only a few weeks or months?

VIGNETTE

"For 2 years I've struggled to meet deadlines for term papers, nursing care plans, and examinations," sighed Leslie. "Now that graduation is almost here, I'm scared that I don't know enough to be a 'real nurse.' And I'm confused about where to begin and what kind of nursing position I should seek. This first job seems so important."

Questions to Consider While Reading this Chapter:

1. How should the new graduate in the scenario decide where to apply for that first position?
2. What kinds of questions should the applicant ask about a prospective position?
3. How can the applicant demonstrate knowledge, skills, and experience to the recruiter?

CHAPTER OVERVIEW

This chapter helps student nurses prepare to successfully negotiate their first employment as professional nurses. It discusses the importance of networking, researching available opportunities, and examining their personal aptitudes, interests, lifestyle priorities, and long-term goals to find the best job fit.

Readers are shown how to create and use cover letters and résumés to market themselves in written introductions and how to prepare for and actively participate in a recruitment interview. The chapter describes what can be expected from a recruiter and how to obtain the information needed to make thoughtful and rewarding job choices. Putting these recommendations into practice will ensure the new graduate of the best chance for finding a good job match as an entry-level nurse practicing in a suitable work environment.

EXPLORING OPTIONS

The job market for graduate nurses is extensive. There are many opportunities in urban as well as rural areas. Health care economics ride a roller coaster from robust to lean times, but the high demand for the skills of professional registered nurses (RNs) remains constant, and the potential for finding suitable employment is good. Trends in health care delivery direct today's health care providers to change their orientation from disease to health and from inpatient to outpatient services, leading to a growing need for professional nurses in nonacute community-based care settings, such as primary care clinics, ambulatory surgery centers, and home, school, and work environments. However, although rapid changes in health care delivery systems continue to create new and varied opportunities outside the acute care settings where nurses have traditionally practiced, hospitals remain the most likely starting place for new graduates to acquire general experience that will be helpful in opening career path doors. In fact, with a nursing shortage there is an increased demand for nurses to work in acute care settings.

Numerous marketing strategies have been tried in an effort to aggressively attract bright, energetic new graduates in times of demand and short supply. For some institutions in selected areas of the country, cost seems irrelevant. Sign-on bonuses, promises of tuition reimbursement for continued education, and student loan repayment, just to name a few, have been offered as enticements. However, in other areas of the country, for the first time in several years, it is taking graduates longer to find employment than in the past, when it was common for new graduates to have promises of employment prior to graduation. Ultimately, being aware of one's own qualities and taking advantage of networking opportunities are more important keys to finding just the right match in today's job market.

Knowing Oneself

The choice of a first nursing position deserves careful study. For some, the opportunities seem to be a smorgasbord of possibilities, all of them attractive. The neophyte nurse should carefully explore any job under consideration and its responsibilities in light of his or her own personal qualities. Some students find it helpful to consult an instructor or a trusted nursing mentor for objective input and perspective. An experienced nurse can see the pros and cons that may not be visible to a new nurse.

A thoughtful review of one's general interests, abilities, and strengths (especially those pointed out by clinical instructors) and awareness of the types of patients who have provided the greatest emotional reward are essential.

Other important considerations are one's physical and emotional stamina, energy level, and responsibilities to others—spouse, children, and other family members; volunteer commitments; and social activities—all of which make legitimate demands on one's schedule. Long-term goals must be factored into the first job choice as well. Is the first job a stepping-stone to an advanced degree, to a narrowly specialized area of nursing, to a traveling nurse position, or to a management role? Selection of a position that fits one's abilities, lifestyle, and career aspirations will affect job satisfaction, career advancement, and overall sense of success and happiness.

Finding the right practice environment is essential to long-term success and job satisfaction. The American Association of Colleges of Nursing (AACN, n.d.a) developed a white paper titled *Hallmarks of the Professional Practice Environment*. On the basis of this paper, a brochure for nursing school graduates was developed, titled "What Every Nursing Student Should Know When Seeking Employment" (AACN, n.d.b) This brochure, which can be downloaded from the website, identifies eight key characteristics, or hallmarks, of the professional practice setting and suggests that applicants ask the following questions about the employer they are considering. Does the potential employer:

- Manifest a philosophy of clinical care emphasizing quality, safety, interdisciplinary collaboration, continuity of care, and professional accountability?
- Recognize the value of nurses' expertise on clinical care quality and patient outcomes?
- Promote executive-level nursing leadership?
- Empower nurses' participation in clinical decision making and organization of clinical care systems?
- Demonstrate professional development support for nurses?
- Maintain clinical advancement programs based on education, certification, and advanced preparation?
- Create collaborative relationships among members of the health care team?
- Use technologic advances in clinical care and information systems?

Box 27.1 provides other statistics and information to request from a potential employer. The numbers of hospitals seeking and receiving Magnet hospital credentialing

> **BOX 27.1   Statistics and Information that Applicants May Request from a Potential Employer**
>
> Registered nurse (RN) vacancy rate and turnover rate
> Patient satisfaction scores (preferably a percentile ranking)
> Employee satisfaction scores
> Average tenure of nursing staff
> Education mix of nursing staff
> Percentage of registry or travelers used
> Key human resources policies (e.g., reduction in work-force; tenure versus performance criteria)
> Copy of the most recent The Joint Commission report on the institution, and the number of contingencies cited
> Information about whether the nurses are unionized
> Copy of the contract
>
> From American Association of Colleges of Nursing. (2002). *What every nursing school graduate should consider when seeking employment.* Washington, DC: American Association of Colleges of Nursing.

are growing, and where these work environments are available, the nurse may wish to consider these organizations. Generally, hospitals with Magnet status have demonstrated excellence in areas such as low RN turnover rates, adherence to standards of nursing care as defined by the American Nurses Association (ANA), and mechanisms in place for staff participation in decision making. A study by Renter and Allen (2014) found that Magnet hospitals had a more positive nurse work environment and outcomes and were more likely to have specialty-certified nurses and a higher percentage of baccalaureate-prepared nurses. The American Nurses Credentialing Center (ANCC) lists all Magnet hospitals on its website (https://www.clinicalmanagementconsultants.com/ancc-list-of-magnet-recognized-hospitals--cid-4457.html).

Many graduate nurses have discovered that working in an environment that did not match well with their personal attributes and long-term goals not only made them unhappy but also damaged their future employment options. Poor job fits lead to frequent job changes, which could lead to poor references and the attachment of the label "job hopper."

Appropriate job choice is critically important and can be costly to the new graduate. Accordingly, an ineffective hiring decision can also be expensive for the employer. Hospitals routinely pay for drug testing and criminal background checks. The preemployment costs alone can tally close to $2000 before the person even steps in the hospital door to begin employment. Class-room and hospital **orientation** includes the salary of the graduate nurse (GN) and the nursing instructors. Additionally, various other paid employees teach mandatory classes, such as infection control and fire safety, and the GN gets an official welcome from the organization's chief executive officer.

Following the classroom orientation is approximately one full month of classroom and clinical instruction before the nurse arrives on the patient care unit. This month of one-on-one instruction to review basic nursing skills incurs the cost of not only the graduate nurse's salary but the salaries of nursing educators.

Subsequently, assignments are made for the graduate nurse to follow a preceptor for the next 8 to 20 weeks, depending on how quickly the nurse achieves competency in each area. This phase of the training process costs the hospital the graduate nurse's salary and the preceptor's salary.

In addition, the clinical nursing instructor, who follows the nurse through completion of orientation to eventual competency, is also paid for the duration of the process. The additional time it takes to teach is another consideration in adding up the cost, a cost to which it is difficult to assign a dollar value. Other nonspecific cost considerations include the cost of provision of space required for the education of new staff. Included in this category would be building utilities, engineering staff that support the operation, housekeeping costs, and general administration costs associated with the procurement of new graduate nurses.

Some estimate the cost of recruiting, placing, and orienting a new nurse to be from two to two and a half times the average RN salary—but the costs are more than financial. It causes hard feelings between employers and the school of nursing and the recruit when a new nurse goes through orientation and then leaves. The cost of nurse turnover can have a huge impact on a hospital's profit margin. According to the survey, the average cost of turnover for a bedside RN is $49,500 and ranges from $38,000 to $61,100 resulting in the average hospital losing $4.4M – $7.0M. Each percent change in RN turnover will cost/save the average hospital an additional $337,500 (Nursing Solutions, Inc., 2018).

Critical to effective selection is high-level nurse leader competency in resource management processes and attention to creation of an effective, healthful practice environment. A great decision on the part of the new graduate and the nurse leader will have better outcomes for the individual nurse in areas of job satisfaction and retention and for overall organizational outcomes in terms of employee engagement and retention and patient outcomes.

Networking

The investigative process of researching potential employers begins with networking at school, in the community, and within student nurse organizations. One may question other nurses, employees, and former employees, especially alumni of one's own school, who have worked in various settings. Faculty will have pertinent observations based on their experiences with clinical sites in the community. It is also valuable to listen to neighbors, friends, and family members who have been patients.

Some employers now offer "phone-a-thons," in which they invite nurses to speak directly with recruiters or nursing department supervisors. Websites, open houses, health care job fairs, and virtual online career events are great places to pick up information about institutions. Recruitment materials and brochures often contain interesting facts about the organization, such as the mission, vision, values statements and goals, available services, and information about associate benefits.

The Internet offers links to actual jobs and information on career planning. Most hospital and large health care systems maintain websites to post their employment needs and invite applications online. The Internet is a cost-effective recruiting method, and larger health care systems expect early communications to take place by fax and e-mail. Applicants who use this method to follow up on a job posting should pay particular attention to the application and **résumé** that is sent electronically, being sure to follow the online prompts correctly, making sure there are no errors before submitting materials online. To make sure one's online information is secure, one should never share the username or password with anyone. If there is no response to Internet inquiries within a week, applicants should follow up with a phone call.

Internet sites are helpful for exploring job opportunities, writing résumés, and preparing for employment interviews. If a new graduate is seeking a position in a large community with multiple job choices available, this informal research will help narrow the list to the best place to begin the job application process. Later in the interview, the applicant may wish to describe to the recruiter how his or her search resulted in this employer's being the number-one choice over others for the graduate's first job. This process of researching potential employers will continue through the interview process. Assessing the climate of the work environment is a valuable tool in "finding a match" and is discussed more thoroughly later in this chapter.

WRITTEN INTRODUCTIONS

Three of the most important steps in a job search are writing a cover letter, preparing a professional résumé, and assembling a professional **portfolio**. These tools introduce the applicant to a prospective employer. The first impression should be persuasive; there may not be a second chance. Presenting oneself on paper can make a difference, perhaps the difference between getting a desired interview and being passed over in favor of someone else. These written introductions should present a conscientious, mature, competent, committed professional who would be an asset to an agency that prides itself on its nursing services.

How to Write a Cover Letter

The cover letter is a chance for an applicant to sell himself or herself and make the recruiter look forward to meeting an attractive candidate (Box 27.2). A convincing cover letter will show how this candidate is different and convey to the recruiter why he or she is the best fit for the position. The letter should also address why this institution is the applicant's first choice.

A cover letter should reflect the nurse's own style of writing, should never appear to have been copied from a book, and should be tailored to the particular job. Like any business document it should be clean, direct, and letter perfect. It should be attractive and effortless to read. There must be no typing errors and no grammar or spelling mistakes. Everything should fit on a single page of 8.5 by 11–inch white heavyweight bond paper with ample margins on the top, bottom, and sides.

The letter should be addressed to a specific person. If the person's name or title is unknown, the applicant should refer to a marketing brochure or call the recruitment office to ask for correct title and spelling of the appropriate person's first and last names.

If spelling is not one's strength, one should use the spell-check tool on the computer, but should not

---

BOX 27.2 Cover Letter

April 8, 2018

Ms. Donna Henderson, MS, RN
Director of Nurse Recruitment
Charleston Memorial Hospital
1600 Beckley Avenue
Memphis, TN 38104

Dear Ms. Henderson:

I would like to apply for a new graduate position on a cardiology nursing unit at Charleston Memorial Hospital. After graduating from Smith College with a BSN on June 6, I will be ready to start work immediately. I plan to take the RN licensing examination in early July.

Through reading about your hospital and my own personal experience in a recent clinical rotation at Charleston Memorial, I have learned that your institution is a modern, professional one with an emphasis on quality patient care. For this and many other reasons, I am convinced that Charleston Memorial is where I want to work as a nurse.

I will be in Memphis from April 20 to April 25 and will call to schedule an appointment to see you then. My home phone number is 555-912-3120; my cell phone number is 555-200-9999.

I look forward to meeting you and discussing how I can contribute to Charleston Memorial Hospital.

Sincerely,
(Name signed here in pen)

Bonnie McCray Pino
Enclosure

---

depend on its accuracy. Using a dictionary and asking a competent friend to proofread the final copy is also a good idea. Poor typists would be well served to pay someone to type for them. A sloppy letter will cast doubt on one's abilities to practice as a professional.

The body of the letter should be single-spaced, three or four block paragraphs long, with blank lines between paragraphs, and organized as follows:

- Paragraph 1 should be a statement of purpose that tells the recruiter what kind of position is being sought, the writer's expected date of graduation, state licensing status, and the date the writer will be ready to begin work.
- Paragraph 2 should emphasize the writer's suitability. The implied message should be "I'm just the person for the job" without going into all the details that will be included in the résumé. A sentence

should describe past work or educational experiences that relate to the agency's particular needs and philosophy. The more homework the nurse has done in learning about the institution, the more persuaded the recruiter will be. The final sentence should refer to the enclosed résumé.

- Paragraph 3 should request an interview appointment and give a range of dates of availability. It is a good idea for the writer to promise a phone call "next week" or "soon" to schedule a meeting time and to provide a phone number by which the writer can be reached, if the number is different from the permanent phone number listed on the résumé.
- The letter can end with a "written handshake," such as, "I look forward to meeting with you to discuss available nursing positions in your institution"—a cautiously optimistic note.
- The letter closes with "Sincerely," and after four lines of space for a signature, the writer's name is typed. A line is skipped, and "Enclosure" is typed on the left margin to indicate that a résumé is enclosed.

The letter should be proofread carefully, signed, and copied; and the copy filed. If the nurse has chosen to use different approaches with different institutions, it would be wise to review the appropriate cover letter before each interview.

One week later the writer should follow up by phone to be sure the letter was received. This attention to detail and follow-through will impress the recruiter or personnel office and improve chances of getting an interview soon. These phone calls usually become mini-interviews, and the applicant should be extra courteous, aware that it usually is the secretary who controls the interview schedule. By keeping a written list of all contacts made, the new graduate will be able to add the flattering personal touch of acknowledging previous phone contacts when meeting them for the first time during the interview process.

The cover letter serves as the foundation on which all other follow-up is built: résumé, call for appointment, and interview. What is presented in the letter should prompt the person responsible for hiring to take a close look at the enclosed résumé.

How to Prepare a Résumé

A résumé is a short compilation of one's education, work experience, credentials, and accomplishments. In many cases, the résumé is the first document a hiring manager will look at when reviewing the application, and therefore is a true "first impression." Accordingly, it is important to put time and effort into developing and maintaining an updated, accurate résumé (Box 27.3). The résumé is different from a curriculum vitae (CV), which is a chronologic account of one's entire educational and professional work experience, usually required by academic institutions for educator positions. The résumé is the most appropriate format for the new graduate and will complement the cover letter by filling in important details about educational and

---

BOX 27.3   Résumé

Bonnie McCray Pino
416 Melody Avenue
Bristol, TN 37620
555-912-3120 (Home)
555-200-9999 (Cell)
E-mail: bpino@xyz.com

Professional Objective:	**Staff Nurse Position (Cardiology)**
Licensure:	Eligible to take NCLEX examination after June 6, 2018 Anticipated date of NCLEX: July 2018
Education:	
2014 to 2018	Smith College School of Nursing, Bristol, TN BSN, June 6, 2018
2011 to 2014	Oakview High School, Nashville, TN Diploma, June 2014
Experience:	
May 2016 to August 2016	St. Mary's Hospital, Knoxville, TN Patient Care Assistant: Assisted RNs in providing basic nursing care including feeding, bathing, assisting with ADLs, and patient teaching in a pediatric setting
June 2017 to August 2017	Drs. Smith and Jones OB/GYN office, Bristol, TN Office Assistant: Accompanied patients to treatment area; weighed patients and recorded vital signs
Honors:	Sigma Theta Tau International, 2017 *Who's Who Among American High School Students*, 2014
Professional Organizations:	Tennessee Student Nurses Association, 2014-2018
References:	Provided on request

work experiences. It is important to provide accurate information because inaccurate information on a résumé or application can lead to dismissal later. An effective résumé should compress education and employment history into an attractive, easy-to-read one-page summary. A wealth of valuable information can be communicated simply and straightforwardly by saying more with less. The key is writing concisely. For example, "BSN with high honors" speaks for itself. Citing exact grade point average or "dean's list" standing adds little. Succinct ways to convey a message can be found by experimenting with phrases and word choices. The writer should avoid pompous language and use of the passive voice, instead using active verbs, such as *improved, established, trained, administered, prepared, wrote,* and *evaluated.*

A basic résumé contains three essential sections: (1) identifying information; (2) education; and (3) work experience. In addition, optional information may include professional objectives, honors, achievements, and memberships in professional organizations. A well-designed résumé marks the writer as a career-minded professional, just what recruiters are seeking. A succinct, well-organized résumé indicates that the applicant is focused and organized in other areas as well.

The first section of the résumé, the identifying information, contains the applicant's name, address, and home and work phone numbers, followed by licensure information. The states of licensure and license numbers are listed. Graduating students should indicate when and where they have taken or will take the National Council of Licensing Examination (NCLEX).

If the résumé writer opts to include a professional objective, it should come next. Some interviewers like to see this because it shows that the nurse has put some thought into career planning. The writer should keep in mind, though, that it is limiting to put forth a singular objective that ties the nurse to only one particular clinical area. If there is no such opening available in that department, the recruiter will consider the applicant an unlikely candidate to pursue. It is better to have an objective statement that is broad and general.

The second section should include details about education, including degrees and diplomas awarded, names and locations of schools, and graduation dates, starting with the most recent graduation and degree and going in reverse chronologic order.

The third section presents the information apt to be the greatest help in obtaining a job: work experience

and employment history. Many recruiters are nurses themselves, so a detailed description of what a routine job entails is not needed. Instead efforts should be directed toward illustrating any special knowledge or contributions. The new graduate's résumé might reflect student accomplishments or elaborate on jobs in which he or she has demonstrated skills also applicable to nursing responsibilities, such as organization of tasks, time management, delegation to subordinates, and ability to work well with others. The summary should start with the current or most recent position and work chronologically backward, including places of employment, job titles, dates worked, and responsibilities. Accomplishments during employment should be listed, including number and type of patients cared for, any special techniques used, or any participation in the development of programs, policies, or forms pertinent to the position.

This section closes with optional information, such as seminars attended, honors received, and memberships in professional organizations. It is not advisable to list community activities or activities from more than 5 years ago unless it can be clearly shown that they are pertinent to a nursing career. Similarly, personal information, such as marital and health status, age, number of children, and hobbies, should be excluded. This information is not job related and should not be used by the employer to screen applicants.

References do not need to be included in the résumé but should be ready for presentation in a neatly typed list when requested from any future employer. The résumé should conclude with the simple statement "References provided on request" or "References available." When someone agrees to be listed as a reference, the applicant should take time to discuss with him or her what prospective employers may want to know. Former instructors or former employers may require written permission before releasing information. As the job search continues, the nurse should keep references informed of the names of employers who may be inquiring.

The résumé should be produced neatly and inexpensively, on a computer, because a good résumé will be used repeatedly with revisions, and the nurse will want to be able to produce an up-to-date version without completely rewriting it. Production methods should be kept as simple as possible. Many tools and templates are available in most word processing software programs for résumé building and formatting. It is not necessary to go to the added trouble and expense of having the résumé professionally typeset and printed. Having it neatly typed and reproduced using good-quality photo-copying services suffices. These resources as well as laser/color printers are available at public or university libraries. To make the text easy to read, one style of serif font should be used throughout, in 11- or 12-point size. Again the applicant should have someone review the final copy for typing errors, then use a photocopying service for "quick copying" onto good-quality white or ivory paper. It is important to remember that when it comes to résumés, appearances do count. A well-formatted résumé that is properly organized and neatly typed makes a great first impression.

How to Prepare a Portfolio

The nursing **portfolio** contains more information than a résumé and provides documentation to support the résumé. As health professionals, nurses are responsible for staying abreast of current professional knowledge and managing their own careers, professional growth and development, and ideally, practices to support these activities should start during their student years. Professional development is a lifelong and continuous process, which is essential to the maintenance of clinical skills and knowledge required in today's ever-changing health care environment. By creating a professional portfolio, a professional may showcase personal and professional development, practice excellence, and clinical leadership. Portfolio compilation gives one an opportunity to assess abilities, identify learning goals, and devise a plan for further personal and professional development. In addition to validating accomplishments and highlighting milestones, this tool may illustrate a professional's progression along the continuum from novice to expert.

The portfolio introduces the professional nurse to recruiters, employers, admissions committees, and potential supervisors in a visual and tangible way. It includes traditional documents, such as a résumé, license to practice and certifications, educational documents (e.g., diplomas, transcripts), and examples of significant professional, community, and student activities (Box 27.4).

The simplest way to build a portfolio is to start with an attractive three-ring binder. A table of contents gives interviewers a map to guide their review of the information. Dividers can separate sections, each with its own cover page, and plastic sleeves or pocketed pages work well to hold loose items. Appropriate documents are

---

BOX 27.4 Documents for Professional Portfolio

Professional Credentials
Résumé
Licenses
Certifications
Specialty practice certifications
Basic cardiac life support (BCLS)
Advanced cardiac life support (ACLS)

Educational Credentials
Diplomas
Transcripts
Continuing education certificates
Honors and awards (including program from awards ceremony, letters regarding awards, newspaper articles)

Research and Scholarly Activity
Publications
Teaching materials for patients, staff, handouts
Case studies
Photo of poster sessions, classroom presentations
PowerPoint outline of presentation
Student papers and projects

Professional Activities
Membership cards
Evidence of service as an officer or leader in student organizations
Community involvement and volunteer activities
Performance evaluations
Letters of recommendation

---

assigned to each section. Copies should be made of important originals, such as diplomas, certifications, and licenses that would be difficult to replace. Samples of letters from grateful patients, congratulations from peers, and complimentary notes from supervisors, should be included. Sentences in longer letters or performance appraisals that address the information considered to be most important for the reader to note should be highlighted. The graduate nurse may want to include supervisor evaluations from non-nursing positions to demonstrate leadership qualities, dependability, and attention to detail, characteristics also relevant to the nursing work setting.

Interest in electronic portfolios or e-portfolios is gathering momentum as a strategy for fostering lifelong learning and enhancing ongoing personal and professional development. The e-portfolio can represent an authentic means of assessing cognitive, reflective, and affective skills. Furthermore, e-portfolios provide a means through which nurses can record and provide evidence of skills, achievements, experience, professional development and ongoing learning, not only for themselves but also for the informing and scrutiny of registration boards, employers, managers, and peers (Birk et al, 2016).

Graduation is the perfect time to create a career portfolio, one that will be easy to build on and update as one's nursing career evolves. If documents are created on the computer, updates and revisions will be easy when the nurse pursues new and different professional roles and responsibilities. Many baccalaureate educational programs require students to create such a portfolio as part of their preparation for graduation and entry into the first job. Nurses who present portfolios to the recruiter may have a competitive edge over nurses who do not; increasingly, boards of nursing and many specialty organizations are making portfolios (or other methods of documenting evidence of competency) mandatory for relicensure and recertification. Continuing education and testing provide a limited picture of an individual's knowledge and/or skill acquisition in a limited area at one point in time. However, portfolios promote critical thinking, self-assessment, and individual accountability. A portfolio is a portable mechanism for evaluating competencies that may otherwise be difficult to assess.

HOW TO INTERVIEW EFFECTIVELY

No matter how qualified and self-confident a person may feel, sitting across the desk from an interviewer can be intimidating. One's conduct in the recruiter's office may determine whether a job offer is made. Being a little anxious is normal, but panic is not. When the applicant has made a good first impression in the cover letter and résumé, he or she can expect to be called for an interview. The graduate's task then becomes to enter the interview prepared to answer and ask questions that will help determine whether this organization, with its available job opportunities, is a good match.

Every agency has its own hiring and interviewing policies. Generally the smaller the organization and the more decentralized the nursing department, the more involved the lower-level manager is in the recruitment and hiring process. The same person who interviews nurse applicants also may be the manager, staff development instructor, quality assurance director, employee health nurse, or chair of the product standards committee. A large organization with many employees may have a separate human resources department with a nurse recruiter on staff. Within such large organizations, the hiring process becomes more complicated and more formal; applicants are more tightly screened, and the hiring decisions are further removed from the actual work position.

Increasingly hospitals are conducting panel interviews. A panel interview can be more efficient because several people can be in the room together and all have the same experience. The interviewers learn from the responses to one another's questions. Some organizations find this approach to be the easiest way to reach consensus on job candidates. If the applicant knows a panel interview is a possibility, he or she should learn as much as possible about the panel members and the departments they represent (Bauer, 2013).

Some "nurse recruiters" are not nurses themselves, a situation that may make a difference in the kind of information exchanged in the interview. A non-nurse is not likely to be able to fully discuss questions that pertain directly to a nurse's job description, patient care workload, and nursing responsibilities. Also, the applicant does not have to answer questions that are not job related. In fact some questions are not legally allowed to be asked (Box 27.5). After a job offer is made, the prospective employer may ask certain non–job-related questions, but not before. They should not be a part of deciding whether the applicant is offered a position.

BOX 27.5   Legal and Illegal Areas of Questioning

Some questions are inappropriate to be asked of an applicant before a job offer is made.

Legal	Illegal
Educational preparation	Race
Licensure status	Creed
Work experience	Color
Reasons for leaving previous jobs	Age
	Nationality
Reasons for applying to this institution	Marital status
	Sexual preference
Qualifications for this job	Religious beliefs
Strengths and weaknesses	Number of children or dependents
Criminal convictions	Financial or credit status

How to Prepare: Planning Ahead

It is recommended that interview appointments be made as early as possible and that senior students not wait until graduation day. Ideally interviews should be scheduled at least 2 months prior to graduation. Job hunting takes time, and appointments are not easily scheduled near nursing school graduation dates, times that tend to be busy weeks for recruiters.

How to Prepare: Self-Talk

As the day approached, Mary obsessed about the interview, thinking to herself, "What if they ask me something I cannot answer, and I go blank like I used to do in clinicals when the instructor quizzed me about my patient's medicines? I will look like an idiot, and maybe even start to cry." The night before the appointment, Mary could not sleep.

One's thoughts dictate one's reality. Nurses, especially new nurses, should be aware of what they are saying to themselves. The applicant who thinks, "Why would anyone want to hire a graduate nurse with no practical experience like me?" will project a lack of self-trust that may be interpreted by the recruiter as a lack of enthusiasm or even incompetence. However, a confident graduate's self-talk may be something like this: "I have successfully completed a difficult nursing course of study. I am now ready to take on the responsibilities of a professional. With orientation, on-the-job training, and the support of experienced nurses, I can succeed as an RN. I have everything I need to begin practice." This reality-based self-talk is an important internal dialogue for establishing feelings of confidence before the job interview.

The reality is that all graduates have met the criteria for graduation from a nursing education program and have been deemed ready by that credentialing body for entry-level positions as RNs. The final test of competence to practice, the NCLEX examination, will provide further proof. Graduate nurses who fear failure of this final test must remind themselves of those now successfully practicing who preceded them from the same educational program with the same preparation.

How to Prepare: Rehearse

A simple visualization of how the graduate wants to appear to the recruiter can bring about the self-assurance needed to create an attractive candidate. It is helpful to mentally review and to be prepared to describe pride in any past work experiences, especially the parts of any job that relate to what is required of a nurse. Even baby-sitting jobs can validate a worker as a responsible adult if that person worked consistently for the same family and showed stability and good judgment as a trusted caretaker for children. Applicants tend to discount minimum-wage, part-time, adolescent, or summer employment, but these experiences often reveal a great deal about the applicant: Would attendance records attest to the worker's dependability? Was the worker given greater responsibility over time? Was the worker allowed to open or close the business? Handle the cash receipts? Consider Case Study 27.1.

Remember that it is not only the graduate's academic standing or honors and awards that measure success as a student. Perhaps the student was not in the top 10% of the class but was active in student affairs. Perhaps the student was chair of a student government committee or a contributor to the campus newspaper. The graduate should be prepared to describe other areas of student accomplishments.

Unfortunately, many nurses are not accustomed to selling themselves and are uncomfortable in situations in which they need to discuss their best attributes and market their qualifications. Therefore, after rehearsing in one's own mind how to present these qualifications to interviewers, it would be wise to rehearse with another person, role-playing the expected interview dialogue. The nurse should role-play with another student or an experienced nurse (even better), rehearsing answers to questions the interviewer is expected to ask and practicing descriptions of the key points of past employment. A few minutes spent in rehearsing with another person will contribute to composure and self-confidence in the actual situation.

Finally, it is important for the graduate to remember that the job interview is not an examination to pass or fail, nor is it an interrogation. It is an exchange of information—the

---

CASE STUDY 27.1

The only job Sam had before nursing school had been working at the customer service desk at a large children's toy store, where he scheduled and supervised the cashiers. His title was "designated key carrier," which he listed on his résumé. The interviewer reasonably interpreted this to be a position that demonstrated the employer's trust in Sam.

recruiter hoping to find a potential employee to fill a staff vacancy and the applicant hoping to find employment as a nurse in this organization. Each has responsibilities for informing the other, and each has rights to obtain information from the other (Box 27.6).

How to Prepare: The Interview Itself

Dress Appropriately. Business-appropriate clothing, such as a neat dress, suit, or pantsuit, projects a professional attitude. Casual attire projects a casual attitude. Jeans are not acceptable, nor are shorts, tennis shoes, flip-flops, or any clothes that are too short, too tight, too revealing, or too trendy. Conservative and simple are always best. When people are dressed to look their best, their attitudes improve and levels of self-confidence increase. Makeup should be light, and the use of perfume or cologne should be avoided. Most institutions are fragrance free because of patients' and employees' allergic reactions to perfumes. Large, distracting jewelry should be avoided. Applicants who have lots of piercings should wear only earrings; tattoos should be covered. Smartphones should be muted or put on vibrate during the interview. Applicants should also avoid distracting behavior such as chewing gum and drinking coffee or other beverages.

Arrive on Time. Arriving late for a job interview creates a poor first impression. The applicant should be considerate of the interviewer's time and agenda. If delayed, he or she should call to reschedule. Arriving too early can make the interviewer feel rushed or the applicant appear overanxious; however, 10 to 15 minutes early is a reasonable target.

Bring a Résumé. Even if a résumé has already been submitted, the applicant should bring extra copies. The recruiter may have routed the mailed copy to a manager for review. Applicants probably will be asked to complete an employment application, and the résumé is a ready reference for past employers and dates of employment. A Social Security card, driver's license, and nursing license, if available, also will be requested as necessary parts of the identification process. Some agencies request that a current cardiopulmonary resuscitation card be made available to photocopy. These documents will be easy to produce if the applicant has also brought a professional portfolio folder.

The Phone Interview

Phone interviews are becoming a standard first step to narrowing down the applicant pool, and they minimize travel expenses for out-of-town applicants. The purpose of the phone interview is to screen applicants and determine which ones to invite for a face-to-face interview. The applicant should be prepared for the interview just as if it were an in-person interview. Many job applicants have found it helpful to dress in business attire for the interview because it makes them feel and act more professionally. The applicant should control the surroundings by eliminating distracting background noise. Whether the interviewer is calling the applicant, or vice versa, the applicant should be ready before the appointed time, anticipate any time zone differences, and respect the employer's time constraints. The applicant should also eliminate any possible distractions from the phone room by (1) making sure children and pets are quiet; (2) putting a "do not ring or knock" sign on the door; and (3) turning off call waiting, cell phones, music, and television sets. The résumé should be printed out, a pen and paper should be ready for note-taking, and a glass of water should be nearby in case of a dry throat. Standing may make the applicant sound more confident, and smiling can be heard in the voice (Pagana, 2012).

In preparation for a phone interview or a call from a potential employer, it is wise to make sure one's voicemail message sounds professional. Although friends may enjoy listening to a favorite band or sarcastic message, the potential employer might find it unprofessional (Pagana, 2012). The same caution goes for social media. It is important to remember that the messages and pictures posted on YouTube, MySpace, Facebook, Twitter, or other Internet websites are generally not private. Potential employers often research applicants' social media presence during the screening phase of the employment process.

Video Interviewing

Skype and Zoom, online phone and video Internet services, are being used to conduct long-distance initial interviews. Advance preparations should include the following (Doyle, 2018b):

- Downloading software
- Conducting a quick test the morning of the interview to make sure the camera and the microphone are working.
- Considering your appearance: It is important to choose colors that look good on video, such as blue, rather than colors that may look too bright, like red. Patterns can be less attractive than solids so think about a pattern that will not be distracting to your viewer. During the video interview it is important to remember to smile and focus direct eye contact.
- Remembering the background that the viewer will see. Are you in sitting so that a blank wall is behind you or is there a cluttered bookshelf behind you? Set up the webcam accordingly.
- Having a few notes written down about what you would like to talk about and a pen handy to jot down thoughts for additional comments you think of to add during the conversation.

The Face-to-Face Interview

The in-person interview is the most time-consuming and subjective part of the employment process. For professionals, it is appropriate for interviews to be unstructured, using open-ended questions (see Box 27.8); both recruiter and applicant will have questions. The initial interview can be expected to last 30 minutes to 1 hour. It is important to maintain professional communication with direct eye contact and to avoid casual chatter about things that are unrelated to the job. Being prepared is the key, and planning answers to the

questions most likely to be asked is the best way to prepare. Nine of the most frequently asked questions follow. Mentally reviewing practiced responses to these questions will give the applicant confidence.

1. What Positions Interest You? The interviewer needs to know whether there are positions available in the applicant's area of interest and whether the applicant has the required qualifications to fit the vacant positions. If there is no fit in interest or qualifications with jobs available, neither applicant nor recruiter needs to waste more time in the interview.

Because titles and position names vary from organization to organization, it is better to answer the question with favorite clinical experiences. Applicants might share short- and long-term goals and how they visualize laying the groundwork today for tomorrow's professional roles. A good response might be, "I'm interested in a position that will help me grow as a professional and give me opportunities to develop greater competency as a nurse. Ultimately, I would like to work as a critical care clinical nurse specialist." If interest, qualifications, and the available positions match, the interviewer will want to start planning secondary interviews and tours.

2. Tell Me About Your Work History. Even if previous jobs were not nursing related, the applicant can highlight the responsibilities carried out, the skills acquired, and how these skills can transfer to the professional nursing role. This is the point at which the interviewer will get an idea of motivation, drive, energy level, and reliability. No new graduate will be expected to have all the knowledge and skills of an experienced RN; however, when answering, the graduate may stress other aptitudes, such as verbal skills or interpersonal skills. It is best to start with the current or most recent job and proceed backward. A new graduate might discuss student clinical experiences, which clinical areas were favored, and why.

3. How Did You Choose to Apply for a Job Here? Any previous investigative homework done on the institution is useful and helps form honest responses. For example, an applicant might say, "This hospital has a reputation for its quality care, and I like that," or "I am interested in research and have heard you have a nursing research committee for staff nurses."

4. Do You Want a Full-Time or Part-Time Position, and Which Shift Do You Prefer?

If there is a need or desire for a particular schedule, the nurse should be honest and ask for that schedule. If the recruiter does not have that schedule available, ask what is available so that a decision can be made. Can the nurse be flexible to accept an undesirable shift until a preferred one becomes available? Part of one's investigation of an institution should include looking at a current list of posted positions. Particularly with smaller agencies, if what the nurse desires is not posted, it may be beneficial to ask for a particular schedule but, if willing, express an interest in working a schedule that is posted. For example, "I'm willing to work the evening shift posted for the medical-surgical unit; however, I'm most interested in moving into a day position in labor and delivery."

5 and 6. What Are Your Strengths/Weaknesses?

Sometimes these questions may be asked in less direct ways, such as, "What are some of the areas you know you need to improve?" or "How have your skills developed in your advanced nursing courses?" Honesty always is best. In asking this question, the interviewer may only be trying to pinpoint the special skills and preferences of the nurse. For example, with what kind of patients has the nurse been most effective, and which ones proved most difficult? The clearer the applicant can be in articulating specific talents and deficiencies, the more closely the recruiter will be able to match the candidate to a position suited to his or her abilities. The closer these match, the more likely the employee will flourish and be able to use special talents.

It is not advisable to avoid the issue of weaknesses. Everyone has them. It is better to admit them, but to present them in a positive way. In addition, it may be helpful to tell the interviewer what is being done to correct weaknesses. For example, "Sometimes I tend to see the big picture and have to remind myself to pay more attention to the details. I've started keeping lists, and they seem helpful." Another suggestion might be, "I have limited bedside nursing experience, but I am excited about building on the clinical skills I have learned in school."

7. What Would You Do If . . .?

The recruiter probably will ask some situational questions related to decision making and critical thinking skills. The nurse will be asked to explain how to assess a particular situation, set priorities, decide what should be implemented first for a patient, and what can be delegated. Rather than fabricate an answer about unfamiliar circumstances, one can honestly say, "I've never been in that situation, but I think I would . . . ." or "I was in a similar situation in which . . . occurred, and this is what I did in that circumstance."

When an interviewer says, "Tell me about a time when . . ." or "Give me a specific example of . . .," he or she is conducting a behavioral interview. The applicant must be prepared to respond to these questions because many employers use a behavioral interview as part of the hiring process for nursing positions (LaMaster and Larsen, 2010). This type of job interview is based on the logic that past behavior predicts future behavior and seeks previous experience of required job-related behaviors. If the job requires the ability to analyze and find solutions to problems, then the candidate may be asked to provide an example of when he or she previously found solutions to a difficult problem. The question might be: "Tell me about a time when you faced a difficult problem. What steps did you take to solve that problem?" Examples may be taken from any context as long as they include the required behavior. The applicant should remember that there are no right or wrong answers to this question.

8. Why Should We Hire You?

This question gives the applicant an opportunity to share his or her special assets that the applicant would bring to the employer's institution. Without embellishment or selling oneself short, it is important to convey pride in being a nurse and conviction that one has something special to offer.

9. What Questions Do You Have?

Usually the interview ends with the interviewer asking whether the applicant has any questions. This is an opportunity for the applicant to demonstrate initiative, and he or she should take advantage of it, although not to excess. In an effective interview with an experienced interviewer, most questions regarding salary, benefits, and human resource policies will have been addressed (Box 27.7). If they have not been addressed, this is the time they should be asked about. Should a tour of the nursing unit and a meeting with the supervisor be arranged, many such concerns will be answered then.

Further Questions. Box 27.8 presents an additional list of open-ended interview questions that the applicant

BOX 27.7   What to Expect a Recruiter to Communicate

Recruiters should inform applicants of basic human resource policies regarding job descriptions, compensation, benefits, and staff development, including:

- Conditional period
- Job descriptions
- Shift rotation
- Weekend rotation
- Salary
- Staff development
- Parking
- Security
- Health insurance and other insurance benefits
- Preemployment physical examinations
- Credit union
- Overtime
- Scheduled paydays
- Paid time off
- Leaves of absence
- Employee discounts
- Transfer and promotion policies
- Resignation policies
- Preemployment policies
- Pay increases

BOX 27.8   Open-Ended Interview Questions

Applicants may expect to be asked a series of open-ended questions such as the following:

- How do you evaluate success?
- How would you describe yourself?
- Tell me about yourself.
- Tell me about something that's not on your résumé.
- What is your greatest strength?
- How will your greatest strength help you perform?
- What challenges are you looking for in a position?
- What are your goals for the future?
- How do you handle conflict?
- What is your greatest weakness?
- Why are you leaving your job?
- How do you handle stress and pressure?
- What motivates you?
- What do you find are the most difficult decisions to make?
- What are you passionate about?
- Why are you the best person for the job?

From Doyle, A. (2018b). Open-ended job interview questions and answers. The Balance: careers. Retrieved from https://www.thebalancecareers.com/open-ended-interview-questions-and-answers-2061635. Accessed July 26, 2018.

may be asked, and Box 27.9 lists questions appropriate for the applicant to ask. The more information gathered, the easier it will be to make a decision, and the more likely it is that the nurse will be happy in the long term.

BOX 27.9   Appropriate Questions for the Applicant to Ask

1. May I see the job description for the position we are discussing?
2. What is the nurse-to-patient ratio?
3. What support staff are available on the unit to assist nurses?
4. What about clerical help and support services? What nursing care delivery systems or models are practiced here (e.g., team nursing, primary nursing, centralized, decentralized)?
5. How available are physicians? Admitting physicians and house staff?
6. How often are nursing care conferences held on this unit?
7. What type of nursing documentation is used?
8. How long is the orientation program? What does the program include? What continuing education programs are available after my initial orientation?
9. How will my performance be evaluated? How often, and by whom?
10. What exact schedule or shift will I be working in this position?
11. What will my salary be? Is there a shift differential?
12. Are there differentiated practice levels or roles and differentiated pay scales for nursing congruent with differences in educational preparation, certification, and other advanced nursing preparation?
13. How are pay increases decided?
14. What other benefits are there (e.g., health, life insurance, vacation time, tuition reimbursement, retirement plan)?
15. What input do staff nurses have in decision making about nursing practice?

THE APPLICANT'S TASKS

Assess the Climate of the Work Environment

As mentioned in the discussion of researching potential employers, there are ways other than direct questioning to learn a lot about the institution. Every organization has its own personality and atmosphere. The first impression probably came from the secretary who answered the phone when the applicant called for an appointment with the recruiter, followed by the greeting on arrival at the recruiter's office. A tone of respect and pride in being associated with the organization may have been communicated in the first encounter. Every subsequent encounter builds on the first.

In the hallways of the agency, how do people acknowledge each other? A visit to the employee cafeteria to buy a cup of coffee or a sandwich at mealtime can be enlightening. Are nurses eating there? Does it seem that the staff members are enjoying themselves? The applicant should pick up for later reading any available in-house publications, such as employee newsletters or bulletins.

Ask for a Tour

If the interviewer does not automatically offer a tour of the unit, the applicant can request to see it and will certainly want to meet with the person who would be the immediate supervisor. Some employers arrange for the recruit to actually shadow a staff nurse for part of a shift. To get an accurate feel for the unit, the applicant should pay close attention to the pace, the tone of the staff interaction, and the morale. Is this a group the prospective employee would like to join? Are the manager's philosophy and management style similar to the applicant's own?

The astute applicant can get an accurate feel for the nursing unit's culture and personality by observing the manager's interactions with staff. Is the manager accessible to the staff and supportive in response to them? How are phone calls and other interruptions handled? How well do people seem to be getting along? The applicant should pay attention to the way people on the unit relate to each other—nurses to physicians, nurses to families, nurses to nurses. How are the patients responded to on the intercommunication system? The efficiency with which staff work should be noted. How rushed are they? Also, bulletin boards and any public displays of staff recognition (e.g., "employee of the month" plaques or brag boards) should be examined. Even a second visit to the unit might be requested before a final decision is made. The more information gathered, the easier it will be to make a decision (DeLuca and DeLuca, 2010).

Some managers offer opportunities for the applicant to meet with staff, and formal interviews with staff nurses may be scheduled as a routine part of the hiring process. Such experiences gives the applicant a closer view of the actual work organization and enables representative staff members a chance to have a voice in selecting new coworkers. Staff nurses provide bedside care to patients and best understand the qualities appreciated in a good team member. Whether the introduction to staff is a formal interview or a casual conference room encounter, the applicant can be made to feel welcome and wanted, while learning about the real work and the real workers of the agency. Now that firsthand knowledge has been obtained, if the applicant confers again with these employees and former employees are consulted before applying, he or she can ask more informed questions.

Follow-up

Thank-You Letter. A follow-up letter thanking the recruiter is a courtesy and a reminder of the nurse's interest in receiving a timely response. It is also a final chance for the applicant to make the case for being chosen for the role and to inquire about when a hiring decision will be made (Box 27.10). If the nurse does not hear from the employer within a reasonable length of time (1 to 2 weeks) after the interview, it is appropriate to inquire by phone about the status of a hiring decision.

Avoid Impulse Decisions. If offered a position and time is needed to make a decision, the applicant should postpone a decision and should not feel pressured into acceptance while still unsure. An offer to phone the recruiter with an answer within an agreed-on time is appropriate.

If there are other job opportunities, certainly comparisons need to be made by weighing the pros and cons

---

BOX 27.10   Interview Follow-up Letter

April 24, 2018

Ms. Donna Henderson, MS, RN
Director of Nurse Recruitment
Charleston Memorial Hospital
1600 Beckley Avenue
Memphis, TN 38104

Dear Ms. Henderson:

It was a pleasure meeting with you on Monday. I now have a clear picture of what I might expect as a new graduate nurse in your hospital. Everyone on the units I visited was very friendly.

I look forward to hearing from you with good news about a position at Charleston Memorial. I can be reached in the afternoons at 555-912-3120 or on my cell, 555-200-9999.

Thank you again for your time and interest.

Sincerely,
(Name signed here in pen)

Bonnie McCray Pino

of each position and each organization. How do benefits compare? What are the possibilities for lateral and vertical movement within the systems? How available are continuing education opportunities to staff nurses? How do observations of the work culture fit with the nurse's ideas of what is needed to support professional success? Does the schedule that is offered fit the applicant's lifestyle? When a decision has been reached, a phone call should be made promptly to the recruiter, whether the answer is yes or no.

Weighing Options. Applicants should take time to weigh options, especially if they have applied to several different organizations. It is not professional to accept a position while knowing one would resign if a more appealing offer came along. Employers invest significant resources in orienting a new nurse and should expect a commitment rather than the casual attitude of "I'll keep this job until the job I really want becomes available." What questions might one ask oneself while weighing the merits of one position against others? Remembering that no job is perfect, the following four questions should be considered. Box 27.11 further helps applicants evaluate potential employment opportunities.

BOX 27.11   Assessment Tool for Decision Making

When weighing options for employment, those measures of a professional work climate that are evident in written documentation and visible in the patient care areas should be considered. The following observations should guide the new graduate in making an informed decision.

- Standards of nursing practice are evident and are an integral part of patient care.
- Nurse-to-patient ratio is adequate and adjusted for patient acuity.
- Orientation is structured, individualized, and adequate for new graduates.
- Opportunities for horizontal transfer and advancement exist within the system.
- The salary is competitive and reasonable.
- Benefits are competitive.
- Continuing education is available, and staff members are encouraged to attend.
- A nurse administrator is responsible for delivery of nursing services.

Does the position match the nurse's qualifications? Although it is flattering to receive a job offer for a position for which a nurse has little or no preparation, one should not be influenced by such a compliment. When there is a nursing shortage, a position that is beyond an applicant's present skills and experience may sound wonderfully challenging, but in actuality it may be overwhelming and a disastrous beginning for a new graduate. Being overzealous, overconfident, and overeager to please can only lead to feelings of guilt and inadequacy if the job is not appropriate. It is wiser to accept a position in which adequate orientation and clinical support exist, which would allow the graduate to gain the experience and preparation necessary to accept a position requiring more skills at a later time.

What are the actual responsibilities of the job? The newly hired nurse has the right to completely understand what will be expected in the position offered, including the overall and daily responsibilities and the length and nature of on-the-job training that will be provided. What will be the supervisory responsibilities? How many and what skill level of employees will be under the RN's leadership? What orientation is planned to prepare the RN for practicing independently? Are there arrangements for a preceptor to guide the graduate through the difficult transition of entering a first nursing job? Reality shock can be anticipated, and the more assistance a new graduate receives in adjusting to the new role of the nurse, the more likely the beginner is to be successful and satisfied.

Does this position lead the nurse in the direction of projected career goals? Is the offered job a step toward meeting long-term career objectives? For example, a graduate who wants to be a nurse-midwife would be wiser to accept a position in postpartum if labor and delivery is not available, rather than a position in neurosurgery just because it offers a slightly higher salary or a few more weekends. No position or job change should be accidental or the result of a snap decision. Wise career moves result from deliberate planning and purposeful preparation.

How will the work be compensated? Experienced nurses often advise novices that money, although important, is not the only reward associated with a job. However, money does matter, especially to a new graduate who may have subsisted on a limited income while in school. It is common for loans to have accumulated, along with unpaid bills. Inadequate salary can be a real source of job dissatisfaction, of course, but because of the 24-hour responsibilities in health care, nurses traditionally have basic salaries that include other income-contributing factors, such as shift differentials, weekend differentials, holiday pay, paid vacation days, and expected salary increases over time. Compensation comes in other packages besides paychecks. There are policies that allow for maternity leaves, medical leaves, tuition reimbursement, sick days, discounts on prescriptions and health insurance, retirement benefits, and malpractice insurance coverage, all of which affect income in indirect but important ways. As is true in other areas of consideration, the better the total compensation package fits one's needs, the greater the likelihood that one will remain satisfied with the job.

Well-prepared job applicants will have listed those benefits they consider essential, and these vary with individual circumstances. For example, the essentials for someone who is the sole family breadwinner probably include health insurance, paid time off, and an employer-provided retirement plan. Available child care would be especially important for parents of preschool children.

THE EMPLOYER'S TASKS

In any agency providing nursing services, its nurses are the indispensable employees. The selection of new nurse employees is a critically important responsibility, and it is the recruiter's duty to make sure the best selection is made.

First, the nurse must meet the minimal requirements for the position desired. For example, 1 year of experience might be required for a nurse to work a weekender program or in a critical care area. Operating room (OR) experience may be required for OR nursing positions, and perinatal nursing experience may be required for labor and delivery positions. A secondary consideration is the nurse's suitability for contributing to the mission of the health care delivery system. The recruiter is selling the organization to the applicant and measuring the skills and aptitudes the applicant would bring to the organization.

The bottom line for any employer who provides health care services to the public is to ensure that its nursing staff practices safely. Recruiters are looking to uncover anything that would impair a nurse applicant's ability to provide safe nursing care, such as incompetence, unprofessional conduct, unreliability in attendance, chemical dependency, or record of criminal activity. For screening, recruiters have four primary sources of information: the application, interview impressions, test results, and references.

Applications are validated. Work history and references are checked to ensure accuracy. Many employers are checking credit history because they may assume that an individual who has good credit is reliable and accountable and will likely be a dependable nurse. Previous supervisors are asked about attendance, dependability, performance, attitude, ability to get along with others, integrity, and eligibility for rehire. The applicant's stated reason for termination is compared with information obtained from work references. The employer has a right to obtain reasonable information about the people who are hired. Most employment applications ask whether the applicant has ever been convicted of a crime other than a minor traffic violation. The question is about convictions, not arrests, and the response is verified by a background or criminal record check. Response to this or any other question in the application process must be honest and truthful. Each institution has its own policies regarding convictions, but most are vitally concerned about their responsibilities regarding negligent hiring. The applicant is rejected if he or she committed a crime that, if repeated while in the employ of the institution, would cause harm to patients, families, other employees, or the institution.

A physical examination is often required. It usually is performed on-site and at the employer's expense. It may involve obtaining the applicant's full medical history and vital signs, routine blood tests, a urine drug screen, and sometimes a chest radiograph. The purpose of the examination is to provide protection for patients and to ensure that the caregiver can carry out the necessary physical responsibilities of the job. For example, are illegal mood-altering substances evident that would impair the nurse's abilities and judgment? Are there physical limitations the institution should know about to determine whether any special accommodations are necessary to allow the candidate to perform the usual duties associated with the position? Employers may do job function matching, a process to determine whether the applicant has the physical capability to perform functions such as bending or stooping required by a specific job. Psychological testing is also frequently part of the preemployment screening process.

Even with a job offer made and a date for employment set, actual start dates are contingent on receipt of documentation of these final screenings, plus a reference check to verify the résumé; these items establish the practitioner's safety and reliability. Other parts of screening for safety might include paper-and-pencil testing, such as skills tests, pharmacology tests, and, in some cases, personality testing and psychological testing for specialty areas.

Although a preemployment pharmacology test is becoming less common than in past years, many institutions still give such a quiz to determine basic knowledge of routinely administered medications, their purposes, and their side effects. Simple dosage questions and calculation methods may be asked. Some questions may be situational ones, such as, "What would you do in this case?" or "The first nursing action in this scenario should be . . . ."

A few larger institutions also may administer a clinical skills test. Such a test might be conducted in a simulated laboratory setting, where frequently used patient care equipment is set up. Usually a staff development instructor accompanies the nurse through a series of stations where the nurse is asked to plan and perform the appropriate nursing actions. Examples might be starting cardiopulmonary resuscitation on a simulated patient, demonstrating the proper procedure for starting an intravenous line, and talking through the assessment of a patient.

It is far better to be prepared and even better to be proactive and to offer to produce some of the documentation required. For instance, the nurse may be able to get a written reference from a former employer or a statement from a physician sooner than the institution can. The employment start date depends on the receipt of all necessary information, so it will expedite the process if the candidate volunteers to initiate some of the documentation gathering or even has references in hand with other documentation at the time of interview.

Once an applicant is selected, the agency has committed itself to costly training, orientation, and additional benefits that may cost as much as 30% to 40% of the employee's salary. A major element of control, which any organization possesses, is its ability to choose its employees. A thorough selection process is a sign to the committed professional that this is a reputable employer.

SUMMARY

If not offered a position, the new graduate should still feel good about himself or herself. There may have been several candidates for that same position. Perhaps it was not the best match for one's skills or preferences. There is victory in having had an opportunity to practice interview skills. Preparation, practice, and perseverance will reward the nurse with a job that is best suited to his or her personality, values, qualifications, and skills. New graduates have internalized standards of practice from their nursing education experience. On graduation, they must decide where to begin to put these standards to work in real-life terms handling real responsibilities with real patients. The question becomes, "Can school and work values be reconciled in this nursing environment?" When adequate groundwork in pursuit of a job has been laid, the answer should come easily.

REFERENCES

American Association of Colleges of Nursing Task Force on Hallmarks of the Professional Practice Setting. (n.d.a). *Hallmarks of the professional practice environment.* Retrieved from http://www.aacnnursing.org/News-Information/Position-Statements-White-Papers/Hallmarks-Practice. Accessed April 2018.

American Association of Colleges of Nursing. (n.d.b). *What every nursing student should know when seeking employment.* Retrieved from *http://www.aacnnursing.org/Portals/42/Student/what-every-nursing-student-should-know-when-seeking-employment.pdf?ver=2017-07-28-083316-627.*

Bauer, J. (2013). *The essential interview handbook.* Prompton Plains, New Jersey: Career Press.

Birks, M., Hartin, P., Woods, C., Emmanuel, E., & Hitchins, M. (2016). Students' perceptions of the use of eportfolios in nursing and midwifery education. *Nurse Education in Practice, 18,* 46–51.

DeLuca, M., & Deluca, N. (2010). *Stand out and get hired: Best answers to the 201 most frequently asked interview questions* (2nd ed.). New York: The McGraw Hill Companies, Inc.

Doyle, A. (2018a). *Tips on using skype for video job interviews.* Updated September 09, 2016. Retrieved from https://www.thebalance.com/video-interviewing-with-skype-2061627. Accessed January 17, 2018.

Doyle, A. *The Balance.* (2018b). Updated 2018. Retrieved from http://www.aacnnursing.org/Portals/42/Student/what-every-nursing-student-should-know-when-seeking-employment.pdf?ver=2017-07-28-083316-627. Accessed January 17, 2018.

LaMaster, M. A., & Larsen, R. A. (2010). Prepare for a behavioral interview, then ace it! *American Journal of Nursing,* *40*(1), 8–10.

Nursing Solutions, Inc. (2018). *Permanent Nurses, Permanent Solutions! National Healthcare Retention & RN Staffing Report.* Published by: NSI Nursing Solutions, Inc. Retrieved from http://www.nsinursingsolutions.com/Files/assets/library/retention-institute/NationalHealthcareRNRetentionReport2018.pdf. Accessed July 26, 2018.

Pagana, K. (2012). Ten tips for handling job interviews by phone. *American Nurse Today,* *7*(1), 40–41.

Renter, M., & Allen, A. (2014). How Magnet® designation affects nurse retention: an evidence-based research project. *American Nurse Today,* *9*(3). Retrieved from https://www.americannursetoday.com/how-magnet-designation-affects-nurse-retention-an-evidence-based-research-project/.

28

The NCLEX-RN® Examination

Tommie L. Norris, DNS, RN

Adequate preparation for the NCLEX-RN examination can reduce panic and ensure success.

ⓔ Additional resources are available online at: *http://evolve.elsevier.com/Cherry/*

LEARNING OUTCOMES

After studying this chapter, the reader will be able to:

1. Explain the purpose of the NCLEX-RN examination.
2. Evaluate various methods of preparation for the NCLEX-RN examination.
3. Create a personal plan for preparing for the NCLEX-RN examination.
4. Analyze the relationship between the nursing process and client needs as they relate to NCLEX-RN test items.
5. Compare various review courses designed to aid in review for the NCLEX-RN examination.
6. Use the NCLEX-RN Test Plan to plan review and remediation strategies.

KEY TERMS

Computer adaptive testing (CAT) A type of testing taken on a computer, in which a person is given a test question to answer, followed by a subsequent question the level of which depends on whether the candidate correctly answered the first question.

National Council of State Board of Nursing An independent not-for-profit organization that supports boards of nursing by monitoring trends in nursing practice and develops the licensing examination for both registered and practical nursing.

NCLEX-RN NCLEX stands for National Council Licensure Examination for Registered Nurses, an examination taken by qualified graduates of approved schools of nursing. Graduates who pass the NCLEX-RN are granted licenses to practice as RNs.

PROFESSIONAL/ETHICAL ISSUE

Jamie Wilcox, senior nursing student, just left a meeting with the director of her Bachelor of Science in Nursing (BSN) program. Jamie was devastated. She just learned that she would not graduate in a few weeks as planned because her score on the final standardized exam was not high enough and, according to the program director, was a predictor that she might not pass the NCLEX. Jamie did not realize there was so much at stake when she took the standardized exam, and she admitted to herself that she really did not prepare or take the exam seriously. After all, she had passed every course in the nursing program; her grades were not outstanding, but they were passing. She wondered, can this be fair? Was this high-stakes testing even ethical?

Over the next week Jamie learned more about standardized exams. She learned they were used at various points throughout the nursing school curriculum to provide students and faculty with insight into how a student's performance compares with other student's at other schools. These exams also provide individual assessment by noting a student's strengths and weaknesses and are used to develop remediation plans. Standardized exams are often used by nursing schools to predict the chance for being successful on the NCLEX-RN and to determine whether a student will graduate, so they are considered "high stakes." However, she also learned that standardized exams are just "predictors" or, at best, estimates of future performance. Standardized exams lack the sophistication of computerized adaptive testing, so comparing them to the NCLEX may prevent qualified students from graduating or taking the NCLEX. Although Jamie was determined to be successful in completing her remediation plan and performing well on the next standardized exam, she still had many questions about such "high-stakes" testing.

- What responsibility belongs with the nursing program that progressed a student through the program but then deemed a student ineligible to graduate because of his/her performance on a standardized exam?
- What responsibility lies with the student who had poor performance on a standardized exam?
- Should standardized exams become the "standard" that determines whether a student should graduate from nursing school? Why or why not?

VIGNETTE

Consider for a moment how nursing and licensure examinations have changed as society has changed. Nursing is a reflection of society's values, knowledge, and needs. Test items or questions found on the NCLEX-RN examination today have little resemblance to questions asked on state board examinations administered during the early part of the twentieth century. The examinations of that era dealt with practical issues and consisted mainly of knowledge-based questions that had little to do with assessment, application, evaluation, or need. Consider, for instance, the following questions taken

from the 1919 state board questions and answers for nurses (Foote, 1919):

- What are the advantages of fireplaces?
- How would you sterilize silkworm-gut and silk sutures?
- What care regarding nourishment would you give a gynecological patient to prevent a common discomfort?
- Give some general rules for preparing meats.
- Give three common complaints that the public makes about graduate nurses.

Questions to Consider While Reading this Chapter:

1. What is the purpose of the NCLEX-RN examination?
2. What type of questions can I expect on today's NCLEX-RN examination?
3. What is the best way to prepare for the examination?

CHAPTER OVERVIEW

This chapter helps student nurses prepare to successfully pass the NCLEX-RN examination. The purpose of the NCLEX-RN is discussed, and an overview of the format and content is given. Various strategies for preparing for the examination are given, and students are encouraged to develop a personal plan of study.

ARE YOU PREPARED FOR THE NCLEX-RN EXAMINATION?

You are pursuing a degree in nursing and plan to take the NCLEX-RN licensure examination after graduation. Do you know what to expect on the examination itself? Do you feel you have the knowledge necessary for NCLEX-RN examination success? If not, you should be interested in this chapter, which offers an overview of the format and content you can expect on the test and strategies for success.

THE NCLEX-RN EXAMINATION

The NCLEX-RN examination and licensure to practice nursing go hand in hand. To receive a license to practice as a registered nurse (RN) in the United States and its territories, candidates must furnish evidence of competency to provide safe and effective nursing care by successfully completing the NCLEX-RN examination

(National Council of State Boards of Nursing [NCSBN], 2016a).

There are three types of RN programs: (1) 2-year associate degree programs usually found in community or junior colleges, (2) hospital-based diploma programs, and (3) baccalaureate degree or higher programs found in 4-year colleges and universities or academic health centers. Graduates from all programs take the same NCLEX-RN examination. The examination content common to all of these programs is job related and reflects current entry-level nursing practice (NCSBN, 2016a). Individuals taking the examination must have graduated from approved schools of nursing.

In January 2015, the NCLEX-RN became the licensure/registration examination for Canadian provinces and territories (NCSBN, 2014). Prior to 2015, Canadian RN applicants were required to take the Canadian Registered Nurse Examination (CRNE). The pass rate for Canadian graduates on the NCLEX-RN January to June 2016 was 81.2%, surpassing that on the 2014 CRNE, which was 79.0% (College of Nurses of Ontario, 2017).

Purpose of the NCLEX-RN Examination

The purpose of the NCLEX-RN examination is to:
1. Safeguard the public from unsafe practitioners.
2. Assist state boards of nursing in determining candidates' capabilities for performing entry-level RN positions.

To keep the NCLEX-RN examination current, the NCSBN conducts a practice analysis on a 3-year cycle by investigating current practice that entry-level nurses are performing in various health care settings in the United States. In the most current practice analysis completed in 2014, newly licensed nurses (n = 3699) were asked to prioritize 139 nursing care activities and state how often they perform them (NCSBN, 2015). The survey was sent by either paper version or web-based survey, with participants evaluating between 46 and 70 activities. Results showed that the greatest amount of time was spent in management of care (17.6%), psychologic adaptation (13.8%), and pharmacologic and parenteral therapies (13.2%). Most care was provided for clients with acutely ill conditions (50%), clients with unstable chronic conditions (29.0%), and clients with behavioral conditions (25.3%). Care for older clients, aged 65 to 85 (54.3%), was most often reported. The majority of respondents (72%) continue to work in hospitals. A panel

of 12 RNs serving as subject matter experts (SMEs) helped to create the practice analysis survey; nurses on this panel worked with or supervised RNs within the first 6 months of practice or were themselves new RNs (NCSBN, 2015). The SMEs created a list of activities performed by newly licensed nurses using job descriptions, activity logs kept by newly licensed RNs, performance evaluation documents, and their own knowledge of newly licensed RN practice. This list of activities eventually became the 139 items used in the practice analysis survey. To view the latest practice analysis, visit the NCSBN website (https://www.ncsbn.org/nclex) and click on Practice Analyses.

Characteristics of the NCLEX-RN Examination. The NCLEX-RN examination is a pass-fail examination and has been computerized since 1994. Before that time, it was a paper-and-pencil examination requiring 2 days to complete. Today the examination is offered at Pearson Professional Centers throughout the United States, American Samoa, Guam, Northern Mariana Islands, and the U.S. Virgin Islands. International scheduling is also available. It can be taken at the candidate's convenience and can be completed in 6 hours or less, which includes examination instructions and breaks. The official results of the examination are sent to candidates within 6 weeks after they have taken the examination. Unofficial results are available on the NCLEX candidate website (www.pearsonvue.com/nclex) after 2 business days for an additional fee if the candidate's board of nursing participates in "Quick Results Service." Candidates may also check their state board's website for licensure verification.

Computer Adaptive Testing. The NCLEX-RN examination uses computer adaptive testing (CAT), a test-administering technique that uses computer technology and measurement theory. As a candidate answers questions on the examination, CAT adapts to the level of the candidate's knowledge, skills, and ability. After a candidate answers a question at a particular level of difficulty, the computer selects the next item that the candidate should have a 50% chance of answering correctly. All examinations are consistent with the NCLEX-RN examination Test Plan, which controls inclusion of nursing content. Candidates have ample opportunity to demonstrate their competence because the examination does not end until stability of the pass or fail result is certain or time runs out (NCSBN, 2018).

Candidates taking the examination answer a minimum of 75 questions to a maximum of 265 questions. The NCSBN (2018) advises that the length of an NCLEX-RN examination be based on the performance of the candidate on the examination and has established a goal to be 95% sure of pass-fail decisions. The computer determines whether a candidate passes or fails according to the following three rules:

1. *95% confidence interval rule:* 95% certainty that the candidate's ability is obviously above or below the passing standard.
2. *Maximum-length examination rule:* When the candidate is very close to the passing standard, the computer continues to give test items until the maximum number of items is reached; at this point, the computer disregards the 95% confidence rule and considers only the final ability estimate.
3. *Run-out-of-time rule:* The candidate runs out of time, and the 95% confidence interval has not been determined. If the candidate has not answered the minimum number of questions, then he or she fails; if the candidate has answered the minimum number of questions, the computer analyzes the last 60 questions to determine whether these questions were above or below the passing standard.

It is important for students to understand that the goal of CAT is to determine competency based on the difficulty of questions answered correctly rather than on the number of questions answered correctly. The CAT is individualized, and two people taking the examination at the same time will not have the same questions. The candidate moves from easy to difficult questions and then defaults back to easy questions if a harder question is missed. The point at which the candidate has answered half the questions correctly is identified, and the competency level is determined on the basis of the difficulty level of those questions. To learn more about CAT, view a short video, NCLEX Using CAT, on the NCSBN website (https://www.ncsbn.org/1216.htm).

A tutorial is administered before the examination actually begins, providing candidates with experience in using the computer in CAT situations and explaining various question formats that may be presented in the exam. Candidates should carefully read an entire question and all possible answer options before selecting an answer. Candidates may request assistance regarding the use of the computer at any point, even during the NCLEX-RN examination. In addition, they may find it helpful to view the valuable information about NCLEX and CAT found on the NCSBN website (https://www.ncsbn.org).

Skipping Questions and Changing Answers. Candidates taking the NCLEX-RN examination are not allowed to skip questions and return to them at a later time or to change the answer to a question once the answer has been selected and entered into the computer. These actions would defeat the purpose of adaptive testing, because CAT selects questions according to the examination taker's knowledge, skills, and abilities.

Question Format

All of the information needed to answer a particular question appears on one computer screen, so candidates do not need to see the previous or next screen to determine the answer. Questions are presented in traditional top-down format, in which the question is presented, followed by the potential answers to it. Candidates receive test items in a variety of formats, including traditional multiple choice, multiple response, ordered response, fill-in-the-blank calculations, and/or hot spots. Recently items have also included charts, graphics, sound, video, tables, and multimedia.

Traditional Format: Multiple-Choice, One Option. With this type of format, the candidate is presented with a question followed by four possible responses. The candidate is asked to select the one option that best answers the question. Multiple-choice, one-option format is the style most commonly used on the examination. See the following example.

*The nurse has received the following information about assigned clients. The nurse should assess which client **first**?*
a) A 64-year-old client who had a total knee replacement 3 hours ago and has 15 mL of serosanguineous drainage in the collection device.
b) A 32-year-old client who had closed reduction of a fractured right malleolus 5 hours ago and has swelling of the right toes.
c) A 9-month-old client admitted 6 hours ago with vomiting; whose vital signs are temperature, 37.6° C (99.7° F); pulse, 124; respirations, 26.
d) A 6-week-old client who was admitted 2 hours ago with nasal flaring and has a pulse oximetry reading of 90%.
(Answer: d)

Alternate Item Formats

Because of the nature of CAT, the type of item presented to the candidate will depend on the content area.

- *Hot spot (questions based on illustrations and charts):* With the hot spot item, the candidate is asked to identify one or more area(s) on a picture or graphic and answer using the mouse button when the cursor is over the area identified. See the following example:

The nurse palpates the point of maximum impulse as part of the assessment exam. Where would the nurse locate the point of maximal impulse (PMI)?
1. A
2. B
3. C
4. D
   (Answer: D)

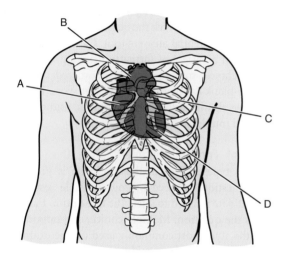

- *Multiple-response, multiple-choice:* The candidate is presented with a question followed by five or more responses. The candidate is asked to check all responses that are correct; partial credit is not given. See the following example:

A nurse is caring for a 47-year-old female client who has been diagnosed with hypothyroidism. Which manifestations might the nurse expect the client to report? (Select all that apply.)
a) Intolerance to heat
b) Periorbital edema
c) Weight loss
d) Menorrhagia
e) Constipation
f) Fatigue
   (Answer: b, d, e, and f)

- *Fill-in-the-blank:* The candidate is presented with a question to which the answer must be typed, instead of selecting from among a set of four options. The candidate may be asked to calculate values, such as dosages. A drop-down calculator is available for the candidate to use. See the following example:

A nurse is completing the intake and output record for a client who had a left total knee replacement 1 day ago. The client has had the following intake and output during the shift:
Intake:
3 oz apple juice
½ serving oatmeal
8 ounces water
1 cup fruit-flavored gelatin
½ cup beef broth
800 mL of 0.45 sodium chloride (half-strength saline), IV
Output:
1200 mL of urine
50 mL from the drainage tube
   How many milliliters should the nurse document as the client's intake?
   (Answer: 1490 mL)

- *Ordered response "Drag and drop" (prioritize):* The candidate is presented with a set of responses to a question and asked to place them in logical order or to prioritize them. See the following example:

A nurse is preparing to perform a sterile dressing change. In what order would the following steps be performed?
1) Gather supplies.
2) Set up the sterile field.
3) Assess the wound.
4) Explain the procedure to the patient.
5) Remove the soiled dressing.
6) Document the dressing change.
   Candidates will be asked to click on the steps and drag items in the correct order.
   (Answer: 1 4 5 3 2 6)

- *Chart exhibit:* The candidate is asked to seek additional information in a patient's chart to answer the question. See the following example, in which the candidate must look in the chart to find pertinent information to report:

A patient is ordered Lanoxin 0.25 mg daily. The nurse assesses the patient's heart rate as 48 beats per minute. Prior to calling the physician, what additional information is needed?
a) Potassium 2.8 mEq/L
b) Arterial blood gases (Pao₂) 95
c) History of kidney stones
d) Diet: 1800 calorie
   (Answer: a)

- *Audio:* Each candidate is furnished with earphones and listens to an audio clip. The candidate is asked to identify specific assessment findings. See the following example:

Candidate listens to an adventitious breath sound such as crackles.
   Candidate is asked to identify the abnormal finding.

- *Graphic option identification:* The candidate is presented with options that are either pictures or graphic images rather than text.

Candidates should note that any of the item formats, including standard multiple-choice items, may include tables, graphic images, or charts. More information about alternate item formats can be found on the NCSBN website.

COGNITIVE DOMAINS AND THE NCLEX-RN EXAMINATION

NCLEX-RN examination questions use Bloom's original cognitive levels—knowledge, comprehension, application, and analysis; however, the revised taxonomy—remember, understand, apply, analyze, evaluate, and create (Anderson and Krathwohl, 2001; Bloom et al, 1956)—can be applied. One primary difference between the two versions is that the original version uses nouns whereas the revised version uses verbs (Table 28.1). These levels may be viewed as consecutive steps, with knowledge (remembering) being the lowest, most fundamental step and analysis (analyzing) being the highest, most highly evolved of the steps. Because nursing requires application of knowledge, skills, and abilities, the majority of NCLEX-RN examination questions are written at the application or higher cognitive and critical thinking skills levels (NCSBN, 2016a).

TABLE 28.1 Comparison of Original and Revised Versions of Bloom's Taxonomy

Original Bloom's Taxonomy	Revised Bloom's Taxonomy
Evaluation	Creating
Synthesis	Evaluating
Analysis	Analyzing
Application	Applying
Comprehension	Understanding
Knowledge	Remembering

Knowledge Questions *(Remember)*

Knowledge is the lowest and simplest level of learning within the cognitive domain, and it is demonstrated by remembering or recalling information. This may include knowing selected facts, such as normal range of laboratory values, or common terminology, such as dyspnea. Giving definitions and examples are common skills at this cognitive level because this level requires no understanding or judgment. Following is an example of a knowledge level question:

The nurse reviewing a patient's laboratory values identifies which report as the normal range for serum potassium measured in mEq/L?
a) 0.5 to 2.5
b) 3.5 to 5.5
c) 6.0 to 8.0
d) 10.0 to 12.0
   (Answer: b)

Comprehension Questions *(Understand)*

Comprehension, the second level of Bloom's cognitive domain, is the fundamental level of understanding or the ability to grasp or summarize information or material or to restate it in one's own words. Following is an example of a comprehension level question:

A patient is ordered a clear liquid diet. The nurse can offer the patient which items on the food tray?
a) Orange juice
b) Lime Jell-O
c) Skim milk
d) Tomato soup
   (Answer: b)

Application Questions *(Apply)*

The third cognitive level, application, refers to the ability to use learned information in new situations. This level involves applying abstract theories and principles in new concrete or practical situations, solving mathematical problems, constructing charts and graphs, and making inferences. Information learned is applied to deliver safe and effective nursing care. The following is an example of an application level question:

> *An adult patient with a history of alcoholism, 24 hours after gastric resection surgery, is complaining of pain rated as 9 on a scale of 1 to 10, with 10 being most severe. The nurse reviews the orders and prepares to administer morphine 2 mg intramuscularly. Before administration of pain medication, which assessment is a priority that must be completed by the RN?*
> a) Bowel sounds and degree of nausea
> b) Respiratory rate and level of consciousness
> c) Heart rate and ambulatory status
> d) History of addiction to narcotics and potassium level
> *(Answer: b)*

Analysis Questions *(Analyze)*

The highest cognitive level used on the NCLEX-RN examination, analysis, requires complex thought processes and involves the ability to reduce material into its fundamental parts so that relationships may be understood. Examination questions at this level are questions that require drawing conclusions, setting priorities, forming hypotheses, and creating something new. The majority of items are written at the application level or higher because the practice of nursing necessitates that nurses apply knowledge, skills, and abilities to problem solve. The following is an example of a question written at the analysis level:

> *A patient exhibits tetany and the presence of Trousseau sign. The following lab values were reported: sodium 140 mg/dL, potassium 5 mEq/mL, calcium 8 mg/dL, and magnesium 3 mg/dL. These clinical manifestations and laboratory findings are consistent with which electrolyte disorder?*
> a) Hyponatremia
> b) Hypomagnesemia
> c) Hypocalcemia
> d) Hypokalemia
> *(Answer: c)*

COMPONENTS OF THE NCLEX-RN TEST PLAN

The Test Plan for the NCLEX-RN examination is based on the current nursing practice of entry-level RNs. According to the NCSBN (2016a), "The NCLEX assesses the knowledge, skills and abilities that are essential for the entry-level nurse to use in order to meet the needs of clients requiring the promotion, maintenance or restoration of health (p. 3)." The NCLEX-RN Test Plan is framed by four major categories of client needs, which are further subdivided into a total of six subcategories, as follows (NCSBN, 2016a):

1. Safe, effective care environment
   - Management of care
   - Safety and infection control
2. Health promotion and maintenance
3. Psychosocial integrity
4. Physiologic integrity
   - Basic care and comfort
   - Pharmacologic and parenteral therapies
   - Reduction of risk potential
   - Physiologic adaptation

Each of these will be examined individually here, followed by a discussion of several processes that are fundamental to nursing and integrated throughout the client needs categories and subcategories.

Client Needs

"The goal of nursing for client care in any setting is preventing illnesses and potential complications; alleviating suffering; protecting, promoting, restoring, and facilitating comfort and health; and dignity in dying" (NCSBN, 2016a, p. 4). The organizing framework of the NCLEX-RN examination is client needs, a broad component that "provides a universal structure for defining nursing actions and competencies, and focuses on clients in all settings" (NCSBN, 2016a, p. 4).

Safe and Effective Care Environment. The category safe and effective care environment pertains to the provision and direction of nursing care delivery to safeguard clients, their families or significant others, and health care providers. It is further divided into two subcategories, management of care, from which 17% to 23% of the Test Plan is constructed, and safety and infection control, from which 9% to 15% of the Test Plan is constructed (NCSBN, 2016a). Within this section, the nurse should have the knowledge, skills, and ability to meet the client's needs for a safe and effective environment.

Health Promotion and Maintenance.

The health promotion and maintenance category pertains to the provision and direction of nursing care that takes into consideration the projected growth and development principles, early detection and prevention of health problems, techniques of physical assessment, and plans to realize best possible health care outcomes. Six percent to 12% of NCLEX-RN examination questions are related to this category.

Psychosocial Integrity.

In the psychosocial integrity category, "The nurse provides and directs nursing care that promotes and supports the emotional, mental, and social well-being of the client experiencing stressful events, as well as clients with acute or chronic mental illness" (NCSBN, 2016a, p. 7). Psychosocial integrity is addressed in 6% to 12% of NCLEX-RN examination questions.

Physiologic Integrity.

The physical aspects of health and wellness are the focus of physiologic integrity. This category is further divided into four subcategories:

Basic care and comfort, accounting for 6% to 12% of examination questions, is directed at the provision of comfort and assistance in performing activities of daily living. A new addition under this category for the 2016 Test Plan was the inclusion of complimentary therapies, including their contraindications.

The pharmacologic and parenteral therapies subcategory, to which 12% to 18% of NCLEX questions are devoted, is concerned with administration of medications and parenteral therapies. For 2016, handling and maintaining medication in a safe controlled environment were added.

Reduction of risk potential, addressed in 9% to 15% of the questions, correlates with reducing the risk of development of complications related to clients' current conditions or treatments. Providing intraoperative care was deleted from the 2016 Test Plan.

Physiologic adaptation, accounting for 11% to 17% of examination questions, is the management or coordination of care for clients with acute or chronic and life-threatening disease processes (NCSBN, 2016a).

Integrated Processes

Processes that are fundamental to nursing are integrated throughout the previously noted client needs categories and subcategories (NCSBN, 2016a):

- Nursing process
- Caring
- Communication and documentation
- Teaching and learning
- Culture and spirituality

For example, a health promotion and maintenance question also involves assessment or a psychosocial integrity question that also addresses implementation. All questions relate to some activity in which an entry-level nurse may engage when caring for or managing a patient. A more complete overview of these integrated processes follows.

Nursing Process.

Success on the NCLEX-RN examination relies on a sound working knowledge of the nursing process. The NCSBN (2016a) defines the nursing process as "a scientific, clinical reasoning approach to client care that includes assessment, analysis, planning, implementation, and evaluation" (p. 5). The nursing process is applicable to all situations in which the nurse and patient interact and may be used with any theoretic framework.

Assessment. The first step of the nursing process, assessment establishes a database for the client. Just as the nursing process provides a foundation for nursing practice, assessment provides the foundation for the nursing process. Assessment consists of gathering information or data about an identified client. Depending on the nurse's focus, the client may be a person, a family, a group of people, or a community.

Information about a client comes from a variety of sources, including the client, the family and significant others, laboratory or radiographic reports, physician records, hospital or clinic records, and other caregivers. Client data are typically classified as subjective and objective. Simply put, subjective data are the client's perception or understanding of a specific event or phenomenon. It is his or her opinion, such as the degree of pain experienced during an episode of angina. Objective data are observable and measurable by the nurse and come from various patient records. Blood pressure, heart rate, and the presence or absence of edema are examples of objective data.

Assessment also includes verification and communication of data. Seeking additional client-related information, such as laboratory work or talking with the family, may confirm data. Communication of data may be accomplished by verbal report to other health care workers or by written or computerized record.

Analysis. Analysis is the second step of the nursing process. Client-related data gathered during assessment provide the basis for analysis. During this step, the nurse classifies or groups assessment data and identifies actual or potential client problems. During classification, data also are validated and interpreted, and additional data may be required.

Planning. Planning, the third step of the nursing process, consists of setting realistic and measurable mutual goals, developing interventions to meet or resolve identified patient needs or problems, and modifying goals as necessary. Included in planning of care are ranking nursing diagnoses, documenting expected outcomes for each goal, and setting realistic target dates for the accomplishment of each goal. Goal setting should include the collaboration of members of the interdisciplinary health care team, the client, his or her family, and significant others as indicated. As with the previous steps of the nursing process, the plan must be communicated to other members of the health care team to ensure continuity of care.

Implementation. The fourth step of the nursing process is implementation. It includes initiating and carrying out nursing interventions or nursing actions to achieve the goals set in the planning stage of the nursing process. The nurse implements interventions that will allow the patient to achieve goals and outcomes to support or improve the patient's health status (Potter and Perry, 2013).

Evaluation. To evaluate, data must be collected to document the progress the patient has made, or not made, in relation to the stated goal. Once data have been collected and analyzed, the nurse must decide what action to take or what modification to make regarding the goal. Using evidence, the nurse makes a judgment to determine whether the established outcome has met the actual response.

Caring. The NCSBN defines caring as "the interaction of the nurse and client in an atmosphere of mutual respect and trust. In this collaborative environment, the nurse provides encouragement, hope, support and compassion to help achieve desired outcomes" (NCSBN, 2016a, p.5).

Communication and Documentation. The NCSBN defines communication and documentation as "the verbal and nonverbal interactions between the nurse and the client, the client's significant others and the other members of the health care team. Events and activities associated with client care are validated in written and/or electronic records that reflect standards of practice and accountability in the provision of care" (NCSBN, 2016a, p. 5).

Teaching and Learning. The NCSBN defines teaching and learning as "facilitation of the acquisition of knowledge, skills and attitudes promoting a change in behavior" (NCSBN, 2016a, p. 5).

Culture and Spirituality. The NCSBN defines culture and spirituality as the regard for the unique and personal preferences for care, the applicable standard of care, and legal requirements (NCSBN, 2016a).

PREPARING FOR THE NCLEX-RN EXAMINATION

NCLEX is a "high-stakes" examination to evaluate nursing competence and protect the public. There is much debate concerning the use of similar high-stakes examinations used in nursing schools for progression, graduation, or eligibility to take the NCLEX. Because there are no universally accepted standards on using predictive tests, schools are debating best practices. The National League for Nursing and the American Association of Colleges of Nursing have heard the concerns of the nursing community related to the use of standardized exit examinations and suggest that a better understanding of this practice is needed.

There is no one best method for preparing to take the NCLEX-RN. Success depends on a candidate's nursing knowledge and ability to use that knowledge, test-taking skills, and confidence level. The best preparation any candidate can have is what the candidate brings from his or her nursing program.

Some measure of preparation for the NCLEX-RN examination after graduation from nursing school is a must for all candidates seeking success on the examination. Candidates should NOT convince themselves that they do not need to review because they made average or above-average grades in their academic and nursing coursework, nor should they decide that review will serve no purpose because they made average or below-average grades in their coursework.

In preparation for the NCLEX-RN examination, it is important to remember that review is a personal undertaking. What works for one candidate may not work for another, and vice versa. Each candidate should use the study and review methods that have proved successful in the past. It is estimated that most students study for 2 for 3 months prior to the examination. International students typically begin much earlier, studying for approximately 6 months prior to the examination.

Build Your NCLEX Study Plan

Use the following tips and strategies to build your own study plan and increase the likelihood of passing the NCLEX-RN examination:

- *Review the NCLEX Candidate Bulletin* (find the most current Bulletin at https://www.ncsbn.org).
- *Become familiar with the test plan* (find the most current Test Plan at https://www.ncsbn.org).
- *Locate your test site early.* Be sure to obtain an Authorization to Test (ATT). Remember: You must apply to your board of nursing or regulatory body before registering with Pearson Vue (http://www.pearsonvue.com/nclex) to take the examination. Be certain you have acceptable identification as stated on the NCSBN website. You may need to order replacement identification before testing. If you have changed your name, the only identification documents accepted are a marriage license, divorce decree, or legal court name change documents.
- *Perform a needs assessment.* Determine content areas of strengths and weaknesses. Look at previous academic and nursing coursework, class notes and handouts, examination grades, and grades made on nursing care plans or process papers. If your school uses nationally normed assessment examinations, use their report to determine areas of strengths and weaknesses. The rationale provided

when reviewing these exams provides a wealth of information and validates the correct answers. Talk with faculty in courses in which you had weakness or difficulty. Determine where the greatest amount of review is needed. Be honest in performing the needs assessment. The foundation for success or failure on the NCLEX-RN examination may be determined here.

- *Analyze standardized examinations.* If your school uses standardized examinations to compare you with your peers and the national population of test takers, look at where you rank in comparison with both groups. Again, do not be overconfident if you scored higher than either group. This fact should give you positive affirmation that you have a high chance of passing the NCLEX—not that you can delete your NCLEX-RN study plans. Even when students score at the highest level, many miss some questions. The "focused review" provided by the standardized examination describes the area of the nursing process, and the specific content area should be used to remediate. Remember, these exams cannot test all content matter, so always consider that you received only what is highly tested on the NCLEX-RN.
- *Determine the number of days or weeks necessary for review.* Candidates with a strong nursing knowledge base may need less time than candidates with weaknesses. As with the needs assessment, you should be realistic in planning the amount of review time you need.
- *Decide what method of review will be used.* Both individual and group study methods have strong and weak points. Strong points of individual study include having total control over content and time spent in review. Weak points include having no immediate resources to explain or assist with understanding difficult concepts. Candidates with weakness in disciplining themselves may have problems sticking to review schedules and focusing on specific content with individual study. Strong points of group study include the support that members can give one another and learning from others in the group. Also, many minds working together are stronger than one working alone. Weak points of group study include lack of preparation by some group members, the group being held back by

weaker members, and a tendency of the group to focus on socialization rather than review. If you use a study group, get the others to agree that all members coming to sessions must be prepared to work.

- *Decide what materials or resources will be used during review.* Textbooks and class notes from nursing or nursing-related courses, such as anatomy and physiology, psychology, and nutrition, are helpful. It has been suggested that rereading your nursing school notes may not be the best use of time. Computer-assisted instructions used during the nursing program may be available. Numerous NCLEX-RN examination review books are available. Many review books include a CD or online resources to be used during review. Before purchasing any, make sure that these computer aids are compatible with the type of computer you will be using during review.
- *Structure review time.* Schedule review during your times of peak performance. Learning is enhanced when reviewing for short blocks of time, around 50 minutes, instead of for several unbroken hours at a time. Remember that you are reviewing for an examination, not cramming for one.
- *Control the review environment.* Keep noise and distraction at a minimum. Have adequate space and lighting for review. Control the room temperature when possible; if not possible, dress for the environment. Have all materials needed for review, including soft drinks and snacks, close at hand so as not to waste time gathering these items during review time. Make sure that friends and family know not to interrupt you during review time.
- *Have a game plan for each review session.* Develop a review schedule complete with subject matter to be considered and specific tasks to be completed during each session. Stick to the schedule.
- *Learn concepts and principles, not isolated facts.* The NCLEX-RN examination tests a candidate's ability to apply, analyze, and evaluate nursing knowledge and does not focus on isolated events. Candidates whose past test-taking success has been based on memorization rather than actual learning have an increased risk for failure on this examination.
- *Use learning techniques that have proved successful in the past.* People have different learning styles and

therefore benefit from different learning techniques. You might choose to use flash cards, underscore key points, take notes or outline material, or record pertinent information for later playback. Quiz yourself or ask others to pose questions. Many people find downloading application software (i.e., an "app") to practice NCLEX-style questions is helpful. Examples include NCLEX Mastery (https://app.nclexmastery.com/).

- *Seek qualified help when reviewing information that is particularly difficult.* Faculty members are an excellent resource. If you invest in an external course review, ask for help during the question and answer sessions or determine whether an open forum to ask questions extends beyond the actual review class. Be cautious when asking peers for assistance because they may not understand the material as well as they think they do.
- *Practice taking NCLEX-RN–type examinations, paying particular attention to the rationales or reasons provided for correct and incorrect answers.* Successful test takers know why a specific option is correct or incorrect. Even though candidates may spend as much time as they want on a question when actually taking the examination, you should get into the habit of taking about 1 minute for each question. Poor time management may cause a candidate to not have enough time to complete the test and therefore to be unsuccessful on the NCLEX-RN examination. Practice also will help reduce test anxiety. NCLEX-RN–type examinations are commonly found in NCLEX-RN review books.
- *Use the Internet.* It provides numerous sources that may aid in preparation for the NCLEX-RN examination.
- *Avoid excessive stimulants* (e.g., caffeine) *to increase review time.* The best learning takes place when your head is clear.
- *Maintain a healthy, positive attitude toward reviewing and taking the NCLEX-RN examination.* Have confidence in your abilities to be successful on the examination. Remember that even practicing nurses with years of experience do not know everything there is to know about every aspect of nursing and that your goal on the NCLEX-RN examination is to demonstrate minimal competency for an entry-level RN position, not competency required for an advanced RN position.

Food for Thought when Selecting an NCLEX-RN Review Course

Just as there is no one best method for preparing to take the NCLEX-RN examination, there is no one best review course for a candidate to take in preparation for the examination. The most important thing to remember is that a review course is exactly what it says it is—a review course. Such courses are designed to reconsider or reexamine content common to the three types of nursing programs.

The purpose of a review course is to enhance or polish what candidates already know from their nursing programs. Review courses are not intended to teach totally new concepts. For a candidate who has an extreme weakness in one or more content areas, the review course may not provide enough content to bring him or her up to speed on the topic.

Numerous companies and people offer review courses. Each review offering has strong and weak points, and what appeals to one candidate may not appeal to another. Some companies offer financial discounts or other incentives if more than one candidate from a school of nursing registers for their course.

Review courses can be expensive and may last from 1 or 2 days to a complete week. Some courses provide books, CDs, or other written materials. Others may offer additional materials for a fee. Some companies will refund a part or all of the cost of the review course if a candidate who takes it does not pass the NCLEX-RN.

Investigate who is teaching the review course you are considering. Are the credentials and nursing background of those teaching the course available? And do they appear to be competent to teach the course? A review course is no better than the person or people teaching it. The decision to take a review course in preparation for the NCLEX-RN examination is a personal one. Some candidates find the structure and schedule of a review course helpful in preparation. Other candidates may find the structure and schedule restrictive and overly time-consuming.

Candidates seriously interested in taking an NCLEX-RN examination review course should look to the faculty at their school of nursing for guidance. Many faculty have had experience with review courses or may teach them. Candidates should also talk to peers who have recently graduated about recommendations for review courses. Serious candidates also should obtain written information from several different offerings and compare and contrast them. Selection of a review course should be based on more than the cost—it should meet the candidate's unique needs.

The NCSBN's online course, Review for the NCLEX-RN Examination, offers 3-, 5-, 8- and 15-week subscriptions (https://learningext.com/students/p/nclex-rn). Student testimonials describe the course as extremely helpful in passing the NCLEX. New items are continually added, ensuring the review is current with the latest Test Plan. It allows candidates to practice alternate format items. Immediate instructor feedback is available through the "Ask the Instructor" feature. The site offers a timeline for interested candidates; for example, if one registers for the 3-week subscription, 27 hours per week are needed for review; by comparison, 5 to 6 hours per week are needed with the 15-week subscription.

The NCSBN website offers tips for the actual examination date, such as dressing comfortably, arriving 30 minutes early, and being prepared to provide your signature, photograph, and palm vein scan. Be sure to watch the "NCLEX Using CAT" video on the NCSBN website if you have any questions about how this type of testing works.

▌ S U M M A R Y

Success on the NCLEX-RN examination is needed to obtain a license and practice as an RN. Most candidates taking the NCLEX-RN examination pass it. Of the 157,073 first-time, U.S.-educated candidates taking the examination during 2016, approximately 84.57% were successful (NCSBN, 2016b). The pass rate was somewhat higher for those testing for the first time in the first three quarters of 2017, with an average of 87.78% of the candidates passing (NCSBN, 2017). The key to success on the NCLEX-RN examination is sound preparation from the nursing program, adequate preparation for the examination, and confidence in oneself.

REFERENCES

Anderson, L. W., & Krathwohl, D. R. (Eds.), (2001). *A taxonomy for learning, teaching, and assessing: A revision of Bloom's taxonomy of educational objectives*. New York: Addison-Wesley.

Bloom, B. S., Englehart, M. D., & Furst, E. J. (1956). *Taxonomy of educational objectives: The classification of educational goals. Handbook I. Cognitive domain*. New York: David McKay.

College of Nurses of Ontario. (2017). *2016 mid-year NCLEX-RN results: Ontario graduates applying to CNO*. Retrieved from http://www.cno.org/en/news/2016/july-2016/2016-mid-year-nclex-rn-results-ontario-graduates-applying-to-cno/. Accessed January 3, 2018.

Foote, J. (1919). *State board questions and answers for nurses*. Philadelphia: Lippincott.

National Council of State Boards of Nursing. (2014). *Transitional NCLEX examination candidate bulletin for Canadian NCLEX candidates*. Retrieved from https://www.ncsbn.org/Transitional_NCLEX_Candidate_Bulletin_2014.pdf. Accessed January 3, 2018.

National Council of State Boards of Nursing. (2015). *2014 RN practice analysis: Linking the NCLEX-RN® examination to practice, NCSBN Research Brief 62*. Retrieved from https://www.ncsbn.org/15_RN_Practice_Analysis_Vol62_web.pdf. Accessed January 3, 2018.

National Council of State Boards of Nursing. (2016a). *NCLEX-RN examination detailed test plan for the National Council Licensure examination for registered nurses*. Retrieved from https://www.ncsbn.org/2016_RN_DetTestPlan_Educator.pdf. Accessed January 3, 2018.

National Council of State Boards of Nursing. (2018). *2018 NCLEX examination candidate bulletin*. Retrieved from https://www.ncsbn.org/089900_2018_Bulletin_Proof2.pdf.pdf. Accessed January 3, 2018.

National Council of State Boards of Nursing. (2016b). *NCLEX pass rates*. Retrieved from https://www.ncsbn.org/Table_of_Pass_Rates_2016.pdf. Accessed December 2017.

National Council of State Boards of Nursing. (2017). *NCLEX pass rates*. Retrieved from https://www.ncsbn.org/Table_of_Pass_Rates_2017.pdf. Accessed December 2017.

Potter, P. A., & Perry, A. G. (2013). *Fundamentals of nursing*. St. Louis: Mosby Elsevier.

A

A Manual of Nursing, 9
AACN. *See* American Association of Colleges of Nursing
AAN. *See* American Academy of Nursing
AANA. *See* American Association of Nurse Anesthetists
ABC approach, time management and, 437
Abdellah, Faye, nursing theory of, 83t
Abstract, definition of, 88, 102
ACA. *See* Affordable Care Act
Academic Center for Evidence-Based Practice (ACE), 44
Accommodation, conflict resolution and, 341
Accountability, 119, 122, 161, 169
    challenge of, 176–177
    definition of, 345
Accreditation
    consensus model for, 73–74
    definition of, 62
    patient safety improved with, 385–386
    quality improvement through, 378–379
Accreditation Commission for Education in Nursing (ACEN), 10,
Accreditation, staffing affected by, 363
Accuracy, in communication, 331–332
ACE. *See* Academic Center for Evidence-Based Practice
ACEN. *See* Accreditation Commission for Education in Nursing
ACRL. *See* Association of College and Research Libraries
Active listening, 322, 341–342t
Active shooter, 274, 286, 286t
Activities, scheduling of, time management and, 438
Acuity, patient
    definition of, 359
    level of, 361–362
Acupuncture, 6, 202–203
Acute care setting, nursing care delivery model for, 369
Ad hominem abusive, 330
Adaptation model, 85, 85f
Administrator, nurse as, 460
Advance care plan, 228
    definition of, 216
Advance directives, 119, 151, 217, 228
    definition of, 216
Advanced practice nurse (APN), definition of, 62, 73

Advanced practice nursing, 457–460
    definition of, 445
Advanced practice registered nurses (APRNs), 30
    regulation of, 73–74
Adverse event, preventable, 147
Advices, Nightingale's theory of practice and, 82
Aesculapius, 5
Affordable Care Act (ACA), 17–18
African-Americans
    nursing schools for, 9
    poverty rate of, 182
    syphilis study of, 103
Agency for Healthcare Research and Quality (AHRQ), 44, 92–93
Aggressive communication, 335
AHRQ. *See* Agency for Healthcare Research and Quality
Airline industry, opportunities for nurses in, 454
Alcott, Louisa May, 9
Alexander technique, 208b
Algorithm, health care protocols described with, 382, 383f
All-hazards approach, 277
    definition of, 274
Alternate item format, 486–487
AMA. *See* American Medical Association
Ambulatory care, nursing care delivery model, 369
American Academy of Nursing (AAN), 14, 56b
American Association of Colleges of Nursing (AACN), 56b, 423–424, 465
American Association of Nurse Anesthetists (AANA), 29–30
American Association of Occupational Health Nurses, 246–247
American Indians, poverty rate of, 182
American Medical Association (AMA), 396
American Nurses Association (ANA), 3–4b, 56b, 93, 403, 465
    Code of Ethics for Nurses, 219
    collective bargaining and, 254
    description of, 62
    health policy development of, 397
    history of, 65
    Nursing: Scope and Standards of Practice, 351
    Principles of Delegation, 353–354
    workplace advocacy by, 234–235

American Nurses Credentialing Center (ANCC), 62, 71, 72b, 247, 453
American Nursing Information Association (ANIA), 453
American Red Cross, 3–4b
    founding of, 9
Americans with Disabilities Act of 1990, 125
ANA. *See* American Nurses Association
Analysis
    of health policy issues, 400
    questions, in NCLEX-RN examination, 488, 490
    as stage of nursing process, 303
ANA's Code of Ethics for Nurses with Interpretive Statements, 49
ANCC. *See* American Nurses Credentialing Center
ANIA. *See* American Nursing Information Association
Antidumping law, 124–125
Antiestablishment
    definition of, 21
    era, nursing in, 26
APN. *See* Advanced practice nurse
Application questions, in NCLEX-RN examination, 488
Appraisal of Guidelines for Research and Evaluation (AGREE) Instrument, 102
APRNs. *See* Advanced practice registered nurses
Arbitration, definition of, 251
Art
    definition of, 21
    nursing in, 24–29
Assault, 148–149
Assertive communication, 335
Assertiveness skills, novice nurse development of, 420–421
Assessment
    function of, delegation of nursing tasks and, 347–348
    of health policy issues, 400
    NCLEX-RN examination and, 489–490
    in nursing education, 43–45
    as stage of nursing process, 303
Assessment tool, for decision making, 478b
Assignment, definition of, 345
Associate degree programs, 52
Association of College and Research Libraries (ACRL), 269

Association of perioperative Registered Nurses, 246–247
Attitude, verbal communication affected by, 326
Audio, as alternate item format, 487
Authority
    definition of, 288, 290
    leadership and management use of, 291
Autonomy, 161, 170
    challenge of, 176
Avoidance, conflict resolution and, 341
Ayurveda, 203–204

B

Baby boomers, in communication, 336–337
Baccalaureate degree nursing programs, 53
Balanced Budget Amendment, 396–397t
Balancing science and morality, 166–167
Barton, Clara, 9
Basic Guide to the National Labor Relations Act, 254
Battery, 148–149
Behavior model, 424f
Beliefs, cultural
    on sickness and cures, 194, 195b, 195t
    systems for, 189
Beneficence, 161, 170–171
Benefits, employment, job interview process and, 476b
Best practices, process improvement with, 381–382
Biculturalism
    definition of, 409
    novice nurse and, 422
Bioethical concerns, nursing education affected by, 48–49
Bioethical dilemmas, 173–177
Bioethics, 161, 163–165
    dilemmas, 165
Biofeedback, 204
Biologic agent
    definition of, 274
    terrorism with, 279t
Biologic variation, as cultural phenomena, 189
Bioterrorism, emergency management plan for, 277
Blind review, 102
Blocking, in negative communication techniques, 329
Bloodborne pathogens, exposure to, 244–245
Bloom's taxonomy, NCLEX-RN® examination and, 487t
Board of nursing, duties of, 68
Body language, in positive communication techniques, 328

Bodywork, 208b
Breach of duty, 119, 134
Breakthrough thinking, quality improvement with, 382–384
Breckenridge, Mary, 11
Budget
    assumptions used in, 309
    basic functions of, 311–313
    capital, 314–315
    definition of, 309
    development of, 315–316
    labor, 314
    methods for, 315
    operational, 313–314
    overview of, 311
    types of, 313–315, 313b
    variance in, sample report for, 318t
Budgeting
    cost concepts related to, 317–320
    improving skills in, 317b
    incremental, 310, 315
    management and, 303
    methods for, 315
    performance evaluation in, 313
    zero-based, 310, 315
Bullying
    addressing and preventing, 306
    novice nurse affected by, 421
    workplace, 245–246
Business agent, 255–256

C

CAB. See Computer at bedside
California, nursing staffing regulations in, 239–240
CAM. See Complementary and alternative medicine
CAPC. See Center to Advance Palliative care
Capital budget, 314–315
Capital expenditures, definition of, 309
Care
    ethics of, 166–167
    right to refuse, 154
    standard, 121, 134
Care coordination, health care cost management and, 116
Care delivery systems, 363
Care maps, 369
Care provider, nurse as, 447
Career opportunities, for nurses, 445–462
Caregiver, family, definition of, 226
Caretaker, need to be, time management and, 434
Caring
    environment of, 305–306
    NCLEX-RN examination and, 490

Case law, 119, 123–124
Case management, 367–369
Case manager
    functions of, 368b
    nurse as, 455
Case nursing, 364
CAT. See Computer adaptive testing
Cause-and-effect diagram, 381
    definition of, 372
    example of, 381f
CBRNE, terrorism categorization by, 278, 279t
CCNE. See Commission on Collegiate Nursing Education
CDC. See Centers for Disease Control and Prevention
Center for Nursing Advocacy, 28
Center to Advance Palliative care (CAPC), 223–224
Centers for Disease Control and Prevention (CDC), 282
Centers for Medicare and Medicaid Services (CMS), 106, 110, 386, 386b
    electronic health record and, 263
Certification, 62–74
    consensus model for, 73–74
    cultural competence and, 191
    definition of, 62
    history of, 71–72
    issues in, 73
    licensure compared to, 71
    organizations, 72b
    purpose of, 72–73
    steps to, 73
Certified nurse-midwife, 459–460
Certified registered nurse anesthetist (CRNA), 25–26, 458–459
Chamomile, facts about, 205–206b
Change agent
    nurse as, 447
    nurse manager as, 304–305
Change, stages of, 304–305
Chaos, conquistador of, time management and, 434
Chaos theory, 295
Chaplain, as interprofessional health care team member, 448–449b
Charge nurse, delegation and supervision by, example of, 354
Chart exhibit, as alternate item format, 486–487
Chemical agents
    definition of, 274
    terrorism with, 279t
Child abuse reporting statutes, 131
Children's Health Insurance Program (CHIP), 395

China, ancient, health care in, 5–6
CHIP. *See* Children's Health Insurance Program
Chiropractic medicine, 204
CINAHL. *See* Cumulative Index to Nursing and Allied Health Literature
Civil law, 119, 133–146
Civil war period, health care in, 8–9
Clance Impostor Phenomenon Scale, 424
CLAS. *See* Culturally and linguistically appropriate services
Classroom orientation, 465–466
Cleanliness, Nightingale's theory of practice and, 82
Client
   cultural assessment of, 193–194
   needs of, NCLEX-RN examination and, 488–489
   nutrition of, 194
Client advocate, nurse as, 447
Client education, nurse's role in, 448
Clinical care, improving cost and quality of, 320
Clinical consultant, nurse manager as, 305
Clinical indicator
   definition of, 372
   process improvement and, 379–381
Clinical nurse leader (CNL), 3–4b, 54
   role of, 98
Clinical nurse specialist (CNS), 97–98
   definition of, 88
   description of, 458
   transcultural nursing, 192
Clinical pathways, 369, 382
   components of, 369
   definition of, 359
Clinical practice guidelines (CPGs), 100, 101–102
   clinical pathway and, 369
   definition of, 88, 359
Clinical protocols, 382
Clinical research nurse (CRN), 98
Clinical situation, delegation and, 351
Clinical skills, novice nurse development of, 419, 427
Clinical skills test, job application process and, 480
CMS. *See* Centers for Medicare and Medicaid Services
CNL. *See* Clinical nurse leader
CNS. *See* Clinical nurse specialist
Coaching
   effective, 301b
   performance evaluation and, 301
Cochrane Collaboration, 100
Code for Professional Nurses, 3–4b
Code of ethics, 161, 163

Coercive power, 291
Cognitive domain, NCLEX-RN examination and, 487–488
Collaboration, conflict resolution and, 341
Collective bargaining, 251–260
   definition of, 251
   development of, 253–254
   early activities of, 253
   federal legislation affecting, 253–254
   in nursing, 254
   process of, 254–257
Colonial American period, health care in, 7
Commission on Collegiate Nursing Education (CCNE), 3–4b, 10, 56b
Commissioned Corps, emergency preparedness and response and, 281–282
Common law, 119, 132–133
Communication
   aggressive, 335
   assertive, 335
   as barrier to palliative care, 227
   as budgeting function, 312
   cultural diversity and, 337–338
   as cultural phenomena, 190
   definition of, 324
   details in, 332–333
   effective, 322–344, 353b, 356–357
   electronic, 331–334, 332b, 333b
   electronic health record for, 265–266
   and gender differences, 335–336
   generational differences and, 336–337
   within health care facility, during emergency response, 283
   interprofessional team, 338
   listening and, 330–331
   NCLEX-RN examination and, 490
   negative techniques for, 322, 328–330
   nonverbal, 326
      vs. verbal, 325–326
   online etiquette, 339
   open, 328
   passive, 335
   passive-aggressive, 335
   of performance expectation, 299–300
   positive techniques for, 322, 326–328
   process, 324–325
   special influences on, 335–338
   styles of, 335
   verbal, 325–326
      vs. nonverbal, 325–326
   written, 331–334, 332b, 333b
Communication barriers, and informed consent, 153–154
Community, emergency preparedness and response by, 281f
Community-focused interprofessional approaches, 46–47

Community Mental Health Centers Act, 13
Compact state, definition of, 62
Comparative negligence, 119
Compassion fatigue, 409, 413–414, 414f
Compensation, job application process and, 478–479
Competency
   definition of, 345
   delegation and, 350
Competency outcomes
   definition of, 37
   practice-based, 42–43
Competency program, continued, 71
Complementary and alternative healing, 199–215, 212b
Complementary and alternative medicine (CAM)
   consumers' desire, 201
   in conventional settings, 211
   definition of, 199
   examples of, 202b
   facilitating use of, 211
   legal considerations, 213
   nursing and, 210–213
   overview of, 200–201
   principles of, 201–202
   use of, 201
   used competently, 213
Complexity compression, 436
Comprehension questions, in NCLEX-RN® examination, 487
Compromise, conflict resolution and, 341
Computer adaptive testing (CAT)
   definition of, 482
   NCLEX-RN® examination through, 484–485
Computer at bedside (CAB), 268
Computer on wheels (COWs), 268
Computerized provider order entry (CPOE), 263–264
Concept, definition of, 75, 79t
Conceptual framework, 78
Conceptual model
   definition of, 75, 79t
   description of, 78
Conceptual practices, in leading and managing, 293b
Conceptual skills, 293
Conciseness, in communication, 333–334, 333b
Conditions of participation for hospitals in Medicare (CoPS), 123–124
Confidentiality
   communication and, 338
   patient, electronic health record and, 266

Conflict
  definition of, 322
  nature of, 340
  understanding and managing, 340–343
  verbal, response to, 342b
Conflict resolution, 340–343
  effective communication and, 322–344
  procedures for, 248
Conflicting messages, in negative
    communication techniques, 329–330
Connection power, 291
Consensus model, for APRN regulation,
    73–74
Constituent, definition of, 392
Constituent/State Nurses Association
    (C/SNA), definition of, 392
Consumer empowerment, 117, 117b
Contemporary issues, 50–51
  definition of, 37
Context, communication process and,
    324
Continued competency program, 62, 71
Continuous process improvement, 376
Continuous quality improvement (CQI),
    376
Continuum approach, priority setting with,
    time management and, 438
Control
  implementing for, 440–443
    attacking the priorities, 440
    avoiding procrastination, 440–441
    controlling interruptions, 441–442
    delegating appropriately, 441
    finding "extra" time, 440
    learning the art of saying no, 442
    rewarding yourself, 442
    using technology, 442–443
  organizing for, 439–440
  planning for, time management and,
      437–439
Control group, definition of, 88
Controlling
  interruptions, time management and,
      441–442
  as management function, 295, 296f,
      300–301
Conventional medicine, 199
Coordination, as budgeting function, 312
Coordinator positions, for nurse, 452–453
Coprimary nursing, 363–364, 367
CoPS. See Conditions of participation for
    hospitals in Medicare
Core competencies, definition of, 37
Core measures, 378–379
Corporate liability, 145–146
Corporate supporter, nurse leader as,
    305

Cost
  direct, 317–320
  fixed, 320
  full, 320
  indirect, 320
  variable, 320
Cost shifting, 112
Counselor, nurse as, 447
County Health Rankings Model, 405–406, 405f
Cover letter, 467–468, 467b
COWs. See Computer on wheels
CPGs. See Clinical practice guidelines
CPOE. See Computerized provider order
    entry
CQI. See Continuous quality improvement
Creativity, fear of losing, time management
    and, 434
Crimean War, 7
Criminal law, nurse and, 151
Criminal negligence, 119, 137–138
Criminal record check, job application
    process and, 479
Crisis standards of care, 274, 280
Critical paths, 369
Critical pathway, 382
Critical thinking, in nursing education, 43
CRN. See Clinical research nurse
CRNA. See Certified registered nurse
    anesthetist
Crossing the Quality Chasm: A New Health
    System for the 21st Century, 375
Cruise ship industry, opportunities for
    nurses in, 454
Cultural belief systems, 189
Cultural competency, 179–198
  assessment of, 193–194
  in nursing education, 188–189
  practice issues related to, 191–193
Cultural diversity
  communication and, 337–338
  nursing education affected by, 45–46
Cultural humility, definition of, 179
Cultural phenomena, 189–191
  biologic variations, 189
  communication, 190
  environmental control, 189
  social organization, 190
  space, 190
  time, 190–191
Cultural sensitivity, definition of, 179
Culturally and linguistically appropriate
    services (CLAS), 192–193
Culture
  assessment of, 193–194
  definition of, 179
  NCLEX-RN examination and, 490
  phenomena in, 189–191

Culture shock, reality shock and, 416
Cumulative Index to Nursing and Allied
    Health Literature (CINAHL), 270
  Information Systems, 99
Cures, cultural beliefs and, 194, 195b, 195t
Curriculum vitae (CV), 468–469
Customer
  definition of, 372
  perspective of quality by, 376–377
  satisfaction of, staffing affected by, 363
Customer service provider, nurse leader as, 302

D

Damages, 120, 133
  punitive, 120, 130, 136
Data collection, definition of, 88
Data management, electronic health record
    and, 265–266
Data mining, 267
Death, two roads of, 222
Decision maker, nurse manager as, 303–304
Decision making, assessment tool for, 478b
Decision-making capacity, definition of, 216
Decision support tools, 265
  definition of, 261
Decision tree, for delegation, 349f
Declaration of Helsinki, 103
Defamation of character, 149–150
Defendant, 120, 133
Delegation, 345–358
  assigning vs, 355–356
  barriers of, 441
  building, 356–357
  clinical situation and, 351
  competency of delegates and, 350
  decision making, 352b
  decision tree, 349f
  definition of, 345, 347–348
  description of, 347–348
  evaluation after, 357
  excellence in practice, 355b
  explain the task and outcomes, 352–353
  in health care system, 347
  high-risk, 354
  job descriptions and, 350
  knowing the staff member, 352
  knowing the tasks, 352
  nurse practice acts and, 348–350
  nursing assessment and, 351
  organizational policies and, 350–351
  parameters of, 348
  patient needs and, 350
  procedures and, 350–351
  responsible action from delegate, 353
  safe practices for, 351–354
  skills for, novice nurse development of,
      420, 428

Delegation of authority, 70
Deontology, 161, 170
Deployment flowchart, 379–380, 380f
Depression, nursing during, 11–12
Diagnosis
    of health policy issues, 400
    as stage of nursing process, 303
Diagnosis-related groups (DRGs), 106, 110,
    396–397t
    reimbursement and, 15
Diagnostic testing, right to refuse, 154
Diet
    alternative, healing and, 204
    Nightingale's theory of practice and, 82
Dietitian, as interprofessional health care
    team member, 448–449b
Dilemmas
    in between, 174–175
    bioethical, 173–177
    created by technology, 165
    for health professionals, 165
Direct costs, 317–320
Directing, as management function, 295,
    296f, 299–300
Disaster
    major, definition of, 275
    nursing education affected by, 48
    phases of, 278–283
Disaster condition, definition of, 274,
    277–278
Disaster medical assistance team (DMAT),
    definition of, 281
Discharge planning, 448
Disclosure, 120
    of error, 140
Disease trajectory, definition of, 216
Distance-learning, 54–56
Diversity
    cultural
        attitude towards, 182–183, 182f
        nursing education affected by, 45–46
    in health care workforce, 183–186, 183f,
        184f
    nursing education affected by, 51–54
Dix, Dorothea, 8
DMAT. See Disaster medical assistance
    team
DNP. See Doctor of nursing practice
Do not resuscitate (DNR) orders, 152
Doctor of nursing, 54
Doctor of nursing practice (DNP), 54
    role of, 98
Doctoral programs, in nursing education, 54
Documentation
    accuracy in, 331–332
    detail in, 332–333
    NCLEX-RN examination and, 490

Domestic abuse, nursing practice affected
    by, 45
Domestic violence, 182
    nursing education affected by, 48
Double effect, 228
    definition of, 216
Downtime, fear of, time management and, 434
Dress, appropriate, for job interview, 473
DRGs. See Diagnosis-related groups
Durable power of attorney for health care,
    152

E
Ebola, 285–286
Echinacea, facts about, 205–206b
Economics
    health care and, 181–182
    nursing education affected by, 45–46
Ecosystem model, for workplace advocacy,
    234b, 234f
Education
    change implementation and, 305
    description of, in résumé, 469
    for nurses, 243
Education trends, definition of, 37
Educational mobility, definition of, 37
Educator, nurse as, 447
Effectiveness, 106, 116
Efficiency, 106, 116
Egypt, ancient, health care in, 5
EHR. See Electronic health record
Electronic communication, 331–334, 332b,
    333b
Electronic health record (EHR), 263–267,
    331, 442–443
    adoption of, 263
        opportunities in, 267
    barriers to use of, 267
    certification of, 266–267
    data capture in, 265
    data management in, 265–266
    definition of, 261
    description of, 263
    example of, 264f, 265f
    functions of, 263–264
    Health Insurance Portability and
        Accountability Act and, 267
    information communication in, 265–266
    information presentation in, 266
    information processing in, 265
    interoperability of, 261
    meaningful use of, 261, 266–267
    security of, 266
    storage of, 265
Electronic portfolios, 470–471
ELNEC. See End-of-Life Nursing Education
    Consortium

EMAC. See Emergency Management
    Assistance Compact
E-mail
    effective communication through, 332b,
        333b
    management of, 439–440
Emergency, definition of, 274
Emergency Management Assistance
    Compact (EMAC), 274
Emergency management plan, 277
Emergency Medical Treatment and Active
    Labor Law, 124–125
Emergency Nurses Association, 246–247
Emergency operating plan, mass casualty,
    incident and, 280
Emergency operations center, 285–286
Emergency preparedness and response, for
    today's world, 274–287
    basics of, 277–278
    national imperative for, 276–277
    preparedness phase of, 278–282
    relief response phase of, 282–283
Emerging roles, 98–99
Emotion, appeal to, 330
Emotional distress, intentional infliction of,
    150
Emotional energy, 435
Emotional intelligence, 435
Empathy, 340
    in positive communication techniques,
        328
Empirical, definition of, 88
Empirical outcomes, 247
Employer
    information applicants may request from,
        465, 465b
    liability, 145
    task of, 479–480
Employment history, description of, in
    résumé, 469
End of life, 174
End-of-Life Nursing Education Consortium
    (ELNEC), 216, 223
    curriculum, on palliative care, 224
Energy
    distractions of, 436, 436b
    emotional, 435
    mental, 435
    physical, 435
    spiritual, 435
Energy management, 435–436
    definition of, 431
Energy therapy, 209
    definition of, 199
    example of, 202b
Engagement, patient-centered care and,
    47–48

Environment, communication process and, 324

Environmental control, as cultural phenomena, 189

Equality, 340

Error, definition of, 120

Ethical decision-making model, 171–173, 172b

Ethical issues, 120

Ethical theory, 169–170

Ethics, 122, 161, 163
   of care, 166–167
   challenge in, 175
   nursing education affected by, 48–49
   in nursing research, 103
   professional, 45

Ethics acculturation, 161, 163, 168

Ethnicity, definition of, 179

Ethnocentrism, definition of, 179

Ethnography
   definition of, 88
   description of, 95t

Evaluation
   delegation of nursing tasks and, 354
   of health policy, 400
   methods, nurse reality shock and, 417–418, 418b
   in NCLEX-RN examination, 490
   as stage of nursing process, 304

Evidence
   levels of, 100–101
   strength of, 101
   types of, 100–101

Evidence-based practice, 88–105
   advancement of, 96–97
   clinical practice guidelines and, 101–102
   competencies, 97t, 98t
   definition of, 88, 90
   description of, 99
   evolution of, 102–103
   nurse roles in, 97–99, 99b
   steps of, 96b
   summaries for, 99–100

Evidence hierarchy, 101, 101f

Examining trends, 267

Excelsior College, 55

Executive, nurse as, 460

Exemplary professional practice, 247

Expense
   definition of, 309
   in health care organizations, 314, 314b

Experimental design, definition of, 88

Experimental study, description of, 94t

Expert power, 291

Explosive agent, terrorism with, 279t

Eye contact, in positive communication techniques, 327

F

Face-to-face interview, 474–476

Faculty, shortage of, 49–50

Failure, fear of, time management and, 434

Failure mode and effects analysis (FMEA), 379
   definition of, 372

Faith community nurse (FCN), 456

Faith, healing and, 210

Fallacies, logical, in negative communication techniques, 330

False assurances, in negative communication techniques, 329

False imprisonment, 150

Family caregiving, in palliative care, 226

Family, definition of, 46, 190

Fatigue, 246

FCN. *See* Faith community nurse

Federal government
   branches of, 398t
   emergency preparedness and response by, 281f

Federal health policy, 395–396

Federal Register, 399

Federal statutes, 123–126

Feedback
   in communication process, 325
   performance evaluation and, 301

Feedback loop, 325

Feldenkrais method, 208b

Feverfew, facts about, 205–206b

Fidelity, 161, 172

Field representative, 255–256

Fill-in-the-blank question, as alternate item format, 486

Filtration
   in communication process, 325
   definition of, 322

Financial resources, staffing affected by, 362–363

Fiscal year, definition of, 309, 315–316

Fishbone diagram, 381

Fixed costs, 320

Flexible education programs, 54–56

Flight nurse, 455

Floating, description of, 242

Flowchart, 379–380
   definition of, 372
   deployment, 379–380
   processes described with, 379–380
   top-down, example of, 379f

FMEA. *See* Failure mode and effects analysis

FNS. *See* Frontier Nursing Service

Folk healer, 192

Force, conflict resolution and, 341

Foreign nurses, 69

Forensic, opportunities for nurses in, 455

Frontier Nursing Service (FNS), 11

FTE. *See* Full-time equivalent

Full cost, 320

Full-time equivalent (FTE)
   budget development and, 316
   definition of, 309

Functional nursing care delivery model, 364–365, 365f

G

Garlic, facts about, 205–206b

GDP. *See* Gross domestic product

Gender differences, communication and, 335–336

Generalizability, definition of, 88

Generation X, in communication, 336, 337

Generation Y, in communication, 336

Generational differences, communication and, 336–337

Ginger, facts about, 205–206b

Ginkgo biloba, facts about, 205–206b

Ginseng, facts about, 205–206b

Global health, 47

Goal, definition of, 431

Goals and objectives, management and, 297, 297b

Goals and priorities, unclear, time management and, 434

Good Samaritan immunity, 139

Governance, shared, models for, 247

Government, federal, branches of, 398t

Government nurses, 68

Governmental immunity, 139

Graduation, portfolio and, 471

Grandfathered, definition of, 62

Grant, definition of, 88

Graphic option identification, as alternate item format, 487

Grassroots lobbying, definition of, 392

Grassroots political strategies, 400–403

Greece, ancient, health care in, 5

Green tea, facts about, 205–206b

Grievance, definition of, 251

Gross domestic product (GDP), 106, 110

Gross negligence, 120, 136

Grounded theory
   definition of, 88
   description of, 95t

Guidelines for Preventing Workplace Violence for Health Care and Social Service Workers, 425–426

H

H1N1 virus, 285

H5N1 virus, 285

HACs. *See* Hospital-acquired conditions
Hallmarks of the Professional Practice Environment, 465
Hand off report, 334–335
HCAHPS. *See* Hospital Consumer Assessment of Healthcare Providers and Systems
Healing, complementary and alternative, 199–215, 211b, 212b
  in conventional settings, 211
  facilitating use of, 211
  legal considerations for, 213
  overview of, 200–201
  principles of, 201–202
  use of, 201
  used competently, 213
Healing touch, 208b
Health and Human Services Administration (HRSA), 450
Health as expanding consciousness theory, 86
Health care, 433
  bioethical issues in, 161–178
  community, description of, 46
  cultural competency in, 179–198
  ethical issues in, 161–178
  facilities
    communication within, during emergency response, 283
    on cultural care, 192
  global, 47
  information technology in, 261–273
  legal issues in, 119–160
  partial-task system, 417, 417b
  patient-centered, 47–48
  payment of, 106–115, 113t
  quality improvement in, 372–391
  relationship-based, 370
  resources of, allocation of, 174–175
  right to, 174
  social issues in, 179–198
  value of, 320
  whole-task system for, 417, 417b
  workforce, diversity in, 183, 183f, 184f
Health Care and Education Affordability Reconciliation Act, 17–18
Health care delivery systems, trends in, 451t
Health care financing
  history of, 109–111, 109t
  revolution of the 1980s, 110
Health care law, 120
Health care organization, definition of, 288
Health care reform, 404–405
Health care system, delegation and supervision in, 347
Health, culture of, 405–406
Health information, cultural competence and, 191

Health information technology, 263.
    See also Information technology
  consumer, 269–272
  definition of, 261
  future trends in, 272
  point-of-care, 267–269
  in United States, 263
Health Insurance and Accountability Act of 1996, 126
Health insurance exchange, 106, 113
Health insurance, lack of, 404
Health Insurance Portability and Accountability Act (HIPAA), 47–48
  electronic health record and, 267
Health Ministries Association (HMA), 456
Health policy
  current issues in, 404–407
  definition of, 392
  description of, 394–396
  development of, 397–399
    legislation and, 397
  federal, 395–396
  local, 395
  nurses' involvement in, 394
  nursing process and, 400
  private, 394–395
  public, 394–395
  regulation and, 399
  state, 395
  that have influenced professional nursing practice, 396–397t
Health promotion, NCLEX-RN examination and, 489
Healthcare Information and Management Systems Society (HIMSS), 42
Healthy People 2000: National Health Promotion and Disease Prevention Objectives, 16
Healthy People 2010, 46
Healthy People 2020, 46
Henderson, Virginia, nursing theory of, 83t
Henry Street Settlement House, 10
Herbs, complementary and alternative healing and, 204
Heroine, nurse as, 25–26
HICS. *See* Hospital incident command system
High-risk delegation, 353–354
Hill-Burton Act, 12–13, 396, 396–397t
HIMSS. *See* Healthcare Information and Management Systems Society
HIPAA. *See* Health Insurance Portability and Accountability Act
Hippocrates, 5
HMA. *See* Health Ministries Association

Home health agency, nursing care delivery model for, 370
Home health care, nursing roles in, 460
Homelanders, in communication, 336, 337
Homeopathy, 206–207, 207b
Honeymoon phase, of reality shock, 413
Hopes, chattering, Nightingale's theory of practice and, 82
Horizontal hostility, 409
Hospice and Palliative Nurse Association (HPNA)
  areas of expertise, 227
  on palliative nurse, definition of, 219
Hospice care
  definition of, 216
  vs. palliative care, 220t
Hospice, nurse role in, 453
Hospital
  Magnet, 247
    working environment in, 465
  nursing opportunities in, 451–453, 451t
  Pathway to Excellence recognition program and, 247
Hospital-acquired conditions (HACs), 123, 124b
  definition of, 372
Hospital Consumer Assessment of Healthcare Providers and Systems (HCAHPS), 302
Hospital diploma programs, 52
Hospital incident command system (HICS), 282–283
Hospital Survey and Construction Act, 12–13
Hostility, horizontal, definition of, 409
Hot spot, as alternate item format, 486, 486f
HPNA. *See* Hospice and Palliative Nurse Association
HRSA. *See* Health and Human Services Administration
Human practices, in leading and managing, 293b
Human skills, 293
Hypnotherapy, 207

I

"I" messages, in positive communication techniques, 327
ICN. *See* International Council of Nursing
ICS. *See* Incident command system
IENs. *See* Internationally educated nurses
IHI. *See* Institute for Healthcare Improvement
Illness, natural course of, 219–223

Image, of nursing, 22–23
  as Angel of Mercy, 25
  in antiestablishment era, 26
  antiquity of, 25
  early twentieth-century, 25
  as heroine, 25–26
  importance of, 23–24
  in sexual revolution, 26
  Victorian, 25
Imagery, 207–208
Immunity, 131
  definition of, 120
Implementation
  for control, 440–443
  of health policy, 400
  in NCLEX-RN examination, 490
  as stage of nursing process, 304
Incident command system (ICS), definition
  of, 275
Incident reports, 147–148, 148b
Incremental budgeting, 310, 315
India, ancient, health care in, 5
Indirect costs, 320
Individual citizen preparedness, 282
Individual membership, 13
Industrial unionism, definition of, 251
Infection control, nurse role in, 452
Influenza, pandemic, 284–285
  emergency management plan for, 277
  mass casualty incident caused by,
    284–285
Informatics, 41–42
  nurse role in, 453
Information, 322, 340
  clarifying, communication and, 328
  identification of, in résumé, 466
Information literacy (IL), 269
Information power, 291
Information processing, electronic health
  record for, 265
Information technology, 261–273.
    See also Health information
    technology
  definition of, 262
  nursing education use of, 41–42
  point-of-care, 267–269
Informed consent, 152–154
  communication barriers and, 153–154
  definition of, 216
  in palliative sedation, 229
Informed voting, 401
Injury, ergonomic, 245
Institute for Healthcare Improvement (IHI),
  384
  quality improvement model of, 384f
Institute for Safe Medication Practices
  (ISMP), 384–385

Institute of Medicine (IOM), 15, 29, 372,
  375, 451
  electronic health record functionality
    described by, 264t
  future of nursing report and, 406–407
Institutional licensing laws, 131–132
Institutional review board (IRB), 103
Institutional review, nursing research and,
  103
Insurance
  private, 114
  public, 114
Integrative Research Review (IRR),
  definition of, 89
Intentional infliction, of emotional distress,
  150
International Council of Nursing (ICN), 62
Internationally educated nurses (IENs),
  68–69
Internet
  accuracy of information on, 269–272
  authority of information on, 270–272
  consumer use of, for health information,
    269
  currency of information on, 270–272
  evaluation of information on, 270–272
  finding information on, 270
  job searching on, 466
  nursing education use of, 41–42
  objectivity of information on, 270–272
  usability of information on, 270–272
Interoperability, electronic health record
  and, 261
Interpersonal relations, as a nursing process,
  84
Interpersonal skills, novice nurse
  development of, 418, 427–428
Interpretation, 322
  communication process and, 324–325, 324f
Interpreters, for nurse/client communication,
  190
Interprofessional team, 224
  communication and, 338
  definition of, 217, 445
  members of, description of, 448–449b
    case study, 450b
  nurse as coordinator, 448–450
Interruptions, controlling, in time
  management, 441–442
Interview
  face-to-face, 474–476
  job searching and, 471–476
  legal and illegal questions in, 471b
  phone, 473–474
  preparation for, 473
  questions in, 474, 476b
  thank-you letter after, 477, 477b

Intimate partner violence (IPV), 182
Intuition
  definition of, 409
  of nurse, 422
Invasion of privacy, 150–151
Involvement, change implementation and,
  305
IOM. *See* Institute of Medicine
IPV. *See* Intimate partner violence
IRB. *See* Institutional review board
IRR. *See* Integrative Research Review
ISMP. *See* Institute for Safe Medication
  Practices

J

Jewish Chronic Disease Hospital, 103
Job applicant
  information requested from employer by,
    465b
  interview follow-up by, 477–479, 477b
  rights of, 473b
  tasks of, 476–479, 476b
Job descriptions, delegation and, 350
"Job hopper," 465
Job interview, 471–476
  face-to-face, 474–476
  phone, 473–474
  questions in, 474, 476b
  thank-you letter after, 477, 477b
Job satisfaction
  and dissatisfaction, factors influencing,
    299b
  nurse retention and, 236
  union representation and, 258
Job search, 463–481
  applicant's task in, 476–479
  cover letter in, 467–468, 467b
  employer information requested in, 465b
  exploring options in, 464–467
  interview, legal and illegal areas of
    questioning in, 471b
  knowing oneself in, 464–466
  written introductions in, 467–471
    cover letter, 467–468, 467b
    portfolio, 470–471, 470b
    résumé, 468–470, 468b
Johnson, Dorothy, nursing theory of, 83t
Justice, 161, 168

K

Kapha, Ayurveda and, 203, 203t
Karnofsky Scale, on prognostication,
  220–222, 221t
Keeping Patients Safe: Transforming the
  Work Environment of Nurses, staffing
  and, 361

King, Imogene, nursing theory of, 83t
Knowledge
    nursing, expansion of, 41–42
    questions, in NCLEX-RN® examination, 487

L

Labor budget, 314
Labor, definition of, 251
Language, health care and, 192–193
Laptop computer, point-of-care technology with, 268
Lateral hostility. *See* Horizontal hostility
Lavender, facts about, 205–206b
Law
    case, 119, 123–124
    civil, 119, 133–146
    common, 119, 132–133
    federal, for collective bargaining, 253–254
    institutional licensing, 131–132
    licensing, 120, 131
    and patient rights, 151–156
    right-to-work, definition of, 252
    sources of, 122
    statutory, 121, 122, 123–132
Lead agency, definition of, in emergency preparedness and response, 275
Leader, nurse as, 447
Leadership, 288–308, 294f
    definition of, 288, 290
    formal, 291–292
    informal, 291–292
    practices of, 293b
    resources for, 307b
    roles in, 302–305
    skills for, 293
    theory of, 292–293
    trait theory of, 292
    transactional, 292b
    transformational, 292–293, 292b
    vs. management, 291
Lean Methodology, 379
Lean Six Sigma, 379
Learning
    in NCLEX-RN examination, 490
    performance-based, 43–45
Legal liability, 120
    reducing, 146–148
Legislation, health policy development and, 397
Legitimate power, 291
Leininger, Madeline, nursing theory of, 83t, 85
Levine, Myra Estrin, nursing theory of, 83t

Liability, 134–135, 141
    corporate, 145–146
    definition of, 120
    employer, 145
    personal, 142b, 145
    strict, definition of, 123–124
    vicarious, definition of, 136
Licensing laws, 120, 131
Licensing regulations, staffing affected by, 363
Licensure, 62–74
    activities
        current, 70–71
        early, 65–66
    advanced practice nursing, 67
    certification compared to, 71
    consensus model for, 73–74
    by endorsement, 63, 67
    entry into practice, 67
    history, 64–66
    mandatory, 66
    mutual recognition model in, 70–71
    purpose of, 65
    renewal of, 67–68
    requirements for, in nurse practice act, 67
    special cases of, 68–69
Life, definition of, 173–174
Light, Nightingale's theory of practice and, 82
Listening, 330–331
    active, 331
Literature
    definition of, 21
    nursing in, 24–29
Living wills, 151–152
Lobbying, definition of, 392, 400–401
Local health policy, 395
Logical fallacies, in negative communication techniques, 330
Loners, novice nurse as, 414
Long-term care
    nursing care delivery model for, 369
    nursing role in, 460–461

M

Magnet hospital, 247
    working environment in, 465
Magnet Recognition Program, 247
Magnet therapy, 208
Malpractice, 120, 123–124, 134
    elements essential to prove, 134–135, 135b
Malpractice insurance, nursing, 140–141
Managed care, development of, 110–111, 111t

Management, 288–308, 294f
    authoritarian, 293, 294b
    definition of, 251, 288, 290–291
    democratic, 293, 294b
    functions of, 295–301, 296f
    laissez-faire, 293, 294b
    leadership *vs.*, 291
    participative, 293, 294b
    practices of, 293b
    of resources, 303
    roles in, 302–305
    styles of, 294b
    theory of, 293–295
    by walking around, 300
Manager, nurse as, 447
Mandatory continuing education, 63, 68
Mandatory licensure, 66
Mandatory overtime, 242
    safe staffing levels and, 240b
Manipulative and body-based methods, 199
Marginal, definition of, 107, 109
Mass casualty event (MCE)
    definition of, 278
    human causes of, 286
Mass casualty incident (MCI)
    definition of, 275, 278
    lessons learned from, 284
Master's degree nursing programs, 53–54
MCE. *See* Mass casualty event
MCI. *See* Mass casualty incident
Media
    campaigns, for nursing, 28–29
    definition of, 21
    millennial, nurses on, 27
    social, nurses on, 27–28
Medicaid, 107, 110, 112
    cost of, 15
    creation of, 17–18
    funding, 395
Medical advice, leaving against, 154–155
Medical directives, 152
Medical error, increase in, 48
Medical Reserve Corps (MRC), 280
Medicare, 108, 110
    cost of, 15
    creation of, 17–18
Medicare Modernization Act, 396–397t
Medicare program, 396–397t
Medication Errors Reporting Program (MERP), 384
Medication Safety Self Assessments, 384–385
Medicine
    chiropractic, 204
    conventional, definition of, 199
Meditation, 209
MEDLINE, 99
    scientific information in, 270

Meetings, time management and, 442
Mental energy, 435
Mental Health Parity and Addictions Equity Act (MHPAEA), 396–397t
Mentor
  characteristics of, 423b
  novice nurse use of, 422
  nurse leader as, 305
Mentoring, definition of, 409, 422
MENtorship Program, 423
Meridians, acupuncture, 202, 203f
MERP. *See* Medication Errors Reporting Program
Meta-analysis
  definition of, 89
  description of, 94t
Metasynthesis
  definition of, 89
  description of, 100–101
Methodologic design
  definition of, 89
  description of, 94t
Metropolitan Medical Response System (MMRS), 280
MHPAEA. *See* Mental Health Parity and Addictions Equity Act
Middle ages, health care in, 6
Midwifery, 459–460
Military nurses, 68
Millennial media, nursing in, 27
Millennials, in communication, 337
Mind-body interventions, 199
  example of, 202b
Mind-body-spirit, harmony of, 201–202
Mining data, 267
Minority
  definition of, 179
  group
    attitudes towards, 182–183, 182f
    federally defined, 181
  percentage of, 181
  recruitment and retention of
    in health care, 186
    in nursing, 184–186
  violence and, 182
Mishel, Merle, nursing theory of, 86
Mishel's uncertainty in illness theory, 80–81b, 86
Mission, management functions and, 295–296
Mission statement, 295–296
  sample, 297b
Mitigation, definition of, in emergency preparedness and response, 275
MMRS. *See* Metropolitan Medical Response System
Mobile point-of-care (MPOC), 268

Mobility program, 54–56
Monitoring, as budgeting function, 312–313
Moral courage, 169
Moral development, 167
  theory, understanding, 168
  values and, 167–169
Moral maturity, 168–169
Moreno, Jennifer, 23f
Mosaic Code, on health care, 5
Motivating climate, creating a, 300
Movement therapy, 199
Moving stage, of change, 305
Moxibustion, 202–203
MPOC. *See* Mobile point-of-care
MRC. *See* Medical Reserve Corps
Multiple-response, multiple choice questions, as alternate item format, 485
Musculoskeletal disorder, nurse affected by, 245
Mutual recognition model, 63, 70–71

N

NACGN. *See* National Association of Colored Graduate Nurses
National Alliance for Caregiving, 226
National Association of Colored Graduate Nurses (NACGN), 13, 185
National Center for Nursing Research, 3–4b
National Consensus Project (NCP), 223–224
National Council of State Boards of Nursing (NCSBN), 56b, 63, 65, 412, 482
National Database for Nursing Quality Indicators (NDNQI), 243, 386–387
National Disaster Medical System (NDMS), 280–281
National Hospice and Palliative Care Organization (NHPCO), 228
National Hospital Quality Measures, 378–379
National Incident Management System (NIMS), 282–283
National Institute for Occupational Safety and Health (NIOSH), 244
National Institute of Nursing Research (NINR), 92
National Labor Relations Act (NLRA), 253
National Labor Relations Board (NLRB), 253
National League for Nursing (NLN), 10, 42–43, 56b
  on cultural competence in nursing education, 188
  description of, 66
National League for Nursing Accreditation Commission (NLNAC), 10

National Nurses United (NNU), 254
National Nursing Council, 12
National Organization of Nurse Practitioner Faculties (NONPF), 42, 56b
National patient safety goals, 385, 385b
National Response Framework, 280
National Sample Survey of Registered Nurses (NSSR), 29
National Student Nurses Association (NSNA), 33, 56b, 424
Natives, nurse, 413
Natural disaster, emergency response to, 276
Natural products, 199
Naturalistic paradigm, definition of, 89
Naturopathy, 209–210
Navigating the Work Environment: Embracing a Zero Tolerance for Bullying, 421
NCLEX-RN examination, 482–494
  alternate item format in, 486–487
  analysis questions in, 488
  application questions in, 488
  Bloom's taxonomy used in, 487t
  characteristics of, 484
  cognitive domains and, 487–488
  components of, 488–490
    client needs, 488–489
    integrated processes, 489–490
  comprehension questions in, 487
  computer adaptive testing for, 484–485
  culture and, 490
  definition of, 482
  description of, 483–487
  history of, 66
  integrated processes in, 489–490
  knowledge questions in, 487
  multiple choice questions in, 485
  nursing process in, 489–490
  preparation for, 490–493
  purpose of, 484–485
  question format in, 485
  review course for, 493
  spirituality and, 490
  study plan for, 491–492
NCP. *See* National Consensus Project
NCSBN. *See* National Council of State Boards of Nursing
NDMS. *See* National Disaster Medical System
NDNQI. *See* National Database for Nursing Quality Indicators
Needlestick Safety and Prevention Act, 244
Needs assessment
  definition of, 89
  description of, 94t
Negative communication techniques, 322, 328–330

Negligence, 120, 134
  claims of, 136–137
  comparative, 119
  criminal, 119, 137–138
  defenses against claims of, 138
  elements essential to prove, 134–135, 135b
  gross, 136
  res ipsa loquitur and, 135–136
Networking, job searching and, 466–467
Neuman, Betty, nursing theory of, 83t, 84
Never events
  Centers for Medicare & Medicaid Services and, 386, 386b
  definition of, 372
  health care costs and, 320
New Grad Transition Stages, 416f
New knowledge and innovation, 247
Newman, Margaret, nursing theory of, 83t, 86
NHPCO. *See* National Hospice and Palliative Care Organization
Nightingale, Florence, 1–2, 3–4b, 7–8
  image of nursing and, 23
  as nursing theorist, 81–82
  nursing theory of, 83t
Nightingale's theory of practice, 82
NIMS. *See* National Incident Management System
NINR. *See* National Institute of Nursing Research
NIOSH. *See* National Institute for Occupational Safety and Health
NLC. *See* Nurse Licensure Compact
NLN. *See* National League for Nursing
NLN Accreditation Commission (NLNAC), 56b
NLNAC. *See* National League for Nursing Accreditation Commission
NLRA. *See* National Labor Relations Act
NLRB. *See* National Labor Relations Board
NNU. *See* National Nurses United
"No detourism," time management and, 439
NOA. *See* Nurses of America
Noise, Nightingale's theory of practice and, 82
Nonmaleficence, 161, 170–171
NONPF. *See* National Organization of Nurse Practitioner Faculties
Nonverbal communication, 326
  vs. verbal communication, 325–326
Notes on Nursing, 8
Novice nurse, definition of, 409
NPA. *See* Nurse practice act
NSNA. *See* National Student Nurses Association

NSSR. *See* National Sample Survey of Registered Nurses
Nuclear agent, terrorism with, 279t
Nuremberg Code, 103
Nurse
  as administrator, 460
  as Angel of Mercy, 25
  average age of, 26
  baccalaureate prepared, 236–237
  bioethical issues in, 161–178
  on boards, 406–407
  budgeting basics for, 309–321
  burn out of, 413
  career goals of, 478
  as case manager, 455
  as certified registered anesthetist, 458–459
  as change agent, 304–305, 447
  as client advocate, 447
  as clinical consultant, 305
  coordinator positions for, 452–453
  as corporate supporter, 305
  as counselor, 447
  and criminal law, 151
  cultural self-assessment and, 193
  educational level of, 31
  as educator, 447
  ergonomic injury to, 245
  ethical issues in, 161–178
  as ethical profession, 29
  as executive, 460
  faith community, 456
  fatigue, 246
  flight, 455
  foreign, 69
  forensic, 455
  future of, 460–461
  government, 68
  health policy involvement by, 394
  as heroine, 25–26
  hospice, 453
  hospital floor, duties of, 9b
  implications for, 115–117, 116b
  infection control, 452
  information literacy for, 269
  international marketplace for, 191
  internationally educated, 68–69
  as interprofessional health care team coordinator, 448–450
  as interprofessional health care team member, 448–449b
  job growth in, 450–457
  job satisfaction and dissatisfaction of, 299b
  leadership role of, 302–305
  licensed practical
    competencies of, 350b
    delegation and, 346

Nurse *(Continued)*
  education programs for, 51–52
  registered nurse partnered with, 361
  licensed vocational, education programs for, 51
  male, percentage of, 184
  malpractice insurance, 140–141
  mandatory overtime for, 242
  as mentor, 305
  military, 68
  in millennial media, 27
  musculoskeletal disorder and, 245
  new image of, 33–34
  new, on the block, 414
  novice
    assertiveness for, 420–421
    clinical skills for, 419, 423b, 427
    definition of, 409
    delegation skills for, 420, 428
    to expert, 418
    interpersonal skills for, 419, 427–428
    keys to transition for, 426
    organizational skills for, 420, 426–427
    priority-setting skills for, 420, 428–429
    self-mentoring of, 423
    special needs of, 418–421, 426–429
    stages of competency of, 418
    strategies to ease transition of, 422–426
  older, recruitment and retention of, 237–238
  palliative
    areas of expertise, 227
    certification, 227–228
    definition, 219
  parish, 456
  participation in budget process by, 312
  performance evaluation for, 301
  physician interaction with, 31–32, 32b
  political action involvement by, 394
  "primary," 366
  profession, definition of, 1
  professional, 447b
    patient safety as responsibility of, 386–387
    student nurse transition to, 409–430
  in professional organizations, 33
  in quality improvement, role of, 390
  quality indicators, 386–387, 387b
  quality management, 452
  as quality manager, 454–455
  quality safety and educations for, 243
  reality shock for, 412–413
  real-life scenario, 411, 411–412b
  recruitment of, 236

Nurse *(Continued)*
  registered
    competencies of, 350b
    demographics for, 451
    educational preparation of, 236–237
    employment opportunities for, 235–236
    facts about, 29–31
    licensed practical nurse partnered with, 361
    retention of, 237
    supervision of unlicensed assistive personnel by, 347
    as team leader, 365–366
  as researcher, 447
  as role model, 300
  roles of, 445–462
    in evidence-based practice, 97–99
    other, 457
  school, 455–456
  shortage of, 15, 49–50, 235–239
    work environment and, 236
  social media and, 27–28
  as staff developer, 305
  staff, reality of, 29
  staffing assignment for, 241b
  staffing issues in, 242
  supply of, 24
  as team builder, 302–303
  telehealth, 455
  travel, 456
  as whistle-blower, 243–244, 244b
Nurse anesthetist, certified registered, 25–26, 458–459
"Nurse champions," 96
Nurse Licensure Compact (NLC), 70
Nurse manager, 302. *See also* Management
  role modeling and, 300
  unionization and, 258–259
Nurse-midwife, 459–460
Nurse-patient ratio, 129–130
  staffing levels affected by, 363
Nurse practice act (NPA)
  components of, 66–68
  definition of, 63
  model, 65
  nursing defined in, 66–67
  purpose of, 66
  revision of, 69–70
  sunset provision in, 69–70
  violations of, 128–129, 128t, 129b
Nurse practitioner
  description of, 457–458
  salary of, 18
Nurse staffing plan, nursing staffing levels, 239
Nurse Training Act, 12–13, 396–397t
Nurses of America (NOA), 28

Nursing
  advanced practice, 457–460
  aging workforce in, 237–238
  appropriate staffing level in, 242
  in art, 24–29
  assessment in, delegation and, 350
  care provider role in, 447
  career opportunities in, 445–462
  case, 364
  collective bargaining in, 254
  complementary and alternative medicine and, 210–213
  conceptual model of, 78
  concerns with, 29
  coprimary, 367
  cultural competency in, 179–198
  definition of
    Nightingale's, 82b
    in nurse practice act, 66–67
  in early civilization, 5–6
  expansion of knowledge in, 41–42
  functional nursing care delivery model for, 364–365, 365f
  future of, 460–461
  gains for, 257–258
  and health-related journals, 100b
  history of
    from 1900 to World War I, 10
    in 1960s, 13–14
    in 1970s, 14
    in 1980s, 15
    in 1990s, 16–17
    during Civil War, 8–9
    in colonial American period, 7
    during Great Depression, 11–12
    in post-World War II period, 12–13, 13b
    in twenty-first century, 17–18
    World War I to 1920s, 10–11
    World War II, 12
  holistic, 210–211
  image of, 21–36
    in 1960s, 26
    in 1970s, 26
    in 1980s, 26–27
    in 1990s, 26–27
    as angel of mercy, 25
    antiquity, 25
    as heroine, 25–26
    in twentieth-century, 25
    in twenty-first century, 31
    in Victorian era, 25
  important events in evolution of, 2, 3–4b
  Institute of Medicine (IOM) on, 29
  leadership and management, 288–308
  legal issues in, 119–160
  in literature, 24–29
  look of, 33

Nursing *(Continued)*
  media campaigns for, 28–29
  in Middle Ages, 6
  minorities in, recruitment and retention of, 184–186
  modular, 366
  mutual recognition of, 70–71
  new image of, 33–34
  pod, 366
  in prehistoric period, 2
  primary, 366–367
  professional
    contemporary image of, 21–36
    unionization and, 257
  professional organizations for, 33
  in promoting positive work environment, 258
  public opinion of, 29
  relationship-based, 370
  in Renaissance and Reformation, 6–7
  response of, 28
  roles in, 445–462
    definition of, 445
    professional, 447b
  safe staffing in, 239–242
    mandatory overtime and, 242
    nurse acceptance of, 241b
  salaries, 238
  scope of practice in, 66–67
  shortage of, 235–239
  social issues in, 179–198
  social media and, 27–28
  staffing schedules in, 298
  state board of, 63
  team, 365–366
  telehealth, 363–364
  transcultural, 191
    literature in, 191–192
  union, 251–260
  in United States, 8–18
  variations on traditional roles in, 453–457
  workforce, diversity in, 183–186
Nursing assistive personnel, decision tree for delegating, 349f
Nursing cap, 64
Nursing care, cultural competence in, 186–188, 187t
Nursing care delivery models, 359–371
  case management related to other, 368
  choosing, 369–370
  definitions of, 359
  description of, 363–367
  future of, 370
  newer models of, 368–369
  total patient care delivery model for, 364, 364f
Nursing case law, 120, 132

Nursing education
    assessment in, 43–45
    associate degree programs in, 51t, 52
    baccalaureate degree nursing programs
        in, 53
    bioethical concerns in, 48–49
    for clinical nurse leader, 54
    community-focused interprofessional
        approaches in, 46–47
    consensus model for, 73–74
    cultural competence in, 188–189
    diploma program in, 51t
    distance-learning in, 54–56
    diversity in, 51–54
    doctoral programs in, 51t, 54
    ethics in, 48–49
    flexible, 54–56
    global health in, 47
    hospital diploma programs in, 52
    issues in, 40–41t, 41–51
        influence of, 37–61
    licensed practical programs, 51–52
    master's degree nursing program in, 51t,
        53–54
    mobility programs in, 54–56
    patient-centered care in, 47–48
    performance-based learning in, 43–45
    personal responsibilities in, 50–51
    practical nursing program in, 51t
    practice-based competency outcomes in,
        42–43
    professional responsibilities in, 50–51
    shortage of nurses and faculty in, 49–50
    trends in, 40–41t, 41–51
        influence of, 37–61
    types of, programs in, 49f, 51t
    vocational nurse programs in, 51–52, 51t
Nursing educator, 456–457
Nursing ethics, 163, 164–165b, 164b
Nursing faculty
    opportunities as, 456–457
    shortage of, 49–50, 237
Nursing informatics (NI), 453
Nursing malpractice, 120
Nursing organization, 401
Nursing pin, 64
Nursing practice
    definition of, in nurse practice act, 66–67
    health policies affecting, 394, 396–397t, 400
    holistic, 210–211
    intentional torts in, 148–151
    international, 69
    professional standards of, 351
    shared governance and excellence in, 247,
        247b
    sources of, 122
    theories of, 75–87, 75f

Nursing practice act, 120
Nursing process
    as guide for decision making and
        problem solving, 303–304
    NCLEX-RN examination and, 489–490
Nursing research, 88–105
    components of, 93, 93b
    critical appraisal of, 102
    definition of, 90–91
    ethical issues related to, 103
    evolution of, 91
    nursing organizations providing funding
        for, 93
    priorities of, 91–93
    publication of, 99–100
Nursing schools
    beginning of, 12–13
    enrollment and recruitment in, nursing
        shortage and, 236
    segregation of, 185
Nursing science, 78
    definition of, 75, 77–79
    description of, 78
Nursing student
    exploring options for, 464–467
    job search of, 463–481
    minority, recruitment and retention of,
        184–186
    percentage of minorities in, 184
    rights of, in job interview, 473b
    transition of, to professional nurse, 409–430
Nursing theory, 78
    definition of, 75, 77–79
    future of, 86
    language of, 79t
    levels of, 79
    summary of, 83t
    survey of, 82–86
Nursys, 70–71
Nutrition, of client, cultural assessment of,
    194
NY Regents External Degree Program
    (NYREDP), 55
NYREDP. See NY Regents External Degree
    Program

O

Obesity, nursing practice affected by, 46
Objective Structured Clinical Examinations
    (OSCE), 44
Occupational health, opportunities for
    nurses in, 453–454
Occupational Safety and Health
    Administration (OSHA), 244
Occupational therapist (OT), as inter-
    professional team member, 448–449b
Occupational unionism, definition of, 251

Office of Alternative Medicine, 202
Older adult, percentage of, in United States,
    180
Omnibus budget reconciliation act of 1990,
    125–126
Oncology Nurses Society (ONS), 93
Online etiquette, 339
ONS. See Oncology Nurses Society
Openness, 340
Operational budget, 313–314
Operational planning, 297–298
Order of the Visitation of St. Mary, 7
Ordered response "Drag and drop," as
    alternate item format, 486
Orem, Dorothea, nursing theory of, 83t, 85
Organizational chart, 298
    definition of, 288
Organizational factors, 234, 234f
Organizational skills, novice nurse
    development of, 420, 426–427
Organizational theory, 294–295, 294f
Organizations, nursing research funded by,
    93
Organizing
    as management function, 295, 296f, 298
    time management and, 437
Orientation, definition of, 463
Orlando, Ida Jean, nursing theory of, 83t
ORYX®, performance measurement with,
    378
OSCE. See Objective Structured Clinical
    Examinations
OSHA. See Occupational Safety and Health
    Administration

P

PAC. See Political action committee
Pacific Islanders, poverty rate of, 182
Palestine, ancient, health care in, 5
Palliative care, 216–231, 218t
    barriers to, 226–227
    benefits, 224–226
    common challenges in, 227
    continuum model for, 219, 219f
    criteria for, 222–223
    definition of, 217
        World Health Organization, 219
    double effect in, 228
    End-of-Life Nursing Education
        Consortium (ELNEC) on, 223
    ethical concerns in, 228–229
    family caregiving in, 226
    illness, natural course of, 219–223
        prognostication in, 220–222, 221t
    key elements o, 223–224
    legal concerns in, 229–230
        right to refuse treatment, 229

Palliative care *(Continued)*
  medically futile care in, 229
  National Consensus Project (NCP) on, 223–224
  National Hospice and Palliative Care Organization (NHPCO) on, 228
  pain and symptom management in, 225
  professional issues in, 227–229
  quality assessment and improvement in, 228
  research in, 228
  sedation in, 229
  suffering, and, 225–226
  SUPPORT study in, 225
  vs. hospice care, 220t
Palliative Performance Scale (PPS), on prognostication, 220–222, 221t
Pandemic, definition of, 275
Pandemic influenza, 284–285
Paperwork, management of, 439
Pareto chart, 380, 381f
  definition of, 373
Pareto principle, time management and, 437–438
Parish nurse, 456
Parse, Rosemarie Rizzo, nursing theory of, 83t
Partial-task system, health care in, 417, 417b
Participative management, 293
Partnership nursing care model, 367
Passive-aggressive communication, 335
Passive communication, 335
Past experiences, communication process and, 325
Pastoral representative, as interprofessional health care team member, 448–449b
Paternalism, 161, 172
  challenge of, 175–176
Pathway to Excellence, recognition program, 247
Patient
  delegation of nursing tasks and, 351
  needs of, 350
    NCLEX-RN® examination and, 488–489
    staffing and, 361–362
  satisfaction of
    nurse leader and, 302
    staffing affected by, 363
Patient acuity
  definition of, 359
  level of, 361–362
Patient advocacy, 242–244, 242f
  definition of, 232, 242–243
Patient care delivery models, 363
Patient care protocols, 369
Patient-centered care, 367

Patient classification system
  definition of, 359
  description of, 361–362
Patient-days, budget development and, 316
Patient education, nurse's role in, 455
Patient navigators, 368
Patient outcome, definition of, 359
Patient Protection and Affordable Care Act (PPACA), 3–4b, 17–18, 107, 108, 112–113, 395
  health care reform in, 404
Patient safety, 243, 372–391
  advocacy for, 243
  health care system redesign and, 384–386
  interprofessional teamwork and, 387
  national goals for, 385
  nurse staffing levels and, 386
  professional nurse and, 386–387
  regulatory agencies and, 385–386
Patient Self Determination Act (PSDA), 125–126, 228
  definition of, 217
Payment modes, effect of, 114
Peer review, 89
Pennsylvania Hospital, 7
Peplau, Hildegard
  nursing theory of, 83t, 84
  psychodynamic nursing model, 84f
Perception, 322, 325
  personal, communication process and, 325
Perfection, need for, time management and, 434
Performance
  delegation of nursing tasks and, 353
  evaluation, 301
    budget process and, 313
  standards for, 301
Performance-based learning, 43–45
Performance examinations, definition of, 37
Performance expectation, communicating of, 299–300
Performance improvement, 376
Performance standards, establishing, 301
Personal and social factors, 234, 234f
Personal liability, 141–142, 142b
  for charge nurses, 143–145
  in delegation, 145
  with floating and cross-training, 142–143
  for managers, 143–145
  and supervision of team members, 145
  for team leaders, 143–145
Personal perception, communication process and, 325
Personal protective equipment (PPE), 283
Pharmacist, as interprofessional health care team member, 448–449b

Pharmacology test, job application process and, 480
Phenomenology
  definition of, 89
  description of, 95t
Philosophy
  definition of, 79t
  management functions and, 295–296
  statement of, 297b
Phone, job interview through, 473–474
"Phone-a-thons," networking and, 466
Physical energy, 435
Physical environment, 234, 234f
Physical examination, job application process and, 479
Physical restraints, use of, 155–156
Physical therapist, as interprofessional health care team member, 448–449b
Physician
  as interprofessional health care team member, 448–449b
  nurse interaction with, 31–32, 32b
Physician assistant, as interprofessional health care team member, 448–449b
Physician directives, 152
Physiologic integrity, NCLEX-RN examination and, 489
Picketing, definition of, 252
Pilot study
  definition of, 89
  description of, 95
Pitta, Ayurveda and, 203, 203t
Plaintiff, 120, 133
Plan-do-check-act (PDCA) cycle, 384
Planning
  as budgeting function, 311–312
  of health policy, 400
  interview process and, 472
  as management function, 295–298, 296f
  mission and philosophy, 295–296
  in nursing process, NCLEX-RN examination and, 490
  operational, 297–298
  as stage of nursing process, 303–304
  strategic, 296, 297b
  time management and, 437–439, 437f
Platform, definition of, 392
Pod nursing, 366
Point-of-care technology, 267–269
  definition of, 262
Policy process, 394
Policymakers
  communication with, through e-mail, fax, and telephone, 402–403
  definition of, 392
  visiting, and staff members, 401–402
Political action committee (PAC), 401

Politics
 candidates' campaigns in, 401
 grassroots strategies in, 400–403
 nurses' involvement in, 394
 nursing education affected by, 45–46
Population
 minority percentage in, 181
 older adults, percentage of, 180
 trends in, 180–181
  federally defined minority groups, 181
Portfolio
 definition of, 463
 preparation of, 470–471, 470b
Positive communication techniques, 322,
  326–328, 338
Positiveness, 340
Poverty, 181–182
 minority population and, 182
Power, leadership and management use of, 291
Power of attorney, durable, for health care, 120
Power outage, emergency preparedness and
  response and, 284
PPACA. See Patient Protection and
  Affordable Care Act
PPE. See Personal protective equipment
PPS. See Palliative Performance Scale
Practice analysis, NCLEX-RN® examination
  changes through, 484
Practice-based competency outcomes, 42–43
Practice guidelines, definition of, 89
Practice protocols, 369
Practice test, NCLEX-RN examination
  preparation with, 492
Prayer, healing and, 210
Preceptor, definition of, 409
Preceptorships, novice nurse use of, 423
Precipitating event, communication process
  and, 324
Preconceived ideas, communication process
  and, 325
Prejudice, definition of, 179
Preparedness
 definition of, in emergency preparedness
  and response, 275
 phase, 278–282
Preprofessional organization, novice nurse
  participation in, 424
Preventable adverse event, 120
"Primary" nurse, 366
Primary nursing care model, 366, 366f
Prioritizing, definition of, 431, 437–438
Priority-setting skills, novice nurse
  development of, 420, 428–429
Privacy
 communication and, 338
 patient, electronic health record and, 266
 patient-centered care and, 47–48

Private foundations, nursing research
  funded by, 93
Private health insurance, 107, 110
Private insurance, 114
Problem solver, nurse manager as,
  303–304
Process
 definition of, 373
 improvement, clinical indicators and,
  379–381
 variation in
  definition of, 373
  types of, 377
Procrastination
 avoiding of, 440–441
 definition of, 431
Productivity
 definition of, 288
 measurement of, 314
 staffing and, 298
Professional objective, definition of, 463
Professional organization, novice nurse
  participation in, 424
Professional/ethical issue, 108, 121, 162
Professional/legal issue, 121
Prognostication, 220–222
 definition of, 217
 Karnofsky Scale on, 220–222, 221t
 Palliative Performance Scale (PPS) on,
  220–222, 221t
Progressive relaxation, 209
Promises, keeping, in positive
  communication techniques, 327–328
Proposition, definition of, 75
Prospective payment system, 107
Protégé, characteristics of, 423b
Provider, 107, 110–111
PSDA. See Patient Self Determination Act
Psychodynamic nursing model, 84f
Psychosocial integrity, NCLEX-RN
  examination and, 489
Public insurance, 114
Punitive damages, 120, 130, 136

Q
QI. See Quality improvement
Qi, acupuncture and, 202
QSEN. See Quality and Safety Education for
  Nurses
Qualitative analysis, budget variance
  analysis with, 317
Qualitative designs, 95
Qualitative research, 94
 definition of, 89
 methodologies, 95t
Quality and Safety Education for Nurses
  (QSEN), 42, 387–390, 388–389t, 416

Quality improvement (QI), 372–391
 accreditation and, 378–379
 breakthrough thinking and, 382–384
 definition of, 373
 principles of, 376–378
 regulation and, 378–379
 scientific approach to, 377
 team and, 377
Quality improvement model, of Institute
  for Healthcare Improvement, 384f
Quality management, nurse role in,
  452
Quality manager, nurse as, 454–455
Quality, patient perspective of, 376–377
Quantitative analysis, budget variance
  analysis with, 317
Quantitative designs, 94–95
Quantitative research, 94
 definition of, 89
 methodologies, 94t
Quasi-experimental research
 definition of, 89
 designs, description of, 94t
Questions
 analysis, 488
 answering difficult, 166
 application, 488
 comprehension, 487
 format of, 485
 interview, 474, 476b
  legal and illegal areas of, 471b
 knowledge, 487

R
Radiologic agent, terrorism with, 279t
Randomization, definition of, 89
RCA. See Root cause analysis
Readmission, 115
Reality shock, 413–415
 causes of, 416–418
 definition of, 409
 honeymoon phase of, 413
 inventory for, 415b
 recovery phase of, 414
 resolution phase of, 414
 shock (rejection) phase of, 413–414
Recovery, definition of, 275
Recovery phase, of reality shock, 414
Recruiter, communication with, 476b
Recruitment
 Internet for, 466
 of minorities
  in health care, 186
  in nursing, 184–186
 of older nurses, 237
 of younger nurse, 237
Red herring, 330

References
    inclusion of, in résumé, 469
    validation of, by employer, 479
Referent power, 291
Reflexology, 208b
Reformation period, health care in, 6–7
Refreezing stage, of change, 305
Regulation
    definition of, 392, 399
    health policy through, 399
    patient safety improved with, 385–386
    quality improvement through, 378–379
Regulatory board, role of, 68
Rehearsal, interview process and, 472–473, 472b
Reiki, 208b, 209
Relief response phase, 282–283
Renaissance, health care in, 6–7
Renal Disease Program, 396–397t
Report sheet, organization with use of, 426, 427b
Reporting statutes, 130–131
Res ipsa loquitur, 120
Research
    components of, 93, 93b
    definition of, 90–91
    nursing role in, 447
    in palliative care, 228
    unethical, 103
Research utilization, 95–103
Researcher, nurse as, 447
Residency programs, novice nurse use of, 423–424
Resolution phase, of reality shock, 414
Resource manager, 303
Resources, definition of, 288
Respiratory therapist, as interprofessional health care team member, 448–449b
Respondeat superior, 120
Response, definition of, in emergency preparedness and response, 275
Response resources, 282
Résumé
    definition of, 463
    description of, 468–470
    example of, 468b
Retention
    aging workforce and, 237–238
    of minorities
        in health care, 186
        in nursing, 184–186
    of older nurse, 237
    of younger nurse, 237
Retrospective payment system, 107, 110
Revenue
    definition of, 310
    in health care organization, 314b

Review course, NCLEX-RN examination preparation with, 493
Reward power, 291
Richards, Linda, 3–4b
Right and wrong, 167–168
Rights of conscience, 161, 168–169
Right-to-work law, 255
    definition of, 252
Risk management, 120, 132
    system, 146–147
Robert Wood Johnson Foundation, 93
Rogers, Martha, nursing theory of, 83t, 84
Role model
    definition of, 409
    novice nurse use of, 422–423
    nurse manager as, 300
Rolfing, 208b
Rome, ancient, health care in, 6
Root cause analysis (RCA), 373, 385
Roy, Sister Callista
    adaptation model of, 85f
    nursing theory of, 83t, 85
Run charts, 381, 382f
    definition of, 373
Runaways, nurse, 413
Rutters, nurse, 413

S

Safe Patient Handling and Mobility Interprofessional National Standards, 245
Safety
    for nurses, quality, 243
    patient-centered care and, 47–48
    personal, in mass casualty response, 283
    workplace, 244–247
Salaries, wages, and benefits (SWB), definition of, 310
Saw palmetto, facts about, 205–206b
Scene assessment, definition of, 275
Schematic model, 75, 79
School nurse, 455–456
Science, description of, 77–79
Science of unitary human beings, 84
Scientific process, steps of, 77b
Search strategy, effectiveness, illustration of, 270t
Second-degree graduate nursing programs, 53
Secondary analysis
    definition of, 89
    description of, 94t
Secret ballot elections, definition of, 252
Security
    of health care data, 272
    patient, electronic health record and, 266

Sedation, in palliative care, 229
Self-assessment, cultural, 193
Self-care deficit model, 85
Self-confidence, novice nurse development, 424–425
Self-esteem
    novice nurse development of, 424–425
    questionnaire, 425b
Self-mentoring, novice nurse use of, 423
Self-talk, interview process and, 472
Sentinel event, 120, 137
    definition of, 373
Sentinel Event Database, 421
Sentinel event standard, 385
Setting priorities, 437–438
Sheppard-Towner Act, 3–4b, 396, 396–397t
SHIEs. *See* State Health Insurance Exchanges
Shock (rejection) phase, of reality shock, 413–414
Sickness, cultural beliefs about, 194, 195b, 195t
Sigma Theta Tau International (STTI), 93
"Signing cards," 255
Simulation, in nursing education, 44
Single payer system, 107, 110
Sisters of Charity, 7
Situation assessment procedure, 171–172
    identify and analyze available alternatives for action, 172
    justify the selection, 172
    select one alternative, 172
    usefulness and application of, 172–173
Slander, 149
Smartphone, point-of-care technology with, 268
Social change, health care and, 181–182
Social distancing, pandemic influenza control and, 285
Social media
    code of ethics for use of, 41–42
    communication and, 338–339
    issues in, 27–28
    job application process and, 473–474
Social organization, as cultural phenomena, 190
Social Security Act, 12
Social worker, as interprofessional health care team member, 448–449b
Socialization, 418
    definition of, 409
Sociodemographics, nursing education affected by, 45–46
Soy, facts about, 205–206b

Space, personal, as cultural phenomena, 190
Specific client services, of nurses, 452
Speech-language pathologist, as interprofessional health care team member, 448–449b
Spiritual energy, 435
Spirituality, NCLEX-RN examination and, 490
St. John's Wort, facts about, 205–206b
St. Vincent de Paul, 7
Stacked-desk syndrome, time management and, 439
Staff developer, 305
Staff member, delegation of nursing tasks and, 352
Staff satisfaction, staffing and, 362
Staffing, 234, 234f, 240b, 359–371
    definition of, 360
    description of, 361–363
    level of staff preparation and experience as factor in, 362
    as management function, 295, 296f, 298–299
    mix of, 360
    organizational needs and, 362–363
    patient needs and, 361–362
    patient satisfaction and, 363
    staff satisfaction and, 362
Stakeholders, 397
    definition of, 392
Standard of care, 121, 134
    in emergency situations, 138–139
Standardization
    definition of, 373
    process improvement and, 381–382
Standards of Professional Nursing Practice, 351
State board of nursing, 63
    duties of, 68
    membership of, 68
State government, emergency preparedness and response by, 281f
State Health Insurance Exchanges (SHIEs), 395
State health policy, 395
State Nurse Practice Act
    and Board of Nursing Rules and Regulations, 126–127
    delegation of tasks and, 348–350
    delegation policies in, 348b
State statutes, 126–129
Statistical process control, 376
Statistics, 25
Status quo, fear of disrupting, time management and, 434

Statute
    child abuse reporting, 131
    of limitation, in malpractice cases, 139–140
    mandatory overtime, 129–130
    reporting, 130–131
Statute law, 121
Statutory law, 121, 123–132
STEEEP, health care quality through, 375–376
Stereotype, definition of, 21
Stereotyping, definition of, 179
Strategic National Stockpile, 282
Strategic planning, 296, 297b
Strict liability, 121, 123–124
Strike
    definition of, 252
    nurses participating in, 259
Structural empowerment, 247
STTI. See Sigma Theta Tau International
Study designs, 94–95
Study plan, for NCLEX-RN examination, 491–492
Subluxation, in chiropractic medicine, 204
Success, fear of, time management and, 434
Suffering, definition of, 225–226
Sunset legislation, 69–70
    definition of, 63
Supervision, 345–358
    definition of, 345
Supplies
    budgeting for, 311
    definition of, 310
SUPPORT study, 225
Supportiveness, 340
Survey
    definition of, 89
    description of, 94t
Swedish massage, 208b
Synergy Model for Patient Care, staffing level and, 362
Synergy, team builder and, 302
System model, 84
Systems theory, 294–295, 295b

T

Tablets, point-of-care technology with, 268
Taft-Hartley Act, 252
Tai chi, 210
Task Force on Education and Regulation (TFER), 54
Taylor, Susie King, 9
Teaching, NCLEX-RN examination and, 490
Team builder, nurse as, 302–303
Team nursing model, 365, 365f

Technical practices, in leading and managing, 293b
Technical skills, 293
Technology
    expansion of, 116
    time management and use of, 442–443
Technology management, definition of, 431
Telehealth
    nursing, 363–364
    opportunities for nurses in, 455
    point-of-care technology and, 268–269
Telephone call, time management and, 439
Telephone triage nurse, 455
Terrorism
    categories of, 278
    nursing education affected by, 48
Terrorist incident
    definition of, 275
    examples of, 276
Test plan, NCLEX-RN examination, 488–490
Texas Nurse-Friendly Program, 247
TFER. See Task Force on Education and Regulation
The Essentials of Baccalaureate Education for Professional Nursing Practice, 42–43
The Future of Nursing, 29
The Future of Nursing: Leading Change, Advancing Health, 55, 406
The House on Henry Street, 10
The Joint Commission (TJC), 373, 378, 453
    description of, 373
    national patient safety goals of, 385, 385b
Theory. See also Nursing theory
    criteria for acceptance of, 77b
    definition of, 77–79, 79t
    description of, 78
Theory of cultural care diversity and universality, 85
Theory of human caring, 85–86
Theory of unpleasant symptoms, 80f
Third-party payer, 107, 113–114
Thoroughness, in communication, 333, 333b
Time
    finding "extra," 440
    perspectives on, 434–435
Time management
    continuing to succeed, 443
    controlling interruptions in, 441–442
    definition of, 431
    distractions and, 436, 436b
    implementing, 437
    organizing, 437
    planning, 437–439, 437f
    strategies for, 436–443
    tips for, 443b

Time Management from the Inside Out, 434
Time, orientation to, as cultural
    phenomena, 190–191
TJC. *See* The Joint Commission
*To Err Is Human: Building a Safer Health
    System,* 384
To-do list, time management with, 438–439
Top-down flowchart, 379f
Tort, 133
Total patient care delivery model, 364, 364f
Total quality management (TQM), 376
Touch, in positive communication
    techniques, 328
Tour, job application process and, 477
Town hall meetings, political participation
    through, 402, 402b
TQM. *See* Total quality management
Trade unionism, 253
Traditional format, question, 485
Traditionalists, in communication, 336
Trager approach, 208b
Training, change implementation and, 305
Trait theory, of leadership, 292
Transcultural nursing, 191
    clinical nurse specialists (CNSs) in, 192
Transculturalism, definition of, 179
Transformational leadership, 247
Transition
    definition of, 410
    novice nurse, keys to, 426
Transition shock, definition of, 410
Transitional care, nursing care delivery
    models for, 368–369
Translation science, 96
Transmission, style of, communication
    process and, 325
Transparency
    disclosure of error and, 140
    health care system redesign and, 376
Travel nurse, 456
Treatment, right to refuse, 154
Triage, definition of, 275
Triangulation
    definition of, 89
    description of, 95
Trigger, clinical pathway and, 369
Trust
    definition of, 410
    developing, in positive communication
        technique, 326–327
Truth About Nursing, 28
Truth, Sojourner, 9
Tubman, Harriet, 9
Tuskegee experiment, 26–27
Tuskegee syphilis study, 103

U

UAN. *See* United American Nurses
UAP. *See* Unlicensed assistive personnel
Uncertainty in illness theory, 80–81b, 86
Underinsured, health care access for, 112
Unemployment, minority population and,
    182
Unfair labor practices, definition of,
    252
Unfreezing stage, of change, 304–305
Uninsured, health care access for, 112
Unintentional tort, 148
Union
    definition of, 252
    election process of, 256
    management and, 258–259
    nurse manager, 258–259
    nursing, 251–260
        interprofessional teamwork and,
            259–260
        questions to answer, 257
    organizing for, 254–256
        allowable actions during, 255–256
        fairness during, 256–257
    post election, 256
    professional nursing and, 257–260
    staff and, 258–259
    strike used by, 259
    vs. professionalism, 257
Union organizer, questions to ask when
    confronted by, 258b
Unionism
    industrial, definition of, 251
    occupational, definition of, 251
United American Nurses (UAN), 254
United States
    government, branches of, 398t
    history of nursing in, 8–18
    population trends in, 180
United States Congress, 399
United States Department of Health and
    Human Services, 399
United States Public Health Service,
    3–4b
Unit-of-service, 316
    budget costs and, 317
Universal Precautions, 16
Unlicensed assistive personnel (UAP)
    definition of, 345, 360
    registered nurse partnered with, 361
    role of, 347
    use of, 347
Unusual occurrence reports, 147–148
Utilitarianism, 161, 169–170

V

Valerian, facts about, 205–206b
Value-based behavior, 169, 169t
Value-based payment models, 114–115
    never events, 115
    reducing readmissions, 115
    value-based purchasing, 115, 115b
Value formation of, moral development
    and, 167–169
Value system, examining, 167
Values, 161, 163
Values clarification, 167
Values statement, 297b
Variable costs, 320
Variance
    analysis of, 310, 313, 317
    clinical pathway and, 369
    definition of, 310
    sample report for, 318t
Variety, Nightingale's theory of practice
    and, 82
Vassar Camp School for Nurses, 11
Vata, Ayurveda and, 203, 203t
Ventilation, Nightingale's theory of practice
    and, 82
Veracity, 161, 171
    challenge of, 175
Verbal communication, 325–326
    vs. nonverbal communication, 325–326
Vicarious liability, 121, 136
Victorian image, of nursing, 25
Violence
    domestic, nursing practice affected
        by, 48
    horizontal, 421
    lateral, 245
    minority population and, 182
    prevention of, 425–426
    workplace, 245–246, 421
        definition of, 410
        types of, 421b
Visiting Nurse Association (VNA), 3–4b
Vizient/American Association of Colleges of
    Nursing (AACN) Nurse Residency
    Program, 423–424
VNA. *See* Visiting Nurse Association
Voting, importance of, 401

W

Wald, Lillian, 10
Warming, Nightingale's theory of practice
    and, 82
"Wastebasketry," time management and,
    439

Watson, Jean, nursing theory of, 83t, 85–86
Website
  accuracy of information on, 270–272
  authority of information on, 270–272
  consumer use of, for health information, 269
  currency of information on, 270–272
  evaluation form for, 270–272
  objectivity of information on, 270–272
  usability of information on, 270–272
Whistle-blower, 124
  description of, 243–244
White Coat Ceremonies, 64
WHO. *See* World Health Organization
Who will keep the Public Healthy?, 15
Whole-task system, health care in, 417, 417b
W.K. Kellogg Foundation, 93
WMD. *See* Weapon of mass destruction

Work habits, productive, time management and, 434
Work history
  description of, in résumé, 474
  validation of, by employer, 479
Workflow design, 234, 234f
Workforce advocacy
  definition of, 232
  ecosystem model for, 234b
  opportunities and challenges for, 235b
  for professional nursing practice environment, 232–250
  promoting, 233–235
  safe staffing and, 239–242
Workplace
  advocacy of a safer, 246–247
  environment of, nursing shortage and, 238–239

Workplace *(Continued)*
  issues in, 232
  safety in, 244–247
  violence in, 245–246, 421
    definition of, 410
    prevention of, 425–426
World Health Organization (WHO), definition of palliative care, 219
World War I, nursing during, 10–11
World War II, nursing during, 12
Written communication, 331–334, 332b, 333b

Y

Yoga, 210

Z

Zero-based budgeting, 310, 315